BASICS OF
PAIN MANAGEMENT

Edited by

Stefan Novevski

ALLIED
HEALTH
PRESS

Basics of Pain Management

Editor **Stefan Novevski**

Allied Health Press
4164 Lakeshore Road
Burlington ON L7L 1A4
Canada
www.alliedhealthpress.com
Email: orders@arclereducation.com

ISBN: 978-1-77956-242-5

Allied Health Press publishes wide variety of books and eBooks. For more information about Allied Health Press and its products, visit our website at www.alliedhealthpress.com

ABOUT THE EDITOR

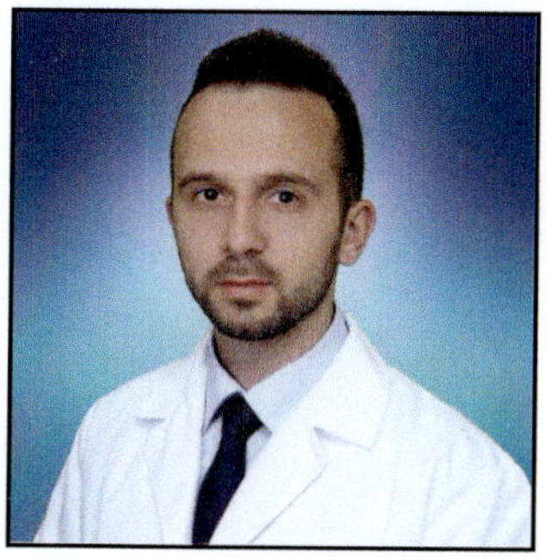

Stefan Novevski is a licensed veterinarian with 4 years of experience as a practitioner, currently working in a new up-to-date veterinary clinic that specializes in working with companion animals. His professional interests and continued education are aimed at working with small animals and he has a passion for reading, writing and researching different topics regarding veterinary medicine. His areas of interests include: internal medicine, obstetrics, pet nutrition, dermatology and animal welfare and behavior. He is dedicated to always staying up-to-date with newest research and is committed to practicing evidence-based veterinary medicine. During his studies and after obtaining his license, he gains first-hand experience in various fields of the veterinary industry through practical work, attending seminars and workshops, and international travel to other universities and private veterinary clinics. From 2023 he is a member of MSAVA (Macedonian Small Animal Veterinary Association).

Word Roots, Prefixes, and Suffixes by Chapter

Chapter 1 Acute and Postoperative Pain

Acute-: Sharp, severe

Pain: Unpleasant sensory and emotional experience

-ive: Pertaining to or characterized by.

Operative: Related to surgery

Chapter 2 Osteoarthritis, Rheumatoid Arthritis, and Muscles Pain

Osteo: From the Greek "osteon," meaning bone.

Arthro: From the Greek "arthron," meaning joint.

-it is: From the Greek "itis," meaning inflammation.

My: From the Greek "mys," meaning muscle.

Algia: From the Greek "algos," meaning pain.

Rheumato-:Relating to a watery discharge or condition affecting joints.

Chapter 3 Chronic Back and Upper Extremity Pain

Chronic: Relating to time, indicating a long-lasting condition.

Back: Posterior part of the body.

Upper: Higher part of the body.

Extremity: Limbs of the body.

Chron-: Time, indicating a long duration.

Chapter 4 Fibromyalgia and Abdominal Pain

Fibro: From the Latin "fibra," meaning fiber. It refers to fibrous tissues in the body, such as muscles and connective tissues.

My: Muscle

Algia: From the Greek "algos," meaning pain.

Abdomen: The part of the body between the chest and the pelvis.

-algia: Pain

Chapter 5 Chronic Pelvic and Obstetric Pain

Chron: From the Greek "chronos," meaning time, indicating a long duration.

Pelv: From the Latin "pelvis," meaning basin, referring to the pelvic region of the body.

Pain: Derived from the Latin word "poena," meaning penalty or punishment, referring to an unpleasant sensory and emotional experience.

Obstetr: From the Latin "obstetrix," meaning midwife, relating to childbirth and the care of women during pregnancy, labor, and postpartum.

Chapter 6 Orofacial Pain Management

Oro: From the Latin "os, oris," meaning mouth.

Facial: From the Latin "facies," meaning face.

Manage: From the Italian "maneggiare," meaning to handle or control.

-ment: From the Latin "-mentum," indicating an action or resulting state.

Oro-: Mouth

Chapter 7 Heart, Vascular, and Hemopathic Pain

Cardi-: Heart

-algia: Pain

Vascul-: Blood vessel

-itis: Inflammation

-pathy: Disease

Hemo- / Hemat-: Blood

Chapter 8 Genitourinary Pain

Genito-: Relating to the genital organs.

Uro-: Relating to urine or the urinary system.

-algia: Pain

-itis: Inflammation

-dynia: Pain

Chapter 9 The Management of Cancer Pain

An-: Without or lack of.

Chemo-: Chemical

-therapy: Treatment

-sic: Relating to.

-induced: Caused by.

Onco-: Relating to tumors.

Carcino-: Relating to cancer.

Table of Contents

3 Chronic Back and Upper Extremity Pain 89

4 Fibromyalgia and Abdominal Pain 133

5 Chronic Pelvic and Obstetric Pain 177

LIST OF FIGURES

LIST OF TABLES

PREFACE

The International Association for the Study of Pain (IASP) defines pain as an unpleasant sensory and/or emotional experience linked to actual or potential tissue damage, or described in terms of such damage. This sensation arises from nerves that transmit signals to the brain, signaling damage or irritation to organs or tissues. In response, the brain sends signals to these organs or muscles, prompting appropriate action.

Chronic pain presents a significant public health challenge in the United States. While healthcare professionals have long recognized pain as a vital biological signal, its management has faced increased scrutiny since being designated as the fifth vital sign. Due to the subjective nature of pain measurement, the optimal approach to its management is not always clear. Various modalities, including interventional procedures and noninvasive techniques, exist for pain treatment.

Acute pain typically resolves on its own when a reversible cause is identified. However, undertreated acute pain can progress to chronic pain, leading to prolonged suffering. Chronic pain can give rise to psychological and social issues that are challenging for both patients and physicians. A multimodal therapeutic approach, with active patient involvement, can effectively manage most pain conditions. Opioids are considered a legitimate medical option for chronic nonmalignant pain. When opioid therapy is deemed necessary, healthcare providers should adhere to recommended guidelines from state licensing boards and professional organizations. Successful pain management can be a gratifying experience for healthcare professionals. The use of drugs for pain management remains a highly controversial subject, especially regarding the use of opioids. The presence of an endogenous opioid system was unknown until the early 1970s. Endogenous opioids include enkephalins, endorphins, and dynorphins. Much of our understanding of drug action is related to receptor specificity, and the pharmacological action of opioids is mediated via specific receptor binding.

This text is a vital resource for pain management students, trainees, and practitioners, covering essential topics in both acute and chronic pain management. Through numerous practical examples, it reinforces fundamental concepts and enhances clinical decision-making skills. Emphasizing a multidisciplinary approach, the text discusses behavioral and physical therapies, along with ethical considerations, making it an indispensable guide for anyone involved in pain management.

The comprehensive coverage in this book includes the latest principles and techniques in acute and chronic pain management. Each chapter brings the topics to life, making the content more engaging and practical. It is specifically designed to benefit all physicians who manage patients in pain, offering valuable insights and strategies applicable to various medical specialties.

While the book targets pain physicians, its content is beneficial for anesthesiologists in their daily practice. Additionally, it is valuable for trainees at any level, providing a solid foundation in pain management principles. Also, this book serves as a comprehensive, up-to-date, and practical guide for understanding and managing pain, catering to the diverse needs of healthcare professionals involved in pain management.

Chapter 1

ACUTE AND POSTOPERATIVE PAIN

Contents

Introduction

Acute pain typically indicates potential or existing tissue damage, allowing the person to prevent additional harm. Additionally, it might stop dangerous movement—like in the event of a fracture. Therefore, decreased mobility brought on by acute pain may promote healing. But the benefit to the organism is fleeting, and if it persists, it will have a negative consequence. In the face of an acute illness or injury, pain also sets off complex neurohumoral reactions that initially aid in maintaining homeostasis; however, if these changes are severe or unduly prolonged, they may result in morbidity or death. When faced with acute pain, psychological reactions could initially help with coping with the physical insult, but if they get too severe or persistent, they could end up being harmful. Because acute pain is complex, treating it safely and effectively requires knowledge of certain guidelines.

Orientation and Directional Terms

Term	Definition	Illustration
Acute pain	Acute pain is a sudden or urgent pain that is usually short in duration and has an obvious cause, such as an injury or trauma.	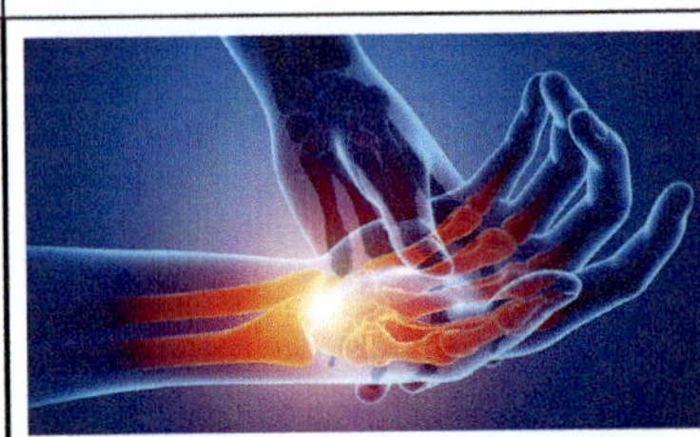
Surgical trauma	Surgical trauma is physical damage to tissues and organs that can occur during a surgical procedure.	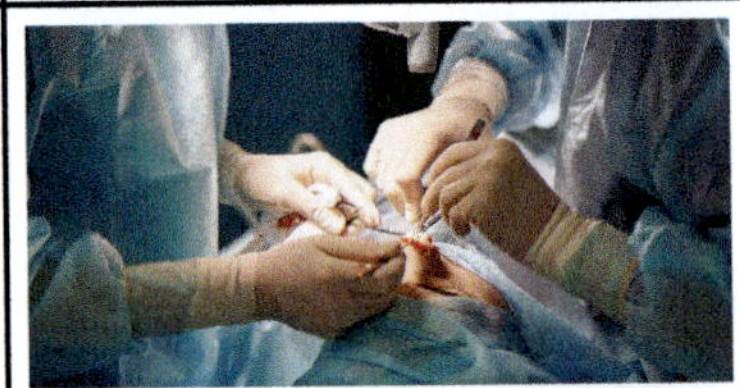
Neurogenic inflammation	Neurogenic inflammation is a form of inflammation (redness, heat, swelling, pain) initiated by activation of peripheral nervous system c-fiber neurons rather than by immunological events	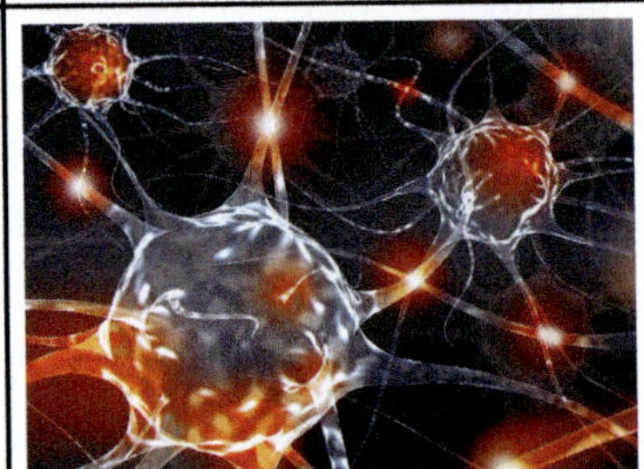
Primary hyperalgesia	Primary hyperalgesia is a type of hyperalgesia that occurs when an injury causes an increase in pain in the injured area of the body.	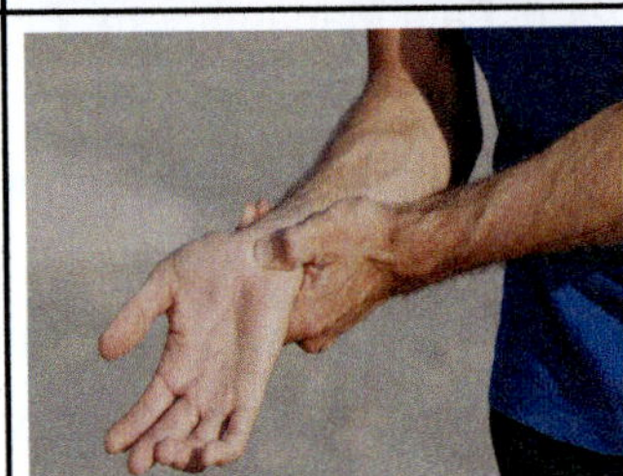
Dorsal horn	The dorsal horns are bilateral structures which form the posterior projection of this shape.	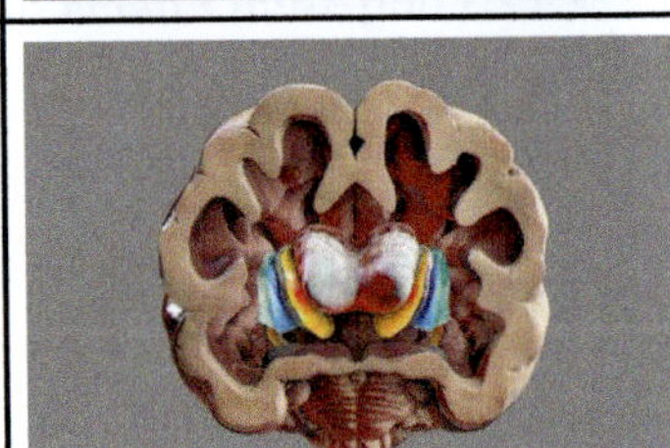

1.1. Acute Pain Mechanisms

Acute pain perception is the result of a complex interplay between behavioral, emotional, and sensory components. A person's emotional and behavioral reactions are psychological factors that should always be taken into consideration when analyzing how they perceive and express acute pain. It is no longer believed that the biological mechanisms underlying our experience of acute pain are a straightforward "hard-wired" system with a "stimulus–reaction" relationship. Any type of trauma to the body, but especially damage to the nerves, can alter other parts of the nervous system, affecting how the body reacts to stimuli in the future. The idea that noxious input can cause long-term changes in the peripheral and central nervous systems is becoming more widely accepted. The "plasticity" of the nervous system then modifies how the body reacts to additional peripheral sensory information.

1.1.1. Peripheral Sensitization

Surgical trauma and other noxious stimuli linked to acute pain are linked to an "inflammatory response," also known as an injury response. The release of intracellular materials from injured and inflammatory cells, including mast cells, lymphocytes, and macrophages, is a component of the inflammatory response. Peripheral sensitization is a phenomenon that arises from nociception-induced neurogenic inflammation and the subsequent release of chemicals that tyrosine nociceptors at high thresholds.

Low-intensity mechanical stimuli that would not typically cause pain are now regarded as painful after sensitization. At the site of injury, there is also a greater sensitivity to thermal stimuli. This area of "primary hyperalgesia" around the injury site is a common post-surgical and post-trauma feature that is brought on by peripheral changes (IASP Task Force on Taxonomy, 1994).

1.2. Non-Steroidal Anti-Inflammatory Drugs

One of the functions of non-steroidal anti-inflammatory drugs (NSAIDs), which are frequently used for "peripheral" analgesia, is to lessen the inflammatory response. By inhibiting the cyclooxygenase pathway, substances like aspirin and other NSAIDs provide their anti-inflammatory effects. There are two types of cyclooxygenase: COX1 and COX2. Although COX1 is consistently found in various tissues, including the mucosa of the stomach, COX2 is activated by inflammation. This offers a chance to create drugs with selective anti-inflammatory properties without adverse effects on the stomach. Drugs that selectively inhibit COX2, e.g., some drugs (e.g., celecoxib, rofecoxib) have been developed that may provide analgesia without antiplatelet effect and with less gastrointestinal toxicity than NSAIDs; however, details regarding renal toxicity, effects in individuals with asthma who are sensitive to aspirin, and long-term cardiovascular effects are still unknown. Besides the peripheral action of NSAIDs, there is increasing evidence that they exert their analgesic effect through central mechanisms.

1.2.1. Peripheral Action of Opioids

Traditionally, opioids have been thought of as centrally acting medications. On the other hand, there is now proof that endogenous opioids act on peripheral sites after tissue damage. Opioid receptors are produced in the dorsal root ganglion, the cell body, and are then transported to the periphery and central terminal in the dorsal horn. When local tissue damage occurs, these peripheral receptors subsequently become active. When opioid receptors are unmasked and immunocompetent cells that have opioid receptors and the capacity to synthesize opioid peptides arrive, this happens. This has sparked interest in the peripheral delivery of opioids, such as topical morphine administration or intraarticular delivery of opioids after knee surgery or arthroscopy. Notwithstanding early enthusiasm for this method, some employees have voiced concerns about the utility and cost-benefit analysis of intra-articular morphine, especially in the wake of an arthroscopy or minor knee surgery. Nonetheless, opioids with physicochemical characteristics that support peripheral action are being developed; if these medications prove effective, they might be helpful for localized use. To prevent systemic absorption, medium-sized peptides are being developed with a localized action in mind.

1.2.2. Peripheral Nerve Injury

Recent research has shown that injury or section of a peripheral nerve causes many morphological, physiological, and biochemical alterations that function as independent pain centers. Modifications in neuroplasticity that sustain sensory input can take place at the spinal or peripheral levels. Contrary to conventional wisdom, neuropathic pain may manifest as early onset within the first 24 hours in patients recovering from surgery or trauma. Additionally, a 10-day delay in onset is possible.

1.2.3. Sympathetic Nervous System

Acute pain states are created and maintained in large part by the sympathetic nervous system. Prostanoids released from sympathetic fibers can sensitize primary nociceptive afferent fibers in the event of inflammation. After a nerve injury, sympathetic nerve stimulation or noradrenaline (norepinephrine) administration can activate primary afferent fibers through α-adrenoceptor action; sympathetic terminals also innervate the dorsal root ganglion. This indicates that aberrant primary afferent fiber activity or responsiveness may result from activity in sympathetic efferent fibers (Levine & Reichling, 1999).

1.3. Dorsal Horn Mechanisms of Importance to Acute Pain

Primary afferents terminate in the dorsal horn, where descending fiber endings from the brain, local intrinsic spinal neurons, and afferent fibers interact intricately. Furthermore, the numerous neurotransmitters and neuromodulators involved in pain processing in the dorsal horn have been identified through pharmacological studies.

1.3.1. Central Sensitization

Primary hyperalgesia and the phenomenon known as "peripheral sensitization" are the results of changes that take place in the peripheral after trauma. However, the modifications in the periphery can only partially account for the sensitization that takes place. After an injury, there is a zone of "secondary hyperalgesia" in the surrounding uninjured tissue that is more sensitive to typically benign mechanical stimuli (allodynia). The threshold to thermal stimuli remains unchanged, in contrast to the zone of primary hyperalgesia. These alterations are thought to be the consequence of processes that take place in the spinal cord's dorsal horn after an injury. This is the central sensitization phenomenon.

The dorsal horn has been shown to undergo several alterations when central sensitization occurs. First, a spinal neuron's receptive field is expanded, allowing it to respond to stimuli outside of its usual response region for nociceptive stimuli. Second, in response to stimuli stronger than the threshold, there is an increase in both the duration and the magnitude of the response. Last but not least, there is a decrease in the threshold, allowing non-noxious stimuli to activate neurons that would typically transmit nociceptive information. These modifications could have a significant impact on the development of chronic pain as well as acute pain states like postoperative pain.

1.3.2. Modulation at a Spinal Level

Numerous levels of the neuraxis, including the dorsal horn, are capable of modulating the transmission of nociceptive information. When afferent impulses enter the dorsal horn, they set off inhibitory mechanisms that reduce the power of incoming impulses. Local inhibitory interneurons and descending brain pathways have the effect of inhibiting. Endogenous and exogenous agents that act on opioid, α-adrenoceptor, GABA, and glycine receptors at pre- and postsynaptic sites in the dorsal horn can modulate incoming nociceptive messages.

Opioids are commonly used and usually effective in treating pain. In the dorsal horn, opioid receptors are present both pre- and postsynaptically, with the majority (roughly 75%) being found presynaptically. The nociceptive primary afferent releases fewer neurotransmitters when presynaptic opioid receptors are activated. On the other hand, inflammatory and neuropathy-related alterations can result in notable modifications to opioid sensitivity through various mechanisms.

When α-adrenoceptors in the spinal cord are activated, the brainstem releases noradrenaline (norepinephrine) naturally through descending pathways. Alternatively, external substances like clonidine are administered spinally to produce an analgesic effect. Moreover, it seems that α-adrenoceptor agonists and opioid agonists work together. Numerous α-adrenoceptor subtypes exist, and the creation of agonists that specifically target specific subtypes of this receptor may yield novel, potent analgesics with fewer adverse effects.

GABA and glycine play a role in the tonic inhibition of nociceptive input; neuropathic pain features like allodynia can arise from a loss of their inhibitory action.

Endogenous opioid peptides and other neurotransmitters, such as serotonin, noradrenaline (norepinephrine), and GABA, play a role in descending inhibition. Numerous established methods for treating acute pain, such as the use of opioids, function by inhibiting these pathways. New methods that seek to activate these inhibitory pathways have been employed as a consequence of the understanding of inhibitory mechanisms. Additionally, it has given a more coherent justification for methods that are currently in use, like epidural/intrathecal opioid and non-opioid drug administration, transcutaneous electrical nerve stimulation, and so forth.

1.4. Etiology And Features of Acute Pain

Visceral, deep somatic, or cutaneous structures can cause acute pain. A thorough mapping of the primary superficial dermatomes is necessary to ensure that neural blockade techniques are applied effectively. Visceral pain differs from somatic pain in that it is more ambiguously localized and has additional characteristics (Table 1.1). Referred pain can be explained by the demonstrated convergence of visceral and somatic afferents. Crucial viscerosomatic reflexes have also been found.

Viscosity nociceptive fibers that travel via the sympathetic chain to the spinal cord must be blocked to relieve visceral pain. Table 1.2 displays the viscera along with the spinal cord segments linked to their visceral nociceptor afferents. Visceral pain is "referred" to the body's surface regions, as Fig1.1. illustrates. It should be highlighted that the different organs have a great deal in common. It follows that the high diagnostic error rate for visceral pain is not shocking. Important somaticovisceral and viscerosomatic reflexes may also complicate diagnosis and treatment.

Potential issues with the interpretation of "diagnostic" local anesthetic nerve blocks arise from the temporary alleviation of visceral pain through blockade of the somatic referred area. It seems that somatic and visceral structures may share the peripheral and central sensitization processes previously discussed in this chapter. This could explain "visceral hyperalgesia," the increased sensitivity of visceral structures to a relatively benign stimulus after inflammation or tissue damage (Cousins & Phillips, 1986).

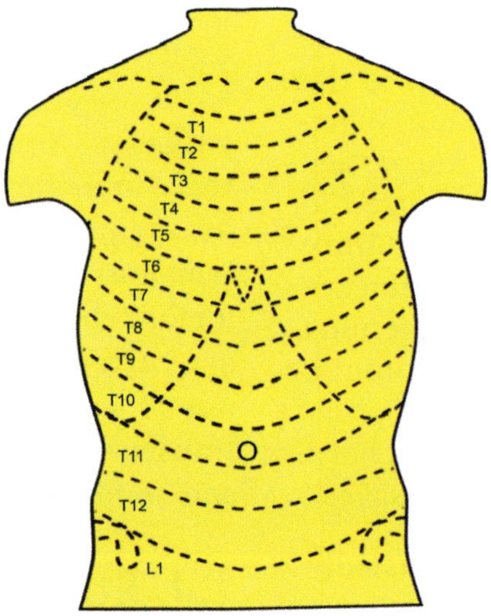

Figure 1.1. *Viscerotomes.*

Source: https://wikimsk.org/w/index.php?curid=2199.

Table 1.1. Main Tetrodotoxin-Sensitive and Tetrodotoxin-Resistant Voltage-Gated Sodium Channels (VGSCs) Related to Visceral Pain

VGSCs	Gene	Tetrodotoxin	Associated Pain	Alteration	References
Nav1.1	*SCN1A*	Sensitive	Irritable bowel syndrome	Upregulation	Levine & Reichling, (1999)
Nav1.5	*SCN5A*	Resistant	Irritable bowel syndrome, cardiac syndrome	Loss of function	Hayes & Molloy, (1997); Jorgensen, Rasmussen, Nielsen, Leffers, & Albrecht-Beste, (1991); Melzack, (1971); Melzack, Wall, & Ty, (1982)

Nav1.6	*SCN8A*	Sensitive	Colorectal pain	Activation	Merry & Power, (1995)
Nav1.7	*SCN9A*	Sensitive	Erythromelalgia, paroxysmal extreme pain	Gain of function or altered functional levels	Inbal, Devor, Tuchendler, & Licblich, (1980); Meert & De Kock, (1994); Merskey, (1986)
Nav1.8	*SCN10A*	Resistant	Chronic jejunitis pain	Change in function or expression	Modig, (1976)
Nav1.9	*SCN11A*	Resistant	Chronic inflammatory pain	Potentiation	Modig, Malmberg, & Karlstom, (1980)

Source: Campos-Ríos, A., Rueda-Ruzafa, L., Herrera-Pérez, S., Rivas-Ramírez, P., & Lamas, J. A. (2021). Tetrodotoxin: A New Strategy to Treat Visceral Pain? *Toxins*, 13(7), 496. https://doi.org/10.3390/toxins13070496.

1.5. Features of Acute Pain

The majority of acute pain types and chronic pain types differ significantly from one another. The nervous system is typically unaffected by acute pain, which can be brought on by trauma, surgery, acute "medical" conditions, or physiological processes (e.g., labor).

Symptoms of pain and discomfort may manifest through facial expressions, increased autonomic activity, and other potentially harmful effects such as hypertension, tachycardia, vasoconstriction, sweating, shallow breathing, muscle spasms, increased gastrointestinal secretions, and other physical symptoms. These symptoms typically subside as the wound heals or the medical condition improves. Patients are usually reassured that the pain will diminish as they recover, providing them with a sense of relief. However, inadequate preparation and information may lead to prolonged discomfort and uncertainty for patients.

Acute pain may occasionally superimpose itself in some chronic pain patients (e.g., if they need additional surgery or experience a fractured bone as a result of metastatic cancer. These patients might not have a healthy nervous system, and they might also have a history of significant psychological issues, opioid tolerance, and other issues.

For some major surgical procedures, acute pain may need to be relieved by extensive somatic and sympathetic blockade. The cervicothoracic sympathetic chain and coeliac plexus (intrathoracic and abdominal viscera); C3, C4 phrenic nerve sensory afferents (pain from incision in central diaphragm referred to shoulder tip); and C3–C4 and T2–T12 sensory nerves (somatic structures in neck, thorax, and abdomen) may be necessary, for example, to treat pain following thoracoabdominal esophagogastrostomy with cervical anastomosis.

In response to acute pain, segmental and suprasegmental reflex responses cause the previously mentioned adverse effects, such as muscle spasms, immobility, and vasospasm. Through many vicious cycles, including increased sensitivity of peripheral nociceptors, this may exacerbate the pain. Unrelieved acute pain leads to anxiety and insomnia, which exacerbates the pain. In addition, pain is increased both before and after surgery by anxiety and a sense of helplessness. Their relief and prevention are beneficial supplements to other therapies. Psychological journals have a lot of information about acute pain. Following a major operation, a traumatic injury, or an excruciating illness (e.g., pancreatitis), severe pain may linger longer than 10 days. In these circumstances, the pain and its aftereffects start to resemble chronic pain. These patients frequently exhibit depression, rage, and other symptoms of chronic pain. Therefore, it's important to exercise caution when making a clear distinction between acute and chronic pain. If acute pain worsens, more attention may need to be given to psychological treatment methods in addition to medical and pharmaceutical ones. Finding patients with new chronic pain issues is a role that acute pain services are playing more and more. These patients are often identifiable by 2–3 weeks following surgery or trauma. Assessing the relative contributions of environmental, psychological, and physical factors, however, may be necessary for a definitive diagnosis (Cousins and Phillips, 1986).

1.6. Pain Management: Clinical Issues

1.6.1. Spinal Administration of Agents

Spinal drug administration is now used as a pain management strategy due to the types of receptors that are present pre- and postsynaptically around nociceptive transmission neurons in the dorsal horn. In the treatment of certain pain issues, the use of comparatively low dosages of drugs that target particular receptor types in the spinal cord while largely avoiding adverse effects has been a significant advancement.

1.6.2. Pre-emptive Analgesia

Attempts to stop these changes from happening have been prompted by the identification of the alterations linked to the central sensitization phenomenon. Early postoperative pain has been shown to be a strong predictor of chronic pain. It was believed that actions taken to lessen or eliminate harmful input to the spinal cord during an unpleasant event, like surgery, would lessen or minimize changes to the spinal cord and, as a result, reduce pain both during the recovery period and in the long run. It is still unknown, though, how long or how much harmful input is necessary to cause these long-term alterations.

Preemptive analgesia is becoming more popular as a result of this idea. Preemptive analgesia has been claimed to reduce postoperative pain, lower the need for analgesics, improve morbidity, and shorten hospital stays in numerous trials. However, Dahl and Kehlet (1993) and Woolf and Chong (1993) conclude that more trials are required before a definitive statement can be made for acute pain, despite studies that seem to indicate the advantages of pre-emptive analgesia.

1.7. Acute Pain and Multimodal Analgesia

Strong evidence suggests that using multimodal, or balanced, analgesia following surgery is beneficial for patients (Table 1.1, point 3). To enhance pain relief, NSAIDs, paracetamol, local anesthetics, other non-opioid analgesics, and opioids are used in combination. In order to provide analgesia while lowering the frequency and intensity of side effects, multimodal analgesia uses a range of medications, possibly administered via various methods. For instance, analgesia following thoracotomy was greatly enhanced by adding routine postoperative injections of the NSAID ketorolac to a regimen previously based on intercostal nerve blocks and patient-controlled (PCA) morphine. Because non-opioid analgesics reduce opioid side effects, such as the inevitable gastrointestinal stasis brought on by opioids, which postpones the patient's return to normal enteral nutrition, they play a critical role in multimodal analgesia and postoperative recovery. Following colon surgery, excellent analgesia and a quicker rate of gastrointestinal function recovery are achieved with multimodal analgesia that includes epidural analgesia using a combination of local anesthetics and low-dose opioids. This is especially true if systemic NSAIDs are used to prevent the need for opioid administration after the epidural has been stopped.

Multimodal analgesia can be used to completely eliminate pain following surgery while significantly lowering overall opioid consumption. Nevertheless, some studies have found disappointing results regarding the effect on 18 morbidity and mortality, indicating that excellent pain management is not always linked to better outcomes. However, recent studies have indicated that using multimodal analgesia following major surgery may enhance recovery and consequently lower costs.

Table 1.2. An Example of Postoperative Pain in Adults: Mean, Standard Deviation (±SD) and 95% Confidence Intervals (CI) of Postoperative Pain Intensity, Measured by the VAS (0–10 cm) and the NRS (0–10 cm), at the ASSESSED time Intervals After Root Canal Instrumentation for Both Groups

Scale	Group	6 h	12 h	24 h	Day 2	Day 3	Day 4	Day 5	Day 6	Day 7	*p* *
VAS	Rotary (PTN) §	1.41 ± 2.35 [a] (0.52–2.31)	1.28 ± 2.05 [a] (0.50–2.06)	1.14 ± 1.36 [a] (0.62–1.65)	1.10 ± 1.32 [a] (0.60–1.61)	1.10 ± 1.42 [a] (0.56–1.64)	1.03 ± 1.84 [a] (0.33–1.74)	0.52 ± 0.91 [b] (0.17–0.86)	0.21 ± 0.62 [c] (−0.03–0.44)	0.14 ± 0.52 [c] (−0.06–0.33)	<0.001
	Reciprocating (R) §	1.00 ± 1.56 [a] (0.34–1.66)	0.96 ± 1.62 [a] (0.29–1.70)	0.71 ± 1.30 [a] (0.16–1.26)	0.71 ± 1.16 [a] (0.22–1.20)	0.54 ± 1.02 [a] (0.11–0.97)	0.42 ± 0.97 [a] (0.01–0.83)	0.25 ± 0.74 [a] (−0.06–0.56)	0.21±0.59 [a] (−0.04–0.46)	0.08 ± 0.41 [a] (−0.09–0.26)	0.001
	p **	0.795	0.903	0.082	0.146	0.052	0.115	0.193	0.845	0.672	
	d	0.21	0.17	0.32	0.31	0.45	0.41	0.33	0.00	0.13	
NRS	Rotary (PTN) §	1.48 ± 2.4 [a] (0.57–2.40)	1.45 ± 2.20 [a] (0.61–2.28)	1.41 ± 1.62 [a] (0.80–2.03)	1.31 ± 1.61 [a] (0.70–1.92)	1.45 ± 1.94 [a] (0.71–2.19)	1.07 ± 2.05 [a] (0.29–1.85)	0.41 ± 0.83 [b] (0.10–0.73)	0.28 ± 0.75 [b] (−0.01–0.56)	0.17 ± 0.54 [b] (−0.03–0.38)	<0.001
	Reciprocating (R) §	1.13 ± 1.78 [a] (0.37–1.88)	1.33 ± 1.76 [a] (0.59–2.08)	0.92 ± 1.47 [a] (0.30–1.54)	0.96 ± 1.40[a] (0.37–1.55)	0.88 ± 1.30 [a] (0.33–1.42)	0.42 ± 0.93 [b] (0.02–0.81)	0.46 ± 1.06 [b] (0.01–0.91)	0.25 ± 0.61 [b] (−0.01–0.51)	0.17 ± 0.48 [b] (−0.04–0.37)	0.002
	p **	0.983	0.770	0.094	0.304	0.188	0.228	0.845	0.841	0.845	
	d	0.17	0.06	0.32	0.23	0.35	0.41	−0.05	0.04	0	

Source: Oliveira PS, Ferreira MC, Paula NGN, Logrcio AD, Grazziotin-Soares R, da Silva GR, da Mata HCS, Bauer J, Carvalho CN. Postoperative Pain Following Root Canal Instrumentation Using ProTaper Next or Reciproc in Asymptomatic Molars: A Randomized Controlled Single-Blind Clinical Trial. *Journal of Clinical Medicine.* 2022; 11(13):3816. https://doi.org/10.3390/jcm11133816.

* Intra-group comparison of all evaluated time intervals—Friedman test. § Comparison by pairs in each group—Wilcoxon test with Bonferroni correction ($p < 0.006$). [a, b, c] For each group, mean scores indicated by the superscript lowercase letters in same line are statistically different. The

comparison was performed between pairs: 6–12 h; 12–24 h; 24 h–2 days; 2–3 days; 3–4 days; 4–5 days; 5–6 days; 6–7 days. ** Inter-group comparison of the same session for each evaluated time interval—Mann–Whitney test. d Effect size: $d \leq 0.20$ (small), d from >0.20 to <0.80 (moderate), $d \geq 0.80$ (large). PTN = ProTaper Next; R = Reciproc.

In a process of acute rehabilitation following surgery, Kehlet suggests that the "pain-free state" be used as a key element of an aggressive regimen of postoperative mobilization and early oral feeding. Undoubtedly, multimodal analgesia that uses non-opioids to reduce the need for opioids has the unique benefit over unimodal systemic opioid administration in that it allows for early mobilization and excellent pain relief upon movement. Furthermore, by avoiding the unfavorable opioid side effects of gastrointestinal stasis, nausea, and vomiting, the patient can return to regular enteral nutrition much faster when non-opioids are used as part of a balanced analgesic plan (Scott, 1988).

1.8. Psychological Factors and Acute Pain

1.8.1. Psychological Response

An individual's behavior may change as a result of severe pain in a variety of ways, such as withdrawing from social interactions and becoming more absorbed in oneself. The main emotional side effects of acute pain are fear and anxiety, which are exacerbated when linked to a fear of dying. Patients who experience severe acute pain and no relief for days at a time may become depressed and feel powerless because they no longer have control over their surroundings. It is now widely accepted that premorbid tendencies for anxiety, hostility, depression, or obsession with health are made worse when severe acute pain goes untreated. In rare instances, an acute psychotic reaction can result from an inability to manage pain. In critical care units, acute pain is a significant factor in the development of delirium.

1.8.2. Psychological Factors Affecting the Acute Pain Response

Significant individual variations in a person's sensitivity to unpleasant stimuli are widely known. Individual differences in pain response to acute injury were first clearly described by Beecher (1946) through clinical observations of injured soldiers. According to his report, 65% of soldiers who suffered severe wounds during combat experienced minimal or no pain. In one study of patients in an emergency room, 30% did not experience any pain at all at the time of the injury, and some patients took up to nine hours to feel any pain at all. "Clearly the link between injury and pain is highly variable: injury may occur without pain and pain without injury," concluded Melzack et al. (1982). According to Peck (1986), the psychological factor most consistently associated with high pain thresholds is anxiety. Acute pain from trauma, surgery, and other causes is linked to fear of dying and general anxiety about one's physical health.

Some important implications for treatment have arisen from knowledge of the psychological factors affecting the acute pain response:

1. Measures to reduce anxiety levels have an important bearing on the acute pain experienced by patients and their need for pain treatment.
2. Approaches that give patients more control are likely to be successful in reducing anxiety and decreasing the requirement for pain and medication. Patient-controlled analgesia (PCA) is a highly successful example.
3. The relief of acute pain is likely to reduce the risks of unwanted psychological sequelae, such as

depression, poor motivation to return to normal activities, antipathy towards further surgical procedures, and, in some situations, psychotic reactions (Yaksh, 1999).

1.9. Pathophysiology and Complications of Unrelieved Acute Pain

Generally speaking, the physiological and psychological reactions to severe acute pain are abnormally enhanced. Therefore, therapy ought to start either before or during the phase of functional impairment brought on by the acute severe pain pathophysiology.

1.9.1. Respiratory System

The most frequent and significant side effect of the pain following surgery or trauma to the chest or abdomen is respiratory dysfunction. A reflex muscle spasm occurs near the tissue injury as well as in the muscle groups cephalad and caudad to the injury site due to involuntary spinal reflex responses to the noxious input from the injured area. Considering that nociceptive afferents typically travel two to three segments above or below their site of entry into the dorsal horn, this is not surprising. Additionally, voluntary muscle atrophy in the thorax and 20 abdominal regions may be brought on by pain. In the clinical context, the outcome is frequently referred to as "muscle splinting," which is defined as contracting the muscles on either side of the injured area to "splint" the area and prevent movement, much like how an external splint is applied to a fractured bone. This splinting is frequently linked to partial glottis closure, which results in a "grunting" sound when breathing. The glottic closure is most likely a part of an ancestral reaction that protects the person from an approaching injury by allowing an increase in intrathoracic and intra-abdominal pressure, which is linked to muscle spasms.

It is necessary to respond to such a response effectively. Alveolar ventilation, functional residual capacity (FRC), and vital capacity all decrease along with the tidal volume. FRC could drop below the volume at which a minor airway closure happens. Individuals with respiratory diseases, smokers, and elderly patients may be at risk for this issue. This condition worsens to the point of regional lung collapse (atelectasis), which is linked to a significant impairment of pulmonary gas exchange due to a change in the lung's ventilation-perfusion relationship (V/Q inequality), which causes hypoxemia. In addition to contributing to hypoxemia, the low ventilation volume also produces hypercarbia. The patient's inability to cough and expel secretions due to the muscle splinting exacerbates lobular or lobar collapse. Pneumonia is frequently the result of infection after this circumstance. Failure to comply with chest physical therapy adds to treatment complications, significantly lengthens the duration of pulmonary complications, and ultimately increases hospital stay.

It is not well known that post-operative lower abdominal and peripheral limb surgery can lead to pulmonary complications in older patients and patients in poor general health due to untreated severe pain that immobilizes them and causes hypostatic pneumonia, which starts at the base of the lung. Modig (1976) provided evidence of this by reporting on a group of elderly patients who had undergone total hip replacement. Patients receiving regular intramuscular opioid therapy had high respiratory rates linked to hypoxemia and low tidal volumes. Since patients receiving epidural analgesia and experiencing no pain at all did not exhibit these abnormalities in pulmonary function, it appeared likely that the hypoxemia was caused by immobility and other adverse reflexes brought on by pain.

A "viscerosomatic" reflex involving the diaphragm has been shown in recent basic and clinical research. This reflex involves changes in the amplitude and pattern of diaphragm activity in response to unpleasant visceral stimuli. Epidural bupivacaine can be used to block this.

The classic clinical picture of a patient experiencing excruciating pain that won't go away and is on the verge of respiratory failure includes obvious splinting of the thoracic and abdominal muscles, grunting upon expiration, a small tidal volume, and a very fast respiratory rate. Unfortunately, this is a very energy- and inefficient way to breathe, and it can lead to high oxygen consumption without a corresponding rise in cardiac output. This could result in mixed venous blood becoming excessively desaturated, which would exacerbate hypoxemia. Effective epidural block pain relief can result in impressive correction of most of these abnormalities in pulmonary function. When a meta-analysis of numerous clinical trials is conducted, the overwhelming evidence shows that epidural opioid administration is superior to systemic opioid administration in terms of reducing postoperative pulmonary morbidity.

1.9.2. Cardiovascular System

Most people agree that sympathetic overactivity in the presence of extreme acute pain raises blood pressure, heart rate, peripheral resistance, and cardiac output. Increased cardiac work and myocardial oxygen consumption are the end results. Heart rate increases significantly cause a decrease in diastolic filling time, which may lead to less oxygen reaching the myocardium. Consequently, there is an imbalance between the oxygen supply and demand in the heart, which increases the risk of hypoxemia. Furthermore, it has been established that strong sympathetic stimulation can cause coronary vasoconstriction in response to α-receptors in the coronary vasculature. This pathophysiology may ultimately lead to myocardial ischemia, which can cause anginal pain or even myocardial infarction. For patients who already have coronary artery disease, this is a more likely scenario. Increased anxiety, elevated catecholamine levels in the blood, and an increased risk of coronary artery constriction are all linked to angina pain.

Sjögren and Wright (1972) have demonstrated the effects of postoperative pain on cardiovascular variables. The fact that epidural analgesia can prevent and reverse these abnormalities indicates that the noxious stimuli were the primary cause of cardiovascular changes. Extensive research on animals has demonstrated that noxious stimulation causes coronary artery vasoconstriction and may even cause myocardial ischemia.

By using thoracic epidural analgesia to prevent these unpleasant stimuli, the myocardium's oxygen supply is significantly improved, and the myocardial ischemia insult is decreased. Additionally, both during and after surgery, the incidence of myocardial ischemia episodes is decreased by epidural blocks. When compared to traditional and less effective pain relief techniques, Yeager et al. discovered an overall reduction in mortality linked to effective pain relief provided by epidural blockade. According to a recent study, patients who have undergone aortic surgery experience an increase in myocardial ischemia when their epidural analgesia is stopped. Thoracic epidural blocks can reduce acute anginal pain in patients who are not surgical candidates while also improving blood flow to the myocardium of patients who are considered to be "at risk" by dilating stenosed coronary artery segments.

It is crucial to understand that there is proof that alternative analgesics can lower the risk of myocardial ischemia following cardiac surgery. Beattie et al. recently observed that adding a continuous infusion of ketorolac (5 mg/h for 24

h) to a PCA morphine regimen decreased pain scores, arterial blood pressure, heart rate, and the length of myocardial ischemia in patients undergoing elective hip or knee arthroplasty. It's unclear if this is a result of better analgesia in and of itself, a side effect of NSAID-induced thromboxane production inhibition, or an inherent cardiac effect.

Acute pain is linked to reduced limb blood flow in the peripheral circulation, and this can be especially dangerous for patients having vascular grafting operations. An improved outcome and a reversal of blood flow reductions linked to surgical trauma and acute pain are the results of epidural blockade-induced pain relief. Reduced arterial inflow and decreased venous emptying may be linked to severe postoperative pain and elevated sympathetic activity. As a result of the patient's immobility and altered blood coagulability, venous thrombosis and pulmonary embolism may develop. While it makes sense that elevated sympathetic activity brought on by pain would lower hepatic and renal blood flow, there is a lack of data demonstrating these modifications in pain patients.

1.9.3. Musculoskeletal System

As mentioned above, a muscle spasm that is triggered by pain can exacerbate it further, creating a vicious cycle of segmental and suprasegmental motor activity in response to pain. This vicious cycle may also cause notable spikes in sympathetic activity, which heightens the sensitivity of peripheral nociceptors. Even in patients with relatively localized nociceptive foci in the long bones or other bony skeleton regions, this condition can cause widespread disruptions. According to recent research, there may be a significant correlation between prolonged postoperative pain and movement restriction, marked impairment of muscle metabolism, and a marked delay in the return of normal muscle function. These alterations seem to be caused by reflex vasoconstriction in response to pain, as well as potential reflex reactions that may be at least partially counteracted by receiving epidural analgesia. Patients treated in this way seem to return to normal function much more quickly.

1.9.4. Gastrointestinal and Genitourinary Systems

While it reduces intestinal motility, increased sympathetic activity raises intestinal secretions and smooth muscle sphincter tone. There could be paralytic ileus and even gastric stasis. Severe pain and the ensuing rise in sympathetic activity are at least partially responsible for these alterations.

On the other hand, delayed gastric emptying may also be significantly influenced by the use of opioid analgesic medications. Neural blockade pain relief may shorten the amount of time that X-ray contrast media takes to pass through the stomach; in a control group, this time could reach 150 hours; however, in a group receiving epidural analgesia, it could only take 35 hours.

Additionally, there is evidence that an epidural local anesthetic, but not an epidural opioid, may be able to relieve the pain-related impairment of intestinal motility. Moreover, systemic intravenous lidocaine (lignocaine) administration decreases pain and shortens hospital stay while hastening the restoration of bowel function following radical prostatectomy.

Urinary sphincter activity is also elevated following surgery due to increased sympathetic activity, which may lead to retention of urine. However, because opioid analgesic medications may cause a significant incidence of urine retention, determining the role of pain is challenging.

1.9.5. General Stress Response to Acute Injury

Increased secretion of catabolic hormones and decreased secretion or action of anabolic hormones are the reasons why surgery and other forms of trauma cause a catabolic state. The patient experiences increased demands on the cardiovascular and respiratory systems, pain, nausea, vomiting, and intestinal stasis; changes in blood flow, coagulation, and fibrinolysis; changes in substrate metabolism; and changes in the body's handling of water and electrolytes. This heightened state following surgery or trauma, coupled with the analgesics' moderating effects.

There are two stages to the reactions to trauma, including surgical trauma. Most physiological processes are slowed down, there is a hypodynamic state, and the metabolic rate is lowered during the first acute "ebb" or "shock phase." This phase is either absent or very brief during the surgical period in cases of surgical trauma.

The hyperdynamic, or "flow phase," is the second stage. Depending on the severity of the surgical or traumatic insult and the occurrence of complications, this phase may extend for a few days or weeks. This phase is characterized by an increase in cardiac output and metabolic rate. There is some evidence to suggest that nociceptive impulses are crucial during the early stages of the flow phase and the ebb phase. But there are a lot of other things that also play a part in the stress response's initiation, and it appears that these things become more and more significant during the flow phase. This is a crucial area for research because the first 48 hours after surgery may yield the greatest benefits from effective techniques for relieving severe postoperative pain.

Surgical trauma causes significant changes to metabolism and endocrine systems. Nonetheless, there is compelling evidence that local anesthetic and opioid neural blockade may result in a significant alteration of the body's reaction to surgical damage. A significant portion of the physiological reaction to surgical or other procedures in the lower abdomen or lower extremities may be diminished by neural blockade using local anesthetics. This usually happens when there is total relief from postoperative pain. The inhibitory effect is significantly less pronounced during and after major thoracic and abdominal procedures, possibly due to the challenge of achieving adequate afferent neural blockade. To achieve a significant decrease in the surgical stress response, pain management with continuous epidural analgesia must be maintained for a minimum of 48–72 hours following surgery.

According to available data, the reduction of stress response is not as effective when opioids are administered intrathecal or epidural for pain relief. Studies on combinations of opioids and local anesthetics, however, suggest that this combination may be able to modify the stress response more effectively. An impressive proof of the effectiveness of continuous epidural neural blockade combined with pain relief to modify the stress response is the notable improvement in cumulative nitrogen balance that results from providing pain relief both intraoperatively and postoperatively.

Pain management with neural blockade may modify changes in coagulation and fibrinolysis related to major surgery. The interpretation of these findings is complicated, though, as variables other than pain might be at play. A neuroblockade-related local anesthetic's absorption may also have an antithrombotic effect. Positively, a clinical trial comparing the effects of general anesthesia versus epidural anesthesia in peripheral vascular surgery discovered that the group receiving epidural anesthesia required five times fewer repeat procedures for graft failure within a month. Acute-phase proteins and immunocompetence changes are frequently linked to surgical trauma. Neural blockade for pain management has a negligible impact on a number of the immunocompetence impairments caused by surgery. The workings of the mechanism are still unclear.

Unrelieved pain can have negative effects that lead to multiple system failures, especially in high-risk surgical patients. Yeager et al. (1987) looked into this issue in a controlled study of high-risk patients having major surgery. Patients were randomized to receive either general anesthesia alone during surgery and parenteral opioid afterward, or general anesthesia and epidural local anesthetic during surgery and epidural opioid afterward. The findings demonstrated a notable disparity in mortality and morbidity in many systems between the two groups. The group receiving epidural analgesia experienced a significant decrease in treatment costs, which was intriguing as well. It is unclear exactly what role pain relief played in achieving these better outcomes with epidural analgesia because intraoperative epidural local anesthesia led to both efferent sympathetic blockade and nociceptive afferent blockade, allowing for a decrease in anesthetic agent dosages. However, pain relief was likely the primary reason for the effects of epidural opioids after surgery. Regrettably, it is difficult to locate supporting data regarding decreased morbidity and mortality after effective pain management techniques.

1.10. Other Forms of Acute Pain

Tissue damage typically, but not always, causes excruciating pain right away. This is followed by neurochemical reactions linked to the inflammatory response. Mechanical factors such as physical distension of joints or fascial compartments, along with ischemia, may play a role in musculoskeletal pain. Distension, obstruction, ischemia, chemical irritation from visceral rupture into the peritoneal cavity, infection, and other factors may also be involved in acute visceral trauma.

Melzack et al. studied patients with more localized and minor trauma (1982). The patients had minor fractures, dislocations, sprains, strains, cuts, and bruises when they arrived at the emergency room. Of the 138 patients examined, 37% experienced no pain at the scene of the injury; of 46 patients with skin-only injuries, 53% experienced no pain for a while, while 86 patients with deep tissue injuries (e.g., only 28% of patients with injuries (fractures, sprains, amputation, bruises, stabs, and crushes) experienced pain-free time. The length of the delays ranged from a few minutes to several hours. By using the McGill Pain Questionnaire, it was discovered that while the affective scores were lower, the sensory scores were comparable to those of patients with chronic pain. The terms used to describe the different types of injuries were very similar: fractures, cuts, and bruises were described as "hot" or "burning," sprains, fractures, and bruises as "sharp," and cuts and lacerations as "throbbing" or "beating."

The pathophysiological reaction to pain after major trauma is probably almost the same as that to pain after surgery. However, anxiety levels are typically very high due to the lack of preparation, the suddenness of the injury, and the severe psychological responses that accompany it. Additionally, CNS responses initiate pronounced versions of the changes in various body systems that have been previously described. One example of an acute medical condition that can cause significant pain and obvious abnormal reflex responses is acute pancreatitis. Severe abdominal muscle spasm, which reduces diaphragmatic movement, and progressive hypoventilation, which raises the risk of hypoxemia and hypercarbia, are typically present in addition to the abdominal pain. Severe pain is linked to the release of substances such as pancreatic enzymes into the peritoneal cavity. It's also possible that toxic depressants are released, which could cause shock and cardiovascular depression. Again, it's unclear exactly how pain plays a part in these happenings. Clinical reports exist of patients whose overall condition improved when epidural local anesthetics or opioids were used to relieve the pain of acute pancreatitis.

The normal reciprocal relationship between the sympathetic and parasympathetic nervous systems, which regulate cardiac function, is disrupted by myocardial infarction, often resulting in overactivity of both systems. These modifications are probably largely brought about by the hemodynamic changes brought on by myocardial infarction.

Nonetheless, pain and the corresponding rises in sympathetic activity, along with an increase in vagal activity, might be part of the issue. Abrupt alterations in vagal activity can lead to several serious conditions, including atrioventricular block, severe hypotension that could lead to cardiogenic shock, peripheral vasodilatation, and bradycardia. As previously mentioned, experimental data on both humans and animals suggests that epidural neural blockade may significantly alter these negative effects. The proportion of this effect attributed to the blockade of afferent nociceptive impulses from the myocardium and efferent sympathetic activity is unknown.

It is not necessary to excessively worry that significant symptoms might be concealed as a result of impeding the pain relief process in emergency rooms. In fact, the early administration of opioids in patients who present with an "acute abdomen" does not impede, but rather may help, the diagnosis of serious pathology. As a result, such patients should not be denied the proper analgesia (Fields and Basbaum, 1994).

1.11. Clinical Syndromes of Acute Pain: Implications for Diagnosis and Treatment

Acute pain can be caused by a wide range of circumstances, including pathological events in chronic pain patients. Patients with cancer who experience sudden episodes of pain due to acute intestinal blockages, pathological long bone fractures, and other issues are notable in this regard. Acute pain episodes can also occur in patients with chronic occlusive vascular disease during a winter exacerbation of their condition. The acquired immune deficiency syndrome (AIDS) is another chronic condition that can cause sudden, intense pain episodes. Visceral, deep somatic, or cutaneous structures can cause acute pain. It's critical to map the exact location of the pain precisely. If the pain is exclusively coming from cutaneous structures, it helps to identify the dermatomes or superficial nerves that are causing the pain. When a person experiences deep somatic or visceral pain, both the classic viscerotome regions and the superficial areas that are associated with visceral pain can provide some guidance regarding the source of the pain. The viscerotomes of different body organs overlap significantly, which surely contributes to a high diagnostic error rate in the case of acute visceral pain. The spinal cord segments linked to nociceptive input from the different viscera should be understood.

There are various general distinctions between visceral and somatic pain. Viscerosomatic and somatovisceral reflexes further impede the distinction between visceral and somatic pain. Acute appendicitis is a classic example of the different neural pathways linked to acute pain. Visceral nociceptive afferents that emerge from the appendix and travel to segment

T10 of the spinal cord transmit pain during the early stages of appendix inflammation. The umbilical area is centrally represented by this viscerotome. As somatic nociceptive afferents in the T10 and L1 regions become involved, the inflammation linked to appendicitis spreads to the parietal peritoneum in the vicinity of the right iliac fossa, localizing pain in this area. However, due to the appendix's anatomical location, the start of the viscerovisceral and viscerosomatic reflexes, and other factors, there may be significant variations in this pattern.

The following factors are crucial in distinguishing between the different causes of acute pain: the pain's onset, its characteristics and intensity, its location and radiation, and its accompanying symptoms. Usually, but not always, one can ascertain if the pain is visceral or somatic in origin based on criteria. When it comes to visceral pain, a sudden onset points to possible causes like organ rupture or embolus-induced artery blockage. A more gradual onset may indicate an infection or inflammation. Intermittent pain may be linked to recurrently elevated pressure in hollow organs as a result of obstruction, while constant pain may be linked to inflammation or ischemia.

The potentially fatal scenario of a ruptured spleen with bleeding beneath the diaphragm serves as a crucial illustration of referred pain since it activates the phrenic afferent fibers (C3 and C4), which in turn causes pain to be referred to the shoulder tip region. Acute trauma to the apical region of the lung can cause pain in the thoracic region, which can then activate somatic afferents in the brachial plexus (C5–T1). This can cause pain to radiate into other arm regions and to the outer aspect of the arm and shoulder. Trauma to the mediastinum can cause pain that is diffusely distributed over the retrosternal region, as well as in the neck and abdomen. Pain may be referred to one or both arms due to the involvement of sympathetic afferent fibers, which may involve segments from at least C8–T5. Acute gallbladder and bile duct disease typically cause diffuse upper abdominal or right upper quadrant pain, which can also radiate to the back, close to the right scapula. Vomiting may help ease this frequently colicky pain that is associated with eating. Additionally, there is diffuse acute pain in the right upper quadrant and epigastrium related to the liver. It might be a sickening pain that never goes away. The typical location of acute pancreatitis pain is high in the upper abdomen or left upper quadrant. It then radiates directly to the back, either to the interscapular region or to the left of the first lumbar vertebra. Most people describe the pain as dull, intense, and continuous.

When the ureter is also affected, as might be the case with a ureter stone (renal colic), pain from the kidney typically travels from the loin region to the groin and, in rare cases, to the penis. It is possible that the reflexive increase in sympathetic activity linked to renal colic exacerbates pain and creates a vicious cycle that stops the stone from passing through the ureter because of severe spasms. When such pain is managed with a continuous epidural block, the stone may occasionally pass through in addition to providing extremely effective pain relief. By inducing local prostaglandin release and consequent smooth muscle spasm, the irritating presence of a stone in the ureter initiates an excruciating cycle of uncoordinated ureteric muscle contraction. NSAIDs work better than opioids to relieve the pain associated with renal colic by inhibiting the production of prostaglandins.

After surgery, acute pain management requires consideration of the underlying cause of the pain. This is since the requirements for the pharmacological treatment of visceral and somatic pain differ. In addition, as previously mentioned, the neural pathways implicated in the pain may have a significant impact on the application of neural blockade techniques. "Incident pain" is defined as pain that manifests itself when not at rest, such as when walking or deep breathing and coughing. It should come as no surprise that the need for analgesia is higher in this type of pain. Opioid tolerance in patients receiving opioid treatment for 7 to 10 days or longer before surgery is another factor contributing to the observed increase in pain levels. Of special significance is that, as opposed to treating pain indiscriminately, certain patterns of pain may indicate the emergence of surgically correctable postoperative complications. It is important to investigate any abrupt increase in the need for local anesthetics, epidural opioid administration, or intravenous opioid infusion because it may indicate the occurrence of a new event. Patients receiving treatment in a critical care unit after experiencing trauma and initially stabilized on an analgesic regimen are in a similar situation. According to one of these authors' experiences, pain that resists a previously effective analgesic regimen is often linked to the emergence of a significant complication.

After surgery, it's important to consider the chance of developing neuropathic pain, which is sometimes overlooked in patients experiencing acute pain and may call for specialized treatment. An injury, illness, or surgical procedure involving the peripheral or central nervous system could be the cause of the pain. Unexpected increases in opioid use following surgery or trauma can be a diagnostic indicator because neuropathic pain may not respond well to opioids.

1.12. Long-Term Effects of Surgical Incision and Acute Tissue Trauma

Surgical incisions are typically thought to be followed by a well-organized healing process with little chance of persistent pain. The division of tiny peripheral nerves and occasionally larger nerves, along with varying degrees of tissue trauma, tissue retraction and compression, and other factors, can complicate surgical incisions. Curiously, there isn't any solid proof that pain issues are less common following elective surgery and the resulting tissue damage than they are following traumatic injuries.

Numerous other chapters in this book address the broad topic of persistent pain after traumatic injury. Among the most notable examples are stump pain, phantom limb pain, complex regional pain syndrome (CRPS types I and II), trauma-related trigeminal neuralgia, trauma-related occipital neuralgia, whiplash syndrome, cervical sprain or whiplash syndrome, acute postmastectomy pain, post-thoracotomy pain, abdominal cutaneous nerve entrapment syndrome, and a wide range of postoperative neuralgias involving peripheral nerves like the obturator, femoral, sciatic, and ulnar nerves.

It is challenging to pinpoint the exact frequency of chronic pain after trauma and surgical incision. But based on our observations, it occurs in at least 10% of surgical procedures. Research on animals has provided compelling evidence that the development of spontaneous activity in neuromas is genetically predisposed. Observations that patients with neuromas and incisional pain often experience similar issues if the neuroma tissue is attempted to be surgically removed provide support for this theory. When operations are performed on other body parts, these patients typically experience comparable complications. As a result, the patient's past medical history is significant and may indicate the necessity of close observation and prompt application of suitable treatment.

Surgery discusses factors that contribute to wound healing, including handling tissues gently, suturing techniques, suture material selection, preventing hematomas and infections, and other factors. On the other hand, it seems that not much research has been done on the variables that significantly affect how different pain syndromes develop after surgery. The general consensus is that incisions that split through rather than along muscle fibers result in greater pain after surgery. One of the few studies to test this theory contrasted the traditional flank approach (muscle-cutting) with a dorsal approach to the kidney (muscle-separating). A shorter hospital stay and less need for postoperative analgesia were linked to the former. Regretfully, there was no patient follow-up to ascertain the relative frequency of pain following incisions.

Based on clinical observation, it appears that the following surgical procedures have a higher likelihood of causing chronic pain at or around the site of the incision: 50% lateral thoracotomy; 50% cholecystectomy; 50% radical mastectomy; vein-stripping (especially long saphenous due to close proximity to saphenous nerve); inguinal herniorrhaphy; episiotomy; various operations on the arm and hand; and facial surgery. Perkins and Kehlet surveyed potential surgical factors. Surgical nerve damage seems to be a major factor. Factors on the patient, such as age, gender, and the existence of untreated pain before surgery, could be significant. The latter is corroborated by studies on animals, wherein injury sustained before a limb was denervated by neurectomy led to a greater tendency toward self-mutilation (autotomy) in comparison to animals that did not sustain injury before neurectomy. According to the study, tissue damage and untreated pain before surgery may increase the risk of chronic pain issues afterward. The clinical finding that patients with pain from occlusive vascular disease who receive neurolytic sympathectomy or epidural block before amputation have a decreased incidence of postamputation pain supports this.

Three general categories can be used to categorize the long-term effects of surgical incisions: deafferentation syndromes, postoperative neuralgias, and complex regional pain syndromes (types I and II) (Levine and Reichling, 1999).

A Closer Look

Hyperalgesia

Hyperalgesia is an abnormally increased sensitivity to pain, which may be caused by damage to nociceptors or peripheral nerves and can cause hypersensitivity to stimulus. Prostaglandins E and F are largely responsible for sensitizing the nociceptors. Temporary increased sensitivity to pain also occurs as part of sickness behavior, the evolved response to infection.

Hyperalgesia can be experienced in focal, discrete areas, or as a more diffuse, body-wide form. Conditioning studies have established that it is possible to experience learned hyperalgesia of the latter, diffuse form.

Hyperalgesia is induced by platelet-activating factor (PAF) which comes about in an inflammatory or an allergic response. This seems to occur via immune cells interacting with the peripheral nervous system and releasing pain-producing chemicals (cytokines and chemokines).

One unusual cause of focal hyperalgesia is platypus venom.

Long-term opioid (e.g., heroin, morphine) users and those on high-dose opioid medications for the treatment of chronic pain, may experience hyperalgesia and experience pain out of proportion to physical findings, which is a common cause for loss of efficacy of these medications over time. As it can be difficult to distinguish from tolerance, opioid-induced hyperalgesia is often compensated for by escalating the dose of opioids, potentially worsening the problem by further increasing pain sensitivity. Chronic hyperstimulation of opioid receptors results in altered homeostasis of pain signaling pathways in the body with several mechanisms of action involved. One major pathway is through stimulation of the nociceptin receptor, and blocking this receptor may therefore be a means of preventing the development of hyperalgesia.

Stimulation of nociceptive fibers in a pattern consistent with that from inflammation switches on a form of amplification in the spinal cord, long-term potentiation. This occurs where the pain fibers synapse to the pain pathway, the periaqueductal gray. Amplification in the spinal cord may be another way of producing hyperalgesia.

The release of proinflammatory cytokines such as interleukin-1 by activated leukocytes triggered by lipopolysaccharides, endotoxins and other signals of infection also increases pain sensitivity as part of sickness behavior, the evolved response to illness

Simple bedside tests include a response (pain intensity and character) to cotton swabs, finger pressure, pinprick, cold and warm stimuli, e.g., metal thermo rollers at 20°C and 40°C, as well as mapping of the area of abnormality.

Quantitative sensory testing can be used to determine pain thresholds (decreased pain threshold indicates allodynia) and stimulus/response functions (increased pain response indicates hyperalgesia). Dynamic mechanical allodynia can be assessed using a cotton swab or a brush. A pressure algometer and standardized monofilaments or weighted pinprick stimuli are used for assessing pressure and punctate allodynia and hyperalgesia and a thermal tester is used for thermal testing.

Hyperalgesia is similar to other sorts of pain associated with nerve irritation or damage such as allodynia and neuropathic pain and consequently may respond to standard treatment for these conditions, using various drugs such as SSRI or tricyclic antidepressants, Nonsteroidal anti-inflammatory drugs (NSAIDs), glucocorticoids, gabapentin or pregabalin, NMDA antagonists, or atypical opioids such as tramadol. Where hyperalgesia has been produced by chronic high doses of opioids, reducing the dose may result in improved pain management. However, as with other forms of nerve dysfunction associated pain, treatment of hyperalgesia can be clinically challenging, and finding a suitable drug or drug combination that is effective for a particular patient may require trial and error. The use of a transcutaneous electrical nerve stimulation device has been shown to alleviate hyperalgesia.

Summary

- Acute pain usually signals impending or actual tissue damage and thus permits the individual to avoid further injury.
- Surgical trauma or other noxious stimuli associated with acute pain are associated with an injury response or 'inflammatory response.'
- Non-steroidal anti-inflammatory drugs (NSAIDs) are commonly used for 'peripheral' analgesia and one of their actions is a reduction in the inflammatory response.
- The sympathetic nervous system also has an important role in the generation and maintenance of acute pain states.
- The dorsal horn is the site of termination of primary afferents, and there is a complex interaction among afferent fibers, local intrinsic spinal neurons and the endings of descending fibers from the brain.
- Acute pain may arise from cutaneous, deep somatic, or visceral structures. Careful mapping of the principal superficial dermatomes is important for the effective use of neural blockade techniques.
- Segmental and suprasegmental reflex responses to acute pain result in muscle spasms, immobility, vasospasm, and other adverse effects.
- The elucidation of the types of receptors present pre- and postsynaptically around nociceptive transmission neurons in the dorsal horn has led to the use of spinal drug administration as a pain management technique.
- Severe pain can cause many changes in an individual's behavior, including increased self absorption and withdrawal from interpersonal contact.
- Surgery and other forms of trauma generate a catabolic state as a result of increased secretion of catabolic hormones and decreased secretion or action of anabolic hormones.
- Tissue trauma usually, but not always, results in immediate sharp pain followed by neurochemical events associated with the inflammatory response.

References

1. Aasbo, V., Raeder, J. C., Grogaard, B., & Roise, O. (1996). No additional analgesic effect of intra-articular morphine or bupivacaine compared with placebo after elective knee arthroscopy. *Acta Anaesthesiologica Scandinavica, 40*(5), 585–588.
2. Ahn, H., Andaker, L., Bronge, A., et al. (1988). Effect of continuous epidural analgesia on gastro-intestinal motility. *British Journal of Surgery, 75*(12), 1176–1178.
3. Applegate, W. V. (1972). Abdominal cutaneous nerve entrapment syndrome. *Surgery, 71*, 118.
4. Attard, A. R., Corlett, M. J., Kidner, N. J., et al. (1992). Safety of early pain relief for acute abdominal pain. *British Medical Journal, 305*, 554–556.
5. Bach, S., Noreng, M. F., & Tjellden, N. U. (1988). Phantom limb pain in amputees during the first 12 months following limb amputation, after preoperative lumbar epidural blockade. *Pain, 33*, 297–301.
6. Bardram, L., Funch-Jensen, P., Jensen, P., Crawford, M. E., & Kehlet, H. (1995). Recovery

after laparoscopic colonic surgery with epidural analgesia, and early oral nutrition and mobilization. *Lancet, 345*, 763–764.

7. Beattie, W. S., Warriner, C. B., Etches, R., et al. (1997). The addition of continuous intravenous infusion of ketorolac to a patient controlled analgesic morphine regime reduced postoperative myocardial ischemia in patients undergoing elective total hip or knee arthroplasty. *Anesthesia and Analgesia, 84*, 715–722.
8. Beecher, H. K. (1946). Pain in men wounded in battle. *Annals of Surgery, 123*, 96.
9. Bennett, G. J., Kajander, K. C., Sahara, Y., Iadarola, M. J., & Sugimoto, T. (1989). Neurochemical and anatomical changes in the dorsal horn of rats with an experimental painful peripheral neuropathy. In F. Cervero, G. J. Bennett, & P. M. Headley (Eds.), *Processing of Sensory Information in the Superficial Dorsal Horn of the Spinal Cord* (pp. 463–471). Plenum.
10. Besse, D., Lombard, M. C., Zakac, J. M., Roques, B. P., & Besson, J. M. (1990). Pre- and postsynaptic distribution of mu, delta and kappa opioid receptors in the superficial layers of the cervical dorsal horn of the rat spinal cord. *Brain Research, 521*, 15–22.
11. Binder, W., Machelska, H., Mousa, S., Schmitt, T., Riviere, P. J. M., Junien, J. L., Stein, C., & Schafer, M. (2001). Analgesic and anti-inflammatory effects of two novel kappa-opioid peptides. *Anesthesiology, 94*, 1034–1044.
12. Blomberg, S., Emanuelsson, H., Kuist, H., Lamm, C., et al. (1990). Effects of thoracic epidural anesthesia on coronary arteries and arterioles in patients with coronary artery disease. *Anesthesiology, 73*(5), 840–847.
13. Bonica, J. J. (1985). Biology, pathophysiology and treatment of acute pain. In S. Lipton & J. Miles (Eds.), *Persistent Pain* (pp. 1–32). Grune & Stratton.
14. Bowler, G., Wildsmith, J., & Scott, D. B. (1986). Epidural administration of local anesthetics. In M. J. Cousins & G. D. Phillips (Eds.), *Acute Pain Management* (pp. 187–236). Churchill Livingstone.
15. Brandt, M. R., Fernandes, A., Mordhorst, R., & Kehlet, H. (1978). Epidural analgesia improves postoperative nitrogen balance. *British Medical Journal, 1*, 1106–1108.
16. Brodner, G., Pogatzki, E., Van Aken, H., Buerkle, H., Goeters, C., Schulzki, C., Nottberg, H., & Mertes, N. (1998). A multimodal approach to control postoperative pathophysiology and rehabilitation in patients undergoing abdominothoracic esophagectomy. *Anesthesia and Analgesia, 86*, 228–234.
17. Chapman, C. R., & Cox, G. B. (1977). Anxiety, pain and depression surrounding elective surgery: a multivariate comparison of abdominal surgery patients with kidney donors and recipients. *Journal of Psychosomatic Research, 21*, 7.
18. Christopherson, R., Beattie, C., Frank, S. M., et al. (1993). The perioperative ischemia randomized anesthesia trial study group: Perioperative morbidity in patients randomized to epidural or general anesthesia for lower-extremity vascular surgery. *Anesthesiology, 79*, 422–434.
19. Coderre, T., Grimes, R. W., & Melzack, R. (1986). Autotomy after nerve section in the rat is influenced by tonic descending inhibition from locus coeruleus. *Neuroscience Letters, 67*, 81–86.
20. Cousins, M. J. (1987). Visceral pain. In S. Andersson, M. Bond, M. Mehta, & M. Swerdlow (Eds.), *Chronic Non-Cancer Pain: Assessment and Practical Management* (pp. 119–132). MTP Press.

21. Cousins, M. J., & Bridenbaugh, P. O. (Eds.). (1998). *Neural Blockade in Clinical Anesthesia and Management of Pain* (3rd ed.). Lippincott–Raven.
22. Cousins, M. J., & Phillips, G. D. (Eds.). (1986). *Acute Pain Management.* Clinics in critical care medicine. Churchill Livingstone.
23. Cousins, M. J., & Wright, C. J. (1971). Graft, muscle and skin blood flow after epidural block in vascular surgical procedures. *Surgery, Gynecology & Obstetrics, 133*, 59.
24. Cousins, M. J., Reeve, T. S., Glynn, C. J., Walsh, J. A., & Cherry, D. A. (1979). Neurolytic lumbar sympathetic blockade: Duration of denervation and relief of rest pain. *Anesthesia and Intensive Care, 7*, 121–135.
25. Craig, D. B. (1981). Postoperative recovery of pulmonary function. *Anesthesia and Analgesia, 60*, 46.
26. Dahl, J. B., & Kehlet, H. (1993). The value of pre-emptive analgesia in the treatment of postoperative pain. *British Journal of Anesthesia, 70*, 434.
27. Dahl, J. B., Rosenberg, J., Dirkes, W. E., Morgensen, T., & Kehlet, H. (1990). Prevention of postoperative pain by balanced analgesia. *British Journal of Anesthesia, 64*, 518–520.
28. Devor, M., & Seltzer, Z. (1999). Pathophysiology of damaged nerves in relation to chronic pain. In P. D. Wall & R. Melzack (Eds.), *Textbook of Pain* (4th ed., pp. 129–164). Churchill Livingstone.
29. Doubell, T. P., Mannion, R. J., & Woolf, C. J. (1999). The dorsal horn: State dependent sensory processing, plasticity and the generation of pain. In P. D. Wall & R. Melzack (Eds.), *Textbook of Pain* (4th ed., pp. 165–182). Churchill Livingstone.
30. Dubner, R., & Ren, K. (1994). Central mechanisms of thermal and mechanical hyperalgesia following tissue inflammation. In J. Boivie, P. Hansson, & U. Lindblom (Eds.), *Touch, Temperature, and Pain in Health and Disease: Mechanisms and Assessments* (pp. 267–277). IASP Press.
31. Egbert, L. D., Battit, G. E., Welch, C. E., et al. (1964). Reduction of postoperative pain by encouragement and instruction of patients. *New England Journal of Medicine, 270*, 825.
32. Fields, H. L., & Basbaum, A. I. (1994). Central nervous system mechanisms of pain modulation. In P. D. Wall & R. Melzack (Eds.), *Textbook of Pain* (3rd ed., pp. 243–257). Churchill Livingstone.
33. Foley, K. M. (1985). The treatment of cancer pain. *New England Journal of Medicine, 313*, 84.
34. Fortin, F., & Kirovac, S. (1976). A randomized controlled trial of preoperative patient education. *Educational Journal of Nursing Studies, 13*, 11.
35. Freiha, F., & Zeineh, S. (1983). Dorsal approach to upper urinary tract. *Urology, 21*, 15–16.
36. Garnett, R. L., MacIntyre, A., & Lindsay, P. (1996). Perioperative ischemia in aortic surgery: Combined epidural/general anesthesia and epidural analgesia vs general anesthesia and IV analgesia. *Canadian Journal of Anesthesia, 43*, 769–778.
37. Groudine, S. B., Fisher, H. A. G., Kaufman, R. P., et al. (1998). *Anesthesia and Analgesia, 86*, 235–239.
38. Hayes, C., & Molloy, A. R. (1997). Neuropathic pain in the perioperative period. In A. R. Molloy & I. Power (Eds.), *International Anesthesiology Clinics. Acute and Chronic Pain* (pp. 67–81). Lippincott–Raven.

39. Haynes, T. K., Appadurai, I. R., Power, I., Rosen, M., & Grant, A. (1994). Intra-articular morphine and bupivacaine analgesia after arthroscopic knee surgery. *Anesthesia, 49*, 54–56.

40. Hetherington, J. W., & Philp, N. H. (1986). Diclofenac sodium versus pethidine in acute renal colic. *British Medical Journal, 292*, 237–338.

41. Hoar, P. F., & Hickey, R. F. (1976). Systemic hypertension following myocardial revascularization: A method of treatment using epidural anesthesia. *Journal of Thoracic and Cardiovascular Surgery, 71*, 859.

42. Hori, Y., Endo, K., & Takahashi, T. (1992). Presynaptic inhibitory action of enkephalin on excitatory transmission in superficial dorsal horn of rat spinal cord. *Journal of Physiology, 450*, 673–685.

43. Hume, D. M., & Egdahl, R. H. (1959). The importance of the brain in the endocrine response to injury. *Annals of Surgery, 150*, 697.

44. IASP Task Force on Taxonomy. (1994). *Classification of Chronic Pain*. IASP Press.

45. Inbal, R., Devor, M., Tuchendler, O., & Licblich, L. (1980). Autotomy following nerve injury: Genetic factors in the development of chronic pain. *Pain, 9*, 327–337.

46. Jänig, W. (1996). The puzzle of 'reflex sympathetic dystrophy': Mechanisms, hypotheses, open questions. In W. Janig & M. Stanton-Hicks (Eds.), *Reflex Sympathetic Dystrophy: A Reappraisal* (pp. 1–24). IASP Press.

47. Jänig, W., & McLachlan, E. M. (1994). The role of modifications in noradrenergic peripheral pathways after nerve lesions in the generation of pain. In H. L. Fields & J. C. Liebeskind (Eds.), *Progress in Pain Research and Management* (pp. 101–128). IASP Press.

48. Jorgensen, L., Rasmussen, L., Nielsen, A., Leffers, A., & Albrecht-Beste, E. (1991). Antithrombotic efficacy of continuous extradural analgesia after knee replacement. *British Journal of Anesthesia, 66*, 8–12.

49. Kam, P. C. A., & Power, I. (2000). New selective Cox-2 inhibitors. *Pain Reviews, 7*, 3–13.

50. Katz, J., Jackson, M., Kavanagh, B. P., & Sandler, A. N. (1996). Acute pain after thoracic surgery predicts long-term post-thoracotomy pain. *Clinical Journal of Pain, 12*, 50–55.

51. Kehlet, H. (1988). Modification of responses to surgery by neural blockade: Clinical implications. In M. J. Cousins & P. O. Bridenbaugh (Eds.), *Neural Blockade in Clinical Anesthesia and Management of Pain* (2nd ed., pp. 145–188). Lippincott.

52. Kehlet, H. (1989). Surgical stress: The role of pain and analgesia. *British Journal of Anesthesia, 63*, 189–195.

53. Kehlet, H. (1996). Effect of pain relief on the surgical stress response. *Regional Anesthesia, 21*(6S), 35–37.

54. Kehlet, H. (1997). Multimodal approach to control postoperative pathophysiology and rehabilitation. *British Journal of Anesthesia, 78*, 606–617.

55. Kehlet, H. (1998). Modification of responses to surgery by neural blockade: Clinical implications. In M. J. Cousins & P. O. Bridenbaugh (Eds.), *Neural Blockade in Clinical Anesthesia and Management of Pain* (3rd ed., pp. 129–178). Lippincott-Raven.

56. Kehlet, H., & Dahl, J. B. (1993a). The value of 'multimodal' or 'balanced analgesia' in postoperative pain treatment. *Anesthesia and Analgesia, 77*, 1048–1056.

57. Kehlet, H., & Dahl, J. B. (1993b). Postoperative pain [Review]. *World Journal of Surgery, 17*, 215–219.

58. Kitzinger, S. (1984). Episiotomy pain. In P. D. Wall & R. Melzack (Eds.), *Textbook of Pain* (1st ed., pp. 293–303). Churchill Livingstone.

59. Klassen, G. A., Bramwell, P. R., Bromage, R. S., & Zborawska-Sluis, D. T. (1980). Effect of acute sympathectomy by epidural anesthesia on the canine coronary circulation. *Anesthesiology, 52*, 8–15.

60. Kumar, B., & Hibbert, G. R. (1984). Control of hypertension during aortic surgery using lumbar extradural blockade. *British Journal of Anesthesia, 56*, 797.

61. Levine, J. D., & Reichling, D. B. (1999). Peripheral mechanisms of inflammatory pain. In P. D. Wall & R. Melzack (Eds.), *Textbook of Pain* (4th ed., pp. 59–84). Churchill Livingstone.

62. Levine, J. D., Fields, H. L., & Basbaum, A. I. (1993). Peptides and the primary afferent nociceptor. *Journal of Neurosciences, 13*, 2273–2286.

63. Lindblom, U. (1979). Sensory abnormalities in neuralgia. In J. J. Bonica, J. C. Liebeskind, & D. L. Albe-Fessard (Eds.), *Advances in pain research and therapy, vol 3* (pp. 111–120). Raven Press.

64. Litwin, M. S. (1962). Postsympathectomy neuralgia. *Archives of Surgery, 84*, 591–595.

65. Liu, S. S., Carpenter, R. L., & Neal, J. M. (1995b). Epidural anesthesia and analgesia. Their role in postoperative outcome. *Anesthesiology, 82*, 1474–1506.

66. Liu, S. S., Carpenter, R. L., Mackey, D. C., et al. (1995a). Effects of perioperative analgesic technique on rate of recovery after colon surgery. *Anesthesiology, 83*, 757–765.

67. Macrae, W. A. (2001). Chronic pain after surgery. *British Journal of Anaesthesia, 87*, 88–98.

68. Mankikian, B., Cantineau, J. P., Bertrand, M., et al. (1988). Improvement of diaphragmatic dysfunction by extradural block after upper abdominal surgery. *Anesthesiology, 68*, 379–386.

69. McLachlan, E. M., Jänig, W., Devor, M., & Michaelis, M. (1993). Peripheral nerve injury triggers noradrenergic sprouting within dorsal root ganglia. *Nature, 363*, 543–546.

70. McMahon, S. B. (1991). Mechanisms of sympathetic pain. *British Medical Bulletin, 47*, 584–600.

71. Meert, T. F., & De Kock, M. (1994). Potentiation of the analgesic properties of fentanyl-like opioids with α2-adrenoceptor agonists in rats. *Anesthesiology, 81*, 677–688.

72. Melzack, R. (1971). Phantom limb pain. *Anesthesiology, 35*, 409.

73. Melzack, R., Wall, P. D., & Ty, T. C. (1982). Acute pain in an emergency clinic: Latency of onset and description patterns. *Pain, 14*, 33.

74. Merry, A., & Power, I. (1995). Perioperative NSAIDs: Towards greater safety. *Pain Reviews, 2*, 268–291.

75. Merskey, H. (1986). Classification of chronic pain. Descriptions of chronic pain syndromes and definition of pain terms. *Pain, 3*(suppl), S1–S225.

76. Modig, J. (1976). Respiration and circulation after total hip replacement surgery: A comparison between parenteral analgesics and continuous lumbar epidural block. *Acta Anaesthesiologica Scandinavica, 20*, 225–236.

77. Modig, J., Borg, T., Karlstom, G., Maripuu, E., & Sahlstedt, B. (1983). Thromboembolism after hip replacement: Role of epidural and general anesthesia. *Anesthesia and Analgesia, 62*, 174–180.

78. Modig, J., Malmberg, P., & Karlstom, G. (1980). Effect of epidural versus general anesthesia on calf blood flow. *Acta Anaesthesiologica Scandinavica, 24*, 305.

79. Moiniche, S., Dahl, J. B., Rosenberg, J., & Kehlet, H. (1994b). Colonic resection with early discharge after combined subarachnoid-epidural analgesia, preoperative glucocorticoids, and early postoperative mobilization and feeding in a pulmonary high-risk patient. *Regional Anesthesia, 19*, 352–356.

80. Moiniche, S., Hjortso, N. C., Hansen, B. L., et al. (1994a). The effect of balanced analgesia on early convalescence after major orthopaedic surgery. *Acta Anaesthesiologica Scandinavica, 38*, 328–335.

81. NHMRC. (1999). *Acute Pain Management: Scientific Evidence*. National Health and Medical Research Council of Australia, Canberra.

82. Nimmo, W. S. (1984). Effect of anesthesia on gastric motility and emptying. *British Journal of Anesthesia, 56*, 29–37.

83. Ollat, H., & Cesaro, P. (1995). Pharmacology of neuropathic pain. *Clinical Neuropharmacology, 18*, 391–404.

84. Peck, C. (1986). Psychological factors in acute pain management. In M. J. Cousins & G. D. Phillips (Eds.), *Acute Pain Management* (pp. 251–274). Churchill Livingstone.

85. Perkins, F. M., & Kehlet, H. (2000). Chronic pain as an outcome of surgery—Aview of predictive factors. *Anesthesiology, 93*, 1123–1133.

86. Power, I., Bowler, G. M. R., Pugh, G. C., & Chambers, W. A. (1994). Ketorolac as a component of balanced analgesia after thoracotomy. *British Journal of Anesthesia, 72*, 224–226.

87. Raja, S. N., Meyer, R. A., Ringkamp, M., & Campbell, J. N. (1999). Peripheral neural mechanisms of nociception. In P. D. Wall & R. Melzack (Eds.), *Textbook of Pain* (4th ed., pp. 11–58). Churchill Livingstone.

88. Reiz, S., Balfors, E., Sorensen, M. R., et al. (1982). Coronary hemodynamic effects of general anesthesia and surgery. *Regional Anesthesia, 7*(suppl), S8–S18.

89. Sabiston, D. C. (1982). *Davis Christopher Textbook of Surgery: The Biological Basis of Modern Surgical Practice* (2nd ed.). Saunders.

90. Scheinin, B., et al. (1987). The effect of bupivacaine and morphine on pain and bowel function after colonic surgery. *Acta Anaesthesiologica Scandinavica, 31*, 161–164.

91. Schulze, S., Roikjaer, O., Hasseistrom, L., Jensen, N. H., & Kehlet, H. (1988). Epidural bupivacaine and morphine plus systemic indomethacin eliminates pain but not systemic response and convalescence after cholecystectomy. *Surgery, 103*, 321–327.

92. Scott, D. B. (1988). Acute pain management. In M. J. Cousins & P. O. Bridenbaugh (Eds.), *Neural Blockade in Clinical Anesthesia and Management of Pain* (2nd ed., pp. 861–864). Lippincott.

93. Scott, N., & Kehlet, H. (1988). Regional anesthesia and surgical morbidity. *British Journal of Surgery, 75*, 199–204.

94. Seibert, K., Zhang, Y., & Leahy, K. (1994). Pharmacological and biochemical demonstration of the role of cyclooxygenase 2 in inflammation and pain. *Proceedings of the National Academy of Sciences of the USA, 91*, 12013–12017.

95. Sivilotti, L., & Woolf, C. J. (1994). The contribution of GABAA and glycine receptors to

central sensitization: Disinhibition and touch-evoked allodynia in the spinal cord. *Journal of Neurophysiology, 72*, 169–179.

96. Sjogren, S., & Wright, B. (1972). Circulatory changes during continuous epidural blockade. *Acta Anaesthesiologica Scandinavica, 46*(suppl), 5.
97. Stein, C. (1993). Peripheral mechanisms of opioid analgesia. *Anesthesia and Analgesia, 76*, 182–191.
98. Stein, C. (1995). Morphine—A local 'analgesic.' *Pain: Clinical Updates, 3*, 1–4.
99. Stein, C., Millan, M. J., & Shippenberg, T. S. (1989). Peripheral opioid receptors mediating antinociception in inflammation: Evidence for involvement of mu, delta, and kappa receptors. *Journal of Pharmacology and Experimental Therapeutics, 248*, 1269–1275.
100. Tasker, R. R., Tsuda, T., & Hawrylyshyn, P. (1983). Clinical neurophysiological investigation of deafferentation pain. In J. J. Bonica, U. Lindblom, & A. Iggo (Eds.), *Advances in Pain Research and Therapy, vol 5* (pp. 713–738). Raven.
101. Tennant, F., Moll, D., & Depaulo, V. (1993). Topical morphine for peripheral pain. *Lancet, 342*, 1047–1048.
102. Thoren, T., Sundberg, A., Wattwil, M., Garvill, J. E., et al. (1989). Effects of epidural bupivacaine and epidural morphine on bowel function and pain after hysterectomy. *Acta Anaesthesiologica Scandinavica, 33*, 181–195.
103. Thorn, S. E., Wattwil, M., Naslund, I., et al. (1992). Post-operative epidural morphine but not epidural bupivacaine, delays gastric emptying on the first day after cholecystectomy. *Regional Anesthesia, 17*(2), 91–94.
104. Tuman, K. J., McCarthy, R. J., March, R. J., et al. (1991). Effects of epidural anesthesia and analgesia on coagulation and outcome after major vascular surgery. *Anesthesia and Analgesia, 73*, 696–704.
105. Urquhart, E. (1993). Central analgesic activity of nonsteroidal anti-inflammatory drugs in animal and human pain models. *Seminars in Arthritis and Rheumatism, 23*, 198–205.
106. Vik-Mo, H., Ottsen, S., & Renck, H. (1978). Cardiac effects of thoracic epidural analgesia before and during acute coronary artery occlusion in open-chest dogs. *Scandinavian Journal of Clinical and Laboratory Investigation, 38*, 737–746.
107. Walker, J. S. (1995). NSAID: An update on their analgesic effects. *Clinical and Experimental Pharmacology and Physiology, 22*, 855–860.
108. Wattwil, M., Thoren, T., Hennerdal, S., Garvill, J. E., et al. (1989). Epidural analgesia with bupivacaine reduces postoperative paralytic ileus after hysterectomy. *Anesthesia and Analgesia, 68*, 353–358.
109. White, J. C., & Sweet, W. H. (1962). *Pain and the Neurosurgeon*. Thomas, pp. 11–49.
110. Wilcox, G. L. (1991). Excitatory neurotransmitters and pain. In M. R. Bond, J. E. Charlton, & C. J. Woolf (Eds.), *Proceedings of the VIth World Congress on Pain*. Elsevier, pp. 97–117.
111. Wilmore, D. W. (1983). Alterations in protein, carbohydrate and fat metabolism in injured and septic patients. *Journal of the American College of Nutrition, 2*, 3.
112. Wilmore, D. W., Long, J. M., Mason, A. D., & Pruitt, B. A. (1976). Stress in surgical patients as a neurophysiologic reflex response. *Surgery, Gynecology and Obstetrics, 142*, 257.

113. Woolf, C. J., & Chong, M. S. (1993). Preemptive analgesia—Treating postoperative pain by preventing the establishment of central sensitization. *Anesthesia and Analgesia, 77*, 362–379.

114. Yaksh, T. L. (1999). Central pharmacology of nociceptive transmission. In P. D. Wall & R. Melzack (Eds.), *Textbook of Pain* (4th ed., pp. 253–308). Churchill Livingstone.

115. Yaksh, T. L., & Reddy, S. V. R. (1981). Studies in the primate on the analgesic effects associated with intrathecal actions of opiates, alpha-adrenergic agonists and baclofen. *Anesthesiology, 54*, 451–467.

116. Yeager, M. P., Glass, D. D., Neff, R. K., & Brinck-Johnson, T. (1987). Epidural anesthesia and analgesia in high-risk surgical patients. *Anesthesiology, 66*, 729–736.

117. Zolte, N., & Cust, M. D. (1986). Analgesia in the acute abdomen. *Annals of the Royal College of Surgeons of England, 68*, 209–210.

Chapter

2

OSTEOARTHRITIS, RHEUMATOID ARTHRITIS, AND MUSCLES PAIN

Contents

Introduction

Both rheumatoid arthritis (RA) and osteoarthritis (OA) are common forms of arthritis that affect the joints and cause pain and discomfort, though they do so in different ways.

The primary cause of osteoarthritis is a degenerative joint disease called cartilage degradation, which affects the tissue that covers the ends of the bones in the joint. As cartilage degrades, bones may grind against one another, causing discomfort, stiffness, and decreased range of motion in the afflicted joint. Although it can also be brought on by overuse or joint injuries, osteoarthritis (OA) usually develops gradually over time and is frequently linked to aging. Osteoarthritis can affect any joint, but it most commonly affects weight-bearing joints like the spine, hips, and knees.

Rheumatoid arthritis, on the other hand, is an autoimmune condition that results in inflammation of the synovium, which lines the joints. Inadvertent immune system attacks on healthy joint tissue result in stiffness, pain, swelling, and eventually joint damage. In addition to affecting several joints at once, rheumatoid arthritis can also result in systemic symptoms like fever, exhaustion, and weight loss. Rheumatoid arthritis is more common in women than in men and can strike at any age, unlike osteoarthritis, which mainly affects older adults.

Myalgia, or pain in the muscles, can be caused by several things, such as overuse, trauma, stress, or specific medical disorders. Muscle pain can be anything from a minor annoyance to excruciating, incapacitating pain, and it sometimes comes with stiffness, weakness, or edema in the affected area. While muscle pain is frequently transient and can be managed with rest, stretching, or over-the-counter painkillers, severe or chronic muscle pain may need to be evaluated by a doctor and treated.

Osteoarthritis, rheumatoid arthritis, and muscle pain are often effectively managed with a combination of lifestyle adjustments, physical therapy, medication, and, in certain situations, surgery. For those impacted by these disorders, early diagnosis and treatment are essential to reducing pain, maintaining joint function, and enhancing overall quality of life.

Orientation and Directional Terms

Term	Definition	Illustration
Osteoarthritis	Osteoarthritis is a degenerative joint disease, in which the tissues in the joint break down over time.	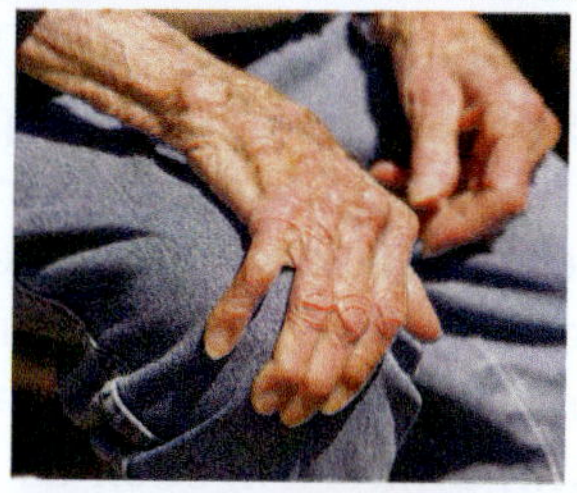
Rheumatoid arthritis	Rheumatoid arthritis (RA) is a chronic (long-lasting) autoimmune disease that mostly affects joints.	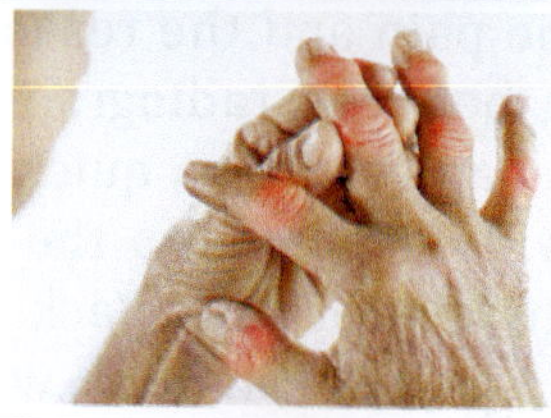
Synovium	The synovium, also known as the synovial membrane, is a soft tissue that lines the inside of joints, tendon sheaths, and bursae.	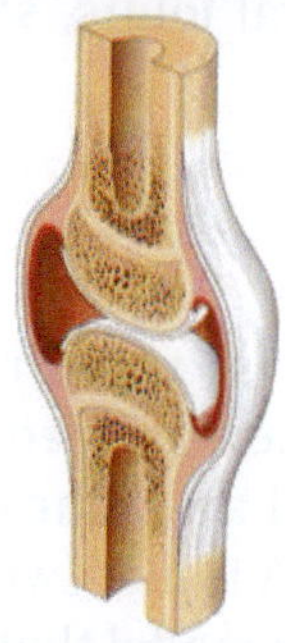
Back pain	Back pain can be pain in the back, neck, middle back, lower back, or coccyx.	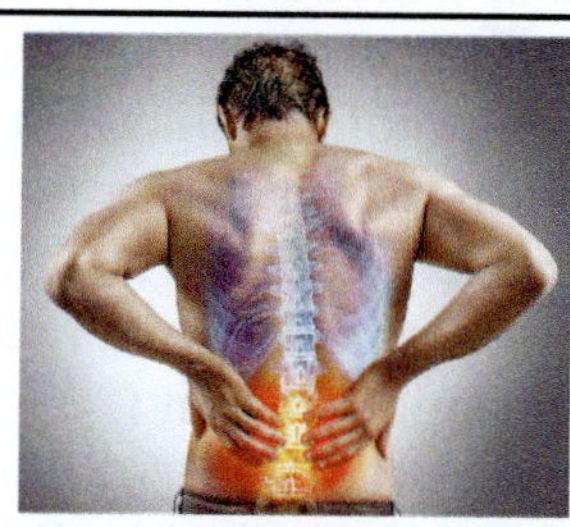
Joint laxity	Joint laxity, also known as joint hypermobility or hyperlaxity, is a connective tissue issue that causes joints to be excessively flexible and unstable.	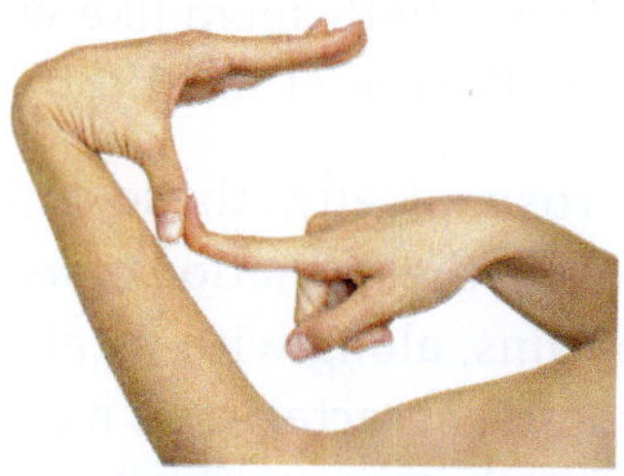

2.1. Osteoarthritis

The most prevalent type of arthritis, osteoarthritis (OA), is linked to increased morbidity, activity limitation, and medical care use (Lawrence et al., 1990). The primary sign of OA is pain, which also serves as the primary motivator for those who experience it to seek medical attention. Another important factor influencing functional loss is pain. Despite its significance, many aspects of OA pain are still unknown, such as the anatomical origin of the pain and the reason for the weak association between radiographic change and pain. This chapter gives a quick synopsis of OA before delving deeper into the nature, causes, and management of pain. Back pain is covered in another chapter; this one will focus on OA of the peripheral joints, specifically the knee.

2.1.1. Etiopathogenesis of Osteoarthritis

Osteoarthritis is a disorder of the synovial joints that is characterized by subchondral bone remodeling and articular cartilage destruction. The idea that OA is just "wear and tear" has been superseded by a model that views OA as an active process that upsets the equilibrium between the production of cartilage and catabolism. An increase in activity on a bone scan, which indicates thickening of the subchondral bone, is another early sign that could indicate the onset of OA in the hand later on (Figure 2.1) and the knee (Dieppe et al., 1993). Although it's unclear which is the main lesion in OA—the bone or the cartilage—both seem like viable targets for treatment (Hutton et al., 1986).

Macroscopically, these alterations cause sclerosis and the formation of osteophytes at the joint margins, along with focal cartilage loss. A few of these characteristics match radiographic alterations that are typically used to diagnose OA.

The term "osteoarthritic disorders" refers to a collection of overlapping, distinct diseases with differing risk factors, clinical characteristics, radiographic features, and outcomes.

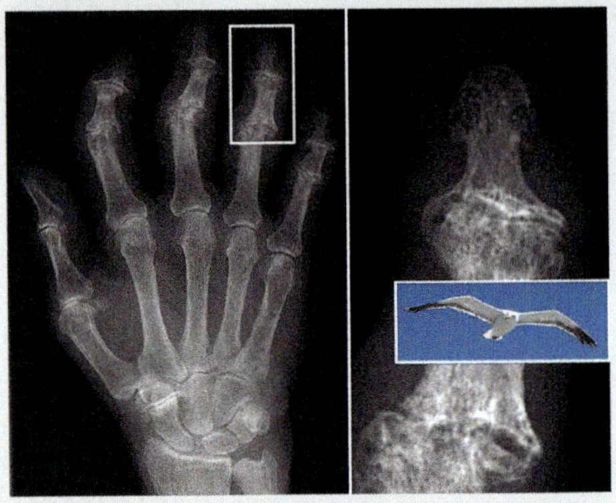

Figure 2.1. X-ray of a patient with hand OA.

Source: By Rennett Stowe and Mikael Häggström – Own work By Rennett Stowe from USA, CC BY 4.0, https://commons.wikimedia.org/w/index.php?curid=76556085.

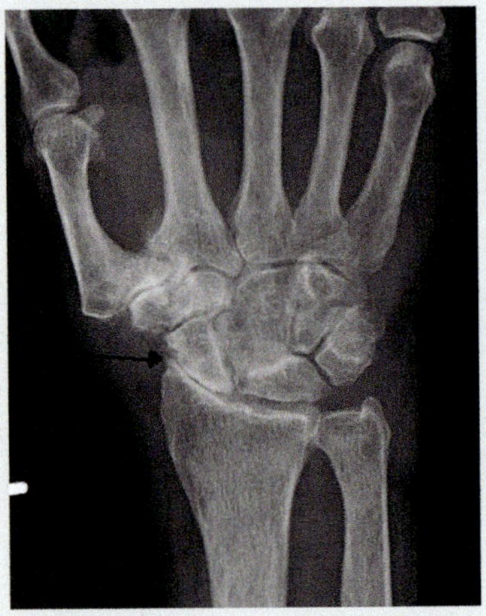

Figure 2.2. Severe osteoarthritis and osteopenia of the carpal joint and 1st carpometacarpal joint.

Source: By James Heilman, MD – Own work, CC BY-SA 3.0, https://commons.wikimedia.org/w/index.php?curid=10385858.

The following variables increase systemic vulnerability to OA: race, age, gender, and nutrition. Misalignment, prior damage, muscle weakness, joint laxity, and proprioceptive defects are examples of local biomechanical factors. Local factors likely influence which joints in a susceptible individual develop osteoarthritis (OA), along with extrinsic factors acting on the joint, such as obesity, physical activity, occupational overuse, and trauma.

2.1.2. Clinical Features of Osteoarthritis

OA most commonly affects the hand's interphalangeal joints (Figure 2.3), the base of the thumb, hips, knees, and cervical and lumbar spine facet joints. When OA does cause symptoms, they include pain, stiffness after inactivity, deformity, swelling, and loss of function. However, most cases of OA appear to be asymptomatic.

Table 2.1. Advantages and Disadvantages of Current in Vitro Models for OA Research

Current In Vitro Models	Advantages	Limitations
Monolayer culture	• Support convenient, high-throughput tests • High reproducibility	• Do not replicate in vivo tissue niche • Chondrocytes undergo dedifferentiation
3D engineered cartilage tissues	• Create a 3D microenvironment enabling cell–cell and/or cell–matrix interactions • Higher chondrogenic potential than 2D culture	• Varying biological relevance for different 3D systems • Other joint tissues not considered
Tissue explant models	• Cells reside in their native environment • Study physiology of cartilage as a whole tissue	• Properties strongly depend on donor and tissue harvest site • Cell death at tissue edges
Microphysiological systems	• Support culture of multiple 3D joint tissues to allow their crosstalk • Controlled cell culture microenvironment • Enable real-time, on-chip analysis • Dynamic medium supply supported by microfluidic flow • Convenient application of insults and drugs/treatments	• Variable biological accuracy due to non-standardized protocols • Limited material selection for chip manufacture

Source: He Y, Li Z, Alexander PG, Ocasio-Nieves BD, Yocum L, Lin H, Tuan RS. Pathogenesis of osteoarthritis: risk factors, regulatory pathways in chondrocytes, and experimental models. *Biology*. 2020; 9(8):194. https://doi.org/10.3390/biology9080194.

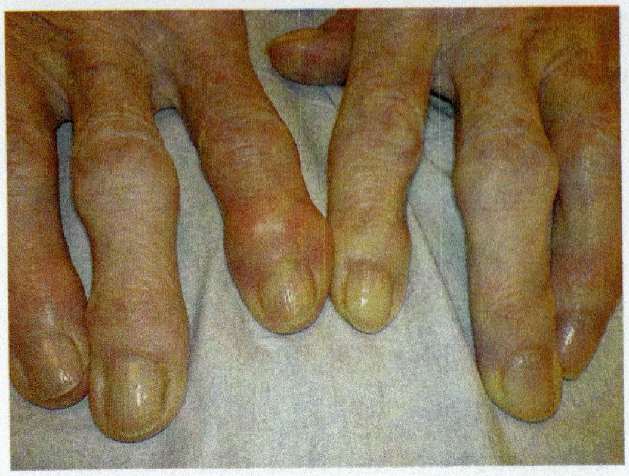

Figure 2.3. Interphalangeal OA.

Source. By Drahreg01 – Own work, CC BY-SA 3.0, https://commons.wikimedia.org/w/index.php?curid=1358952.

Radiographic characteristics such as osteophyte, joint space narrowing, and bony sclerosis are still used to diagnose osteoarthritis. Significant pathological alteration could take place before radiographs show abnormalities (Fife et al., 1991). Direct cartilage visualization is possible with arthroscopy, and scoring systems for uniformly documenting cartilage damage are currently accessible (Ayral et al., 1996). Although magnetic resonance imaging (MRI) is non-invasive and can evaluate non-bony structures, its routine use is impractical due to the cost and expertise involved in its interpretation.

2.1.3. Pathophysiology of Joint Pain

The majority of afferent fibers in articular nerves, which include post-ganglionic sympathetic fibers and C (group IV) fibers, are unmyelinated. Approximately 20% of the total fibers are made up of thinly myelinated Aδ (group III) fibers and heavily myelinated Aβ (group II) fibers (Kidd, 1996). Rich innervation is provided by a combination of free nerve endings and receptors to the periosteum, tendons, ligaments, synovium, and articular capsule. These sensory nerves react to chemical mediators like substance P, lactic acid, histamine, and kinins in addition to mechanical stimuli like stretching of the joint capsule. These inflammatory mediators have the potential to both directly stimulate pain fibers and increase their sensitivity to mechanical stimuli. As a result, there's a chance that an acute injury or inflammation will make nerves more sensitive, making them react even in the absence of the initial stimulus. This "neurogenic plasticity" is likely mediated by the upregulation of particular receptors, such as those for N-methyl-D aspartate (NMDA), and it may function at both the peripheral and spinal levels. These obviously indicate possible therapeutic intervention targets. Peripheral mechanisms are likely more significant, even though there is evidence for a central role in pain production in some patients. For instance, intra-articular local anesthetic effectively and temporarily eliminate pain in many patients with knee OA (Creamer et al., 1996).

2.1.4. Measurement of Pain in Osteoarthritis

A question like "Have you ever had pain in or around the knee on most days for at least a month?" is typically used in community studies to determine whether or not participants have knee pain (Lawrence et al., 1990). A visual analog scale or a basic Likert scale (none, mild, moderate, severe, very severe) can be used to grade the degree of subjective pain. A straightforward "how bad is your (knee, hip, hand) pain?" may serve as the stem question, but it's also helpful to inquire about pain during various activities, such as walking, stairs, resting, and so on. These data are gathered through questionnaires created especially to evaluate OA in the lower limbs; two examples of such questionnaires are the WOMAC (Bellamy et al., 1988) and Lequesne (1991) indices.

Sometimes an attempt is made to use the McGill Pain Questionnaire (MPQ; Melzack, 1975) to evaluate the degree of pain in OA patients. With this tool, participants can choose from 76 different words to best describe their pain. Since the MPQ was not created with arthritis pain in mind, some of the descriptors may actually reflect mood disorders rather than actual pain.

Lastly, by videotaping patients as they participate in a typical activity program, the impact of pain on observed behavior in OA can be evaluated (Keefe et al., 1987a). Independent observers can score actions like guarding, active rubbing, unloading the joint, rigidity, and joint flexing.

2.1.5. Epidemiology of Osteoarthritic Pain

The majority of research on pain in OA has focused on the knee. In the UK, approximately 25.3% of community residents aged 40 to 79 report having knee pain (O'Reilly et al., 1996). Of those reporting pain, 76% had radiographic knee OA. There is less data available for other joints. Carman (1989) defined "mild to severe pain during the last month" and found that 37% of people aged 50–74 reported having hand pain, with 45% having OA.

While the likelihood of reporting pain increases with increasing radiographic severity, there is generally little correlation between pain and structural damage. According to community studies, 7–14% of participants with normal knee X-rays report having knee pain; possible reasons for this include pain sources that are invisible on an X-ray, radiographs that are not sensitive enough, or insufficient views being obtained (e.g., failure to evaluate the knee's patellofemoral joint). Furthermore, only 40–80% of the subjects with clear-cut radiographic knee OA report having pain; this could be because the question isn't sufficiently specific or because the pain might be a phasic process. In outpatients, coping mechanisms and obesity are more important determinants of pain severity than presence, as indicated by previous research (Creamer et al., 1999).

In individuals with osteoarthritis (OA), pain is not solely a consequence of structural alterations; rather, it is the product of a multifaceted interaction involving structural alterations, peripheral and central pain processing systems, and subjective variations in the definition of pain, which are impacted by cultural, gender, and psychological elements. It might be more beneficial to think of radiographic knee OA and knee pain as distinct issues because their risk factors seem to be different (Davis et al., 1992).

Individuals who exhibit clinical characteristics like morning stiffness and crepitus are more likely to report pain. Women are more likely than men to report pain for a given radiographic severity level. Reporting of pain does not seem to be correlated with age. Certain studies have indicated that an increased body mass index is associated with an increased risk of knee OA pain. One of the main risk factors for knee pain and the ensuing disability is quadriceps weakness (McAlindan et al., 1993; Slemenda et al., 1997).

2.1.6. Anatomical Causes of Pain in Osteoarthritis

It's still unknown what anatomical source causes pain in OA. Since there are few pain-sensitive fibers in the main structure involved (articular cartilage), any theory must account for the possibility that pain is coming from other tissues.

Like any other form of chronic pain, OA is influenced by psychosocial factors. Compared to healthy controls, community participants with knee pain had higher rates of anxiety and depression (Dexter and Brandt, 1994). The prevalence is even higher among hospital outpatients: according to Hawley and Wolfe (1993), 33% of patients with hip/knee OA had "possible" depression, compared to 19% of the healthy population. Disparities between hospital and community subjects may be due to the severity of the disease, but patients' decisions to seek medical attention may also be influenced by depression.

Significant relationships between anxiety and depression and the intensity of knee pain in hospital patients have been documented, using the MPQ as a measure of pain severity (Summers et al., 1988). When compared to age-matched pain-free controls from the same community, chronicity and severity of pain were linked to higher psychosocial disability in a community survey of senior subjects reporting episodic, chronic, or sporadic knee pain (Hopman Rock et al., 1996).

Table 2.2. Regulatory Pathways Mediating Chondrocyte Functions

Pathway	Cells Studied	Effects
Wnt/β-catenin	• Mouse and human OA tissues	• Upregulates MMPs and aggrecanases
	• Mouse knee chondrocytes	• Suppresses cartilage degeneration
PI3K/Akt/mTOR	• Rat chondrocytes	• Suppresses PI3K/Akt/mTOR promotes cartilage repair and attenuates inflammatory response
Notch	• Mouse knee chondrocytes	• Induces OA-associated genes and promote OA
		• Required for articular cartilage and joint maintenance
SIRT1/AMPK	• Human and rat knee chondrocytes	• Prevents OA progression by attenuating apoptosis and mitochondrial dysfunction
Hippo/YAP/TAZ	• Human and rat knee chondrocytes	• Alleviates chondrocyte senescence and reduces matrix-degrading enzyme and cartilage degradation
	• Rat knee chondrocytes and human MSCs	• Suppresses YAP, preserves collagen type II expression, promotes chondrogenic differentiation of MSCs, and ameliorates OA development
DOT1L	• Mouse and human knee joints and chondrocytes	• Prevents OA onset and progression

Source: He Y, Li Z, Alexander PG, Ocasio-Nieves BD, Yocum L, Lin H, Tuan RS. Pathogenesis of Osteoarthritis: Risk Factors, Regulatory Pathways in Chondrocytes, and Experimental Models. *Biology*. 2020; 9(8):194. https://doi.org/10.3390/biology9080194.

Personality traits like hypochondriasis, along with "life stress" and "daily hassles," have been linked to increased pain severity in OA of the hip (Lunghi et al., 1978) and knee (Lichtenberg et al., 1986). According to Hannan et al. (1992), there is a correlation between a lower formal education level and an increased risk of both radiographic and symptomatic knee OA.

We are unable to conclude cause and effect from cross-sectional studies, and it is unclear how psychosocial factors are related to knee pain. One of the pathophysiological effects of depression or anxiety is a possible increase in painful muscle tension. Anxiety can cause generalized deconditioning, loss of confidence, and loss of muscle mass when it shows up as a persistent attempt to avoid knee pain. Overly avoiding movement due to knee pain may result in a chronic cycle of inactivity, weakness and muscle wasting, and more pain and inactivity (Dekker et al., 1993). In addition to causing maladapted "coping strategies," depression can also have an impact on a patient's self-perception of their pain management skills, which raises the reported level of pain (Keefe et al., 1987b).

Psychological factors can play a significant role in predicting how patients will respond to therapies and how well they will adhere to treatment. For instance, a study on the effects of exercise on patients with knee arthritis found that baseline anxiety and depression were the strongest indicators of whether patients would continue exercising after 3 months (Minor & Brown, 1993).

2.1.7. The Nature of Osteoarthritic Pain

Osteoarthritis (OA) pain is typically characterized as "aching" or "throbbing," localized, subtle in onset, and unrelated to any systemic disturbance. The intensity of pain from OA is similar to that from RA.

Pain typically worsens when the afflicted joint is used (e.g., knee OA), worse in the evenings, and is alleviated with rest. Nonetheless, a sizable fraction of participants do report experiencing pain at night; these individuals may have more severe illness and have typically had symptoms longer than those without nighttime pain. Some patients exhibit day-to-day variation in addition to diurnal variation, with symptoms being worse on weekends (Bellamy et al., 1990).

Although referred pain is possible, pain from osteoarthritis (OA) typically corresponds to the affected joint; for instance, pain from hip OA may be felt in the knee, while pain from spinal OA may be felt in the hip or buttock. The majority of knee pain is either localized to the inferomedial aspect of the joint or is felt diffusely anteriorly over the patella's surface.

2.1.8. Management of Pain in Osteoarthritis

The most common symptom of osteoarthritis (OA) is pain. As such, therapies for OA are mainly evaluated based on their capacity to alleviate pain, since there are currently no treatments that can alter the underlying disease process. In an ideal world, therapies would be founded on pathogenesis; in reality, though, since the source of pain in OA is unknown, there is some empirical component to treatment. However, four distinct areas can be identified: pharmacological therapy, surgery, central perception of pain modulation, and correction of abnormal mechanical stress.

2.1.9. Correction of Abnormal Biomechanics

The majority of knee OA is a biomechanical condition. By modifying weight distribution through the joint, realigning to correct deformities, and enhancing stability and patient confidence, the biomechanical intervention aims to lessen pain and improve function.

- **Weight Reduction:** Obesity increases the risk of osteoarthritis (OA), especially in women and at the knee. Losing weight is likely to lessen symptoms and is linked to a decreased risk of developing incident radiographic OA and symptomatic OA (Felson et al., 1997). A 6-month program of dietary counseling and exercise led to weight loss in overweight postmenopausal women with symptomatic knee OA (Martin et al., 1996), and this weight loss was associated with a decrease in pain and disability. The lack of additional data may indicate that dieting alone is a difficult way to lose weight, especially for older people who may be less mobile.
- **Orthotics:** With the use of a walking stick and shock-absorbing shoes, symptoms of the affected joint can be reduced by 20–30% when load bearing is reduced. In medial compartment OA with varus deformity, lateral heel wedges can lessen the lateral thrust and alleviate pain (Ogata et al., 1997). Soft neoprene sleeves with extra padding around the patellar tendon may enhance proprioception in addition to patellar tracking. Other orthotic devices are designed to address instability and deformity; these include braces, neck collars, and splints. It has been demonstrated that medial patellar taping is beneficial for patients with knee OA who also have patellofemoral joint disease (Cushnaghan et al., 1994). It is advisable to think about modifying the patient's surroundings with things like elevated chairs, toilet seats, and dressing aids.
- **Quadriceps Strengthening:** Quadriceps weakness is undoubtedly a significant factor in determining function and pain (Dekker et al., 1993; McAlindon et al., 1993), and it may be a risk factor for radiographic OA (Slemenda et al., 1997). Studies lasting three to six months have shown that patients with knee OA can benefit from quadriceps strengthening exercises by feeling less pain and having better function. These exercises can even be taught to patients at home (Fisher et al., 1993; O'Reilly, 1999). Resistance training that is both isometric and isotonic can be used to strengthen the quadriceps.
- **Aerobic Exercise:** For patients with osteoarthritis (OA) of the hip and/or knee, aerobic conditioning exercise—supervised fitness walking or swimming—has been demonstrated to be both well-tolerated and more beneficial than traditional physical therapy or standard medical care. For hip OA, at-home exercises are just as beneficial as outpatient hydrotherapy. A multicenter study (Ettinger et al., 1997) on adults with knee OA who lived in the community and self-reported physical disabilities who were 60 years of age and older showed that aerobic or resistive exercise was preferable to patient education alone.

2.1.10. Central Pain Modification

Cognitive behavioral techniques, which aim to enhance coping mechanisms and self-efficacy, are also advantageous. Through an understanding of how emotions and cognition interact with the behavioral and physical aspects of pain, these interventions emphasize the control of pain. Patients with knee OA who engaged in a program with their spouse showed higher improvements in pain, psychological disability, self-efficacy, and pain behaviors in one study

(Keefe et al., 1996) than patients who engaged in a traditional program without their spouse. They also demonstrated improved marital adjustment and coping skills.

Table 2.3. Osteoarthritis of the Knee Management Recommendations from the Three Societies

Treatment	OARSI	ACR	AAOS
Exercise (Land-based)	Appropriate	Strong recommendation	Strong recommendation
Exercise (Water-based)	Appropriate	Strong recommendation	Strong recommendation
Transcutaneous electrical nerve stimulation	Uncertain	Strong recommendation against use	Inconclusive
Cane (Walking stick)	Appropriate	Strong recommendation	
Weight control	Appropriate	Strong recommendation	Moderate recommendation
Chondroitin or Glucosamine	Not appropriate for disease modification, Uncertain (Sx relief)	Strong recommendation against use	Recommendation against use
Acetaminophen	Without comorbidities: appropriate	Conditional recommendation	Inconclusive
Duloxetine	Appropriate	Conditional recommendation	No recommendation
Oral NSAIDs	Without comorbidities: appropriate; With comorbidities: Uncertain	Strong recommendation	Strong recommendation
Topical NSAIDs	Appropriate	Conditional recommendation against use	Strong recommendation
Opioids	Uncertain	No recommendation	Recommended (only tramadol)
Intra-articular corticosteroids	Appropriate	Strong recommendation	Inconclusive
Intra-articular viscosupplementation	Uncertain	Conditional recommendation against use	Recommendation against use

OARSI: Osteoarthritis Research Society International; ACR: American College of Rheumatology; AAOS: American Academy of Orthopedic Surgeons; NSAIDs: non-steroidal anti-inflammatory drugs.

Source. R Jang S, Lee K, Ju JH. Recent Updates of Diagnosis, Pathophysiology, and Treatment on Osteoarthritis of the Knee. *International Journal of Molecular Sciences*. 2021; 22(5):2619. https://doi.org/10.3390/ijms22052619.

Education is a therapy that works as well. It has been demonstrated that the Arthritis Self-Help Course is beneficial. Six weekly education sessions comprise this course, which covers topics such as joint protection techniques, exercise, relaxation methods, and an overview of the different medications used to treat arthritis. Research conducted by Lorig and associates (Lorig & Holman, 1993) has demonstrated that individuals with OA who take part in this program experience notable improvements in their understanding, pain, and overall well-being. Additionally, they experience a reduction in the number of doctor visits and medical expenses.

Lastly, giving OA patients social support through basic phone calls can help them feel less pain and have a better functional status (Weinberger et al., 1993). The information discussed in the phone calls appears to be significant: according to Maisiak et al. (1996), specific advice and counseling are more effective than symptom monitoring.

2.1.11. Drug Therapy

Testing basic analgesics like paracetamol, coproxamol, or tramadol should be the first line of treatment for osteoarthritis (OA). These medications are well-tolerated, efficient, and safe. Non-steroidal anti-inflammatory drugs (NSAIDs) should not be administered until analgesia and nonpharmacological therapy have undergone thorough testing.

There is not much evidence to support the superiority of NSAIDs over paracetamol, and many patients receiving chronic NSAID therapy for knee OA can stop taking this medication without experiencing a noticeable worsening of their symptoms—at least in trial settings. It is tempting to assume that these patients have a more "inflammatory" form of OA because a small percentage of OA patients do appear to benefit over time from NSAIDs; however, clinical examinations cannot identify which patients will respond (Bradley et al., 1992). NSAID use is linked to significant morbidity, especially in the elderly, who are most likely to have osteoarthritis (OA). This risk can be reduced by co-prescribing gastroprotective medications at the lowest possible dosage, encouraging "intelligent non-compliance" (i.e., taking the pills only in cases of discomfort). While they are not any more effective than conventional NSAIDs, novel, highly selective COX2 inhibitors like celecoxib and rofecoxib likely carry a lower risk of serious gastrointestinal side effects.

NSAIDs can also be administered topically as creams or gels; these forms of administration are safe, well-liked by patients, and productive, possibly because they offer some control over the patient's symptoms. Topical capsaicin, a particular molecule extracted from the pepper plant, has been shown promise, particularly in the treatment of hand OA.

Injections of IA steroids are frequently used. Limited to knee controlled trials, they show some evidence of benefit over placebo, but only for a maximum of 4 weeks (Creamer, 1997). This is in contrast to clinical practice, which indicates that a sustained response of up to six months may be experienced by certain patients. While some studies have suggested that the presence of effusion (Gaffney et al., 1995) or local tenderness (Jones & Doherty, 1996) may be associated with a better response, efforts to identify response predictors have largely proven unsuccessful. According to a recent study (Griffith et al., 1997), hip steroid or anesthetic injections significantly improved the range of motion, pain, and stiffness, but the effects of both injections were similar. Anecdotally, thumb-base OA patients report great benefits from carpometacarpal joint injections. Injections of steroids are remarkably well-tolerated and safe.

A major component of synovial fluid, hyaluronic acid (HA) is the backbone of the proteoglycan molecule. Apart from its functional functions as a lubricant, shock absorber, and buffer between the surfaces of articular cartilage, it could also play a part in binding neuropeptides linked to pain production and inflammatory mediators. For knee OA, HA preparations are available for intra-articular injection. When compared to intra-articular steroids (Jones et al., 1995) or placebo injections (Dougados et al., 1993; Lohmander et al., 1996), many studies indicate a slight benefit. Intra-articular hyaluronic acid may be useful in the treatment of some elderly patients with knee OA, given the reluctance of the elderly to use NSAIDs. These patients may include those in whom surgery is contraindicated and whose pain cannot be adequately managed with oral and/or topical analgesics.

An aminomonosaccaride called glucosesamine is necessary for the articular cartilage's glycosaminoglycans to form. According to Muller-Fassbender et al. (1994), doses of 1,500 mg daily result in more pain relief than a placebo and are equally effective as 1,200 mg of ibuprofen daily with fewer gastrointestinal side effects. A longer study has verified a clinical benefit, but there is still debate regarding a purported disease-modifying effect (Reginster et al., 2001). Finally, low doses of tricyclics at night may improve sleep quality and pain.

2.1.12. Surgical Procedures

For some patients with knee OA who have not responded to standard medical therapy, tidal lavage—the instillation and drainage of 500 ml–2 L of saline—is an effective treatment option. It is especially helpful for patients for whom surgery is either contraindicated or refused (Ravaud et al., 1999). Lavage has historically been done concurrently with arthroscopy, but it can also be done without an operating room or anesthetic by using a "needle" arthroscope or even a sterile disposable 14-gauge cannula. Lavage's exact mode of action is unknown, although theories include stretching the joint capsule, removing inflammatory mediators, and reducing secondary synovitis brought on by crystals or joint debris. It has been shown that lavage improves quadriceps muscle function (Gibson et al., 1992).

Last but not least, total joint replacement (TJR) (Dieppe et al., 1999) is a fantastic treatment for osteoarthritis (OA) and has significantly improved the quality of life for those with severe symptomatic OA in their lower limbs who have not responded to medical management. Three months after treatment, there are noticeable improvements in pain, mobility, social function, and overall health status; these improvements may last up to a year (Hawker et al., 1998).

2.1.13. Future Developments in Osteoarthritis

Better ways to understand OA are being developed; examples include MRI scanning and the use of biochemical markers. These advances will make it possible to evaluate interventions aimed at modifying the disease and logically reducing symptoms. Targeting the enzymes that cause inflammation and degrade cartilage, such as chemically modified tetracyclines and other metalloproteinase inhibitors (Ryan et al., 1996) and interleukin-1 receptor antagonists (Caron et al., 1996), as well as possibly lowering bone turnover with bisphosphonates, may be able to modify the disease. Patients with focal cartilage defects and early disease may benefit from autologous cartilage transplantation (Brittberg et al., 1994). Injuries and mechanical factors are also targets for prevention, such as through altering work procedures in high-risk groups. One should not undervalue the demonstrated ability of straightforward interventions, like losing weight, to modify disease. Better centrally or locally acting analgesics and improved interventions aimed at addressing the patient's emotional and attitudinal response to the illness may lead to a reduction in symptoms.

2.2. Rheumatoid Arthritis

The main issues with rheumatoid arthritis (RA), a complex multisystem inflammatory disease, are with the synovial linings of the joints and tendons. Many patients experience weight loss and generalized malaise during acute illness, and certain complications may have an impact on other organ systems. Sometimes these characteristics are predominant.

Although the exact cause of RA is unknown, the general consensus is that systemic autoimmune reactions trigger a series of inflammatory alterations and that both hereditary and environmental factors play a significant role.

The disease is more likely to recur in families, and monozygotic twins exhibit higher concordance than dizygotic twins. The class II major histocompatibility complex (MHC) antigen HLA DR4 is the most well-established genetic marker for RA that has been found. This hereditary HLA marker indicates a six-fold higher relative risk of contracting the illness. The DR4 antigen is present in about 50% of RA patients. Specifically, it is linked to more serious illness and systemic side effects (Westedt et al., 1986). Although the exact mechanism is still unknown, the existence of this tissue type acts as a susceptibility factor for autoimmune events.

In light of this, it is thought that environmental factors hasten the emergence of this issue. A great deal of work has been done to determine whether there is an infectious basis for RA development in genetically predisposed individuals. Numerous organisms have been linked to the disease, but unlike reactive arthritis and other chronic inflammatory conditions, no clear-cut proof of a particular microbe as the cause has been found.

Many patients attribute a stressful incident to the start of their RA. Although there is little evidence to support this, psychological distress surely makes patients feel that their disease is worse than it actually is.

It is a common misconception that diet has an impact on RA. Individual allergies can cause some patients to experience acute synovitis when they are exposed to particular foods, but this is not the same as the rheumatoid process. There have been many studies on the impact of diet on arthritis, but the findings have not always been encouraging. Excessive consumption of fish oil may have a limited anti-inflammatory effect and result in a reduction in the production of some inflammatory cytokines.

There are significant differences in the disease's prevalence among various populations. Different genetic makeups contribute to this in part, but environmental factors also have an impact. For instance, compared to urban populations, black groups in Africa have a significantly lower prevalence in rural areas (Beighton et al., 1975).

2.2.1. Pathology

Normal diarthrodial joint synovial lining consists of a loosely arranged stroma with connective tissue, microvasculature, and lymphatics, and a delicate tissue layer that can be up to three cells thick. Early active disease causes swelling, hypertrophy, and inflammation of the synovium. Under a microscope, lymphocytes and plasma cells infiltrate on the stroma. On the surface of the hypertrophic synovium, fibrin may deposit. Mesenchymoid transformation causes the local connective tissue cells to proliferate and replace the synovial stroma. Overproduction of synovial fluid causes clinically detectable effusions and swelling in the joints. The predominant cellular component found in rheumatoid synovial fluid is polymorphonuclear leucocytes. The development of pannus, or chronic granulation tissue, that covers the surface of the articular cartilage, is linked to the disease's destructive phase. On an X-ray, cartilage destruction is visible as a loss of joint space and is found on the pannus' deep surface. At the joint margins, where the bone is comparatively unprotected by cartilage and where normal synovial reflection occurs, bone erosions typically first manifest. The breakdown of bone and cartilage is facilitated by neutral proteolytic enzymes (Barrett & Saklatvala, 1981) released by macrophages in the pannus and acidic lysosomal enzymes released by polymorphonuclear leucocytes in the synovial fluid. In severe cases, the disease's ongoing degeneration of bone and cartilage is linked to irreversible deformities and may lead to secondary osteoarthritis, especially in weight-bearing joints.

2.2.2. Clinical Features

Both sexes can get RA, but females are twice or three times more likely than males to get it. Although it can begin at any age, older adults are experiencing it more frequently. Approximately 1% of the population is affected overall. The disease's incidence seems to be declining and its effects seem to be less severe in recent years.

The most noticeable issues with RA, which is a widespread illness, are related to the joints. In addition to articular and extra-articular characteristics, severe forms of the disease may exhibit symptoms and indicators of a systemic disease process. These include low-grade pyrexia, weight loss, and generalized malaise and tiredness. Up to 70% of patients experience a gradual onset of the disease, although it can also happen suddenly and be accompanied by fever and systemic disturbance.

2.2.3. Articular Clinical Features

Generally speaking, established rheumatoid disease is a symmetrical peripheral inflammatory polyarthritis that primarily affects the cervical spine, wrists, ankles, knees, and small joints of the hands and feet. Less frequently, the hips and lumbar spine are affected, but the shoulders and elbows can also be affected. Any synovial joint may be impacted by the disease's severe variants.

Early active rheumatoid arthritis is characterized by stiffness, soft tissue edema, and pain. Active inflammation usually manifests as pain and stiffness that are worse in the morning and get better with activity during the day, though many patients experience worsening symptoms when they get tired in the early evening. Joint stiffness or gelling during inactivity or rest is another hallmark of an inflammatory illness. Upon examination, the warm, tender soft-tissue joint swelling associated with active RA is caused by synovial hypertrophy and effusion. Around painfully swollen joints, muscle wasting develops quickly, and periarticular inflammatory edema can occasionally be seen.

Deformity and loss of function are the most common issues in late-stage destructive RA, with comparatively little active inflammation.

The patterns observed in hands serve as an example of a similar pattern of changes in different joints. Early in the illness, there is pain and swelling along with inflammation in the proximal interphalangeal and metacarpophalangeal joints. Inflammation may also impact the tendon sheaths, which could lead to decreased grip and finger dexterity. Carpal tunnel syndrome symptoms can result from compression of the median nerve caused by synovitis of the wrists and flexor tendon sheaths. Combinations of synovitis, tendon sheath synovitis and rupture, joint erosion and instability, and progressive deformities may result in a range of deformities as the disease progresses. Any synovial joint, but especially those in the feet, ankles, knees, elbows, shoulders, and neck, may experience similar progressive changes.

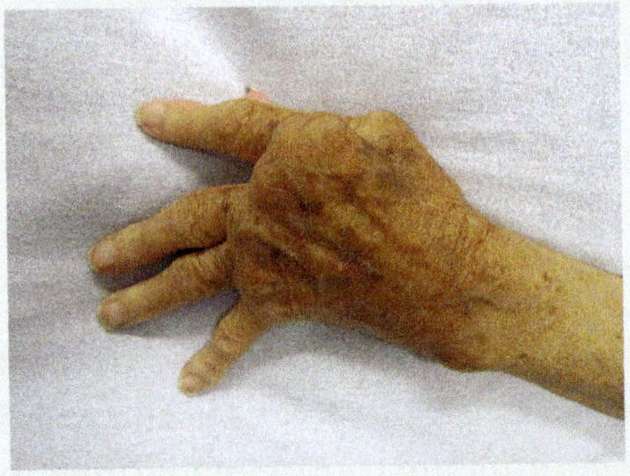

Figure 2.4. Rheumatoid arthritis inflammation of the hand.

Source. By James Heilman, MD – Own work, CC BY-SA 3.0, https://commons.wikimedia.org/w/index.php?curid=11110471.

2.2.4. Extra-Articular Clinical Features

Patients with the most severe forms of articular disease are more likely to exhibit extra-articular features.

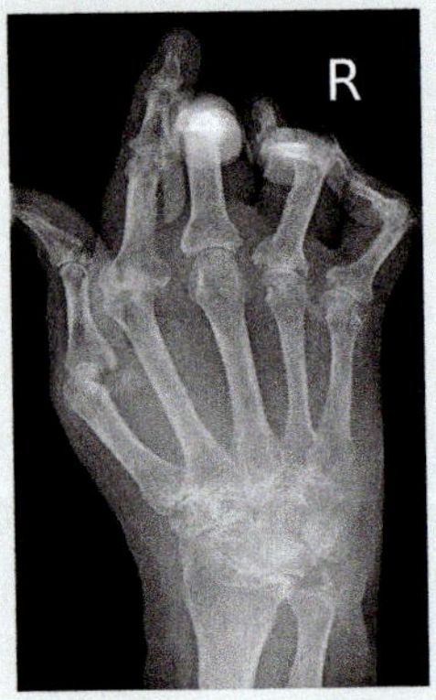

Figure 2.5. X-ray showing the condition.

Source. By Bernd Brägelmann Braegel Mit freundlicher Genehmigung von Dr. Martin Steinhoff – Own work, CC BY 3.0, https://commons.wikimedia.org/w/index.php?curid=3961869.

Numerous systemic characteristics, including vasculitis and nodules, are believed to have a pathogenic relationship with the local deposition of circulating immune complexes that contain IgM and potentially IgG rheumatoid factors.

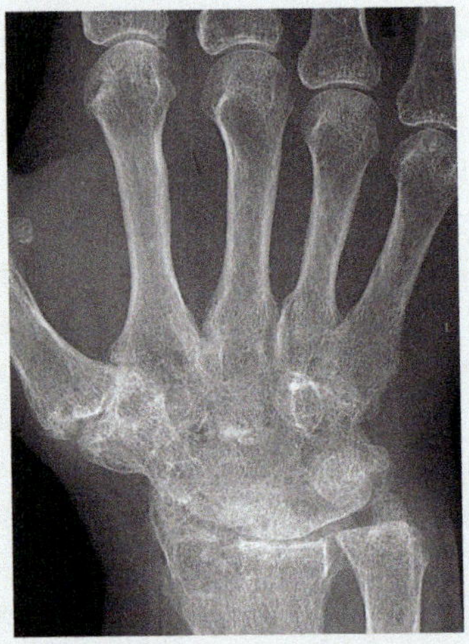

Figure 2.6. Fusion of carpal bones.

Source. By Mikael Häggström – Own work, CC0, https://commons.wikimedia.org/w/index.php?curid=55338793.

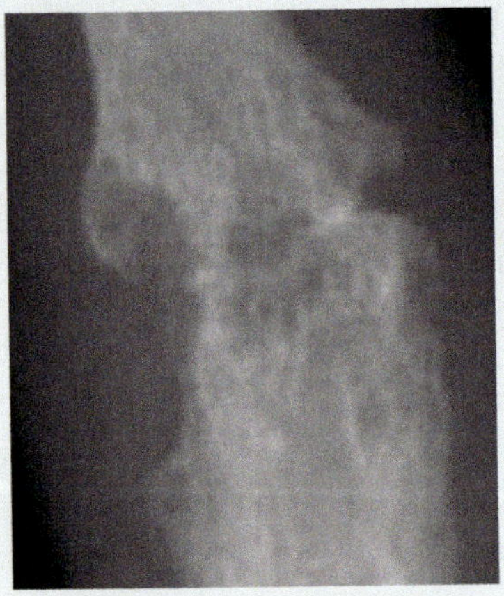

Figure 2.7. Erosion.

Source. By Haruko Ideguchi, Shigeru Ohno, Hideaki Hattori, Akiko Senuma and Yoshiaki Ishigatsubo – (2006). "Bone erosions in rheumatoid arthritis can be repaired through reduction in disease activity with conventional disease-modifying antirheumatic drugs." Arthritis Research & Therapy 8 (3): R76. DOI:10.1186/ar1943. ISSN 14786354. (CC-BY-2.0), CC BY 2.0, https://commons.wikimedia.org/w/index.php?curid=63609849.

2.2.4.1. Nodules

The most common locations for rheumatoid nodules are subcutaneous areas that experience repetitive mechanical stress. Typical locations include the olecranon, frequently in conjunction with an olecranon bursa, the subcutaneous borders of the forearms, and over sites like the sacrum and finger tips. Unlike the tiny nodules of rheumatic fever, rheumatoid nodules in these locations are firm, non-tender, larger, and less ephemeral. Nodules in some places, like over the sacrum, can ulcerate and develop into infected bedsores. They might serve as a target for systemic infections. The sclera, lung, pleura, and myocardium are among the tissues where these nodules can occur, in addition to the subcutaneous regions where they are most commonly found.

The histology of the rheumatoid nodule is nearly unique to RA; it is characterized by a zone of loose connective tissue on the periphery and a central area of fibrinoid necrosis encircled by a palisade layer of histiocytes (Gardner, 1992). The existence of rheumatoid nodules suggests a poor prognosis and may be useful for clinical diagnosis.

2.2.4.2. Vasculitis

This rare but potentially lethal complication only occurs in the most advanced stages of the illness. Blood vessels of all sizes could be impacted. The most common symptom of cutaneous vasculitis is finger nailfold hemorrhages. Although they are more likely to do so, patients with these lesions do not always progress to the more severe forms of vasculitis. Severe cutaneous vasculitis may be linked to chronic cutaneous ulceration, which typically develops in the lower leg and may not respond to therapy. Pulmonary hypertension, small bowel perforation or infarction, and finger gangrene are clinical manifestations of medium- or large-sized blood vessel involvement. Many of the other extra-articular disease features, including peripheral neuropathy and most likely nodule formation, are assumed to be influenced by small-vessel vasculitis.

Rheumatoid vasculitis is characterized by a variety of histological abnormalities, including intimal hyperplasia, an inflammatory response that affects the vessel wall's layers, and occasionally necrosis (Fassbender, 1975). High titers of circulating IgM rheumatoid factors, antinuclear antibodies, and signs of circulating immune complex activity—like lowered serum complement levels and occasionally circulating cryoglobulins—are frequently observed in immunological tests.

Severe vasculitis patients are medical emergencies who frequently need aggressive corticosteroid and immunosuppressive medication treatment.

2.2.4.3. Hematology

The anemia associated with RA is comparable to that of other long-term conditions like uremia, chronic infections, and cancer. Usually normocytic and normochromic, this anemia can also be hypochromic and, less frequently, macrocytic. The erythrocyte sedimentation rate (ESR) and the degree of anemia in rheumatoid arthritis are approximately correlated. Serum ferritin is usually increased and serum iron and total iron binding capacity are usually decreased. The reticuloendothelial system's increased affinity for iron is linked to anemia, and the bone marrow has an abundance of iron reserves. It is important to distinguish between iron deficiency anemia, which is typically caused by gastrointestinal blood loss and is often a consequence of non-steroidal anti-inflammatory drug (NSAID) therapy, and the anemia associated with rheumatoid disease. Serum iron levels are low in iron deficiency anemia, but bone marrow iron stores are decreased and the total iron binding capacity is raised. Two forms of anemia may coexist, and a history of melaena or recent dyspepsia, a sharp decline in hemoglobin, or a hemoglobin level significantly below 9 g/dl may indicate that an iron deficiency is causing the anemia. Oral iron therapy is ineffective in treating RA anemia unless there is a concomitant iron deficiency. Although parenteral iron is occasionally used, suppressing the underlying disease process is the primary treatment for this anemia.

The combination of RA with leucopenia and splenomegaly is known as Felty's syndrome. Thrombocytopenia, lymphadenopathy, pigmentation, cutaneous ulceration, normocytic normochromic anemia, and lymphadenopathy are possible additional symptoms of the syndrome. Recurrent major or minor infection is the condition's main risk factor. In addition to having higher titers of IgM rheumatoid factor and antinuclear factors on serological testing, patients with Felty's syndrome typically have more severe forms of articular disease.

Felty's syndrome leucopenia typically ranges from 800 to 2,500 cells/mm^3 and is linked to a decrease in granulocyte count. A leucopenia of fewer than 800 cells/mm^3 is occasionally observed. Granulocyte maturation arrest is the most commonly discovered abnormality in bone marrow. A splenic humoral factor and circulating immune complexes are two of the multifactorial factors contributing to the pathogenesis of Felty's syndrome: decreased granulopoiesis and increased peripheral destruction. A portion of the apparent decline in circulating cell counts could be explained by the excessive margination of leucocytes in the peripheral circulation.

Only in cases where significant recurrent infection is linked to leucopenia is Felty's syndrome treatment indicated. Corticosteroid therapy may raise the number of peripheral white blood cells, but it also makes people more prone to infection, so its usefulness in treating Felty's syndrome is questionable. Although gold or penicillamine therapy can be very beneficial, these medications should be used with caution due to the possibility of toxic effects on the bone marrow. Splenectomy is effective for some patients with this condition, but there is a significant postoperative mortality rate with the procedure itself. Occasionally, after splenectomy, patients' susceptibility to infection does not improve and they die of fulminating septicemia despite an increase in the peripheral white cell count. It could be due to the elimination of splenic factors that are typically beneficial in the body's defense against infection. It becomes imperative to immunize against illness and to treat infections quickly and aggressively.

When rheumatoid arthritis is active, thrombocytosis, or an increase in the circulating platelet count, may be observed. This is most likely a generalized effect of inflammation. Typically, this thrombocytosis does not have clinical significance.

2.2.4.4. Sjögren's Syndrome

The correlation between RA or other connective tissue disorders and keratoconjunctivitis sicca (KCS) and/or xerostomia is known as Sjögren's syndrome. Lymphocytic infiltration linked to lacrimal and salivary gland dysfunction can lead to fibrosis and total acinar tissue loss. This is not the same as gland dysfunction brought on by age-related simple atrophy. Sjögren's syndrome is thought to affect 13–58% of rheumatoid arthritis patients, depending on estimates (Benedek, 1993).

KCS symptoms include a scratchy sensation or eye irritation. Patients frequently experience difficulty opening their eyes first thing in the morning, making this worse. Tear lysozyme content is decreased, and recurrent infections of the eyes may occur. The best way to confirm the diagnosis of KCS is to use a slit lamp to note the absence of the typical tear film. Thick mucus strands that adhere to the cornea and conjunctiva can also be observed. You can use two drops of 1% rose Bengal injected into the eye to highlight the abnormal epithelium and mucus strands present in the dry conjunctiva. The Schirmer tear test can be used to show that tear production has decreased in the absence of a slit lamp. When less than 10 mm of filter paper is wetted over a 5-minute period, it is deemed abnormal. A strip of filter paper is hooked over the lower lid at the intersection of the middle and outer thirds. Artificial tear drops are routinely injected into the afflicted eyes to relieve the symptoms of KCS. Tarsorrhaphy or lacrimal canal ablation may be necessary on occasion.

There could be a connection between the xerostomia and recurring salivary gland swelling. If the patient reports having a dry mouth and an examination reveals no salivary pool on the mouth's floor, xerostomia may be diagnosed clinically. Once more, it's best to rule out other non-specific causes like medication and anxiety before linking any and all mouth dryness complaints to this illness. A lip biopsy of the small salivary glands may be performed to confirm the diagnosis. Additional studies such as sialography, radioisotope imaging of the salivary glands, and measurement of salivary flow rate after parotid duct cannulation have been employed in the official evaluation of xerostomia. The xerostomia associated with Sjögren's syndrome is not adequately treated.

There is artificial saliva available that might be useful. Patients with the condition are more prone to dental caries, so maintaining good dental hygiene is crucial. In addition to increasing the likelihood that these patients will develop lymphoma, to which they are already more susceptible, local radiation therapy to the affected glands is ineffective.

Dysphagia, dyspareunia, and skin dryness are possible additional symptoms of the condition, as other endothelial surface secretions may also be impacted. Renal tubular acidosis and autoimmune thyroid disease are two immunological symptoms that may be linked to Sjögren's syndrome.

2.2.4.5. Ophthalmic Issues

The most common symptom of rheumatoid arthritis in the eyes is keratoconjunctivitis sicca. Although less common, scleritis (Jayson & Jones, 1971) may be more serious. It could show up nodular or diffuse. Severe necrotizing scleritis is an uncommon occurrence. Scleritis that is left untreated can lead to cataract, glaucoma, and scleritis perforation. Treatment for this condition may involve local steroid drops, systemic steroids at dosages of about 60 mg per day, and occasionally immunosuppressive medications. NSAIDs may be effective against milder attacks.

2.2.4.6. Respiratory Issues

The most typical types of the disease's pulmonary involvement are pleurisy and pleural effusions. In the absence of infection, rheumatoid pleural effusions exhibit decreased glucose content and lymphocytosis. Immunological testing for antinuclear antibodies and IgM rheumatoid factor may be positive when macrophages with IgM inclusions (ragocytes) are present. Occasionally, rheumatoid nodule formation is observed in the histology of the underlying pleura, but most often, non-specific changes of chronic inflammation are seen.

Rarely, progressive dyspnea in seropositive nodular rheumatoid arthritis may be attributed to interstitial fibrosis (fibrosing alveolitis), especially in smokers (Hyland et al., 1983). Finger clubbing, coarse pleural crepitations, and widespread pulmonary shadows on chest X-rays are among the similar symptoms shared by the rheumatoid disease form and the idiopathic form. Although corticosteroid treatment is typically ineffective, immunosuppressive medications sometimes seem to be helpful. Like other connective tissue diseases, rheumatoid disease frequently exhibits asymptomatic impairment of carbon monoxide diffusion capacity in the absence of radiological change, which typically does not progress to symptomatic interstitial fibrosis.

It is important to distinguish rheumatoid nodules from other causes of pulmonary shadowing, such as neoplasms and tuberculosis, because they can manifest in the lungs as nodules of different sizes. Gross forms of pulmonary fibrosis and nodules can occur in seropositive rheumatoid arthritis patients who work as coal miners or are exposed to industrial dust. These lesions were initially reported in coal miners by Caplan (1953).

It has been demonstrated that RA patients have a higher incidence of destructive airway disease than controls who are matched for smoking behavior. In a subset of rheumatoid arthritis patients, an uncommon and increasingly lethal variant of obstructive bronchiolitis has also been reported.

2.2.4.7. Cardiovascular Effects

Echocardiography can be used to identify pericardial effusions. Oftentimes, they exhibit no symptoms. In rare cases, large effusions can cause cardiac tamponade (Hara et al., 1990).

Rarely do clinical manifestations of rheumatoid arthritis impact the heart or the components of the heart valves. Nonetheless, up to 30% of rheumatoid arthritis patients had non-specific valvulitis, according to postmortem investigations. Postmortem investigations have also revealed the presence of rheumatoid granulomas in the myocardium. The aortic and mitral valves of patients undergoing cardiac valve surgery frequently have granulomas in them, although rheumatoid disease is an uncommon cause of persistent valve dysfunction.

2.2.4.8. Neurological Symptoms

Cervical myelopathy and entrapment neuropathies can cause peripheral nerve symptoms in rheumatoid arthritis patients. Appropriate decompression usually relieves the symptoms of entrapment neuropathy. The ulnar nerve at the elbow (ulnar neuritis), the posterior tibial nerve at the ankle (tarsal tunnel syndrome), and the median nerve at the wrist (carpal tunnel syndrome) are among the entrapment sites.

According to Chamberlain and Bruckner (1970), there are two types of rheumatoid peripheral neuropathies: severe sensorimotor neuropathy and milder sensory neuropathy. The former frequently identifies isolated nerves in a mononeuritis multiplex pattern and is linked to an abrupt loss of motor and sensory function. Vasculitis is frequently seen elsewhere, and it is linked to the more severe types of seropositive nodular disease.

Muscle denervation is typically evident in nerve conduction tests, and vasculitis of the vasa nervorum is believed to be the cause of the condition. When sensory neuropathy manifests itself, it typically manifests as a glove-and-stocking pattern of sensory loss. If motor symptoms do arise, they are typically mild. Tests for nerve conduction may reveal normal nerve conduction or a slowdown in motor and sensory conduction.

We have previously addressed the possibility of confounding peripheral neuropathy with cervical myelopathy resulting from atlantoaxial or subaxial subluxation of the cervical spine.

2.2.4.9. Renal and Hepatic Manifestations

Rheumatoid arthritis patients frequently experience mild impairment of renal function (Wish & Kammer, 1993), and approximately 11% of these patients have liver enlargement on a clinical level (Whaley & Webb, 1977). Jayson (1999) discusses these issues.

2.2.4.10. Septic Arthritis

This serious and sometimes fatal complication is more common in rheumatoid disease patients with the most advanced stages of the illness. Acute presentation is possible, characterized by pyrexia and one disproportionately painful and inflamed joint. Sometimes the symptoms of septic arthritis may be less obvious, like feeling sick or even experiencing an apparent flare-up of the condition. The elderly, disabled, and steroid-treated patients who are most likely to develop this condition may not exhibit fever or leucocytosis (Ostensson & Geborek, 1991). The most commonly isolated organism is *Staphylococcus aureus*. To reduce joint damage and maintain life, prompt diagnosis and treatment are crucial.

2.2.5. Laboratory Findings

Rheumatoid arthritis (RA) is primarily diagnosed based on clinical findings, although laboratory tests may also help confirm the diagnosis. These tests can offer objective assessments of disease activity and sometimes provide insight into prognosis. Patients with active RA often exhibit elevated levels of markers such as ESR, plasma viscosity, and C-reactive protein, which can give a general indication of disease severity. Additionally, chronic inflammation may lead to a decrease in serum albumin and an increase in alpha and gamma globulins on protein electrophoresis. Immunoglobulin levels, particularly IgG, IgA, and IgM, may also be elevated in RA. The presence of IgM rheumatoid factor in serological tests may be positive in 75% of patients with RA.

2.2.6. Prognosis

RA has a fluctuating natural history. The majority of patients with the condition have a good prognosis and a mild illness. During a 10-year follow-up, Duthie and colleagues discovered that while only 11% of rheumatoid patients became totally disabled, over 50% of patients who received relatively conservative treatment eventually had satisfactory outcomes (Duthie et al., 1955). Adverse prognostic factors include the following: extra-articular disease features, a persistently high ESR, poor functional capacity early in the disease course, development of erosions within a year of onset, and failure to respond to NSAIDs. According to some research, there could be a connection between severe illness and the histocompatibility antigen DR4 (Westedt et al., 1986).

2.2.7. Therapy

The disease's activity and stage are factors in determining the best course of treatment. The focus is on suppressing inflammation with antirheumatic medications and general measures when there is early active inflammation. As the disease progresses and secondary osteoarthritis takes over, the focus of treatment changes to pain relief through the use of basic analgesics, enhancing joint function, and reconstructive surgery. Most patients have a reasonable prognosis, and the goal of treatment is to suppress the disease process to prevent or limit the development of deformities and disabilities, as well as the onset of erosions.

2.2.7.1. Principles of Management

Rheumatoid arthritis develops a pattern very quickly after it first manifests. In fact, joint erosions appear in the initial few months. As a result, aggressive early treatment seems to be successful in halting the development of long-term alterations and deformities. Early arthritis clinics have been established in many rheumatological centers, resulting in patients receiving aggressive, active treatment at an early stage. This seems to be a good way to avoid harm and permanent disability.

2.2.7.2. General Measures

A management team consisting of rheumatologists, orthopedic surgeons, physiotherapists, occupational therapists, podiatrists, social workers, disablement resettlement officers, and nurses manages patients with RA over the long term. Advice and information about the nature of the illness, the goals of treatment, and its limitations are all included in the program. A longer period of rest during the day is necessary for many patients during active disease phases. Occupational therapists and physiotherapists assist by offering splints to prevent or lessen deformities, providing aids to improve function, and prescribing exercises meant to preserve and restore ranges of motion in the muscles and joints. Short stays in bed during severe disease exacerbations are beneficial, as is splinting, especially inflamed joints. Aspirating synovial effusions and injecting slow-release corticosteroids under very strict aseptic conditions are two ways to manage individual inflammatory joints.

2.2.7.3. Drug Therapy

The drugs used in the treatment of RA can be considered under the following headings:

1. Simple analgesics
2. NSAIDs
3. Second-line antirheumatic drugs
4. Immunosuppressives and corticosteroids
5. TNF-α inhibitors

- **Simple Analgesics:** These include paracetamol, which acts on the central nervous system and is frequently combined with codeine, dextropropoxyphene, and other substances. They are more useful for treating the pain associated with secondary osteoarthritis and as a top-up for patients for whom NSAIDs are insufficient. They are not very effective in relieving the pain associated with acute inflammation. The gastrointestinal side effects of the nonsteroidal anti-inflammatory agents mentioned are absent from these medications. For RA, narcotic analgesics are almost never necessary.
- **Non-Steroidal Anti-Inflammatory Drugs:** This class of drugs relieves pain and stiffness symptomatically. They do not, however, change the disease's natural course or stop progressive joint damage from occurring on their own. While many rheumatoid arthritis patients may find these medications sufficient, second-line antirheumatic medications ought to be the first line of treatment from the outset.

This kind of medication's prototype was soluble aspirin, but more recent medications, like those derived from propionic acid, have essentially replaced it. They are not appreciably more effective, but they are better tolerated.

Studies on osteoarthritis have shown some evidence that certain anti-inflammatory medications, like indomethacin, may actually make articular cartilage damage worse. In vulnerable patients, all of these medications may result in bleeding and gastrointestinal ulcers. Given that the drug is absorbed more slowly and has lower peak levels in the peripheral blood when used as a suppository in patients with dyspepsia, it may be possible to successfully administer the medication in this setting.

Other options include using prodrugs, like benoxaprofen, which are administered inactively and only become active after passing through the intestinal muscosa, or using antiulcer medications as a preventative measure. The cyclo-oxygenase enzymes involved in prostaglandin synthesis are inhibited by these agents, which contributes to their gastrointestinal adverse toxicity as well as their anti-inflammatory effects.

We now understand that cyclooxygenase enzymes come in two varieties (COX1 and COX2). While inhibition of COX2 mediates the anti-inflammatory effects, inhibition of COX1 is more likely to cause gastrointestinal toxicity. A new class of anti-inflammatory medications has emerged that targets COX2 exclusively. These seem less likely to induce dyspepsia and other gastrointestinal issues, but they still have anti-inflammatory effects comparable to those of conventional anti-inflammatory drugs (Emery et al., 1999). There are currently numerous methods for lowering the dangers of gastrointestinal toxicity (Wolfe et al., 1999).

- **Second-Line Antirheumatic Drugs:** Most units now treat active RA aggressively, and if there is evidence of active inflammation, second-line antirheumatic medications are started right away. These medications are administered over an extended period of time, with a typical two- to three-month wait between the start of treatment and the start of action.
- **Sulfasalazine:** This medication works well to put RA into remission. The standard protocol calls for starting the enteric-coated form at 0:5–1:0 g per day and increasing it by weekly increments up to a maximum of 1 g three times a day. While nausea and other gastrointestinal side effects are possible, more severe issues like blood dyscrasias are uncommon. Rarely, sulfasalazine may result in hepatotoxicity and a decrease in sperm count in men. It is necessary to regularly check the liver function, urea, creatinine, and blood count.
- **Antimalarials:** The anti-disease effects of chloroquine and hydroxychloroquine are well-established. A minor chance of developing retinopathy and vision impairment exists, but it can be reduced with careful daily dosage management and ophthalmologist supervision. These medications don't often cause gastrointestinal issues, and they don't have the same negative effects on the kidneys and blood cells as many more powerful antirheumatic medications.
- **Gold Therapy:** Since the 1930s, gold salts have been used to treat RA. The gold salt that is most frequently used in the UK is intramuscular sodium aurothiomalate, or Myocrisin; however, an oral preparation has also been made available. In a widely used regimen, the drug is injected intramuscularly at a rate of 50 mg per week up to a maximum of 1 g, or until toxicity or disease remission occurs, following incremental test doses. After the onset of remission and the appearance of maximal benefit, the usual course of action is to decrease the dosage to a monthly maintenance regimen and extend the time between injections. Most doctors stop using the drug if a cumulative dose of 1 g of gold has not produced any results, but you could try increasing the weekly injection dose (Rothermick et al., 1976).

Minor skin rashes, itching, exfoliative dermatitis, stomatitis, renal issues, blood dyscrasias, hepatotoxicity, and pneumonitis are among the potential side effects of gold therapy. Skin, blood, and urine monitoring is necessary regularly for all patients undergoing gold therapy.

- **D-Penicillamine:** First, Wilson's disease was treated with this medication as a chelating agent. Other than being administered orally, its benefits and drawbacks are comparable to those of gold salts. The recommended starting dose for this medication is 125 or 250 mg per day. It is crucial to take this medication well away from food because it may mix with the nutrients in it. Some patients respond to such low doses, but if no improvement occurs, the dosage is gradually increased up to a maximum of 750 mg per day by comparable amounts spaced out over time. The final dosage is typically 375 mg once a day. Skin rashes, blood dyscrasias, and renal issues are examples of adverse effects. Immunological syndromes like myasthenia gravis and systemic lupus erythematosus brought on by drugs are examples of uncommon side effects. It is crucial to regularly check the skin, blood, and urine for toxicity.
- **Levamisole:** This antirheumatic medication, which is second-line, seems to be useful in the long run for managing the condition. It is crucial to closely monitor liver function, urea, creatinine, and blood count (Smolen et al., 1999).
- **Immunosuppressives and Corticosteroids:** When more conservative measures fail to control a patient's severe persistent disease, immunosuppressive agents—methotrexate in particular—are often used. Methotrexate is an antagonist of folic acid with immunosuppressive qualities. It is administered once a week at a dose of 5 mg initially, with weekly increases usually to a maximum of 15 mg, though occasionally higher. Compared to second-line antirheumatic medications, it seems to be far more effective (Ward, 1985). Usually, it takes at least a month after starting treatment for the benefits to become apparent. Although they are rare, adverse effects can affect the blood, liver, and lungs. Patients who consume large amounts of alcohol should not use this medication. It is crucial to closely monitor liver and blood functions. Folic acid co-prescription, typically given the third day following methotrexate, may lower the incidence of gastrointestinal issues.

In very severe individual cases, alternative immunosuppressive medications like cyclophosphamide are used, and they are occasionally administered as bolus infusions. They are typically saved for patients who have complications, like severe vasculitis, or who have not improved with more conservative therapy. An immunosuppressive medication called cyclosporin is used after transplant surgery. In cases of severe and resistant RA, it works well. Renal function impairment and the emergence of hypertension are frequent treatment-related issues. Extensive observation is necessary.

Prednisolone and other oral corticosteroids significantly reduce symptoms. Regretfully, patients typically find it extremely difficult, if not impossible, to stop taking steroids once they have begun. Over time, patients undergoing steroid therapy often experience severe side effects such as osteoporosis, hypertension, and dermal atrophy. These effects may ultimately outweigh the benefits of the therapy in terms of reducing the symptoms of arthritis. Starting corticosteroids is a big decision that should only be made after giving it considerable thought. Patients on steroids should have their bone mineral density evaluated. Bone-strengthening agents like biophosphates, estrogens, calcium and vitamin D are added if needed.

When there is persistent inflammation in one or two joints or tendon sheaths, local steroid injections can be beneficial. The synovial fluid should be aspirated, and cultured, and a steroid injection should be administered later if there is any suspicion of infection. Preparations of slow-acting steroids are typically utilized. Since fluorinated steroids are more likely to cause dermal atrophy than other steroid preparations, they should be avoided for very superficial injections.

- **TNF-a Inhibitors:** The molecular mechanisms underlying chronic inflammation have been the focus of research. Tumor necrosis factor-α (TNF-α) in particular has been demonstrated to be important for the inflammatory process. Rheumatoid arthritis has been successfully treated with specific inhibition of TNF-α (Moreland, et al., 1999). There are two medications: inflixamab and etanercept. The former is administered twice a week by subcutaneous injection, while the latter is administered intravenously. Immunosuppressive medications can be used alone or in conjunction with etanercept, while inflixamab requires them. For patients with severe illnesses, these medications have shown to be very effective. In fact, there is now proof that they can stop joint erosion and damage from starting and progressing (Bathon et al., 2000).

The main worry is that these medications decrease resistance to infection and should not be used when an infection is present. Concerns have been raised regarding prolonged use and a potential propensity for cancer. Additionally, etanercept may cause localized skin reactions.

These medications are proving to be very beneficial and effective, but their high cost makes them difficult to obtain. They are becoming more widely accessible over time.

2.2.7.4. Surgery

When non-medical measures fail to relieve pain or prevent function loss, surgery becomes necessary. The best way to organize the program is for the orthopedic surgeon and rheumatologist to work together in a combined clinic.

Synovectomy may be beneficial symptomatically in the early stages of the disease if the synovial swelling is restricted to one or two joints and there are no discernible erosions. When tendon sheaths are affected by synovial hypertrophy, impairing hand function or raising the risk of tendon rupture, tenosynovectomy may be helpful. In some cases, decompression is necessary to relieve nerve entrapment syndromes.

In more complex situations, joint replacements are now offered for a range of joints and are always being enhanced. The most successful replacements are those for the hip and knee. Ankle, elbow, and shoulder replacements are available. Other surgical techniques that are occasionally employed include tendon rupture repair, fusion, and excision arthroplasty.

2.3. Muscles, Tendons, and Ligaments

Muscles, tendons, and ligaments make up musculoskeletal soft tissue. It can be challenging for a patient and a clinician to determine which of these three components is causing pain, and multiple parts are frequently impacted at once. The primary indicators of harm to the non-contractile soft tissues are discomfort, soreness, edema, and diminished functionality. Muscle-skeletal pain typically resolves on its own and is clearly related to trauma or exercise, but myalgia can result from many pathological conditions. Although connective tissue and collagen disorders are uncommon, they frequently have disastrous consequences (Pope, 1998).

2.3.1. Muscle Pain

2.3.1.1. Association with Exercise

Although there is usually a clear correlation between muscle soreness and exercise, there can be two completely different time courses. In one instance, commonly referred to as ischemic pain, the pain starts during exercise and intensifies quickly until the contractions cease and blood flow is restored, at which point it quickly goes away. On the other hand, pain might not start for hours and last for days.

- **Ischemic Muscle Pain:** Two well-known instances of this kind of pain that develop in muscles whose blood supply is unduly compromised are intermittent claudication and angina pectoris. When contractions cease in normal subjects, they quickly go away and leave no lasting effects. Even though the exact stimulus or combination of stimuli is unknown, the accumulation of metabolites is the cause. Since patients with myophosphorylase deficiency (McArdle's syndrome) cannot produce lactic acid, lactic acid is not the primary algesic substance (Schmid & Hammaker, 1961; Cady et al., 1989). Instead, these patients experience particularly intense pain during exercise. Moreover, the elimination of intramuscular lactic acid occurs more slowly than the reduction of pain. Potential triggers include histamine, acetylcholine, serotonin, and bradykinin, either acting alone or in combination. In this regard, adenosine (Sylven et al., 1988) and potassium (Lendinger & Sjogaard, 1991) are currently gaining a lot of attention.
- **Delayed-Onset Muscle Pain:** Muscle pain that develops approximately 8 hours after intense or unfamiliar exercise may last for days. Unusual eccentric contractions are especially linked to it (Newham et al., 1983c, 1988; Stauber, 1989; Clarkson & Newham, 1995). They have the lowest metabolic cost per unit force (Curtin & Davies, 1973; Menard et al., 1991) and produce the greatest force per active fiber (Katz, 1939; Abbott et al., 1952). Therefore, mechanical rather than metabolic factors are most likely to be the cause. According to structural (Newham et al., 1983b, Friden, 1984; Jones et al., 1986; Newham, 1988), biochemical (Newham et al., 1983a, 1986a, b; Stauber, 1989), and radioisotopic changes (reviewed by Clarkson & Newham, 1995) studies, it is linked to significant muscle damage. However, according to Jones et al. (1986) and Newham et al. (1986b), none of these damage markers correspond with the pain's temporal course. There is growing evidence of both inflammatory processes and connective tissue damage (Brown et al., 1997). The afflicted muscles feel swollen and are often tender. Muscles in noncompliant compartments have been found to have higher intramuscular pressures (Friden et al., 1986), but not in other muscles (Newham and Jones, 1985).

The effects of steroidal and non-steroidal anti-inflammatory drugs on pain with a delayed onset are inconsistently reported in the literature (Janssen et al., 1983; Kuipers et al., 1983; Headley et al., 1986).

2.3.1.2. Clinical Myalgia

- **Signs and Symptoms:** Patients who present with myalgia typically have a limited vocabulary. Common terms include tenderness, spasms or cramps, aching, stiffness, and soreness. Rather than greater compliance, the symptom of stiffness typically refers to discomfort during muscle movement. The most common description of muscle pain is that it hurts dull and dull. Although acute tenderness from a "trigger point" (Travell & Simons, 1998) may happen, sharp, lancinating pain is not common. Voluntary contraction typically makes muscle pain worse, though this is not always the case.

  Although they have precise definitions, the terms cramp, contracture, spasm, and tetanus or tetany are frequently used incorrectly (Simons & Mense, 1998). Strong, quickly starting, involuntary contractions that cause excruciating pain are known as cramps. The electromyographic signals associated with cramps are comparable to those of a typical voluntary contraction (Mills et al., 1982b). A contracture is an incredibly uncommon type of electrically silent involuntary contraction caused by a deficiency of muscle adenosine triphosphate (ATP). It indicates uncommon metabolic illnesses (e.g., a lack of myophosphorylase). A spasm typically indicates a reflexive contraction of the muscles around an inflammatory or injured area. Tetany is characterized by an involuntary contraction that typically occurs in the carpopedal muscles and is linked to hypocapnia or hypocalcemia (Layzer & Rowland, 1971). Myotonia and dystonia are less common.

- **Associated Signs and Symptoms:** Myalgia patients frequently report weakness, fatigue, or intolerance to exercise (see '2.3.1.5. Investigation of Muscle Pain' for more information on these symptoms). Muscle soreness is frequently reported but rarely verified. If so, it occurs in polymyositis, dermatomyositis, myophosphorylase and phosphofructokinase deficiencies, acute alcoholic myopathy, and almost always implies serious underlying pathology. It is important to inquire about fasting, diet, and alcohol. An alcoholic's binge drinking can cause myoglobinuria and acute alcoholic myopathy. Osteomalation, which results in pain in the muscles and bones, is linked to a diet low in vitamin D (Smith & Stern, 1967). When carnitine palmityltransferase is deficient, attacks of pain and weakness happen, especially after a high-fat, low-carb meal or after prolonged exercise following fasting (Di Mauro & Di Mauro, 1973; Bank et al., 1975). For this condition, fasting may be employed as a provocative test (Carroll et al., 1979).

- **Differentiation of Muscle Pain from Pain in Other Tissues:** Skeletal muscle has poor localization of pain, and patients may not be able to distinguish it from pain originating in nearby noncontractile tissues. Finding the source of the pain is crucial, but it can be challenging because of poor localization and referred pain. For example, pain from an arthritic hip can refer to the thigh or knee joint, carpal tunnel syndrome can refer pain to the forearm muscles, and cervical spondylosis can refer pain to the arm muscles.

  Compared to myalgia, pain from joints and their capsules is typically more localized, and passive joint movement can exacerbate arthralgia. Pain in the capsular region may only occur in particular joint positions (e.g., a painful case of shoulder arc syndrome). Unlike myalgia, bone pain typically has a deep, boring quality, but it also tends to be poorly localized. It typically gets worse at night and doesn't usually go away with movement or muscle use.

- **Myalgia, Exercise, and Rest:** When they first arrive with myalgia, many patients talk about their relationship to exercise. Some discover no connection at all, or even that modest exercise helps them feel better.

Intermittent claudication is the classic example of muscle pain associated with exercise; it is characterized by pain in the calf muscles during exercise and goes away after a period of rest. This pathological type of ischemic muscle pain is felt distal to the feeding artery stenosis and is brought on by the stenosis. Thus, forearm pain is caused by the narrowing of the axillary artery by a cervical rib, buttock pain is caused by thrombosis of the terminal aorta (Leriche's syndrome), and pain in the masticatory muscles during chewing may be caused by arteritis of the cranial arteries. Increased blood viscosity can also result in decreased blood supply (e.g., macroglobulinemia Waldenström).

A compromised energy supply to a contracting muscle is present in other conditions where myalgia is unmistakably linked to exercise; the mechanism involved is probably the same as that of ischemic muscle pain. Exercise-related myalgia with cramps and contracture is a common symptom of myophosphorylase deficiency (Schmid and Mahler, 1959), glycolytic disorders of muscle (McArdle, 1951), and phosphofructokinase deficiency (Tarui et al., 1965). Due to the irreversible muscle breakdown caused by contracture and the potential for significant myoglobin release to cause renal cast formation and failure, contracture is a potentially dangerous occurrence. There is a discernible correlation between physical activity and myalgia in multiple mitochondrial myopathies (Land and Clark, 1979) as well as in carnitine palmityltransferase deficiency (Bank et al., 1975).

The relationship between pain and exercise or rest appears to have no diagnostic or prognostic significance in those individuals where failure of energy or blood supply has been eliminated (Mills & Edwards, 1983).

2.3.1.3. Etiology

- **Primary Infective Myositis:** Bacteria directly infecting muscle is rare. Staphylococcus aureus infection, known as tropical myositis (Taylor et al., 1976), is most likely a result of viral myositis. It is a tropical illness that primarily affects children and young adults. It is characterized by fever, deep intramuscular abscesses, and muscle pain, which is frequently severe and limited to a single limb. Both surgical drainage and antibiotics typically affect it.

  Sarcosporidiosis (Jeffrey, 1974), trichinosis (Gould, 1970), sparganosis (Wirth & Farrow, 1961), and cysticercosis are examples of parasitic infections of the muscle that result in pain and tenderness in the affected area. Trichinella spiralis infection is widespread worldwide, particularly in the USA, and is typically caused by eating undercooked pork. However, many cases of the infection are asymptomatic. The illness is characterized by periorbital edema and fever. Myalgia and muscle weakness later on intensify, peaking at three weeks. The severity of the infection determines the prognosis; 2–10% of cases are fatal. Steroids and thiabendazole have proven to be an effective treatment.

Table 2.4. Treatment Strategies for RA Therapy

Standard Treatments			
First-Line Treatments	Therapy	Mechanisms of Action	References
	NSAIDs *(i.e., Ibuprofen, Naproxen, Diclofenac, Etoricoxib, Celecoxib)*	Inhibition of COX-1 and/ or COX-2 enzymes, blocked formation of pro-inflammatory prostaglandins from the arachidonic acid metabolism, thereby interrupting the inflammatory cycle.	[Paglia, M.D.G.; et al. 2021, Xie, P.; et al. 2021 Bullock, J.; et al. 2018, Singh, J.A.; et al. 2016]
	Glucocorticoids (GCs) *(i.e., Prednisone, Prednisolone, Budesonide)*	Activation or suppression of protein synthesis, including cytokines, chemokines, inflammatory enzymes, and adhesion molecules by activating the cytosolic glucocorticoid receptor; thus, modification of immune responses and inflammatory mechanisms.	[Czock, D.; et al. 2005, Rhen, T.; et al. 2005, Vandewalle, J.; et al. 2018, Stacy, J.M.; et al. 2021, Kirwan, J.R.; 2006]
	DMARDs *(i.e., Methotrexate (MTX),*	Impedes immune cell proliferation. Relieves symptoms such as joint pain and prevents joint damage.	[Cronstein, B.N. 2005]
	Hydroxychloroquine (HCQ),	Interferes with deoxyribonucleotides metabolism, impairs the antigen presentation, and lysosomal membrane stabilization is increased.	[Mavrikakis, I.; et al. 2003]
	Sulfasalazine,	Anti-inflammatory, immunosuppressive effects, which are attributed to its breakdown products sulfapyridine and 5-aminosalicylic acid.	[Villa-Hermosilla, M.C.; et al. 2021]
	Leflunomide,	Interferes with pyrimidine synthesis, which is needed for lymphocyte activation.	[Weinblatt, M.E.; et al. 1999]
	Azathioprine)	Blocks purine metabolism.	[Mohammadi, O.; et al. 2021]

New/Future Treatment Strategies			
Biological Agents	Therapy	Mechanisms of Action	Refs.
	TNF inhibitors (TNFi) *(i.e., Infliximab, Adalimumab, Golimumab, Certolizumab,*	Selective inhibition of TNF-α, one of the major inflammatory cytokines, by specific binding to both its soluble subunit and its transmembrane precursor, leading to prevention of pro-inflammatory cell recruitment. Given the risk of developing Abs to the murine components of the molecule and the decreasing efficacy of monotherapy, RA therapy is only recommended in combination with MTX.	[Bullock, J.; et al. 2018, Catrina, A.I.; et al. 2005, Keystone, E.C.; et al. 2004, Lipsky, P.E.; et al. 2000, Miyazaki, Y.; et al. 2021, Smolen, J.S.; et al. 2017, Subedi, S.; et al. 2019, Voulgari, P.V.; et al. 2006]
	Etanercept)	A biological TNF antagonist inhibiting the interaction of TNF-α and lymphotoxin (TNF-β) with cell-surface receptors, whereby TNF-mediated cellular responses and the activity of other pro-inflammatory cytokines are modulated.	[Mou, X.Y.; et al. 2021, Ngoufack, C.; et al. 2021, Roongta, R.; et al. 2021, Strusberg, I.; et al. 2021]
	IL-inhibitors *(IL-1: i.e., Anakinra, IL-6: i.e., Tocilizumab, Sarilumab, IL-17: i.e., Secukinumab, IL-21 Abs)*	Acting as IL-antagonists, thereby inhibiting cytokine binding to its receptors. Consequently IL-mediated signaling and its pro-inflammatory effects are suppressed.	[Aboobacker, S.; et al. 2021, Cohen, S.; et al. 2002, Fleischmann, R.; et al. 2021, Maini, R.N.; et al. 2006, McGeachy, M.J.; et al. 2019, Ramírez, J.; et al. 2018, Ren, H.M.; et al. 2021]
	CXCL chemokine inhibitors *(i.e., CXCL-10, -12, -13)*	Inhibition of chemokines and chemokine receptors, which are found in inflamed synovia, to reduce the synovial migration of B-cells and the formation of ectopic germinal centers.	[Elemam, N.M.; et al. 2020, Szekanecz, Z.; et al. 2016]
	Co-stimulation blockers *(i.e., Abatacept)*	Modulation of T-cell co-stimulation by binding to CD80 and CD86 receptors, thereby suppressing T-cell activation and B-cell stimulation.	[Bonelli, M.; et al. 2018, Kremer, J.M.; et al. 2005, Rubbert-Roth, A.; et al. 2020, Schiff, M. et al. 2015]

	Anti-B-cell-agents	The monoclonal Abs cause depletion of B-cells through various mechanisms, i.e., apoptosis, complement-dependent cytotoxicity, and mediation of antibody-dependent cellular cytotoxicity.	[Clark, E.A.; et al. 2005, Emery, P.; et al. 2014, Geh, D.; et al. 2018, Giltiay, N.V.; et al. 2017, Milani, C.; et al. 2009, Payandeh, Z.; et al. 2019]
	(CD20: i.e., Rituximab, Ofatumumab, Veltuzumab, Ocrelizumab, CD22: i.e., Epratuzumab,		
	CD79 Abs,	Targeting CD79 leads to inhibition of BCR signaling pathway, thereby depleting B-cells and ectopic germinal centers.	[Li, R.; et al. 2013]
	CD40/CD154 Abs,	Blockade of complex formation leads to attenuation of CD154-mediated T-cell co-stimulation, inhibition of CD40-mediated B-cell stimulation, and supports CD4+ T-cells' conversion to Tregs, mediating immunosuppression.	[Lai, J.-H.; et al. 2019]
	TLR7/9 Abs	Inhibition of the binding between BCR and TLR (dominantly TLR7/9) leads to inactivation of B-cells.	[Huang, Q.-Q.; et al. 2009]
	BAFF: Belimumab	Selective inhibition of BAFF (B-cell activating factor) prevents B-cell differentiation, thus leading to B-cell depletion.	[Blair, H.A.; et al. 2018, Liu, Z.; et al. 2011, Navarra, S.V.; et al. 2011]
	BAFF/APRIL: Atacicept,	Dual inhibitor of BAFF and APRIL (proliferation inducing ligand) by binding soluble BAFF and APRIL, thus interfering the interaction of these cytokines to their related receptors leading to B-cell depletion.	[Kaegi, C.; et al. 2020, Xu, S.; et al. 2020]

	PTK/Syk: i.e., Fostamatinib)	Inhibition of Syk, which is a vital non-receptor-type protein tyrosine kinase (PTK) activating downstream MAPKs and the PI3K signaling pathway, leads to anti-inflammatory effects.	[Kang, Y.; et al. 2019]
Synthetical Agents	**JAK-inhibitors** *(i.e., Tofacitinib, Baricitinib, Upadacitinib, Filgotinib)*	Reducing the production of inflammatory cytokines by suppressing the JAK signaling pathway. Either as monotherapy or in combination with MTX for the treatment of active RA. Ensuring optimal use of JAK inhibitors in the treatment of RA in practice.	[Hodge, J.A.; et al. 2016, Zhang, X.; et al. 2017, Pavelka, K. 2021, Kim, E.S.; et al. 2021, Iwamoto, N.; et al. 2021]
Cell Therapy	**Plasma cell therapy** *(i.e., Anti-thymocyte-globuline (ATG),*	The polyclonal Abs with T-cell-depleting properties can modulate the immune response by affecting the function of various immune effectors including B-cells and Tregs.	[Mohty, M. 2007]
	Bortezomib, Carfilzomib)	Proteasome inhibitor that suppresses activation of the pro-inflammatory transcription factor nuclear factor kappa B (NF-κB) by blocking degradation of the NF-κB inhibitor, thereby secretion of pro-inflammatory cytokines is reduced.	[Lassoued, S.; et al. 2019, Lee, S.W.; et al. 2009, Durkin, A.; et al. 2020, Mahévas, T.; et al. 2020, Woodle, E.S.; et al. 2017]
	Mesenchymal stem cell (MSC) therapy	Modulation of the immune response via cell-to-cell communication and MSC-secreted cytokines. For example, MSCs are able to directly inhibit T-cell function and differentiation or shifting them to functional Tregs.	[Ghannam, S.; et al. 2010, Weiss, A.R.R.; et al. 2019, Hwang, J.J.; et al. 2021]

Combination Therapy	**Combination of biologics and methotrexate**	There is much evidence that treatment with a combination of biologics and MTX is significantly more effective than treatment with biologics or MTX alone in some patients. Combination therapy is usually the treatment of choice when monotherapy with DMARDs is not effective.	[Gabay, C.; et al. 2015, Teitsma, X.M.; et al. 2016, Westhovens, R.; et al. 2021]
	(i.e., Tocilizumab and MTX Filgotinib and MTX)		
Epigenetic Therapy	**DNA-methyltransferase (DNMT) and Histone-deacetylase (HDAC) inhibitors**	Modification of epigenetic marks such as hypomethylation and histone marks as the main treatment goal to restore abnormalities that contribute to the development of RA back to normal levels. Moreover, HDAC inhibitors' effects are related to immune cell apoptosis.	[Hammaker, D.; et al. 2018, Khan, N.M.; et al. 2018, Lohman, R.J.; et al. 2016]
	(i.e., Givinostat, Vorinostat, Panobinostat, Romidepsin)		
	Polyphenols	Therapeutic efficacy in the treatment of arthritis in CIA rats, reduction of inflammatory response by inhibition of NF-κB pathway resulted in significant relief of arthritic symptoms, by epigenetic regulation.	[Alghadir, A.; et al. 2020, Wang, Q.; et al. 2019, Yang, M.; et al. 2019, Escobedo-Martínez, C.; et al. 2019, Sana, E.; et al. 2021, Javadi, M.; et al. 2019]
	Curcumin		
	Curcumin and Prednisolone, or MTX or diclofenac, or Vitamin D3	Combination therapy showed significantly higher therapeutic efficacy than simple treatment alone in patients with active RA and also in rats, by epigenetic regulation.	[Banji, D.; et al. 2011, Chandran, B.; et al. 2012, Hemshekhar, M.; et al. 2021, Poonia, N.; et al. 2020, Sankrityayan, H.; et al. 2016, Singh, P.; et al. 2020, Yan, F.; et al. 2019]

Targeting Autophagy	**Autophagy inhibitors** *(i.e., Rapamycin,*	Activation of autophagy by inhibiting mTOR.	[Levy, J.M.M.; et al. 2017, Wang, T.; et al. 2021]
	Chloroquine (CQ), Hydroxychloroquine (HCQ)	Autophagy suppression by inhibiting the lysosome reduces the activity of T-cells and apoptosis resistance.	[Xiu, Y.; et al. 2014, Goel, P.; et al. 2021]
	3-Methyladenine (3-MA)	Inhibition of autophagy at an early stage of autophagosome development by blocking P13K signaling.	[Dai, S.; et al. 2016, Laha, D.; et al. 2019]
Treat-to-Target	**Monitoring of disease activity and adjusting therapeutic drug management**	Establishment of a treatment goal and measuring treatment progress and disease activity regularly, whereby the treatment strategy is adjusted until the goal is reached. The improvement of disease activity achieved in 3 months should be at least 50% by applying new therapeutic strategies, otherwise the treatment should be modified.	[Aletaha, D.; et al. 2016, Solomon, D.H.; et al. 2017]

Source. Mueller A-L, Payandeh Z, Mohammadkhani N, Mubarak SMH, Zakeri A, Alagheband Bahrami A, Brockmueller A, Shakibaei M. Recent Advances in Understanding the Pathogenesis of Rheumatoid Arthritis: New Treatment Strategies. *Cells*. 2021; 10(11):3017. https://doi.org/10.3390/cells10113017.

- **Inflammatory Myopathies:** Idiopathic inflammatory myopathies, polymyositis and dermatomyositis, were classified by Bohan and Peter (1975a, b) and Carpenter and Karpati (1981). These conditions have undergone a great deal of review (Currie, 1981; Mastaglia, 1988; Dalakas, 1988; Pachman, 1998; Targoff, 1998). Muscle weakness is typically the presenting feature, though in a few cases, muscle pain may be a prominent feature. Females are more likely to experience limb girdle weakness, dysphagia, muscle soreness, and skin involvement when they have acute or subacute onset of dermatomyositis. Other systems, including the heart and lungs, are frequently affected, and in 20% of cases, an associated carcinoma may be present. Pathologically, immunoglobulin deposits on vessel walls that result in microinfarcts are indicative of microangiopathy in dermatomyositis. There may be noticeable perivascular atrophy on a muscle biopsy. On the other hand, respiratory muscle involvement is uncommon, muscle tenderness is rare, and polymyositis manifests equally in males and females and has a chronic course. Neither the skin nor any other systems are involved. Muscle biopsy reveals pathological endomysial lymphocyte infiltration with cytotoxic T cells predominating.

Diagnosis rests on the findings of:

1. A muscle biopsy showing muscle cell necrosis, lymphocyte infiltration, phagocytosis, and variation in size of both fiber types and basophilic fibers reflecting regeneration.
2. Electromyography (EMG) showing brief, small amplitude polyphasic potentials and fibrillations (Marinacci, 1965).
3. Plasma creatine kinase (CK), which is raised in the acute phase but may be normal in 30% of cases.
4. Raised inflammatory markers.

A common belief is that steroid therapy is clinically useful. Long-term steroid therapy complications are rare (Riddoch & Morgan-Hughes, 1975; Bunch et al., 1980; Currie, 1981), but they should always be considered (Carpenter et al., 1977; Edwards et al., 1981). Although other immunosuppressive medications like immunoglobulin infusions, whole body irradiation, plasmapheresis, azathioprine, cyclophosphamide, methotrexate, and cyclosporin have been tried, the advantages and disadvantages are not entirely evident.

2.3.1.4. Polymyositis in Association with Connective Tissue Disease

Systemic lupus erythematosus (Tsokos et al., 1981), progressive systemic sclerosis, mixed connective tissue disease, rheumatoid disease (Haslock et al., 1970), polyarteritis nodosa, Sjögren's syndrome, and occasionally myasthenia gravis are all associated with polymyositis. Although the changes of steroid myopathy are frequently superimposed, the findings in the other conditions are similar to those in idiopathic polymyositis. In polyarteritis nodosa, muscle changes are most likely the result of infarction.

- **Viral Polymyositis:** The majority of acute viral infections cause myalgia; the agents typically involved are coxsackie virus A or B or influenza viruses A or B. The causative agent of epidemic myalgia, also known as Bornholm disease, is the coxsackie B virus. This virus causes fever, headaches, and abdominal and chest muscle pain. Like benign acute childhood myositis, which can occur after contracting the influenza A or B virus, the illness quickly resolves on its own.
- **Polymyalgia Rheumatica:** Patients over the age of 55 are affected by this condition, which is characterized by proximal muscle pain and stiffness, particularly in the shoulder girdle (Hamrin, 1972). Malaise, weight loss, and mild anemia are possible. The first hour's erythrocyte sedimentation rate is usually more than 50 mm, but electromyography (EMG), creatinine kinase (CK), and muscle biopsy are all normal. This illness and giant cell, cranial, or temporal arteritis appear to be closely related. Steroids typically produce an instantaneous and dramatic response (Bird et al., 1979), with the majority of authorities recommending a high initial dose of 40–60 mg daily.
- **Myalgia of Neurogenic Origin:** Appearing to be restricted to the muscles, pain could be a common feature of several neurogenic diseases. Pain radiating into the myotomal distribution of the roots due to cervical radiculopathy or nerve compression (e.g., carpel tunnel syndrome), which can cause discomfort that travels up

the arm muscles. Pain can be caused by peripheral neuropathies, particularly if they impact small fibers. Any source of spasticity can result in flexor muscles.

- **Muscle Cramps:** In addition to the benign "ordinary" cramps that most people experience, cramps can also occur as a result of glycolytic disorders (see below), dehydration, uremia, certain medications (such as salbutamol, phenothiazine, vincristine, lithium, cimetidine, and bumetanide; these types of cramps can also occur after hemodialysis (Layzer, 1994).

The "stiff man" syndrome was initially identified by Moersch and Woltman in 1956 and was later reviewed by Gordon et al., in 1967 and Layzer in 1994. The syndrome is typified by paroxysms of severe cramping, a continuous board-like stiffness of the muscles, abolition of the muscle stiffness during sleep, and a normal motor and sensory examination. There have been reports of diazepam being used to treat stiffness, frequently in very high dosages.

Widespread fasciculation, generalized stiffness, profuse perspiration, and continuous motor unit activity are characteristics of neuromyotonia (Isaacs syndrome), which lasts through anesthesia and sleep (Isaacs, 1961; Newsom-Davis & Mills, 1992). The defect is believed to be in 52 spinal cord or motor axons in all of the aforementioned conditions.

2.3.1.5. Impaired Muscle Energy Metabolism

- Cytosolic Enzyme Defects
    - **Myophosphorylase Deficiency (McArdle's Disease):** McArdle first reported a patient with contractures and pain in the muscles brought on by exercise in 1951, and he proposed a problem with muscle glycolysis. In additional cases, Mommaerts et al. (1959) and Schmid and Mahler (1959) proved myophosphorylase deficiency. Early adolescence is typically when the symptoms first appear, causing excruciating muscle stiffness, cramps, contractures, and weakness brought on by intense exercise. After some rest, the symptoms go away, but contractures could last for several hours. Long stretches of moderate exercise may be completed without experiencing any symptoms; however, should symptoms arise, more exercise may help to relieve the discomfort. This phenomenon, known as the "second wind" (Pernow et al., 1967), is assumed to result from a combination of increased blood flow to the muscles and the liver's mobilization of glucose and free fatty acids. The illness progresses in a fairly benign manner, with symptoms lessening after the age of 40. While at rest, patients frequently exhibit no physical symptoms; however, quantitative testing may reveal quadriceps weakness. When contractures resolve, CK rises to extremely high values from elevated levels at rest. The definitive investigation is a muscle biopsy that demonstrates excessive glycogen deposition and a reduction in or absence of myophosphorylase. The EMG may be normal or exhibit myopathic changes. Acute attack biopsies may also reveal necrosis of the muscle cells.
    - Phosphofructokinase deficiency et al., Although contractures are less common and symptoms can start in early childhood, this condition is very similar to McArdle's disease. The diagnosis is established by showing that muscle glycogen accumulation and phosphofructokinase (PFK) activity

are absent (Tarui et al., 1965).

- **Other Enzyme Deficiencies:** There have been reports of several other enzyme deficiencies that result in muscle fatigue, exercise-induced muscular aches, and exercise intolerance. A small number of cases have been reported for phosphoglycerate kinase deficiency (type 9 glycogenesis; Di Mauro et al., 1983), phosphoglycerate mutase deficiency (type 10 glycogenesis; Di Mauro et al., 1982), and lactate dehydrogenase deficiency (Kanno et al., 1980).
- **Lipid Storage Myopathies:** the carrier molecule carnitine and the enzyme carnitine palmityltransferase (CPT), which is found on the inner membrane, are required for the transport of long-chain fatty acids into the interior of the mitochondrion. Once intramuscular glycogen stores were exhausted, a deficiency in either one would be expected to cause a block in the flow of energy.

Systemic carnitine deficiency, characterized by low levels of both muscle and plasma carnitine, manifests in childhood with symptoms such as nausea, vomiting, encephalopathy, and muscle weakness. On the other hand, muscle carnitine deficiency, with normal plasma carnitine levels, presents in young adults with proximal muscle weakness and pain. Elevated CK levels are typical, along with a myopathic EMG. Muscle biopsy reveals lipid accumulation under the plasma membrane and between myofibrils, as well as reduced carnitine levels (Karpati et al., 1975; Willner et al., 1979).

Adolescents with CPT deficiency typically experience episodes of muscle pain, weakness, and myoglobinuria, which are often brought on by prolonged exercise, particularly following a fast or a diet high in fat and low in carbohydrates (Bertorini et al., 1980). Between attacks, CK is often normal; however, it significantly increases both during and after pain episodes. When an attack is at its worst, a muscle biopsy may reveal lipid buildup and/or necrosis of the muscle cells, and the CPT assay reveals extremely low levels.

- **Mitochondrial Myopathies:** This is a diverse group of conditions that are characterized by the presence of abnormal mitochondria in terms of size, shape, or number, frequently with crystalline inclusions. They are typically accompanied by muscle weakness and/or pain that is exacerbated by exercise. The modified Gomori trichrome stain may show "ragged red fibers" in a large number of patients. Metabolic abnormalities linked to specific cytochrome chain segments can now be identified thanks to increasingly complex biochemical investigations (Petty et al., 1986; Morgan-Hughes et al., 1987; Holt et al., 1989). According to a review by Petty et al. (1986), retinitis pigmentosa (Kearns-Sayre syndrome), growth retardation, deafness, myoclonus, encephalopathy, ophthalmoplegia, and several other mitochondrial cytopathies have been linked to an astounding array of additional abnormalities.

- **Drug-Induced Myalgia:** Muscle pain has now been linked to a wide range of substances (Lane & Mastaglia, 1978). D-penicillamine has the potential to cause polymyositis, which manifests as myopathic features on electromyography, necrosis of muscle cells, and an inflammatory infiltrate in muscle biopsy samples. Acute severe rhabdomyolysis, phencyclidine, alcohol, amphetamine, and myoglobinuria can all cause severe acute rhabdomyolysis and pose a risk to renal function.

- **Myalgic Encephalomyelitis/ Chronic Fatigue Syndrome:** Myalgic encephalomyelitis (ME), a well-known syndrome, is characterized by diffuse muscular pain that is made worse by muscle activity, marked exercise intolerance, weakness, and fatigue. Disturbance in sleep and loss of focus are additional symptoms. The term post-viral (fatigue) syndrome originated from the observation that a certain percentage of cases link the onset of symptoms to a viral illness. A consensus on diagnostic criteria has been reached, although diagnosis is frequently challenging due to the variety of potential symptoms (Dawson, 1990). It is most common in young and middle-aged women, though it can occur occasionally or in epidemics (Behan & Bakheit, 1991). The question of whether the etiology is psychological or physical is currently hotly debated (Wessely, 1990). Whatever the underlying mechanisms, a great number of people are affected by the symptoms; some will recover for months or years, while others become chronic invalids (Wessely & Newham, 1993). Several expert reviews on the diagnosis, etiology, clinical findings, and management of the syndrome were presented by Behan et al. (1991).

  Regarding whether the patients exhibit immunological signs of persistent viral infections, opinions differ. According to reports, hyperventilation is a frequent finding that improves symptoms when treated. Neurophysiological evidence of impaired attention and slowed information processing has been reported (Prasher et al., 1990). When compared to normal people and people with muscle diseases, these patients seem to have a higher incidence of psychiatric disorders (Wessely & Powell, 1989; Wood et al., 1991).

  Objective muscle testing reveals no signs of abnormal fatigue, central or peripheral mechanisms causing muscle wasting, weakness (Stokes et al., 1988; Edwards et al., 1991; Lloyd et al., 1991; Rutherford & White, 1991). Other than the general changes brought on by immobility, neither histochemical nor metabolic alterations are consistent. Blood concentrations of cytoplasmic enzymes in skeletal muscle (e.g., CK) are normal and typically elevated in cases of muscle damage.

- **Muscle Pain of Uncertain Cause:** Feelings of vague aches and pains in the muscles are frequently present in patients suffering from depression and in those with obsessive-compulsive disorders. It's important to pay attention to these symptoms though, as the depression might be a result of an organic muscle abnormality.

  Large studies consistently show a subset of patients complaining of muscle pain in whom, despite thorough investigation, no abnormality is discovered (Serratrice et al., 1980; Mills & Edwards, 1983; Simons & Mense, 1998). ESR and CK measurements seem to be reasonable criteria for excluding patients with organic abnormalities. Exercise, muscle biopsy, EMG, and strength testing should be carried out if any of these are abnormal. Nonetheless, a sizable subset of individuals experiencing muscle soreness do not exhibit any discernible abnormalities in their muscles. There are undoubtedly still many distinct muscle abnormalities that need to be identified.

Recently, the phrase "repetitive strain injury" has become more widely used to describe any pain that results from a repetitive job. There has been no concrete evidence of any neurological or rheumatological abnormality, despite reports of changes in muscle biopsy specimens (Fry, 1986; Barton et al., 1992).

The condition known as primary fibromyalgia (Bengtsson, 1986) or "fibrositis" (Bennett, 1981) is characterized by reduced high-energy phosphate levels (Bengtsson et al., 1986b) and histological abnormalities (Bartels and Danneskiold-Samsoe, 1986; Bengtsson et al., 1986a). However, there is still debate over the exact definition of the syndrome (Hazleman, 1998).

2.3.1.6. Investigation of Muscle Pain

- **Muscle Biopsy:** In many cases, this is the final examination in the management of myalgia. For histological, histochemical, electron microscopy, and metabolic characterization, percutaneous muscle biopsy is appropriate. For all of these procedures, needle biopsies (Edwards et al., 1980) are appropriate, and the conchotome modification enables the removal of larger samples (Dietrichson et al., 1987). These treatments can be used repeatedly to monitor improvement and are comparatively non-traumatic. Open biopsy is still used and may be beneficial in "patchy" conditions like focal polymyositis or arthritic conditions (e.g., polyarteritis nodosa); nevertheless, it is needless and unethical in the majority of primary myalgia investigations.

Although there is little correlation between morphology and myalgia, muscle biopsy can be helpful in the diagnosis of inflammatory myopathies by showing muscle cell necrosis and inflammatory cell infiltration. There may be fiber-type grouping associated with neurogenic pain. Histochemistry reveals the absence or reduction of enzymes like myophosphorylase in metabolic disorders. Enzymes like carnitine palmityltransferase and mitochondrial activity can be measured directly. When there is a defect in either electron transport or substrate transport within the mitochondria, it is crucial for the analysis of mitochondrial myopathies (Gohil et al., 1981).

- Biochemical Markers of Muscle Damage:
    - o **Myoglobinuria and Myoglobinuria:** Myoglobinuria is an important sign of muscle disease (Rowland et al., 1964). It may be the presenting complaint in several conditions with exercise-induced pain or a concomitant of severe polymyositis, viral myositis, or alcoholic myopathy.

      Myoglobin leaks into the plasma when muscle fibers degenerate and is small enough to enter the urine. This is critical because acute tubular necrosis can result in oliguric renal failure, a potentially fatal complication (Paster et al., 1975). After prolonged, intense exercise, especially in hot weather, myoglobinuria can also occur in healthy individuals (Demos et al., 1974). It can be observed in less than 74% of myositis cases and may occur before CK elevation during relapses.
    - o **Creatine kinase:** CK exists as three isoenzymes, MM, MB, and BB, with MM predominating (95–99%) in normal skeletal muscle. All three isoenzymes may occasionally be seen, probably because of the regeneration

of immature fibers in various myopathies, but usually, the MM isoenzyme is predominantly elevated. It has been suggested that the MB fraction emanating from heart muscle can be used as an indicator of cardiac involvement in polymyositis. However, it can be elevated in < 28% of patients with polymyositis uncomplicated by cardiac disease.

Although prolonged moderate exercise in healthy individuals can also cause CK to leak into plasma, this is typically interpreted as evidence of muscle damage (Thomson et al., 1975; Brooke et al., 1979). According to Griffiths (1966), outpatients with high levels of habitual activity have higher plasma CK levels than inpatients. Moreover, electromyography and intramuscular injections raise CK.

Muscular dystrophies—particularly Duchenne—have significantly higher levels of calcium homeostasis (CK). It can also be elevated in cases of spinal muscular atrophy, motor neuron disease, post-poliomyelitis muscular atrophy, hypothyroidism, and toxic muscle damage. Acute rhabdomyolysis can cause very high CK levels, which are linked to myoglobinuria. However, because it may be elevated during asymptomatic intervals between attacks, it can be used as a screening test for painful myopathies with less dramatic onsets; e.g., is typically 5–15 times the upper limit of normal in McArdle's disease, but it can increase to 100 times this level during and after a painful cramp or contracture. In myoadenylate deaminase deficiency, CK may be elevated (Fishbein et al., 1978); however, in carnitine palmityltransferase deficiency, CK is normal in between episodes of muscle pain (Morgan-Hughes, 1982). It is typically elevated in polymyositis and dermatomyositis, but it can also be normal in acute myositis. The CK only stays normal for 3% of patients during the whole polymyositis clinical course. It may increase in polymyositis 4–6 weeks before a relapse and fall 3.4 weeks before a strengthening of the muscles (Bohan & Peter, 1975b). In polymyalgia rheumatica, CK is typically normal.

- o **3-Methylhistidine**: This amino acid is excreted unchanged in the urine and may be used as an indicator of muscle breakdown if related to the total excretion of creatinine (McKeran, et al., 1977). However, other actin-containing tissues such as the skin and gut may turn over 3-methylhistidine much faster, and there are uncertainties about interpretation.
- o **Erythrocyte sedimentation rate*:*** Inflammatory myopathies, particularly polymyalgia rheumatica (Panayi, 1998), cause a rise in the erythrocyte sedimentation rate (ESR). This simple investigation is useful as a screening test for active disease and in monitoring progress.

- **Magnetic Resonance Techniques:** *Spectroscopy* At rest, patients with alcoholic myopathy (Bollaert et al., 1989) and those with the metabolic disorders myophosphorylase deficiency (Ross et al., 1981; Radda et al., 1984) and phosphofructokinase deficiency (Chance et al., 1982; Edwards et al., 1982a; Cady et al., 1985, 1989) typically have normal spectra. Except in myophosphorylase deficiency, where there is little to no change in the internal pH, exercise results in abnormally large metabolic changes.

Excessive changes in pH, Pi, and PCr during exercise and occasionally in unexercised, resting muscle (Gadian et al., 1981; Narayana et al., 1989; Matthews et al., 1991a, b) as well as in a variety of neuromuscular diseases (Barany et al., 1989) are linked to mitochondrial myopathies. Both hypothyroidism and peripheral vascular disease (PVD) patients frequently exhibit signs of increased metabolism at rest (Hands et al., 1986; Kaminsky et al., 1992). Those with rest pain have more metabolic abnormalities in PVD (Hands et al., 1990). The metabolic abnormalities are eliminated and the symptoms are eliminated with vascular surgery (Hands et al., 1986). According to De Blecourt et al. (1991), MRS has not been able to identify metabolic abnormalities in fibromyalgia patients' tender points.

Before the onset of pain, normal individuals with delayed-onset muscle pain have an abnormally high Pi concentration in their resting muscles (Aldridge et al., 1986; McCully et al., 1988). Additionally, some patients with primary muscle diseases—which are typically painless—have it (Barany et al., 1989). This finding might not be specific to myalgia (Newham & Cady, 1990).

- **Imaging:** The ability to see specific muscle groups as well as their relative fat and water composition allows for sensitive therapy monitoring (Fleckenstein et al., 1991b). Intramural masses (Turner et al., 1991), abscesses (Stephenson et al., 1991), and abnormal muscles (Paul et al., 1991; Sanger et al., 1991) have all been found in patients presenting with muscle pain.

In cases of referred pain as well as for differential diagnosis, important information can be gathered (Chevalier et al., 1991; Halpern et al., 1997; Stoller, 1997). MRI is more accurate than other imaging techniques in determining the cause of foot pain (Kier et al., 1991) and shoulder pain (Fritz et al., 1992). (Nelson et al., 1991; Kier et al., 1991). It is possible to distinguish pseudomalignant osseous soft-tissue tumors, or myositis ossificans circumscripta, from malignant neoplasms (Ehara et al., 1991). To investigate the location, size, and metabolic properties of tumors, imaging methods can be coupled with spectroscopy (Zlatkin et al., 1990).

It is possible to ascertain the distribution and degree of muscle involvement in each individual (Lamminen, 1990; Fleckenstein et al., 1991b). Additional abnormalities may be discovered through exercise testing (Amendola et al., 1990; Fleckenstein et al., 1991a). Sports and traumatic injuries are easily seen (Fleckenstein et al., 1989; Greco et al., 1991; Farley et al., 1992), but the precise degree and scope of the damage is not always evident. Hemorrhage may accompany them (De Smet et al., 1990). The technique to be used should be carefully chosen, as with other investigations (Erlemann et al., 1990; Greco et al., 1991). Accuracy may be impacted by the operator as well as the subject's obesity (Nelson et al., 1991).

- **Radioisotope scanning:** Numerous muscle diseases, the majority of which are painless, are caused by an excessive uptake of radioisotope-labeled complexes into the muscle (Bellina et al., 1978; Giraldi et al., 1979). According to Buchpiguel et al. (1991), the degree of uptake in patients with polymyositis and dermatomyositis may be predictive of prognosis.

Trauma and sports injuries can reveal affected soft tissues and bone (Elgazzar et al., 1989; Rockett & Freeman, 1990; Halpern et al., 1997). In cases of PVD (Sayman & Urgancioglu, 1991) and ischemic damage (Yip et al., 1990; Rivera-Luna and Spiegler, 1991), muscle involvement may be discerned.

Following exercise, normal, pain-free

individuals have shown increased muscle uptake of isotope (Matin et al., 1983; Valk, 1984). There is a chance that exercise-induced left ventricular dysfunction is mistakenly diagnosed when pectoral muscles are involved (Campeau et al., 1990). The results for muscle pain with a delayed onset are similar (Jones et al., 1986; Newham et al., 1986b). According to Jones et al. (1986) and Newham et al. (1986b), the time course of muscle uptake and blood CK level changes parallel and are likely caused by sarcolemmal changes. The exact mechanism underlying increased isotope uptake is unknown (see Brill, 1981 for a review); additionally, different mechanisms might be at play depending on the circumstances.

- **Exercise Testing:** The energy supply for muscle contraction is held in essentially three pools:
  - o Creatine phosphate and ADP reform ATP, forming an instantly available energy buffer which lasts only a very short time.
  - o Glycogen stores within muscle provide an intermediate energy supply system.
  - o Long-term energy supply is provided by carbohydrate and fat in endurance exercise.

Exercise testing must be customized to assess particular system components. There is a wealth of research on how healthy people respond to exercise, and exercise testing can provide insight into many different disease categories (Jones et al., 1975). Whole-body exercises, like cycle ergonometry, put stress on the cardiovascular, respiratory, and neuromuscular systems. They also require motivation to perform. In addition to evaluating an individual's general level of work fitness, the technique has the potential to elicit symptoms that can subsequently be further examined. In clinical management, it can also help assure patients that exercise won't cause them undue pain.

There are numerous protocols available for increasing exercise tests on a cycle ergometer (McArdle et al., 1991; Jones et al., 1975). Submaximal tests typically last for a predetermined amount of time while being monitored frequently and at a work rate that is a fixed percentage of the maximal rate that was previously established. In cases of myalgia where a metabolic muscle disease is suspected, exercise testing can be helpful. Resting lactate levels are elevated in many mitochondrial myopathies (see below), but they rise noticeably following moderate exercise.

The goal of the prolonged exercise test (Brooke et al., 1979) is to gauge an individual's capacity to transition from glycogen-based oxidation in muscle to fatty acid oxidation.

Ischemic forearm exercise tests are intended to assess the muscle's phosphorylase system (McArdle, 1951; Munsat, 1970; Sinkeler et al., 1986). After three minutes, lactate levels in healthy subjects increase to three to five times their resting levels. There is no increase in lactate in phosphofructokinase deficiency or McArdle's disease. Patients with myophosphorylase deficiency may develop contractures, so they should be done carefully.

2.3.1.7. Electromyography

Muscle electrical activity can be captured using intramuscular recording needles or surface electrodes. The former is helpful in the study of anomalies in the gross pattern of muscle activation because it records activity from a large volume of tissue (e.g., kinaesiological research) as well as in fatigue studies. However, the muscle signal's diagnostic information is effectively filtered out by the skin's electrical characteristics. Needle electromyography (EMG) is necessary for diagnostic purposes (Hayward & Willison, 1973; Daube, 1983; Desmedt, 1983). When separating conditions linked to anomalies in the anterior horn cell or motor axons from those that are primary muscle diseases, electromyography (EMG) is a valuable tool. Motor unit potentials in primary muscle disease are short-amplitude potentials that are recorded using a traditional concentric needle electrode. At moderate activation, these add up to form a crowded recruitment pattern in the muscle. On the other hand, motor unit potentials with a broad simple waveform and high amplitude are observed in muscles that have experienced denervation and reinnervation. These potentials repeat at high rates even when the muscle is generating its maximum force. Motor unit potentials may have a maximum amplitude of 0–1 mV in primary muscle disease, but they may have an amplitude of up to 20 mV in chronic reinnervation brought on by a neurogenic process (Mills & Willison, 1987).

At rest, healthy muscle produces no electrical noise. The most common cause of spontaneous muscle fiber potentials, or fibrillations, is acute denervating processes, though they can also occur in inflammatory muscle diseases and muscular dystrophies.

EMG has a significant role in differentiating between primary muscle and neurogenic diseases, but it can also be helpful in other studies pertaining to muscle pain. It can distinguish between the excessive motor unit activity of a muscle cramp and the electrically silent contracture of McArdle's disease. It can also detect myotonia when clinical myotonia is absent. EMG can be used in conjunction with nerve conduction studies to determine which nerve or nerve roots are involved and to evaluate the distribution of denervation-affected muscles.

- **Measurements of Muscle Force:** The two most typical symptoms associated with force are extreme fatigue and weakness. It is important to distinguish between the two: weakness is the inability to generate the anticipated force, whereas fatigue is an excessive loss of force generation during or following an activity. Maximal voluntary force generation measurements reveal information about longitudinal changes in strength as well as the presence and distribution of weakness (Edwards, 1982; Edwards et al., 1980, 1983). Information about anomalies in the contractile properties of muscles can be obtained through percutaneous electrical stimulation applied via the motor nerve or its intramuscular nerves (Edwards et al., 1977). Individuals who experience both weakness and myalgia are probably dealing with a particular muscle issue. The distribution may provide useful information. Proximal muscle weakness is frequently linked to primary muscle disease, but pain and weakness in the fingers and forearm may simply be a case of nerve entrapment syndrome.

Neuropathic and myopathic conditions are linked to muscle weakness and wasting, which can also be the primary symptom; the former is typically painless. It is possible to distinguish between the two through clinical examination and electromyographic studies. There are two types of myopathies: atrophic and destructive. Some atrophic myopathies (e.g., hypothyroidism, osteomalacia) do not result in muscle pain (e.g., Cushing's, steroids). Destructive myopathies can be further classified as inflammatory (polymyositis and dermatomyositis) and destructive (muscular dystrophies). The association between pain and either category is highly erratic and doesn't seem to be well correlated with any other findings. Muscle soreness and aching, particularly during activity but occasionally during rest, are the two most common descriptions of pain. For unclear reasons, some, but not all, former poliomyelitis victims report experiencing muscle weakness and pain (Agre et al., 1991). The creation of the maximal voluntary force could always be impeded by low motivation or central tiredness. Because additional force is only generated if the voluntary contraction is submaximal and because submaximal efforts can be used to estimate the true strength of the muscle, the superimposition of electrical or magnetic stimulation on a voluntary contraction determines whether it is maximal (Belanger & McComas, 1981; Rutherford et al., 1986; Gandevia et al., 1995). It's interesting to note that activation failure is uncommon in patients with primary myopathy and myalgia (Rutherford et al., 1986). On the other hand, incomplete voluntary activation is closely linked to mechanical joint damage, even though it may not cause any pain at all (Newham et al., 1989).

Despite the muscle being fully activated, peripheral fatigue results in a failure of force generation. In myasthenia gravis and myotonic disorders, excessive fatigability of this kind is observed without pain (Wiles & Edwards, 1977; Ricker et al., 1978). Mitochondrial myopathies are characterized by fatigability and pain (De Jesus, 1974; Edwards et al., 1982b). Excitation and activation can be studied via motor nerve stimulation, compound muscle action potential, and simultaneous force measurements. These methods have shown that a failure of muscle membrane excitation is the primary cause of excessive peripheral fatigue in myophosphorylase deficiency (Wiles et al., 1981; Linssen et al., 1990).

2.3.1.8. Treatment

There are several medications for myalgia. Along with aspirin and numerous other steroidal and non-steroidal anti-inflammatory medications (e.g., naproxen, indomethacin, flurbiprofen, ibuprofen) may be used, however, no particular preparation has been proven to be better. Both baclofen and dantrolene sodium, though the latter may hinder force production, as well as benzodiazepines like diazepam and others may be useful for muscle "spasm."

Quinine sulfate has long been used as a treatment for hemodialyzer cramps and other nighttime cramps. The medication seems to lessen the frequency in the latter instance, but not the severity (Kaji et al., 1976). Some patients with exertional muscle pain have found relief with verapamil (Lane et al., 1986). Many different physical therapies are employed, especially for trauma and sports-related injuries. Ice, transcutaneous nerve stimulation, and various electrical treatments are among the options. Different stages value immobilization and mobilization differently (Lehto & Jarvinen, 1991; Renstrom, 1991). Although reversible, immobilization causes noticeable muscle atrophy that can postpone full rehabilitation (Appell, 1990). Severe or complete muscle tears, severe hemorrhages, and compartment syndromes should all be treated surgically.

As part of behavioral therapy, patients with myalgia of unknown etiology may be offered a range of treatments. Due to inactivity, people with diffuse myalgia may be extremely unfit, and some may even exhibit some degree of postural hypotension (Newham & Edwards, 1979). Offering an exercise program under close supervision makes sense (Edwards, 1986), though each person's reaction to it varies greatly. Excessive exercise is reported to worsen symptoms in most ME patients; however, a carefully graded exercise program may be helpful.

It has been reported that dietary supplements of protein in McArdle's syndrome (Jensen et al., 1990) and essential fatty acids in ME (Behan et al., 1990) improve symptoms.

Vitamin therapy has been reported to affect patients with mitochondrial cytopathies on occasion. The best-known case (Eleff et al., 1984) involves a patient with complex III deficiency who saw quick clinical improvement after taking vitamins K3 and C, which are likely to circumvent the metabolic defect.

2.3.2. Trauma and Sports Injuries

Muscle pain can clearly be caused by direct trauma, which can come from a variety of sources, including sports injuries, severe crush injuries, and intramuscular injections. If enough muscle tissue is lost, myoglobinuria-induced acute renal failure and hypercalcemia could be fatal. Sports-related injuries range from mild sprains to total ruptures (e.g., hamstring rupture), which are more frequent in societies where physical activity is valued (Renstrom, 1991; Harries et al., 1994; de Lee and Prez, 1994). They may also involve direct trauma.

2.3.2.1. Muscle

Pain following traumatic muscle damage is almost always present and can start slowly or come on suddenly. Imaging methods, blood biochemistry, immunohistochemistry (Fechner et al., 1991), and routine histochemical analysis of biopsy samples, as previously mentioned, can all be used to detect it. Damage and immobilization combined cause significant weakness and wasting that can only be reversed by extended periods of rehabilitation (Appell, 1990).

While spontaneous ruptures, especially of the hamstrings and pectoralis major, are common, the cause of injury is often obvious and linked to forced lengthening of active muscle (Kretzler and Richardson, 1989). Tears and ruptures in the muscles of the limbs can resemble compartment syndrome, whereas groin pain can be caused by injuries in the muscles of the abdomen. They frequently accompany muscular spasms, which exacerbate the pain. A potentially incapacitating complication called myositis ossificans can be mistaken for a sarcoma (Booth and Westers, 1989).

Muscle groups with a comparatively inextensible fascial sheath, like the anterior tibial muscles, are susceptible to activity-related compartment syndromes (Vincent, 1994). Pain starts during exercise and gets worse as it goes on. Pain and cramping sensations resembling those of intermittent claudication are among the symptoms. While at rest, they typically go away, though tenderness might linger. Acute cases can cause weakness, paralysis, and numbness, which typically lead to persistent symptoms and elevated intramuscular pressures when at rest (Martens & Moeyersoons, 1990).

2.3.2.2. Ligaments and Tendons

These two structures differ only slightly in their morphology (Oakes, 1994). Tendons need to be more flexible and strong enough to withstand powerful forces. Ligaments are passive structures that can maintain continuous tension better than tendons. Strong structures have a cross-sectional area that determines their strength; the Achilles tendon has been found to withstand forces less than 4,000 N (Komi, 1992). It is believed that repetitive, cumulative microtrauma linked to intense functional use, especially in structures with a small cross-sectional area, causes injuries in addition to overt trauma. On the other hand, immobilization also reduces bone and ligamentous collagen (Amiel et al., 1983).

Microscopic damage, partial tears, and complete ruptures are all examples of injuries. Some bone that is still attached to the tendon or ligament may become detached due to the high forces involved. The rectus femoris and hamstrings, two muscles that act over two joints, seem to be especially vulnerable. This could be because opposing muscle groups require intricate neuromuscular control for co-contraction and relaxation. Determining the precise location and extent of damage is a challenging task in the field of medicine. These lesions are typically accompanied by pain and tenderness, though localization can be challenging. Muscle contraction will exert force on both the tendon and its sheath, which are always involved in palpation. Imaging methods frequently overestimate a lesion's size. The degree of damage will determine whether pain is constant and severe, occurs only during activity, or is absent altogether.

- **Tendon Injuries:** A significant percentage of the theoretical maximum stress placed on tendons occurs during many athletic activities (Alexander and Vernon, 1975). Changes in the type or intensity of exercise may be linked to the occurrence of tendinitis and rupture.

Failure frequently occurs at the musculotendinous junction (Curwin, 1994). Increased folds are seen in a muscle fiber's final sarcomere, which is assumed to boost surface area and lessen stress at the junction (Oakes, 1994). These are most likely not replicated during repair, which could account for the high rate of recurrent injuries. Although the exact cause of the injury is unknown, potential causes include weariness, insufficient muscle or tendon length, or muscle weakness.

Progressive attrition of tendons may result from overuse, microtrauma, and repetitive use. In young individuals, spontaneous tendon rupture is rare and typically results from age-related degeneration. In the absence of a prior illness or injury, it is likewise uncommon under normal loading (Barfred, 1971). An external cause could be compressive forces, like those from the wearer's tight shoes or own anatomy.

- **Ligament Injuries:** These occur frequently, especially in relation to sports-related injuries. The most frequent specific injury is a sprain of the ankle ligament, possibly accompanied by a bone avulsion (McBride, 1994). They could start out slowly or suddenly. Failure of related muscles to activate voluntarily is linked to mechanical joint damage, including ligament damage (Hurley et al., 1994).

Acute knee injuries, which can affect one or more ligaments and menisci, are among the most frequent events that cause a competitive athlete's career to end (Johnson, 1994). Although anterior cruciate ligament damage can result in either normal function or significant symptoms and significant functional disability, meniscal damage always causes pain and functional impairment.

Particularly in sports like baseball, tennis, and swimming, rotator cuff injuries can occur (Bowen and Warren, 1994). Ligaments, tendons, and joint capsules of the teres major, subscapularis, and supra-and infraspinati muscles are possible structures involved (Itio and Tabata, 1992). Perhaps as a result of its relatively weak vasculature, the supraspinatus appears to be extremely vulnerable to injury. Glenohumeral instability often exists to some extent. Poor localization can cause pain that travels down the afflicted arm. Pain at night is not uncommon. Function has a poor prognosis unless early and effective treatment is initiated.

- **Treatment:** Tendons and ligaments heal more slowly and have poor vascularization. Soft-tissue injuries are difficult to treat because injured tissues need minimal stress to heal, while maintaining or gaining mobility is also a requirement (Curwin, 1994). However, since many injuries won't heal on their own and chronic conditions tend to develop, effective treatment is crucial.

Up to a year can pass while connective tissue remodels and mobilizes (Oakes, 1994). Because smaller diameter fibrils are retained and local collagen matrices may shorten the affected area, the area becomes weaker and more prone to repeated injury. Atrophy occurs in both muscle and collagen when activity is reduced; however, regenerating fibers are not strong enough to withstand strong forces. Application of load causes fibrils to grow larger and stronger once they reach sufficient strength (Butler et al., 1978). Connective tissue alterations are most likely another aspect of muscle hypertrophy.

Extravascular bleeding from trauma frequently needs to be stopped. Extravascular blood alone has the potential to cause excruciating increases in tissue pressure. It also irritates the surrounding tissue, which can result in additional pressure increases and even tissue necrosis.

Whether to start with conservative or surgical treatment is the fundamental question. The ability to identify the location and severity of injury has improved due to advancements in imaging techniques (Halpern et al., 1997; Stoller, 1997). Usually, functional loss and symptoms are the criterion. More than a small portion of the structure is involved in a rupture, which frequently results in chronic conditions and is unlikely to spontaneously reunite with any degree of functional improvement.

Generally, the first few days following surgery or an injury are spent using ice, rest, and anti-inflammatory medications. To prevent additional collagen damage, including that to the regenerating fibrils, minimal applied forces are used. To boost collagen regeneration, fibril size, and cross-sectional area and to avoid the negative effects of immobilization and disuse atrophy, gentle movement and stress are introduced starting at approximately day five. To improve cross-linking, size, and strength, the tissue is subjected to increasing stresses starting at three weeks. It is believed that physical therapy is crucial for the best possible healing and rehabilitation results, and it is used extensively (De Lee and Prez, 1994; Harries et al., 1994; Sallis and Massimo, 1997). Preventing recurrent injuries is the main objective, so potential internal and external contributing factors need to be taken into consideration.

2.3.2.3. Overuse

The capacity of training to prevent injuries in sports has received a lot of attention (Safran et al., 1989). However, it is now acknowledged that overtraining can result in a wide range of symptoms, both psychological and physical, for many athletes (Fry et al., 1991). Overuse is linked to immune system depression (Shepherd, 1998).

It is unclear how much individual variation there is in the vulnerability to sports-related injuries (Taimela et al., 1990). Tendons and ligaments are also affected by the syndrome (Renstrom, 1994). It is broad, encompassing both sedentary people engaged in low-intensity, highly repetitive jobs and elite athletes (Simons and Mense, 1998). External factors (intensity, repetition, duration, environment, clothing, footwear, etc.) and internal (disorders from the past, weak muscles, reduced flexibility, and irregularities in anatomy or posture) are categorized as predisposing factors.

These syndromes have virtually become epidemic in the last 10 years, but it is still unknown what the best course of action is in terms of prevention or treatment. However, because of their high frequency and the fact that untreated acute pain often develops into chronic pain and is interpreted differently in the brains, these are significant issues (Hsieh et al., 1995).

A Closer Look

Synovium

Synovium is very variable but often has two layers. The outer layer, or subintima, can be of almost any type: fibrous, fatty or loosely "areolar." The inner layer, or intima, consists of a sheet of cells thinner than a piece of paper. Where the underlying subintima is loose the intima sits on a pliable membrane, giving rise to the term synovial membrane. This membrane, together with the cells of the intima, provides something like an inner tube, sealing the synovial fluid from the surrounding tissue (effectively stopping the joints from being squeezed dry when subject to impact, such as running). The intimal cells are of two types, fibroblasts and macrophages, both of which are different in certain respects from similar cells in other tissues. The fibroblasts manufacture a long chain sugar polymer called hyaluronan, which is what makes the synovial fluid "ropy" like egg-white, together with a molecule called lubricin, which lubricates the joint surfaces. The water of synovial fluid is not secreted as such, but is effectively trapped in the joint space by the hyaluronan. The macrophages are responsible for the removal of undesirable substances from the synovial fluid. The surface of the synovium may be flat or may be covered with finger-like projections or villi, which probably help to allow the soft tissue to change shape as the joint surfaces move one on another. Just beneath the intima, most synovium has a dense net of small blood vessels that provide nutrients not only for synovium but also for the avascular cartilage. In any one position much of the cartilage is close enough to get nutrition direct from synovium. Some areas of cartilage have to obtain nutrients indirectly and may do so either from diffusion through cartilage or possibly by 'stirring' of synovial fluid, although the film is very thin.

Although a biological joint can resemble a man-made joint in being a hinge or a ball and socket, the engineering problems that nature must solve are very different because the joint works within an almost completely solid structure, with no wheels or nuts and bolts. In general, the bearing surfaces of man-made joints interlock, as in a hinge. This is rare for biological joints, although the badger's jaw interlocks. More often the surfaces are held together by cord-like ligaments. Virtually all the space between muscles, ligaments, bones and cartilage is filled with pliable solid tissue. The fluid-filled gap is mostly only a twentieth of a millimeter thick. This means that synovium has certain rather unexpected jobs to do.

Synovium can become irritated and thickened in conditions such as rheumatoid arthritis. When this happens, the synovium can become a danger to the bearing surface structure in a variety of ways. Excess synovial fluid weeping from inflamed synovium can provide a barrier to the diffusion of nutrients to cartilage. The synovial cells may also use up nutrients so that the glucose level in the tissue is almost zero. These factors may lead to starvation and death of cartilage cells. Synovial cells may also produce enzymes that can digest the cartilage surface, although it is not clear that these will damage cartilage with healthy cells.

Summary

- Osteoarthritis (OA) and rheumatoid arthritis (RA) are two common types of arthritis, each affecting the joints and causing discomfort and pain, albeit through different mechanisms.
- Osteoarthritis is a disorder of synovial joints characterized by the destruction of articular cartilage and remodeling of subchondral bone.
- The anatomical source of pain in OA remains unclear. Any theory must take account of the fact that the principal structure involved (articular cartilage) possesses few pain-sensitive fibers: pain must therefore be arising from other tissues.
- Aerobic conditioning exercise, either supervised fitness walking or aquatics, has been shown to be well tolerated and more effective than conventional physical therapy or standard medical care in patients with OA of the hip and/or knee.
- Rheumatoid arthritis (RA) is a complex multisystem inflammatory disorder in which the principal problems affect the synovial linings of the joints and tendons.
- Rheumatoid nodules are found most frequently in subcutaneous regions subject to recurrent mechanical stress.
- Sjögren's syndrome is the association of keratoconjunctivitis sicca (KCS) and/or xerostomia with RA or other connective tissue disorders.
- Musculoskeletal soft tissue is composed of muscle, tendon, and ligament, and it is often difficult for both patient and clinician to distinguish which are the source of pain, and more than one is often affected at the same time.
- Ligaments and tendons are poorly vascularized and heal slowly. Soft-tissue injuries present a challenge due to the conflicting demands of maintaining or increasing mobility and the requirement of injured tissues for low stress for healing.

References

1. Abbott, B. C., Bigland, B., & Ritchie, J. M. (1952). The physiological cost of negative work. *Journal of Physiology, 117*, 380–390.
2. Agre, J. C., Rodriquez, A. A., & Tafel, J. A. (1991). Late effects of polio: A critical review of the literature on neuromuscular function. *Archives of Physical Medicine and Rehabilitation, 72*, 923–931.
3. Aldridge, R., Cady, E. B., Jones, D. A., & Obletter, G. (1986). Muscle pain after exercise is linked with an inorganic phosphate increase as shown by 31P NMR. *Bioscience Reports, 6*, 663–667.
4. Alexander, D. S., & Vernon, P. (1975). The dimensions of knee and ankle muscles and the force they exert. *Journal of Human Movement Studies, 41*, 115–123.
5. Amendola, A., Rorabeck, C. H., Vellett, D., Vezina, W., Rutt, B., & Nott, L. (1990). The use of magnetic resonance imaging in exertional compartment syndromes. *American Journal of Sports Medicine, 18*, 29–34.
6. Amiel, D., Akeson, W. H., Harwood, F. L., & Frank, C. B. (1983). Stress deprivation effect on metabolic turnover of medial collateral ligament collagen; a comparison between 9- and 12-week immobilization. *Clinical Orthopaedics and Related Research, 172*, 265–270.

7. Appell, H. J. (1990). Muscular atrophy following immobilization. A review. *Sports Medicine, 10*, 42–58.

8. Ayral, X., Dougados, M., Listrat, V., et al. (1996). Arthroscopic evaluation of chondroplasty in osteoarthritis of the knee. *Journal of Rheumatology, 23*, 698–706.

9. Bank, W. J., Di Mauro, S., Bonilla, E., Capuzzi, D. M., & Rowland, L. P. (1975). A disorder of muscle lipid metabolism and myoglobinuria. Absence of carnitine palmityl transferase. *New England Journal of Medicine, 292*, 443–449.

10. Barany, M., Siegel, I. M., Venkatasubrananian, P. N., Mok, E., & Wilbur, A. C. (1989). Human leg neuromuscular diseases: P-31 MR spectroscopy. *Radiology, 172*, 503–508.

11. Barfred, T. (1971). Experimental rupture of Achilles tendon: Comparison of various types of experimental rupture in rats. *Acta Orthopaedical Scandinavica, 42*, 528–543.

12. Barrett, A. J., & Saklatvala, H. (1981). Proteinases in joint disease. In W. N. Kelley, E. D. Harris, S. F. Ruddy, & C. B. Sledge (Eds.), *Textbook of Rheumatology* (pp. 195–209). Saunders.

13. Bartels, E. M., & Danneskiold-Samsoe, B. (1986). Histological abnormalities in muscle from patients with certain types of fibrositis. *Lancet, 7*, 755–757.

14. Barton, N. J., Hooper, G., Noble, J., & Steel, W. M. (1992). Occupational causes of disorders in the upper limb. *British Medical Journal, 304*, 309–311.

15. Bathon, J. M., Martin, R. W., Fleischmann, R. M., et al. (2000). A comparison of etanercept and methotrexate in patients with early rheumatoid arthritis. *New England Journal of Medicine, 343*, 1586–1602.

16. Behan, P. O., & Bakheit, A. M. O. (1991). Clinical spectrum of post viral fatigue syndrome. In P. O. Behan, D. P. Goldberg, & J. F. Mowbray (Eds.), *Post Viral Fatigue Syndrome* (pp. 793–809). *British Medical Bulletin, 47*.

17. Behan, P. O., Behan, W. M., & Horrobin, D. (1990). Effects of high doses of essential fatty acids on the post viral fatigue syndrome. *Acta Neurologica Scandinavica, 82*, 209–216.

18. Behan, P. O., Goldberg, D. P., & Mowbray, J. F. (Eds.). (1991). *Post Viral Fatigue Syndrome. British Medical Bulletin, 47*.

19. Beighton, P., Soloman, L., & Valkenburgh, H. A. (1975). Rheumatoid arthritis in a rural South African population. *Annals of Rheumatic Disease, 34*, 136–141.

20. Belanger, A. Y., & McComas, A. J. (1981). Extent of voluntary unit activation during effort. *Journal of Applied Physiology, 51*, 1131–1135.

21. Bellamy, N., Buchanan, W. W., Goldsmith, C. H., et al. (1988). Validation study of WOMAC: A health status instrument for measuring clinically important patient relevant outcomes to antirheumatic drug therapy in patients with osteoarthritis of the hip or knee. *Journal of Rheumatology, 15*, 1833–1840.

22. Bellamy, N., Sothern, R., & Campbell, J. (1990). Rhythmic variations in pain perception in osteoarthritis of the knee. *Journal of Rheumatology, 17*, 364–372.

23. Bellina, C. R., Biachi, R., Bombardini, S., et al. (1978). Quantitative evaluation of 99mTc pyrophosphate muscle uptake in patients with inflammatory and non-inflammatory muscle diseases. *Journal of Nuclear Medicine, 22*, 89–96.

24. Benedek, T. G. (1993). Association between rheumatic diseases and neoplasia. In P. H. Maddison

et al. (Eds.), *Oxford Textbook of Rheumatology* (pp. 1070–1082). Oxford University Press.

25. Bengtsson, A. (1986). Primary fibromyalgia. A clinical and laboratory study. *Linkoping University, Dissertation 224.*
26. Bengtsson, A., Henriksson, K.-G., & Jarson, J. (1986a). Muscle biopsy in primary fibromyalgia. Light microscopical and histochemical findings. *Scandinavian Journal of Rheumatology, 15*, 1–6.
27. Bengtsson, A., Henriksson, K.-G., & Jarson, J. (1986b). Reduced high energy phosphate levels in painful muscle in patients with primary fibromyalgia. *Arthritis and Rheumatism, 29*, 817–821.
28. Bennett, R. M. (1981). Fibrositis: Misnomer for a common rheumatic disorder. *Western Journal of Medicine, 134*, 405–413.
29. Bertorini, T., Yeh, Y. Y., Trevisan, C., Standlan, E., Sabesin, S., & Di Mauro, S. (1980). Carnitine palmityl transferase deficiency: Myoglobinuria and respiratory failure. *Neurology, 30*, 263–271.
30. Bigland-Ritchie, B., Furbush, F., & Woods, J. J. (1986). Neuromuscular transmission and muscular activation in human post-fatigue ischaemia. *Journal of Physiology, 337*, 76P.
31. Bird, H. A., Esselinck, W., Dixon, A. St J., Mowat, A. G., & Wood, P. H. N. (1979). An evaluation of the criteria for polymyalgia rheumatica. *Annals of the Rheumatic Diseases, 38*, 424–439.
32. Bohan, A., & Peter, J. B. (1975a). Polymyositis and dermatomyositis: Part 1. *New England Journal of Medicine, 292*, 344–347.
33. Bohan, A., & Peter, J. B. (1975b). Polymyositis and dermatomyositis: Part 2. *New England Journal of Medicine, 292*, 402–407.
34. Bollaert, P. E., Robin-Lherbier, B., Escanye, J. M., et al. (1989). Phosphorus nuclear magnetic resonance evidence of abnormal skeletal muscle metabolism in chronic alcoholics. *Neurology, 39*, 821–824.
35. Booth, D. W., & Westers, B. M. (1989). The management of athletes with myositis ossificans traumatica. *Canadian Journal of Sport Science, 14*, 10–16.
36. Bowen, M. K., & Warren, R. F. (1994). Injuries of the rotator cuff. In M. Harries, C. Williams, W. D. Stanish, & L. J. Micheli (Eds.), *Oxford Textbook of Sports Medicine* (pp. 442–452). Oxford Medical Press.
37. Bradley, J. D., Brandt, K. D., Katz, B. P., et al. (1992). Treatment of knee osteoarthritis: Relationship of clinical features of joint inflammation to the response to a nonsteroidal anti-inflammatory drug or pure analgesic. *Journal of Rheumatology, 19*, 1950–1954.
38. Brill, D. R. (1981). Radionuclide imaging of non-neoplastic soft tissue disorders. *Seminars in Nuclear Medicine, 11*, 277–288.
39. Brittberg, M., Lindahl, A., Nilsson, A., et al. (1994). Treatment of deep cartilage defects in the knee with autologous chondrocyte transplantation. *New England Journal of Medicine, 331*, 889–895.
40. Brooke, M. H., Carroll, J. E., & Hagberg, J. M. (1979). The prolonged exercise test. *Neurology, 29*, 636–643.
41. Brown, S. J., Child, R. B., Day, S. H., & Donnelly, A. (1997). Indices of skeletal muscle damage and connective tissue breakdown following eccentric muscle contractions. *European Journal of Applied Physiology, 75*, 369–374.
42. Buchpiguel, C. A., Roizenblatt, S., Lucena-Fernandes, M. F., et al. (1991). Radioisotopic

assessment of peripheral and cardiac muscle involvement and dysfunction in polymyositis/dermatomyositis. *Journal of Rheumatology, 18*, 1359–1363.

43. Bunch, T. W., Worthington, J. W., Combs, J. J., Ilstrup, D. M., & Engel, A. G. (1980). Azathioprine with prednisone for polymyositis. *Annals of Internal Medicine, 92*, 365–369.

44. Butler, D. L., Grood, E. S., Noyes, F. R., & Zernicke, R. G. (1978). Biomechanics of ligaments and tendons. *Exercise and Sports Science Reviews, 6*, 125–182.

45. Cady, E. B., Griffiths, R. D., & Edwards, R. H. T. (1985). The clinical use of nuclear magnetic resonance spectroscopy for studying human muscle metabolism. *International Journal of Technological Assessment in Health Care, 1*, 631–645.

46. Cady, E. B., Jones, D. A., Lynn, J., & Newham, D. J. (1989). Changes in force and intracellular metabolites during fatigue of human skeletal muscle. *Journal of Physiology, 418*, 311–325.

47. Campeau, R. J., Garcia, O. M., Correa, O. A., & Mace, J. E. (1990). Pectoralis muscle uptake of thallium-201 after arm exercise ergometry. Possible confusion with lung thallium-201 activity. *Clinical Nuclear Medicine, 15*, 303–306.

48. Caplan, A. (1953). Certain unusual radiological appearances in the chest of coalminers suffering from rheumatoid arthritis. *Thorax, 8*, 29–37.

49. Carman, W. J. (1989). Factors associated with pain and osteoarthritis in the tecumseh community health study. *Seminars in Arthritis and Rheumatism, 18*, 10–13.

50. Caron, J. P., Fernandes, J. C., Martel-Pelletier, J., et al. (1996). Chondroprotective effect of intraarticular injections of interleukin-1 receptor antagonist in experimental osteoarthritis. Suppression of collagenase-1 expression. *Arthritis and Rheumatism, 39*, 1535–1544.

51. Carpenter, J. R., Bunch, T. W., Angel, A. G., & O'Brien, P. C. (1977). Survival in polymyositis: Corticosteroids and risk factors. *Journal of Rheumatology, 4*, 207–214.

52. Carpenter, S., & Karpati, G. (1981). The major inflammatory myopathies of unknown cause. *Pathological Annual, 16*, 205–237.

53. Carroll, J. E., De Vivo, D. C., Brooke, M. H., Planner, G. J., & Hagberg, J. H. (1979). Fasting as a provocative test in neuromuscular diseases. *Metabolism, 28*, 683–687.

54. Chamberlain, M. A., & Bruckner, F. E. (1970). Rheumatoid neuropathy. Clinical and electrophysiological features. *Annals of the Rheumatic Diseases, 29*, 609–616.

55. Chance, B., Eleff, S., Bank, W., Leigh, J. R., & Warnell, R. (1982). 31P NMR studies of control of mitochondrial function in phosphofructokinase deficient human skeletal muscle. *Proceedings of the National Academy of Sciences USA, 79*, 7714–7718.

56. Chevalier, X., Wrona, N., Avouac, B., & Larget, B. (1991). Thigh pain and multiple osteonecrosis: Value of magnetic resonance imaging. *Journal of Rheumatology, 18*, 1627–1630.

57. Clarkson, P. M., & Newham, D. J. (1995). Associations between muscle soreness, damage and fatigue. In S. C. Gandevia et al. (Eds.), *Fatigue: Neural and muscular mechanisms. Advances in Experimental Medicine and Biology, vol 384* (pp. 457–470). Plenum Press.

58. Creamer, P. (1997). Intra-articular steroid injections in osteoarthritis: Do they work and if so, how? (Editorial). *Annals of the Rheumatic Diseases, 56*, 634–635.

59. Creamer, P., Hunt, M., & Dieppe, P. A. (1996). Pain mechanisms in osteoarthritis of the knee: Effect of intraarticular anesthetic. *Journal of Rheumatology, 23*, 1031–1036.

60. Creamer, P., Lethbridge-Cejku, M., & Hochberg, M. (1999). Determinants of pain severity in knee osteoarthritis: Effect of demographic and psychosocial variables using three pain measures. *Journal of Rheumatology, 26*, 1785–1792.
61. Currie, S. (1981). Inflammatory myopathies. Polymyositis and related disorders. In J. N. Walton (Ed.), *Disorders of Voluntary Muscle* (4th ed., pp. 525–568). Churchill Livingstone.
62. Curtin, N. A., & Davies, R. E. (1973). Chemical and mechanical changes during stretching of activated frog muscle. *Cold Spring Harbor Symposia on Quantitative Biology, 37*, 619–626.
63. Curwin, S. L. (1994). The aetiology and treatment of tendinitis. In M. Harries, C. Williams, W. D. Stanish, & L. J. Micheli (Eds.), *Oxford Textbook of Sports Medicine* (pp. 512–528). Oxford Medical Press.
64. Cushnaghan, J., McCarthy, C., & Dieppe, P. (1994). Taping the patella medially: A new treatment for osteoarthritis of the knee joint? *British Medical Journal, 308*, 753–755.
65. Dalakas, M. C. (Ed.). (1988). *Polymyositis and Dermatomyositis* (1st ed.). Butterworths.
66. Daube, J. R. (1983). Disorders of neuromuscular transmission: A review. *Archives of Physical Medicine and Rehabilitation, 64*, 195–200.
67. Davis, M., Ettinger, W., Neuhaus, J., et al. (1992). Correlates of knee pain among US adults with and without radiographic knee osteoarthritis. *Journal of Rheumatology, 19*, 1943–1949.
68. Dawson, J. (1990). Consensus on research into fatigue syndrome. *British Medical Journal, 300*, 832.
69. De Blecourt, A. C., Wolf, R. F., van Rijswijk, M. H., et al. (1991). In vivo 31P magnetic resonance spectroscopy (MRS) of tender points in patients with primary fibromyalgia syndrome. *Rheumatology International, 1*, 51–54.
70. De Jesus, P. V. (1974). Neuromuscular physiology in Luft's syndrome. *Electroencephalography and Clinical Neurophysiology, 14*, 17–27.
71. de Lee, J. C., & Prez, D. (1994). *Orthopaedic Sports Medicine, vol 11*. Saunders.
72. De Smet, A. A., Fischer, D. R., Heiner, J. P., & Keene, J. S. (1990). Magnetic resonance imaging of muscle tears. *Skeletal Radiology, 19*, 283–286.
73. Dekker, J., Tola, P., Aufdemkampe, G., & Winckers, M. (1993). Negative affect, pain and disability in osteoarthritis patients: The mediating role of muscle weakness. *Behavior Research and Therapy, 31*, 203–206.
74. Demos, M. A., Gitlin, E. L., & Kagen, L. (1974). Exercise myoglobinuria and acute exertional rhabdomyolysis. *Archives of Internal Medicine, 134*, 669–673.
75. Desmedt, J. E. (Ed.). (1983). *Computer Aided Electromyography. Progress in Clinical Neurophysiology, vol 10*. Karger.
76. Dexter, P., & Brandt, K. (1994). Distribution and predictors of depressive symptoms in osteoarthritis. *Journal of Rheumatology, 21*, 279–286.
77. Di Mauro, S., & Di Mauro, P. M. (1973). Muscle carnitine palmityl transferase deficiency and myoglobinuria. *Science, 182*, 929–931.
78. Di Mauro, S., Dalakas, M., & Miranda, A. F. (1983). Phosphoglycerate kinase deficiency: Another cause of recurrent myoglobinuria. *Annals of Neurology, 13*, 11–19.
79. Di Mauro, S., Miranda, A. F., Olarte, M., Friedman, R., & Hays, A. P. (1982). Muscle

phosphoglycerate mutase (GAM) deficiency: A new metabolic myopathy. *Neurology, 32*, 584–591.

80. Dieppe, P. A., Cushnaghan, J., Young, P., & Kirwan, J. (1993). Prediction of the progression of joint space narrowing in osteoarthritis of the knee by scintigraphy. *Annals of the Rheumatic Diseases, 52*, 557–563.
81. Dieppe, P., Basler, H. D., Chard, J., Croft, P., Dixon, J., Hurley, M., & Raspe, H. (1999). Knee replacement surgery for osteoarthritis: Effectiveness, practice variations, indications and possible determinants of utilization. *Rheumatology, 38*, 73–83.
82. Dietrichson, P., Oakley, J., Smith, P. E. M., Griffiths, R. D., Helliwell, T. R., & Edwards, R. H. T. (1987). Conchotome and needle percutaneous biopsy of skeletal muscle. *Journal of Neurology, Neurosurgery, and Psychiatry, 50*, 1461–1476.
83. Dougados, M., Nguyen, M., Listrat, V., & Amor, B. (1993). High molecular weight sodium hyaluronate (hyalectin) in osteoarthritis of the knee: A 1-year placebo-controlled trial. *Osteoarthritis and Cartilage, 1*, 97–103.
84. Douglas, J. G., Ford, M. J., Innes, J. A., & Munro, J. F. (1979). Polymyalgia arteritica: A clinical review. *European Journal of Clinical Investigation, 9*, 137–140.
85. Duthie, J. R., Thompson, M., Wier, M. M., & Fletcher, W. B. (1955). Medical and social aspects of the treatment of rheumatoid arthritis with special reference to factors affecting prognosis. *Annals of the Rheumatic Diseases, 14*, 133–149.
86. Edwards, R. H. T. (1982). Weakness and fatigue of skeletal muscles. In M. Sarner (Ed.), *Advanced Medicine, vol 18* (pp. 100–119). Pitman Medical.
87. Edwards, R. H. T. (1986). Muscle fatigue and pain. *Acta Medica Scandinavica (suppl), 711*, 179–188.
88. Edwards, R. H. T., Isenberg, D. A., Wiles, C. M., Young, A., & Snaith, M. L. (1981). The investigation of inflammatory myopathy. *Journal of the Royal College of Physicians, 15*, 19–24.
89. Edwards, R. H. T., Young, A., & Wiles, C. M. (1980). Needle biopsy of skeletal muscle in diagnosis of myopathy and the clinical study of muscle function and repair. *New England Journal of Medicine, 302*, 261–271.
90. Edwards, R. H. T., Young, A., Hosking, G. P., & Jones, D. A. (1977). Human skeletal muscle function: Description of tests and normal values. *Clinical Science and Molecular Medicine, 52*, 283–290.
91. Emery, P., Zeidler, H., Kvien, T. K., et al. (1999). Celecoxib versus diclofenar in long-term management of rheumatoid arthritis: Randomized double-blind comparison. *The Lancet, 354*, 2106–2111.
92. Ettinger, W. H., Burns, R., Messier, S. P., et al. (1997). A randomized trial comparing aerobic exercise and resistance exercise with a health education program in older adults with knee osteoarthritis. *Journal of the American Medical Association, 277*, 25–31.
93. Fassbender, H. G. (1975). Rheumatoid arthritis. In *Pathology of Rheumatic Diseases* (pp. 70–210). Springer-Verlag.
94. Felson, D. T., Zhang, Y., Hannan, M. T., et al. (1997). Risk factors for incident radiographic knee osteoarthritis in the elderly. *Arthritis and Rheumatism, 40*, 728–733.

95. Fife, R. S., Brandt, K., Braunstein, E., et al. (1991). Relationship between arthroscopic evidence of cartilage damage and radiographic evidence of joint space narrowing in early osteoarthritis of the knee. *Arthritis and Rheumatism, 34*, 377–382.

96. Fisher, N. M., Gresham, G. E., Abrams, M., et al. (1993). Quantitative effects of physical therapy on muscular and functional performance in subjects with osteoarthritis of the knees. *Archives of Physical Medicine and Rehabilitation, 74*, 840–847.

97. Gaffney, K., Ledingham, J., & Perry, J. D. (1995). Intra-articular triamcinolone hex acetonide in knee osteoarthritis: Factors influencing the clinical response. *Annals of the Rheumatic Diseases, 54*, 379–381.

98. Gardner, D. L. (1992). *Pathological Basis of the Connective Tissue Disease*. Edward Arnold.

99. Gibson, J. N., White, M. D., Chapman, V. M., & Strachan, R. K. (1992). Arthroscopic lavage and debridement for osteoarthritis of the knee. *Journal of Bone and Joint Surgery, 74B*, 534–537.

100. Griffith, S. M., Dziedzic, K., Cheung, N. T., et al. (1997). Clinical outcomes: A double blind randomized controlled trial to compare the effect of intra-articular local anesthetic and local anesthetic plus steroid in hip arthritis. *British Journal of Rheumatology, 36(suppl 2)*, 21.

101. Hannan, M. T., Anderson, J. J., Pincus, T., & Felson, D. T. (1992). Educational attainment and osteoarthritis: Differential associations with radiographic changes and symptom reporting. *Journal of Clinical Epidemiology, 45*, 139–147.

102. Hara, K. S., et al. (1990). Rheumatoid pericarditis: Clinical features and survival. *Medicine, 69*, 81–91.

103. Hawker, G., Wright, J., Coyte, P., Paul, J., Dittus, R., Croxford, R., & Katz, B. (1998). Health-related quality of life after knee replacement. *Journal of Bone and Joint Surgery, 80*, 163–173.

104. Hawley, D. J., & Wolfe, F. (1993). Depression is not more common in RA: A 10-year longitudinal study of 6153 patients with rheumatic disease. *Journal of Rheumatology, 20*, 2025–2031.

105. Hopman-Rock, M., Odding, E., Hofman, A., et al. (1996). Physical and psychosocial disability in elderly subjects in relation to pain in the hip and/or knee. *Journal of Rheumatology, 23*, 1037–1044.

106. Hutton, C. W., Higgs, E. R., Jackson, P. C., et al. (1986). 99mTc HMDP bone scanning in generalized nodal osteoarthritis. II The four-hour bone scan predicts radiographic change. *Annals of the Rheumatic Diseases, 45*, 622–626.

107. Hyland, R. H., Gordon, D. A., Broder, I., Davies, G. M., et al. (1983). A systemic controlled study of pulmonary abnormalities in rheumatoid arthritis. *Journal of Rheumatology, 10*, 395–405.

108. Jayson, M. I. V. (1999). Rheumatoid arthritis. In P. D. Wall & R. Melzack (Eds.), *Textbook of Pain, 4th edn.* (pp. 505–516). Churchill Livingstone.

109. Jayson, M. I. V., & Jones, D. E. P. (1971). Scleritis and rheumatoid arthritis. *Annals of the Rheumatic Diseases, 30*, 343–347.

110. Jones, A. C., Pattrick, M., Doherty, S., & Doherty, M. (1995). Intra-articular hyaluronic acid compared to intra-articular triamcinolone hex acetonide in inflammatory knee osteoarthritis. *Osteoarthritis and Cartilage, 3*, 269–273.

111. Jones, A., & Doherty, M. (1996). Intra-articular corticosteroids are effective in osteoarthritis but there are no clinical predictors of response. *Annals of the Rheumatic Diseases, 55*, 829–832.

112. Keefe, F. J., Caldwell, D. S., Baucom, D., et al. (1996). Spouse-assisted coping skills training in the management of osteoarthritic knee pain. *Arthritis Care and Research, 9*, 279–291.

113. Keefe, F. J., Caldwell, D. S., Queen, K. T., et al. (1987b). Pain coping strategies in osteoarthritis patients. *Journal of Consulting and Clinical Psychology, 55*, 208–212.

114. Keefe, F. J., Caldwell, D. S., Queen, K., et al. (1987a). Osteoarthritis knee pain: A behavioral analysis. *Pain, 28*, 309–321.

115. Kidd, B. (1996). Problems with pain—Is the messenger to blame? *Annals of the Rheumatic Diseases, 55*, 276–283.

116. Lawrence, R. C., Everett, D. F., & Hochberg, M. C. (1990). Arthritis. In R. Huntley & J. Cornoni-Huntley (Eds.), *Health Status and Wellbeing of the Elderly: National Health and Nutrition Examination I Epidemiologic Follow-Up Study* (pp. 133–151). Oxford University Press.

117. Lequesne, M. (1991). Indices of severity and disease activity for osteoarthritis. *Seminars in Arthritis and Rheumatism, 20(suppl 2)*, 48–54.

118. Lichtenberg, P. A., Swensen, C. H., & Skehan, M. W. (1986). Further investigation of the role of personality, lifestyle and arthritic severity in predicting pain. *Journal of Psychosomatic Research, 30*, 327–337.

119. Lohmander, L. S., Dalen, N., Englund, G., et al. (1996). Intra-articular hyaluronan injections in the treatment of osteoarthritis of the knee: A randomized, double blind, placebo-controlled trial. *Annals of the Rheumatic Diseases, 55*, 424–431.

120. Lorig, K. R., & Holman, H. R. (1993). Arthritis self-management studies: A 12-year review. *Health Education Quarterly, 20*, 17–28.

121. Lunghi, M., Miller, P., & McQuillan, W. (1978). Psychosocial factors in osteoarthritis of the hip. *Journal of Psychosomatic Research, 22*, 57–63.

122. Maisiak, R., Austin, J., & Heck, L. (1996). Health outcomes of two telephone interventions for patients with rheumatoid arthritis or osteoarthritis. *Arthritis and Rheumatism, 39*, 1391–1399.

123. Martin, K., Nicklas, B. J., Bunyard, L. B., et al. (1996). Weight loss and walking improve symptoms of knee osteoarthritis. *Arthritis and Rheumatism, 39(suppl)*, S225.

124. McAlindon, T., Cooper, C., Kirwan, J. R., & Dieppe, P. A. (1993). Determinants of disability in osteoarthritis of the knee. *Annals of the Rheumatic Diseases, 52*, 258–262.

125. Melzack, R. (1975). The McGill pain questionnaire: Major properties and scoring methods. *Pain, 1*, 277–299.

126. Minor, M. A., & Brown, J. D. (1993). Exercise maintenance of persons with arthritis after participation in a class experience. *Health Education Quarterly, 20*, 83–95.

127. Moreland, L. W., Schiff, M. H., et al. (1999). Etanercept therapy in rheumatoid arthritis. *Annals of Internal Medicine, 130*, 478–486.

128. Muller-Fassbender, H., Bach, G. L., Haase, W., et al. (1994). Glucosamine sulfate compared to ibuprofen in osteoarthritis of the knee. *Osteoarthritis and Cartilage, 2*, 61–69.

129. Ogata, K., Yasunaga, M., & Nomiyama, H. (1997). The effect of wedged insoles on the thrust of osteoarthritic knees. *International Orthopaedics, 21*, 308–312.

130. O'Reilly, S. C., Muir, K. R., & Doherty, M. (1999). Effectiveness of home exercise on pain and

disability from osteoarthritis of the knee: A randomized controlled study. *Annals of the Rheumatic Diseases, 58*, 15–19.

131. O'Reilly, S., Muir, K. R., & Doherty, M. (1996). Screening for pain in knee osteoarthritis: Which question? *Annals of the Rheumatic Diseases, 55*, 931–933.
132. Ostensson, A., & Geborek, P. (1991). Septic arthritis as a non-surgical complication in rheumatoid arthritis and relation to disease severity and therapy. *British Journal of Rheumatology, 30*, 35–38.
133. Ravaud, P., Moulinier, L., Giraudeau, B., Ayral, X., Guerin, C., Noel, E., Thomas, P., Fautrel, B., Mazieres, B., & Dougados, M. (1999). Effects of joint lavage and steroid injection in patients with osteoarthritis of the knee: Results of a multicenter, randomized, controlled trial. *Arthritis and Rheumatism, 42*, 475–482.
134. Reginster, J. Y., et al. (2001). Long term effects of glucosamine sulphate on osteoarthritis progression: A randomized placebo controlled clinical trial. *Lancet, 357*, 251–256.
135. Rothermick, N. O., Philips, V. K., Bergen, W., & Rhomas, M. H. (1976). Chrysotherapy. A prospective study. *Arthritis and Rheumatism, 19*, 1321–1327.
136. Ryan, M. E., Greenwald, R. A., & Golub, L. M. (1996). Potential of tetracyclines to modify cartilage breakdown in osteoarthritis. *Current Opinions in Rheumatology, 8*, 238–247.
137. Slemenda, C., Brandt, K. D., Heilman, D. K., et al. (1997). Quadriceps weakness and osteoarthritis of the knee. *Annals of Internal Medicine, 127*, 97–104.
138. Smolen, J. S., Kalden, J. R., et al. (1999). Efficacy and safety of leflunamide compared with placebo and sulphasalazine in active rheumatoid arthritis: A double-blind, randomized, multi-center trial. *Lancet, 353*, 259–266.
139. Summers, M. N., Haley, W. E., Reveille, J. O., & Alarcon, G. S. (1988). Radiographic assessment and psychological variables as predictors of pain and functional impairment in osteoarthritis of the knee or hip. *Arthritis and Rheumatism, 31*, 204–209.
140. Ward, T. (1985). Historical perspective on the use of methotrexate for the treatment of rheumatoid arthritis. *Journal of Rheumatology (suppl I)*, 3–6.
141. Weinberger, M., Tierney, W. M., Cowper, P. A., et al. (1993). Cost-effectiveness of increased telephone contact for patients with osteoarthritis: A randomized, controlled trial. *Arthritis and Rheumatism, 36*, 243–246.
142. Westedt, M. L., Breedveld, F. C., Schrevder, G. M. Th., d'Amato, J., Cats, N., & de Vries, R. R. P. (1986). Immunogenetic heterogeneity of rheumatoid arthritis. *Annals of the Rheumatic Diseases, 45*, 534–538.
143. Whaley, K., & Webb, J. (1977). Liver and kidney disease in rheumatoid arthritis. *Clinics in Rheumatic Diseases, 3*, 527–547.
144. Wish, J. B., & Kammer, G. M. (1993). Nephrological aspects of management in the rheumatic diseases. In P. H. Maddison et al. (Eds.), *Oxford Textbook of Rheumatology* (pp. 179–187). Oxford University Press.
145. Wolfe, M. M., Lichtenstein, D. R., & Singh, G. (1999). Gastrointestinal toxicity of nonsteroidal anti-inflammatory drugs. *New England Journal of Medicine, 340*, 1888–1899.

Chapter 3

CHRONIC BACK AND UPPER EXTREMITY PAIN

Contents

Introduction

People with chronic back and upper extremity pain face many obstacles that negatively affect their quality of life, mobility, and everyday activities. These illnesses include a broad spectrum of neurological and musculoskeletal disorders that cause pain in the arms, shoulders, back, and neck that is either constant or recurrent.

Chronic pain in the back and upper extremities has a complex etiology that frequently combines biomechanical, structural, neurological, and psychosocial factors. Common causes include inflammatory diseases like rheumatoid arthritis or fibromyalgia, repetitive stress injuries, muscle strains or sprains, nerve compression like radiculopathy or neuropathy, and degenerative changes in the spine like osteoarthritis, disc herniation, and spinal stenosis. Depending on the underlying cause, the symptoms of chronic back and upper extremity pain can vary greatly and include localized pain, stiffness, weakness, numbness, tingling, and reduced range of motion. The pain may radiate to other parts of the body, like the arms or legs, and it may be intermittent or continuous. Chronic back and upper extremity pain management call for an all-encompassing, multidisciplinary strategy customized to each patient's requirements. Conservative methods of treatment include physical therapy, exercise, ergonomic changes, heat or cold therapy, and medication (such as muscle relaxants, nonsteroidal anti-inflammatory drugs, or neuropathic pain medications).

Interventional procedures like facet joint injections, nerve blocks, epidural steroid injections, or spinal cord stimulation may be considered for people with more severe or resistant pain. Surgical procedures like discectomy, laminectomy, or spinal fusion might be required in certain situations to treat structural deformities or nerve compression.

Chronic pain is experienced and managed in large part by psychosocial factors like stress, anxiety, depression, and coping techniques. Thus, for best results, a comprehensive strategy that takes into account the mental and physical components of pain is necessary.

Complex and multidimensional conditions like chronic back and upper extremity pain necessitate a thorough and customized approach to diagnosis and treatment. Healthcare professionals can help patients with these difficult conditions live better lives by addressing the underlying causes and combining conservative, interventional, and psychosocial therapies to improve function and reduce symptoms.

Orientation and Directional Terms

Term	Definition	Illustration
Chronic trauma	Chronic trauma is a type of post-traumatic stress disorder (PTSD) that can result from repeated exposure to stressful events.	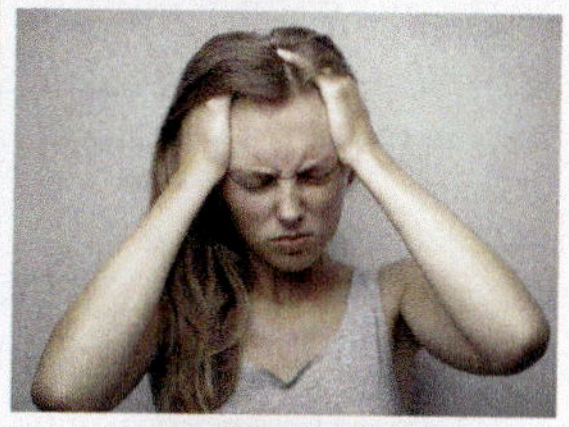
Spinal fusion	Spinal fusion is a surgery procedure that reinforces your back structure and stability by linking two vertebrae together.	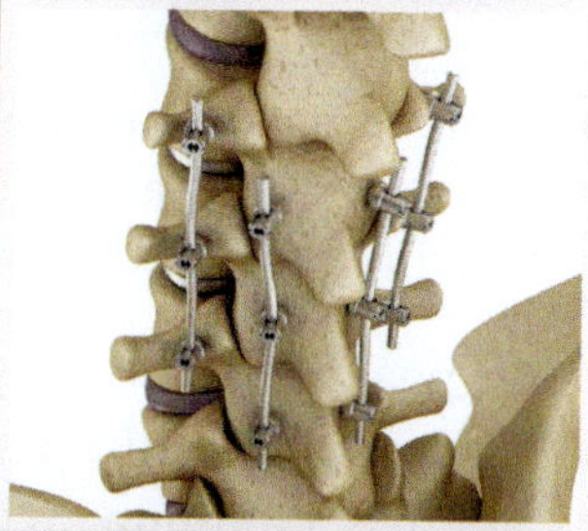
Upper extremity pain	Upper extremity pain can affect the shoulder, arm, elbow, forearm, wrist, and hand.	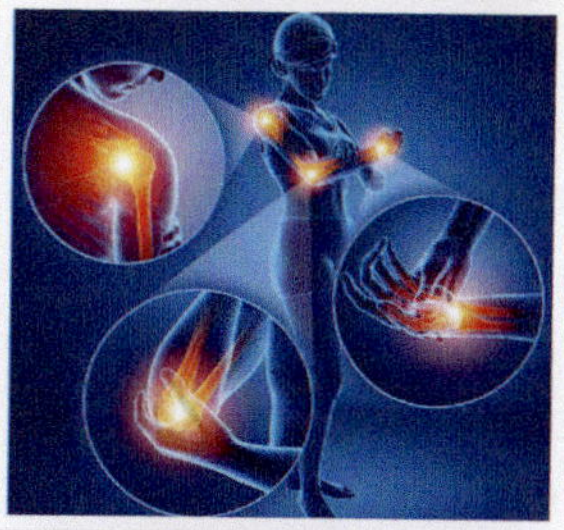
Disc herniation	A condition that refers to a problem with a rubbery disc ruptured between the spinal bones.	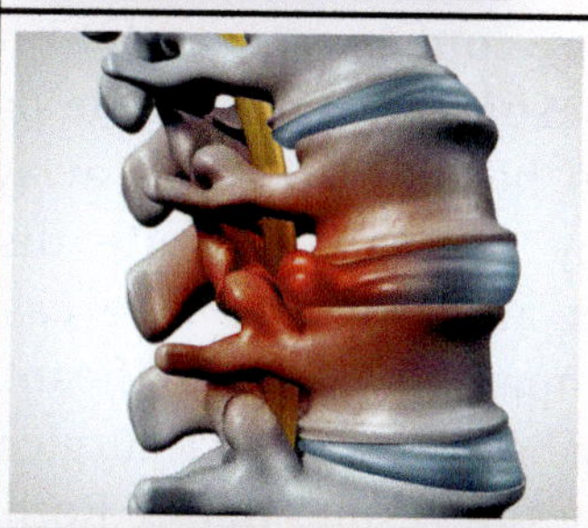
Spondylosis	Spondylosis is a condition in which there is abnormal wear on the cartilage and bones of the neck (cervical vertebrae).	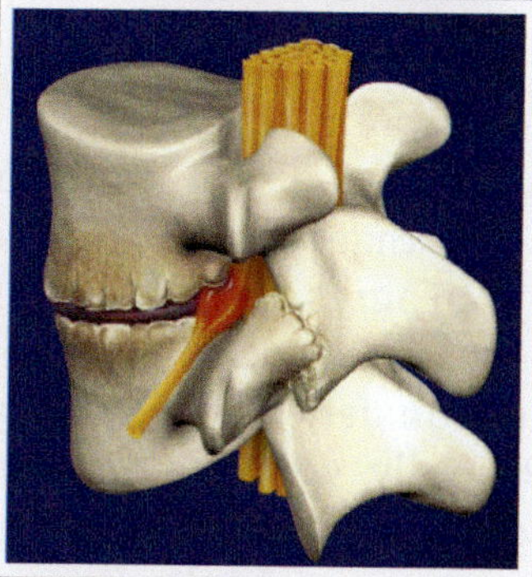

3.1. Classification of the Complaint of Low Back Pain

Low back pain is categorized according to temporal features in the most useful way yet. Since idiopathic low back pain still accounts for a large portion of cases, this classification, albeit imperfect, is helpful (BenDebba et al., 1997). Except for history later, transient low back pain usually passes quickly and does not require medical attention. The patient usually initiates treatment based on their symptoms. The problem's causes are rarely identified, and it has little bearing on practice or disability.

Generally speaking, low back pain that lasts a few days to a few months is classified as acute. Back pain is common, whether or not there is leg radiation. Based on empirical data and some supporting evidence, most of these issues are self-limiting and resolved on their own. According to Long and Zeidman (1994), standard treatments have little effect on the natural history. Short bouts of bed rest, sufficient analgesia, local physical measures, and cautious waiting are common treatment protocols. Some patients experience intractable pain that is too severe to be allowed to go away on its own, especially those with acute disc herniation (Bigos et al., 1994). In rare cases, pain may be accompanied by a significant neurological deficit. In both cases, quick surgical intervention is usually the result (Bell & Rothman, 1984).

3.1.1. Persistent Low Back Pain

According to the most widely accepted schema, pain that lasts longer than six months gradually progresses to the chronic state, which is characterized by pain obsession, depression, anxiety, and disability (Long et al., 1988). Recently, we have discovered a sizable population of patients whose pain lasts longer than six months and who do not also exhibit any symptoms of chronic pain syndrome (BenDebba et al., 1997). 95% of the patients exhibited complaints of pain and dysfunction that diminished but did not significantly impact, all other activities. When they underwent psychological testing, the results showed trends that were typical of any sick normal population. In the entire group, there was a 5% incidence of psychological dysfunction. To distinguish this set from the connotations of the term "chronic" in the context of pain, we have named it the persistent low back pain syndrome. The majority of these individuals had spondylotic illness. These patients did not respond to standard therapy modalities used for them, and there was no discernible worsening or improvement over the course of the longitudinal evaluation (Long et al., 1996).

3.1.2. The Chronic Pain Syndrome

Regarding the symptoms and indicators that characterize a subset of patients who complain of pain on a chronic basis, the consensus has prevailed over the last 20 years (Long et al., 1988; Long, 1991). These patients present with similar complaints and findings almost regardless of the cause of the pain (Waddell et al., 1980). They are hampered because of pain, which is the source of their obsession. A significant portion experience anxiety and depression. A remarkably elevated frequency of mental health diagnoses is observed in them. Even more of them exhibit traits that are typical of personality disorders. While drug addiction is uncommon, drug misuse is a common occurrence. These patients are chronically incapacitated due to pain and heavily rely on medical resources. Around the world, specialized treatment centers have been established to address them.

3.2. Evaluation of Back and Leg Pain

A thorough history that details the location, intensity, and causes of the pain should be taken before beginning any evaluation (Deyo et al., 1992). A physical examination will evaluate any musculoskeletal and neurological abnormalities but is unlikely to be diagnostic (McCombe et al., 1989; Jonsson and Stromqvist, 1993). Keep an ear out for warning signs during these exams, such as persistent pain (cancer or infection), nighttime pain (intraspinal tumor), systemic symptoms (cancer or infection), and signs of other organ or systemic disease. Observe the patient's behavior throughout the examination as well. Are behaviors consistent with complaints, is motor examination reliable (Waddell et al., 1980), and is there a lot of pain behavior?

Imaging is crucial for chronic patients, as opposed to those with acute pain issues. It's crucial to use simple films with flexion and extension. For most screenings, MRI works best. If there is a suspicion of bony pathology, CT can be used to reduce fixator artifacts with 2–3D reconstructions. In patients who have had prior surgery, CT myelograms are most frequently required (Wiesel et al., 1984; Boden et al., 1990; Cavanagh et al., 1993; Ackerman et al., 1997).

3.2.1. Back and Leg Pain as a Manifestation of Unexpected or Intercurrent Disease

Just 3% of patients in our own patient series had an unanticipated systemic disease (Long et al., 1996). All exhibited indications or symptoms that pointed to conditions other than common spondylotic disease. The most typical type of metastases are osseous. Rarely, pancreatitis, acute and chronic renal disease, retroperitoneal inflammatory processes, and chronic gastrointestinal disorders can all lead to back pain. Though differentiation may occasionally be unclear, the signs that these do not represent spondylotic disease are typically clear. Any of these processes typically cause localized pain. Although it is rarely usually sciatic, leg radiation may develop as a result of involvement of the lumbosacral plexus. These pains tend to be persistent, unaffected by activity or rest and frequently coexist with other systemic disease signs and symptoms. Both the leg pain and the physical symptoms linked to plexus infiltration are nonradicular. Intractable pain, unremitting pain, neurological deficit suggestive of involvement of the lumbosacral plexus, history of cancer or inflammatory disease, history of any disease likely to be complicated by infection, and history of significant trauma are signs and symptoms that suggest intercurrent disease. Patients who have any of these should be evaluated, and MRI and plain spine films should be used for diagnosis. Treatment is determined by the reason why the symptoms are occurring.

3.2.1.1. Osteoporosis

The question of whether osteoporosis by itself can cause back pain is still up for debate. Many spinal pain specialists think it is possible. Compression fractures, however, are the most frequent reason for excruciating pain in people with osteoporosis. Compression fractures cause intense, localized pain. Signs and symptoms of individual nerve root compression may appear if the collapse is significant enough. Nevertheless, the pain is usually focal in the back, does not radiate, and is extremely accurate in its localization over the collapsed segment. Postmenopausal women, people with other disorders of the metabolism of calcium and estrogen, heavy smokers, long-term users of steroids, and patients on prolonged immunosuppression are among those who are at risk. A simple X-ray is used to make the diagnosis. The standard course of treatment includes time spent in therapy for the underlying issue, rest, external support, and activity restriction. After suffering a compression fracture, the pain frequently lasts for six months or longer.

Vertebroplasty was introduced as an approach. Using fluoroscopy, the acutely compressed segment is seen during this process. To reinforce the collapse, methyl methacrylate is injected into the vertebral body through a needle inserted through the pedicle. Pain relief can be extremely satisfying and is typically immediate.

3.2.1.2. Spondylitis

Rheumatoid arthritis is most frequently linked to chronic back pain as an inflammatory condition. Back pain is typically not an early sign of the illness, so when it does arise, the diagnosis is made. It can be challenging to determine the diagnosis with clinical certainty if systemic manifestations are not prominent. MR, CT, and plain films all point to inflammatory spondylotic disease. Serological testing confirms the diagnosis. There are three stages to the treatment. Treating the underlying illness comes first. The second is an exercise regimen to maintain axial muscle strength throughout life. The third is surgical treatment for root compression syndromes or spinal instability. Although spinal stenosis in the lumbar region does happen, cervical rheumatoid spinal problems that necessitate surgery make up the majority of cases. Typical neurogenic claudication is the syndrome. Decompression and frequently fusion are necessary during surgery.

A common issue that comes up second is ankylosing spondylitis. This illness primarily affects men. Early-life back pain is typically the first symptom, and a history of progressive, ongoing back pain is common. Symptoms of cord compression or radiculopathy are rare. The characteristic "bamboo spine" appearance on a standard X-ray or MRI is used to make the diagnosis. The usual mode of treatment is symptomatic. The lumbar area experiences a reduction in pain as spontaneous fusion advances up the spine, but the pain gradually returns to higher levels.

An uncommon condition that is similar is psoriatic arthritis. According to Liu et al. (1990), the issue is more facet arthropathy with synovial proliferation. Thus, spinal stenosis is typical and root compression syndromes are common in psoriatic arthritis. It is best to treat back pain symptomatically on its own. Root compression syndromes necessitate surgical decompression and sporadic stabilization.

Untreated cases of acromegaly spondylitis are not uncommon. Thankfully, this issue has become extremely uncommon thanks to the high caliber of treatment now offered for these pituitary tumors. Similar to ankylosing spondylitis, the syndrome causes progressive pain that typically starts in the lumbar area and ends on its own through spontaneous fusion. It is a symptomatic treatment.

3.2.2. Musculoskeletal Pain Syndromes

A subset of individuals with idiopathic pain in their legs and backs do not have any associated underlying abnormalities (Panjabi et al., 1982). The majority report pain and tenderness in their muscles. Most have been linked to loss of range of motion, focal tenderness, and spasms (Pope et al., 1994). No concomitant neurological symptoms exist. Although the back pain is usually localized, it can also radiate upward and into the hips and upper thighs (Mense, 1991). The issue could be specific to the lumbar spine or it could be a component of the more general syndrome known as myofascial pain. The history and non-specific physical findings, which usually include loss of range of motion, localized pain and tenderness in the muscles or at the insertions of the muscles, and the presence of focal areas of myositis, are used to make the diagnosis. The majority of imaging studies show normal or non-diagnostic spondylotic abnormalities. Anti-inflammatories, long-term exercise, and local passive therapy techniques for specific abnormality areas make up the treatment.

3.2.3. Abdominal and Pelvic Disease Causing Low Back Pain

A few particular diseases are significant, but it is uncommon for abdominal pelvic or hip disease to mimic spondylotic or idopathic low back pain. The most frequent is probably lumbar spine metastatic disease, which can be identified with the right imaging. Other identifiable causes include cancer and retroperitoneal inflammatory disease. Leg and low back pain can be caused by endometriosis or chronic pelvic inflammatory disease. Dissection of an aortic aneurysm typically results in acute pain, but it can also cause chronic back pain linked to vascular claudication in patients. Since idiopathic chronic back pain and intraabdominal disease of other organs are so rarely confused, any one of them is unlikely to be significant in the diagnosis process. Diagnosis confusion is unlikely because renal, gallbladder, and bowel diseases are frequently associated with other symptoms.

3.2.4. Back Pain as a Manifestation of Psychiatric Disease

Physicians and many other professionals who treat chronic pain have a strong tendency to assume that all pain that cannot be diagnosed is psychosomatic. This is especially true when it comes to persistent back pain. According to data from the National Low Back Pain Study, back pain patients do not have a higher incidence of psychopathology than would be predicted for any sick population. In that study, 3% of patients had a psychiatric diagnosis that the examiners believed to be the main reason for the complaint (BenDebba et al., 1997). Nonetheless, the incidence of psychopathology was significantly higher in a population of over 2,000 patients admitted to a pain treatment program due to chronic pain syndrome manifestations. It was believed that a primary psychiatric diagnosis, or at least a significant mediator, was the cause of the pain complaint in 15–20% of these patients (Long et al., 1988; Long, 1991).

The most prevalent diagnosis was endogenous depression. The psychiatrists who worked with these patients distinguished between this diagnosis and the far more typical reactive depression. After schizophrenia, somatoform disorder was the next most frequently diagnosed condition. The most common diagnosis is a topic of significant disagreement among pain specialists. In certain cases, personality disorders are to blame. This chapter is not meant to be a comprehensive analysis of these psychological variables. In this case, it's crucial to stress that pain is a significant symptom of psychiatric illness. The possibility that the patient has a diagnosable independent cause is not ruled out even in the presence of psychiatric illness.

Patients with symptoms secondary to psychiatric disease are far less likely to have their symptoms mistakenly diagnosed as organic issues than patients with idiopathic low back pain, who are far more likely to have their symptoms attributed to psychosomatic causes.

3.2.5. Spondylotic Low Back Pain (Idiopathic)

Most patients with low back pain, either alone or in conjunction with leg pain, also have spondylotic spinal disease. Although there is a correlation, it is not very strong, between the complaints and the presence of spondylosis (Boden et al., 1990; Wiesel et al., 1984).

Even in the event that the relationship is causative, little is known about the mechanisms underlying the pain. A significant portion of patients have spondylotic changes without any obvious symptoms, which presents a diagnostic challenge. Spondylotic changes, however, are present in a significant majority of patients complaining of persistent back pain, and they are the only abnormalities that appear to account for the pain.

The most crucial diagnostic tool is the problem's history. Individuals who appear to have spondylitis origin pain typically experience increased pain during standing or weight bearing. Rest helps most of them. Although this is usually restricted to reclining in extension, a minority find that reclining worsens their condition. Simple local modalities like heat and massage can temporarily relieve pain, and non-steroidal analgesics are not very effective. The patient can usually pinpoint the exact location of the pain with a fingertip because it is localized in the lumbar region. Non-radicular leg pain, typically diffuse and aching in the anterior or posterior thighs, is frequently linked to severe back pain. Neurogenic claudication and associated true radicular pain are both 70% common.

3.2.5.1. Diagnosis

Ackerman et al. (1997) state that the diagnosis is made using a plain X-ray, CT scan, or MRI, each of which shows distinct disease characteristics. The disc dissipation is the first alteration. The disc narrows, becomes uneven, and loses water as the nucleus loses its distinct character. Changes in inflammation occur in the bone surrounding the end plate and beyond, initially as acute and subsequently as chronic. Discs cause interosseous herniation by wearing down the end plates. Traction spurs can develop anteriorly or posteriorly, there is a thickening of the ligamentous tissue, and disc bulges can occur. The canal may narrow, and facets with degenerative changes are common. A combination of ligamentous thickening, bony enlargement, facet overgrowth, and synovial hypertrophy results in canal narrowing.

3.2.5.2. Treatment of Spondylitic Back Pain

Only the relief of proven nerve root compression, the correction of a fixed deformity, or the stabilization of an unstable segment are the reasons why surgical procedures are worthwhile (O'Connell, 1951; Hanley et al., 1991; Zdeblick, 1993). Spondylosis-related pain by itself is not a sufficient justification for surgery. For most patients, there is probably no benefit to direct intervention. Therapy only addresses symptoms (Waddell, 1987a). There is compelling new evidence that patients whose symptoms have persisted for six months or more are unlikely to experience spontaneous improvement. There is also strong evidence that standard conservative measures, when used in a typical practice, are ineffective and cannot be distinguished from receiving no treatment at all. Our research has looked at a wide range of treatments, such as acupuncture, back schools, nutritional therapies, pain treatment centers, and cognitive therapies, in addition to many types of conventional physical therapy and manipulation therapy. As these treatments are currently being used in practice, we were unable to find any effect from any of them. Thus, simply referring patients for any of these treatments will not be sufficient. Every patient should have a customized program designed using the best available data (Hsieh et al., 1992; Koes et al., 1992; Meade et al., 1995).

Initially, adequate analgesia should be used. Standard pain relievers are nonsteroidal anti-inflammatory drugs (Bigos et al., 1994). Long-acting opioids are being studied by some researchers as a potential treatment for benign pain. It is worthwhile to try lumbar support because some patients will benefit from short-term bracing, especially when they are active. There is solid evidence that many patients will benefit from a customized exercise program to strengthen the abdominal and paravertebral muscles as well as local therapies to restore painless range of motion. Although the benefits of weight loss have not been established, most intensive rehabilitation programs include weight loss because it makes intuitive sense (Heliovaara, 1987). If these intense physical therapy regimens are to be successful, both the patient and the doctor must be truly committed. Treatment for severe osteoporosis is also necessary.

3.2.6. The Facet Syndrome

It appears that lumbar zygapophyseal joints cause pain in a small percentage of patients (Bogduk and Long, 1980; Moran et al., 1988). These patients typically report localized pain, and they are frequently able to identify the affected joint. Moving hurts. Rest is beneficial, and pain is especially caused by axial loading.

Arthropathy is shown by imaging studies. The joints have hypertrophy. Common are synovial cysts. Around the articular surfaces, there are changes in inflammation that can be either acute or chronic, and the cartilage end plates deteriorate. There are often subluxations.

When pain is relieved by injecting a local anesthetic into a joint or its innervation, the diagnosis is considered confirmed. Most patients who meet the diagnostic criteria experience long-lasting relief from radiofrequency destruction of the innervation. Based on observations, only a very tiny portion of patients—roughly 1 to 2%—present with back pain (Bogduk & Long, 1980).

3.2.7. Spinal Stenosis

Leg pain and claudication accompanied by back pain are symptoms of spinal stenosis syndrome. Usually, patients first show up with a straightforward gait abnormality. That is, after walking for an extended period of time, they find it difficult to walk normally. After that, there is pain, and the diagnosis is confirmed by the painful weakness that walking causes in both legs. These patients are usually relieved when they stop walking, and they frequently sit with their legs bent to expedite the resolution of their symptoms. These characteristics set it apart from vascular claudication, whose symptoms go away as soon as an activity is stopped. Sensory complaints typically resemble stockings and are indicative of metabolic peripheral neuropathy, which is sometimes mistaken for the issue. While the neurological examination might be completely normal while at rest, activity can cause both motor and sensory loss. Imaging studies are used to make the diagnosis. The diagnosis is made by CT or MRI.

When spinal stenosis symptoms are severe, surgical decompression is the recommended course of treatment. The results are very good. The question is whether the symptoms are severe enough to necessitate surgery. Most patients are only mildly to moderately incapacitated and don't necessarily need surgery. Surgery is recommended when symptoms become seriously incapacitating or when significant neurological deficits progress over time.

3.2.8. Foraminal Root Compression Syndrome

Compression of an isolated root in a spondylotic foramen results in a variation of the spinal stenosis problem. Patients complain of acute disc herniation when they first arrive, but the condition takes a long time to develop and usually starts slowly. Within the recognized distribution of a single root, patients report experiencing sciatica or femoral pain. Bilateral root involvement can occur occasionally, affecting multiple roots on one side. That syndrome is not claudication, though. It has to do with continuous root compression. That is to say, even though activity, standing, and axial loading frequently make the pain worse, it usually remains constant. The corresponding changes in reflex, motor, and sensory function are related to the specific root. In contrast to the tension sign of an acute disc herniation, a positive straight leg raising is unusual. MR and CT scans are used to make the diagnosis because they can show the compression of the nerve root and the neural foramina. A comprehensive trial of an individualized exercise activity program is recommended if the pain is manageable and there is no significant neurological deficit (Saal and Saal, 1989). Surgery should be performed if the rehabilitation program is ineffective, the pain is unbearable, or there are concomitant neurological deficits (Saal et al., 1990). Surgery should result in a similar favorable outcome as in cases of acute disc herniation.

3.2.9. Spinal Instability and Progressive Deformity Syndromes

A considerable portion of spondylotic disease patients will experience progressive spinal deformities. Most of these are degenerative in nature, though congenital and traumatic instability can happen and will present similarly. Thankfully, the course of treatment remains largely unchanged, so the etiology has minimal bearing (Cholewicki & McGill, 1996).

3.2.9.1. Degenerative Spondylolisthesis

Of all the issues, this one arises the most frequently. The direction of the slip could be anterior or posterior. It might be demonstrable and actively moving on dynamic films. It might progress gradually and occasionally be fixed. Most often, lumbar back pain is reported by patients, either with or without accompanying root symptoms. Plain X-rays are used for diagnosis, and dynamic films should be included to confirm whether the spine is moving actively.

Unless there is an intractable pain or a significant nerve root compression resulting in a neurological deficit, treatment should be symptomatic. Bracing, lifestyle changes, and tailored active exercise for improving range of motion, leg strength, and axial muscle strength are examples of symptomatic therapies. When radicular pain, axial back pain, or both are severe and incapacitating, surgery should be considered. For stabilization and fusion, most patients with slowly progressing scoliotic deformities of any kind or progressive listhesis will need to use a fixator. When symptoms are evidently severe enough to require surgery, but before severe deformities manifest, it is best to move forward (Raugstad et al., 1982; Zdeblick, 1993).

3.2.10. The Failed Back Syndrome

A broad group of patients who have had lumbar spine surgeries without success are often grouped together under the imprecise term "failed back syndrome" (Waddell, 1987b; Long, 1991). If anything, the evaluation of a patient who has not benefited from one or more operations needs to be more complex than that of a patient who has not had surgery (Fager & Freidberg, 1980). To enable the prescription of a customized treatment plan, the evaluation's objective should be to define abnormalities as precisely as possible. Within this heterogeneous group, patients fit into broad categories that help direct the assessment and the treatment plans (Long et al., 1988). A subset of patients falls into the first of these broad categories, as they are likely not candidates for surgery in the first place. Patients in the second category have obvious signs of needing surgery, but the initial abnormality was not fixed by the procedure. Patients who experienced a major surgical complication 72 that is currently the source of their pain fall into a third category. Another extremely tiny subset of patients has an unrecognized concurrent diagnosis.

No matter what kind of treatment is suggested, it is critical to precisely identify the abnormalities that need to be treated because they are most likely the source of the pain (Frymoyer et al., 1978). In particular, abnormalities that are as well defined as those for the initial surgery should be the focus of any reoperative surgery (Finnegan et al., 1979). Surgery will only help these patients if they have nerve root compression or if their instability is blatantly apparent (Turner et al., 1992).

3.3. Common Post-Operative Pain Syndromes

3.3.1. Inappropriate Patient Selection

Research on patients who don't get better after their first lumbar surgery frequently indicates that most of them didn't meet accepted standards before the procedure and didn't have imaging evidence of either an instability syndrome or root compression syndrome. The availability of prior research and documentation will either support or contradict the initial surgical indications.

Even though the initial surgery was not clearly necessary, this does not mean the patient does not currently have a problem that can be fixed. Reassessment is necessary. It's crucial to keep in mind that a failed first surgery leaving pain behind does not necessarily mean that a second surgery is necessary. Surgery reoperation indications ought to be just as strict as initial ones (Spengler & Freeman, 1979). Stereotypical fusion addition brought about by an unsuccessful initial procedure is not warranted.

3.3.2. Failure to Correct the Initial Pathology

The fact that the initial surgeon did not operate intended to fully treat the initial illness is another frequent issue. Failure to decompress a nerve root or roots through foraminotomy, failing to decompress the spinal canal, incorrect level, complete disc removal, and failing to identify and stabilize unstable segments are common examples. Imaging studies conducted again will typically show the residual abnormality. When the patient's complaints align with these abnormalities, surgical repair is almost as successful as a first-time procedure.

3.3.3. Surgical Complications

There's a long list of potential complications. These include infection, excessive scarring, surgically induced instability, nerve root injury, and pseudomeningocele.

Fixators face a unique set of issues. Pseudarthrosis is a possible outcome of fusions (Steinman & Herkowitz, 1992). Hardware could come loose or even protrude. Occasionally, hardware is positioned incorrectly. Every patient who has had fusion surgery should be examined in order to evaluate the effectiveness of the bony fusion, the stability of the fixators' placement, and the appropriateness of their placement (Kozak & O'Brien, 1990).

Surgery-related issues can arise that are not direct or even immediate aftercare. Degeneration of the segment above may result from the fixation of one or more spinal segments. Usually, this is a chronic issue, though it can occasionally be acute. Stenosis above the fusion and instability are the symptoms.

Many patients have visibly thick scars, which can cause the thecal sac to distort after surgery. These scars may or may not be significant. According to Bandschuh et al. (1990), there is no proof that operating on non-compressive patients is advantageous for them.

3.3.4. Arachnoiditis

If this condition is considered a clinical syndrome rather than a radiological finding, then it is a unique issue. Numerous individuals who have experienced spinal surgery, whether with or without myelography, exhibit nerve root adherence to the dural sac as well as root adhesions. While some of these findings appear to be related to symptoms, the majority do not appear to have any clear clinical significance. On the other hand, persistent adhesive arachnoiditis is rarely progressive and should be taken into account in certain cases. This uncommon syndrome manifests as a slowly progressing loss of function and diffuse, frequently burning, lower extremity pain. Arachnoiditis may be suggested by MRI, but myelography is necessary to determine the exact severity of the condition, especially in cases where spinal stenosis is present. When arachnoiditis was first reported, it was most frequently linked to infection. Later, it was described as a side effect of myelography and surgery. As a consequence of surgery alone, arachnoiditis is now observed in patients who have not undergone myelography. There is minimal doubt about the connection between the myelographic findings of arachnoiditis and the symptomatology when the uncommon progressive problem is present. The connection between arachnoiditis and symptoms is still unknown for most patients, though. The presence of arachnoiditis alone does not indicate that the patient's complaints are related to this pathological process. Spinal cord stimulation is typically used to treat pain (Long et al., 1981).

3.3.5. Theoretical Causes of Low Back Pain

Many studies into potential causes of back and leg pain have been conducted because these types of pain frequently do not present with clearly defined nerve root compression or obvious diagnosable instability. It seems that ligaments and muscles are the primary source of pain in certain patients (Panjabi et al., 1982). At the very least, no other reasons are known. According to researchers, the first of these hypothesizes that the pain may be neuropathic and that it may result from mild degrees of demyelinization and sensitization, most likely coupled with changes in central receptors (Wall & Gutnick, 1974; Calvin et al., 1982; Devor et al., 1991). Numerous elements and potential mechanisms are under investigation. As of yet, none of these are obviously relevant to normal patients who experience persistent leg and back pain.

Another significant line of research contends that the release of inflammatory products as a result of degeneration, spondylotic alterations, and/or surgical trauma is what causes the nerve activation and sensitization (Schwarzer et al., 1995).

A third broad category is named after the micromovement of its founders. This theory states that minute but aberrant movements in the zygapophyseal joints and within and surrounding the disc are the source of the noxious stimuli. These motions would likely trigger nociceptors in muscles, ligaments, and the periosteum (Kuslich et al., 1991; Gracely et al., 1992).

3.3.6. Further Evaluation of the Patient without an Apparent Cause of Pain

Even after all of these particular anomalies have been identified or ruled out, the majority of patients still have unidentified pain that cannot currently be explained. While many of them don't react well to general conservative measures, some of them do. Numerous specialists in spine care have persisted in using physiologic techniques to assess these patients to supplement the anatomical information obtained from imaging studies.

The simple theory underlying the use of temporary diagnostic blockade to support clinical decision-making is that pain being produced should be relieved upon anesthesia of a pain generator. The additions include injecting a placebo to control pain and producing it mechanically by irritating the generator (Bogduk et al., 1995a).

The use of diagnostic blocks to help the clinician identify painful segments or structures in the lumbar spine is arguably the most misunderstood area of spinal disease today. To apply blocks correctly, it is necessary to grasp a few principles. According to recent research, these blocks can effectively identify painful segments, but they may not be specific to the individual structures they block because multiple blocks of various types seem to overlap significantly within the same segment (Knox and Chapman, 1993). Blocks that are controlled by a placebo are more precise than others. Suspicious blocks are those that lack negative control (Bogduk et al., 1995b).

Currently used blocks include provocative disc blockade, individual root blockade, block of the donor site and pseudoarthrosis, and block of zygapophyseal joints. These blocks are currently used to support a clinical opinion regarding the source of the pain complaint. The next significant action hasn't been taken yet. That is, no research has been done that conclusively shows how well any of these building blocks can predict the likelihood of a successful outcome from a carefully considered interventional procedure. However, when administered by a skilled clinician who interprets the results objectively, they can be helpful.

3.3.7. Alternatives for Care of Chronic Low Back Pain

It should come as no surprise that a clinical issue with as little understanding as low back pain should lead to an enormous number of beneficial therapies being developed. Many are backed by established practice, but many are still unproven.

Included in the first general category are all the adjuncts that promise to increase comfort levels. The list is extensive and includes, among other things, whirlpools, chairs, pillows, supports, firm mattresses, and adjustable beds. Patients are free to use the ones that feel comfortable and try those that catch their eye. We don't prescribe any and usually discourage using those that are very pricey.

Many patients are enrolled in active programs that involve massage and manipulation or long-term programs that involve 74 passive therapy techniques like heat, massage, and electrical stimulation. There is insufficient evidence to support the efficacy of any of these in treating chronic back pain. If patients feel they are symptomatically better, I advise them to keep going (O'Connell, 1951).

In addition, patients seek out acupuncture as well as a range of complementary and alternative therapies, such as those that can be ordered through catalogs. None are backed by scientific evidence for chronic back pain, and do not suggest any. This also applies to the numerous herbal remedies that patients purchase.

Back pain is the subject of a vast array of books, audio files, and videos. Some may be harmful, but the majority are beneficial. Instead of giving the patient free reign to select anything they want, it's better to find some you like and suggest them. There are now a lot of minimally invasive procedures available that guarantee patients no-risk relief. The most common ones were and still are percutaneous discectomy (Choy et al., 1987; Kambin, 1988; Onik et al., 1990; Revel et al., 1993), endoscopic laser discectomy, endoscopic discectomy, endoscopic fusion, and microdiscectomy. Steroids in epidural or intradiscal spaces These are all expert-only techniques. A few came and went. A few are undergoing assessment. None have been shown to play a significant part in persistent leg and low back pain (Heyse-Moore, 1978; Berman et al., 1984; Bowman et al., 1993)

3.4. Upper Extremity Pain

Because it can be caused by a wide range of conditions, including degeneration of the cervical spine processes, degeneration of the affected joint, trauma to the cervical spine or affected joint, vascular compromise, nerve impingement, thoracic or abdominal pathology, or any combination of these, upper extremity pain can be mysterious to doctors. Additionally, pain originating from a joint region may involve the capsule, tendons, ligaments, or muscles. The clinical management of upper extremity pain therefore starts with determining, through history and examination, whether the pain is intrinsic to the shoulder area, extrinsic, or of combined etiologies (DePalma, 1973; Bateman, 1978; Calliet, 1981). This is because the etiology of pain is not always evident.

3.4.1. Intrinsic Shoulder Pain

Acute trauma, mild chronic trauma (overuse or strain), arthritides (rheumatoid arthritis is less common than osteoarthritis), local infections or tumors, infectious arthritis, and capsulitis in conjunction with any condition that causes splinting are the most common causes of intrinsic pain. The particular structure is extremely sensitive to touch if the supraspinatus tendon, acromioclavicular joint, sternoclavicular joint, or anterior subacromial area is suspected of being the source of pain (Steindler, 1959; DePalma, 1973). To determine the source of pain referral, more effort and pressure must be applied when examining trigger points (Travell & Simons, 1983).

3.4.2. Extrinsic Shoulder Pain

Shoulder pain is often caused by cervical radiculopathy affecting the C5-T1 roots, a common neurological issue. In some cases, cervical lesions can lead to irritation of multiple nerve roots without radiculitis. Other possible sources of shoulder pain include pathology in the cervical roots, brachial plexus, as well as the axillary, suprascapular, or other peripheral nerves.

Myofascial trigger points in the shoulder and neck muscles, severe temporomandibular joint disease, cervicodorsal ligamental sprains, thoracic outlet syndromes, brachial plexus injuries, and referred pain from visceral disorders like hepatitis, gallstones, cholecystitis, myocardial infarction, pneumonitis, or lung or spinal cord tumors are additional causes of extrinsic pain (Bonica, 1990). The anterior-superior region of the shoulder is frequently the site of pain when it is referred to the shoulder.

Three clues suggest exclusively extrinsic causes:

1. virtual absence of objective findings in the shoulder joint;
2. normal active and passive range of movement (ROM) without pain; and
3. absence of point tenderness with direct pressure on the bicipital tendon, supraspinatus tendon, and the clavicular joints.

Table 3.1. An Example of Shoulder Pain Analysis-Spearman Correlation Coefficients Between the Extent of Pain (Total Area of Pain Extracted from Frontal and Dorsal Body Views) Computed Using Pain Drawings and Measures of Central Sensitization and Clinical Symptoms in Patients with Frozen Shoulder (N = 48)

Measures	**Correlation with Pain Extent (r_s)**
Pain duration (y)	0.195
Direct measures of CS	**Mean (SD) (*N* = 48)**
PPT affected shoulder	−0.118
Temporal summation (TS)	−0.149
Conditioned pain modulation (CPM)	−0.138
Indirect measures of CS	

Central Sensitization Inventory (CSI)	0.358 *
Clinical symptoms	
Current pain (VAS, 0–100)	0.421 *
Pain last 24 h (VAS, 0–100)	0.057
Shoulder Pain and Disability Index (SPADI)	0.182
Pain Catastrophizing Scale (PCS)	0.307 *
Pain Vigilance and Awareness Questionnaire (PVAQ)	−0.252

FS, frozen shoulder; CS, central sensitization; PPT, pressure pain thresholds; VAS, Visual Analog Scale; * correlation is significant at the 0.05 level.

Source. *Balasch-Bernat M, Dueñas L, Aguilar-Rodríguez M, Falla D, Schneebeli A, Navarro-Bosch M, Lluch E, Barbero M. The Spatial Extent of Pain Is Associated with Pain Intensity, Catastrophizing and Some Measures of Central Sensitization in People with Frozen Shoulder. Journal of Clinical Medicine. 2022; 11(1):154. https://doi.org/10.3390/jcm11010154et al.*

When the extremities are affected, a primary or secondary extrinsic cause is suggested because pain referred from the shoulder is rarely felt beyond the insertion of the deltoid. As people age, the pain from a combined intrinsic and extrinsic etiology increases; i.e., shoulder pain in elderly patients is more likely to be exacerbated by spondylosis or multiple nerve root involvement and joint degeneration, especially in the rotator cuff muscles. Myofascial disorders frequently coexist as a secondary disorder with degenerative conditions and acute or non-acute trauma. Finally, the etiology and intensity can be influenced by a variety of factors. These include latent trigger points from prior injuries, physical or psychological stressors, and the patient's physical and mental "interpretation" of the pain and its significance.

3.4.3. Important Elements of the History

Finding out whether upper extremity pain truly stems from the neck, shoulder, forearm, or wrist structures is the primary goal of taking a history. It's critical to observe the patient as a whole. What is the patient's age and overall health status? Does the patient seem ill? Is he or she feverish or reporting recent illness? Does the patient seem tense or report unusual stresses?

Asking the patient what they believe to be the issue is usually helpful in obtaining pertinent information. If leading the patient is required, the examiner should inquire about recent events, any past auto accidents, and any changes to the patient's employment or leisure schedule.

The person taking the patient's history should always ask him or her detailed questions concerning the onset and nature of pain, as well as the chronological progression of the symptoms. What does it feel like? Terms like "pins and needles," "burning sensations," and "shooting pains" are easily understood. Where is it felt? Does it feel deep, like bone pain? When turning their head or neck, does the patient feel a "grating feeling"? Does the patient feel electric-like pain when flexion or extension of the neck? Has the patient had any problems with arthritis, gout, or rheumatism? Does the patient have other aches and pains? Does the patient have trouble swallowing? Does the patient have strange sensations in their hands or fingers? Has the patient had this problem in the past? If yes, what was the diagnosis and course of treatment? It makes sense to inquire about the pain's consequences as well. Does the patient's pain prevent him or her from doing anything that they normally do? Does driving exacerbate the condition? Does the pain cause weakness or limitation of movement? Is the pain worse at night? Does it prevent the 78 patients from sleeping or force them to adopt different sleeping positions?

In addition, recent medical care and drug or medication use should be included in the history. Heavy alcohol consumption may be a significant clue and exposure to industrial chemicals may contribute to upper extremity pain. Has the patient recently been treated by another physician? Were any X-rays taken? Has the patient been hospitalized, particularly because of injury to the back or upper extremity? Is the patient taking any drugs, or antibiotics?

3.4.4. Examination

3.4.4.1. Head, Neck, and Cervical Spine

At the very least, a standard assessment of the head, neck, and cervical spine is usually the first step in a comprehensive screening process to identify the likely cause of upper extremity pain. In the initial assessment, the few procedures listed below are sufficient to rule out these structures as the likely source of pain.

1. Visual inspection, looking for deformities, atrophy, loss of normal contour
2. Palpation of spinous and transverse processes, thyroid gland, and carotid pulse
3. Range of movement of head and neck, with rotation right to left, flexion/extension, and lateral bending
4. Distraction or evaluation of the effect of cervical traction by placing hands on occiput and under the chin
5. Compression: if neural foramina are compromised, this may produce or intensify pain
6. Valsalva maneuver to determine whether straining with breath holding reproduces pain
7. Lhermitte's sign: flexion or extension of the head and neck causes lancinating or 'electric' shock radiating from the neck into hands (Brody and Wilkins, 1969)
8. Adson's test: in the modified Adson's test, the patient's arm is abducted to 90° and externally rotated with the elbow flexed. The patient turns the head towards the abducted arm, takes a deep breath, and coughs. The test is positive if the radial pulse is reduced or absent. This may indicate compression of the subclavian artery (Adson, 1951).

Radiation symptoms, such as loss of reflexes, weakness, and sensory abnormalities, are used to diagnose radiculitis. Cervical tests that stretch the nerve roots, elevate intraspinal pressure (Valsalva maneuver), or reduce spinal foramina (head compression) are implied in the diagnosis if they exacerbate the symptoms.

Particularly in patients over 55, cervical spondylosis can cause multiple levels of nerve root irritation and complicate diagnosis because it causes gradually increasing clinical signs. Cervical herniation-related single nerve root involvement is more common in younger age groups.

In addition to evaluating the extremity itself, additional testing of the cervical spine is necessary if any of these extremity structures exhibit weakness.

3.4.4.2. Local Structures

The body's most complicated motions are found at the shoulder joint (Saha, 1961; Post, 1987).

These are made possible by the fact that the scapulothoracic articulation and the three joints that make up the shoulder girdle—the sternoclavicular, acromioclavicular, and glenohumeral—work in unison to provide extension, flexion, abduction, adduction, and internal and external rotation.

Table 3.2. A Study Analyzed the Relationship Between Neuromuscular Tissue Mechanosensitivity and Neck Pain in Guitarists. Between-Group Differences in Pressure Pain Threshold Measurements (kg/cm2)

Location of Measurement *	**Healthy (*n* = 70)**	**Neck Pain (*n* = 70)**	**Between-Group Differences, Mean (95% CI)**	**Effect Size (95% CI)**
Upper trapezius, dominant side	4.65 (1.82)	3.19 (1.28)	−1.46 ‡ (−1.99, −0.93)	0.93 (0.57, 1.28)
Upper trapezius, non-dominant side	4.35 (1.71)	3.12 (1.06)	−1.23 ‡ (−1.71, −0.76)	0.87 (0.52, 1.22)
Median nerve, dominant side	4.00 (1.52)	2.79 (1.44)	−1.21 ‡ (−1.70, −0.71)	0.82 (0.47, 1.16)
Median nerve, non-dominant side	4.08 (1.73)	2.83 (1.52)	−1.25 ‡ (−1.79, −0.70)	0.77 (0.42, 1.11)

* Data are presented as mean (standard deviation) unless otherwise specified. ‡ Statistically significant ($p < 0.01$). Abbreviations: CI, confidence interval.

Source. Rojas VEA, Pluma AF, Pecos-Martín D, Achalandabaso-Ochoa A, Fernández-Matías R, Martinez-Merinero P, Nuñez-Nagy S, Gallego-Izquierdo T. Relationship between neuromuscular mechanosensitivity and chronic neck pain in guitarists: A cross-sectional study. *International Journal of Environmental Research and Public Health*. 2021; 18(5):2673. https://doi.org/10.3390/ijerph18052673.

The range of motion of any of the three joints may be restricted due to skeletal or soft tissue pathology, pain, or neurological deficits. To compare and characterize the pain pattern, tests for both extremities' active and passive range of motion should be performed. It is important to test ROM against resistance as well. A comprehensive muscle test and grading ought to be conducted if any weakness is identified.

Supraspinatus tendinitis is suggested by pain during abduction between 60° and 120°; rotator cuff involvement due to impingement is suggested by pain during forward flexion up to 90° with internal rotation; and acromioclavicular joint pain is suggested by pain during abduction between 140° and 180°. During range of motion testing, patients can use scapulothoracic motion to compensate for restrictions in their glenohumeral range, which is limited in the first 30° to 40°.

Joint noises, crepitation, or loss of normal gliding motion indicate that intrinsic injury and degenerative changes need to be ruled out. Friction rub, which results from exostoses on the scapula or ribs, is a common condition that causes pain even though the range of motion may be normal. Specialized thoracic and scapular X-ray views are necessary when this is suspected. To identify local pathology, a point tenderness examination of the anterior subacromial region (for impingement syndrome), the supraspinatus tendon, the bicipital tendon, and the two clavicular joints will typically be sufficient Palpation needs to be done carefully because applying too much pressure can hurt and irritate delicate tissues. Yergason's test involves rotating the arm externally to palpate the bicipital groove. The more lateral greater tuberosity and the medial lesser tuberosity are where the groove is located. The insertion of the subscapularis is not palpable, but the passive extension of the shoulder facilitates examination of the bursa and the cuff as it moves these structures forward. Take note of any swelling and unusual warmth. A thorough examination might identify thickening or unusual masses. In a healthy synovial joint, fluid cannot be felt, and its existence indicates joint pathology. A ligament has either been injured or there is pathology at the joint if it is palpably tender or painful. Muscle palpation can be used to locate sensitive trigger points, which could be the main or secondary source of pain.

3.4.5. Supporting Diagnostic Procedures

During the first visit, thorough history taking, palpation, and range of motion examination can frequently identify the precise cause of upper extremity pain. However, two or three evaluation visits may be required for more complex issues or combined etiologies, and the use of supporting diagnostic procedures like electromyograms (EMG) with peripheral nerve conduction studies or special roentgenographs may be beneficial.

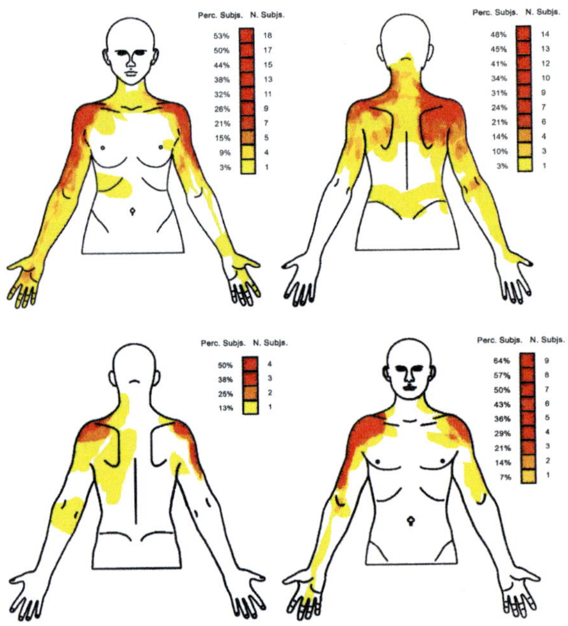

Figure 3.1. Pain frequency and pain location maps in men and women with frozen shoulder. The color grid indicates both the number and the percentage of participants reporting pain in that specific area. Dark red represents the most frequently reported painful area.

Source. Balasch-Bernat M, Dueñas L, Aguilar-Rodríguez M, Falla D, Schneebeli A, Navarro-Bosch M, Lluch E, Barbero M. The Spatial Extent of Pain Is Associated with Pain Intensity, Catastrophizing and Some Measures of Central Sensitization in People with Frozen Shoulder. *Journal of Clinical Medicine*. 2022; 11(1):154. https://doi.org/10.3390/jcm11010154.

3.4.5.1. Diagnostic Radiographic Studies

Joints are the subject of radiographic studies, as the initial work-up indicated. These studies should include oblique views to visualize the neuroforamina as well as anterior/posterior, lateral, and extended views of the neck in neutral, flexed, and extended positions in any situation where the diagnosis is challenging. Abduction, axillary, and bicipital groove views, as well as anterior and posterior views, are all part of standard shoulder films. Keep in mind that pathology is not ruled out by negative results. Even encouraging results may not always account for the origin of pain or other symptoms.

To rule out rotator cuff tears, high-resolution ultrasonography is a particularly useful non-invasive procedure. The most straightforward methods for verifying a tear or raising any doubts are magnetic resonance imaging (MRI) and arthrography.

When it comes to assessing and diagnosing soft tissue injuries, MRI has enormous potential. When diagnosing injuries to tendons, ligaments, and fibrocartilage, as well as tears in the rotator cuff or glenoid labrum, magnetic resonance imaging (MRI) is especially useful.

3.4.5.2. EMG and Peripheral Nerve Conduction Studies

EMG is especially useful in ruling out cervical lesions, discogenic disease, and nerve root entrapment as potential causes of upper extremity pain and dysfunction. It is also useful in identifying peripheral neuropathies. It is the sole trustworthy instrument for diagnosing neurocervical radiculitis in the periphery.

3.5. Rotator Cuff Injuries

3.5.1. Tendinitis

Generally speaking, tendinitis is a non-traumatic lesion that develops as the rotator cuff gradually deteriorates. The tendon may or may not have calcium deposits in conjunction with these alterations. For months, a slight ache or discomfort might persist. When calcific tendinitis occurs, a mild ache that typically affects the top or lateral aspect of the shoulder can suddenly become unbearable and persistent. Typically, the patient will keep the arm pressed immobile against their body. Breathing deeply could make the pain worse. Because calcium can build up in the tendon after an injury and enter the bursal sac, this acute episode may be linked to acute bursitis. The condition is more common after the age of 50 because it is associated with degenerative changes (Calliet, 1981).

3.5.1.1. Signs and Symptoms

With a physical examination that includes a resisted range of motion, a working diagnosis of shoulder tendinitis can typically be made. When the supraspinatus tendon is involved, pain is frequently felt at the humerus's greater tuberosity. Even though the patient might not be able or desire to move their arm, passive range of motion can be fully achieved. Supraspinatus tendinitis is indicated by pain during resisted abduction. Pain at the greater tuberosity is also linked to the involvement of the infraspinatus, but the pain is made worse by resistance to external rotation. Resisted external rotation exacerbates the pain at the greater tuberosity caused by tendinitis of the teres minor. Localized pain at the lesser tuberosity could be a sign of subscapularis tendinitis. If the pain is linked to resisted medial rotation, this is verified further. Most often, bicipital tendinitis affects the long head of the biceps muscle. Localized pain is felt at the attachment site at the superior rim of the glenoid fossa as well as in the bicipital groove.

3.5.1.2. Treatment Course and Prognosis

When calcific tendinitis is in its acute phase, treatment options include local anesthetic injections, steroid injections, oral anti-inflammatory and non-steroidal anti-inflammatory product medication, cold packs, and immobilization of the arm in a sling. Some patients might need to take a narcotic for a few days. Some medical professionals would rather aspirate the joint if this course of treatment fails. Treatment for milder cases is typically conservative. The primary focus of treatment is to mobilize the shoulder as soon as possible, beginning with passive pendular exercises. Active pendular exercises are then performed as soon as tolerated after that.

3.5.2. Bursitis

Regretfully, the word "bursitis" is frequently applied incorrectly to any shoulder pain. In particular, bursitis is an acute inflammatory reaction that is typically linked to the accumulation of calcific material. The bursa enlarges and presses against neighboring structures, causing unbearable pain. Primary bursitis is not common, but it can happen. Bursa inflammation is more likely to result from direct trauma or from a rip or inflammation of a nearby tendon or muscle. Though it can occasionally affect younger patients, it is primarily a disease of middle age, linked to degenerative changes in the rotator cuff, muscle, or tendon.

- **Signs and Symptoms:** Painful passive arc is a characteristic of subdeltoid bursitis. Pain limits passive abduction between about 70° and 110°–115°, after which the pain subsides. Usually, the pain is intense and restricted. Any motion can hurt, but abduction and external rotation significantly intensify the pain. It appears that pain gets worse at night. Roentgenograms can verify if calcific deposits are present. It is noteworthy, though, that only 35% of patients with calcium evidence on X-rays experience symptoms. More than 1.5 cm of calcium deposits are typically accompanied by symptoms.
- **Treatment Course and Prognosis:** The management of bursitis and calcific tendinitis is largely similar. Adhesive capsulitis is a regrettable side effect of bursitis, especially if appropriate care is not received to maintain range of motion.

3.5.3. Bicipital Tendinitis

The long head of the big tendon is attached to the superior rim of the glenoid cavity after passing through the bicipital groove and across the shoulder joint. Chronic irritation over the anterior aspect of the shoulder may arise from degenerative changes. This is frequently connected to motion repetition. Since the location of pain is similar, this condition is often misdiagnosed as bursitis.

- **Signs and Symptoms:** In cases where there is pain and tenderness when applying pressure over the bicipital groove, bicipital tendinitis should be suspected. Both a palpably swollen tendon and Yergason's sign, which is increased pain upon resistance to supination, are positive indicators. Bicipital tendinitis is a pain that can happen after heavy lifting and is linked to unusually high levels of athletic activity in young adults.
- **Treatment Course and Prognosis:** The majority of these patients benefit from conservative treatment, which consists of giving analgesics for pain and resting the arm in a sling. Local injections of steroids are recommended by certain clinicians; however, the author has observed multiple instances where this treatment has

led to tendon rupture. Maintaining the range of motion is essential to avoiding adhesive capsulitis and a "frozen shoulder" during treatment. Until pain is sufficiently managed, this is typically done passively. Only then can active exercises be introduced.

3.5.4. Rotator Cuff Tears

The tendons of the subscapularis, supraspinatus, infraspinatus, and teres minor muscles fuse together around the anatomic neck of the humerus where it inserts into the joint capsule to form the rotator cuff, a band of tendinous-fibrous tissue. A marginal blood supply in this area of the cuff is indicative of early degeneration, which is linked to small tears from everyday activities.

When considering injuries from working with arms overhead, falls involving the shoulder being struck or the force of the fall being broken with an outstretched hand, fractures or dislocations of the shoulder, and greater tuberosity of the humerus, one should take into account the possibility of rotator cuff tears. Loss of range of motion and persistent pain following an earlier injury should also be indicators of a rotator cuff tear. Cervical degenerative disease is a risk factor. It might not be necessary to treat small tears. According to reports, rotator cuff tears are present in 30% of cadavers.

3.5.4.1. Signs and Symptoms

Anterolateral margin of the acromion pain is linked to rotator cuff tears. Except for patients who use the joint frequently, they are uncommon in patients under 40. The patient, who is typically a laborer in his or her 40s or 65s, describes feeling a tear or snap in the shoulder, followed by excruciating pain if the tear is large. Less severe tears may cause the pain to worsen over time, peaking 48 hours later and lasting several days in an acute stage. Pain is usually felt in the shoulder joint, but it can also radiate to the forearm, deltoid, and posterior scapular region when one moves their shoulder. The pain is often described as a throbbing, deep sensation that can make it difficult to fall asleep.

Exceptional tenderness when pressure is applied over the greater tuberosity, decreased abduction or pain when abduction is resisted, and weakness when forward flexion or pain during internal rotation are examples of physical findings. There could be a scapulohumeral dysrhythmia. The arm may drop freely from the patient's grasp if he is unable to control its lowering to his side. This is a helpful guide for rotator cuff tears, however, keep in mind that the same clinical sign can also be caused by lesions of the fifth cervical root, injuries to the supra 82 scapular and axillary nerves, etc. Atrophy of the rotator cuff indicates a supraspinatus or infraspinatus muscle injury that occurred several weeks ago.

A subacromial bursa, which is located directly beneath the acromial arch, is injected laterally with 5 milliliters of local anesthetic to rule out the diagnosis of rotator cuff impingement. Rotator cuff impingement syndrome is confirmed by pain relief and increased shoulder joint strength after injection.

3.5.4.2. Treatment Course and Prognosis

An MRI, ultrasonography, or contrast radiography must be used to confirm suspected lesions. Small tears heal in two months on average when non-surgical treatment is used. Tears are a chronic issue because they are frequently linked to a degenerative process of some kind. An orthopedic surgeon should assess severe tears in order to determine whether they can be repaired (Neviaser, 1975; Post, 1987) (Table 3.3.

3.5.5. Adhesive Capsulitis

The glenohumeral joint is affected by adhesive capsulitis. An inflammatory response results in saturation with a serofibrinous exudate, which leads to the formation of adhesions. It is a frequent finding secondary to heart attacks, general surgery, infections, neoplasms, fractures near the shoulder, immobilization, heavy use, and tendonitis. There are also reports of bicipital tenosynovitis as a common cause. Putting a shoulder through its full range of motion a few times a day, according to McLaughlin (1961), will not result in adhesive capsulitis, suggesting that prolonged dependency is the causative factor. For patients under 40, the condition is uncommon.

3.5.5.1. Signs and Symptoms

Even in the absence of any apparent injuries, the patient may experience gradual onset pain. It frequently occurs in sedentary people who have just started engaging in upper extremity-heavy sports like tennis, bowling, or golf (Neer & Welsh, 1977). The patient will find it challenging to comb their hair, put on a shirt, or put their hand in their back pocket. Even though there might not be much pain when palpated, both internal and external rotation will make it worse. A pain that often occurs at night and appears to be localized in the deltoid, especially at its insertion, is experienced.

To distinguish the inflammatory condition from a simple case of stiff shoulder, arthrography is required to confirm the tentative diagnosis of adhesive capsulitis.

Table 3.3. Current and Proposed Pathways Leading to the Frozen Shoulder Syndrome

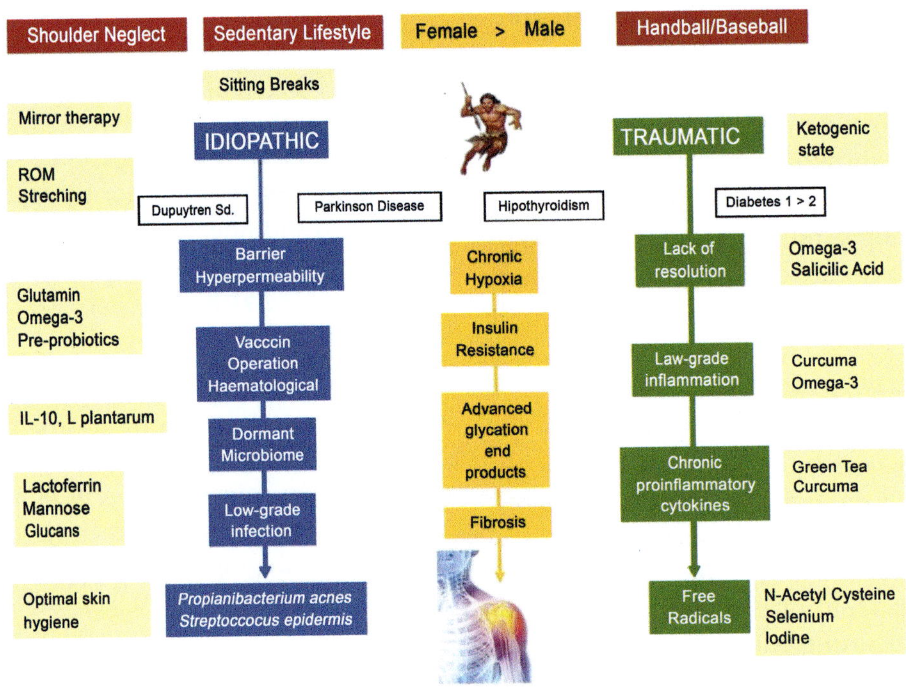

Source: de la Serna D, Navarro-Ledesma S, Alayón F, López E, Pruimboom L (2021). A Comprehensive View of Frozen Shoulder: A Mystery Syndrome. Front. Med. 8:663703. doi: 10.3389/fmed.2021.663703.

Neviaser (1975) categorized patients based on their range of passive abduction and the amount of dye that was injected into the capsule. A mild form is indicated by abduction greater than 90° and dye acceptance of greater than 10 ml. Patients with moderate involvement are those who have a capsular joint space measurement of 5 to 10 ml and are unable to abduct more than 90°. Severe capsulitis is classified into a third category and is typically observed in patients with osteoporosis only after a proximal humerus fracture or after a severe dislocation of the shoulder.

3.5.5.2. Treatment Course and Prognosis

The best way to treat adhesive capsulitis is to prevent it with daily, consistent range-of-motion exercises. Thankfully, a conservative treatment plan that mostly consists of steroid therapy and pain management combined with an intensive physical therapy regimen administered by a licensed physical therapist effectively resolves a lot of cases. When combined with intense physical therapy, the prudent injection of steroids into the intra-articular space and rotator cuff may be beneficial (Sheon et al., 1987).

While local anesthetics might be sufficient to support therapy, it might also be necessary to block a local nerve, specifically the suprascapular nerve. Sometimes, muscle relaxants are beneficial. To lessen the likelihood of a pain cycle, lidocaine or procaine can be injected into trigger points. The use of manipulation is common. Anesthesia may be necessary for manipulation when there is a higher degree of involvement. For two weeks, the arm may be placed in a 90° abduction while on bed rest. A three- to six-month therapy program is then typically necessary to achieve full recovery. It is not advised to use drugs for an extended length of time. These patients frequently experience depression, which needs to be identified and treated as needed.

3.6. Bicipital Lesions

3.6.1. Bicipital Subluxation

The same kind of degenerative process that causes tendinitis can also put elderly patients at risk for tendon subluxation. In younger people, sports-related activities may be linked to this condition.

- **Signs and Symptoms:** Local tenderness is typically felt in the area where the transverse ligament is ripped. When the arm is passively rotated in the abducted position, the clinician might be able to feel the muscle "snap" in and out of the groove.
- **Treatment Course and Prognosis:** Surgery is recommended when a young, active person develops a subluxation. Chronic tenosynovitis can result from bicipital subluxation. Limiting an older person's activities may be the best course of action unless they are in excruciating pain.

3.6.2. Bicipital Rupture

Another ailment commonly associated with degenerative changes in the biceps tendon or muscle is bicipital rupture. The biceps may have totally separated from the supraglenoid fossa or between the muscle belly and the tendon in this painless condition.

- **Signs and Symptoms:** Complete separation can usually be visualized. The flaccid biceps muscle bulges.
- **Treatment Course and Prognosis:** Surgical repair is recommended for younger patients, while older patients may not need treatment if a decrease in upper extremity strength does not

affect their daily activities. However, treatment for cosmetic reasons may still be considered.

3.7. Acromioclavicular Joint Lesions

One of the most common reasons for shoulder and arm pain is lesions of the acromioclavicular joint. Injuries such as sprains, contusions, and separations, as well as tumors—though they are uncommon—can affect the joint in addition to arthritis (DePalma, 1957).

- **Signs and Symptoms:** Acromioclavicular joint pain is typically localized and self-limiting. Shoulder shrugging and complete passive adduction of the arm across the chest exacerbate it. If an arthritic process is the etiology, X-rays are not very helpful for diagnosis, but they can rule out joint separation. A separation typically results in pain radiating throughout the shoulder, which is frequently accompanied by loss of function and weakness in all shoulder motions. Subluxation, in which the clavicle typically shifts upward, may be palpable at the clavicular attachment. Degenerative arthritis is characterized by warmth, swelling, and/or tenderness over the joint (84).
- **Treatment Course and Prognosis*:*** When a joint injury is not too severe, a shoulder elbow strap can be used to immobilize the affected area for one to two weeks. The strap may be worn for up to 4–6 weeks if the injury is more serious (subluxation). If immobilization is unsuccessful, surgery might be required. The range of motion in the shoulder joint must be passively extended as long as pain is tolerated. Furthermore, the necessary precautions need to be taken to avoid injuries to the elbow, wrist, and hand.

3.7.1. Arthritis

Because the shoulder joint is not weight-bearing and is only occasionally used for power-bearing, its susceptibility to arthritis is relatively low. It is largely protected from the damaging degenerative changes brought on by constant stress and trauma.

Athletes are a notable exception to this rule, especially those who put stress on their joints during "bursts." People who play baseball and overhead racquet sports, skiers, and musicians are moderately likely to develop osteoarthritis; this condition is more activity-related than disease-related. However, other patients do develop osteoarthritis and traumatic arthritis, and symptoms such as warm, swollen, and painful joints should prompt a thorough work-up for arthritic involvement.

3.7.2. Hemiplegia

People who have hemiplegia frequently complain of shoulder pain. It can be so bad that it gets in the way of the rehabilitation regimen, which is so important right after a "stroke." Early in therapy, appropriate splinting is required to prevent capsular stretching and the subsequent subluxation of the glenohumeral joint, which should help prevent the complication of pain.

Treatment for the pain is similar to that used for other painful shoulder conditions: oral medications appropriate for the patient's medical condition, suprascapular nerve block, local anesthetic injections, and steroid injections. Physical therapists or other members of a healthcare team with training in rehabilitation should be in charge of these patients.

3.8. Pain of Combined Etiologies

3.8.1. Myofascial Disorders

When treating upper extremity pain, knowledge of myofascial disorders—including their incidence, causes, symptoms, and appropriate interventions—is crucial.

Similar to the lower back, the shoulder and neck region are frequently the "storehouse" of many latent points that can become painful when they are pushed to their limits by physical (and, to some extent, emotional) stressors. The following is a description of the mechanism of pain: a physiological reaction is triggered by an initiating stimulus, such as stress, exhaustion, or trauma, and a specific trigger point (TP) starts to transmit distress signals to the central nervous system. Trigger point-related muscles tense up, and soon after, muscle fatigue sets in. When local ischemia happens, the affected cells' extracellular environment changes, causing the release of analgesics among other things. Other trigger points "flare up," adding to the cycle of increased motor and sympathetic activity that is fueled by these (Zimmerman, 1979). These exchanges have the potential to greatly exaggerate an unpleasant experience relative to the underlying difficulty. Furthermore, even though the stimulus that started the cycle can be controlled, a painful event may continue to occur once it has been established. Therefore, pain relief from a local injury may not result from appropriate and sufficient treatment. Almost everyone is impacted by trigger-point syndromes, which can manifest in two ways: either as a primary function that converts stress reactions into pain, or as a secondary function that intensifies or prolongs pain from another stimulus. Sharp or dull pain can range from mild discomfort to excruciating, constant pain, which is known as trigger-point pain. Additionally, it can mimic the pain associated with visceral disorders that radiate to the shoulder region.

It is noteworthy that while trigger-point pain can occur on either side of the body, it typically affects only one side and is frequently accompanied by ipsilateral hypersensitivity in muscles that appear to be unrelated to the reported issue. For instance, even though the patient may not express overt pain in these muscles, gluteal TPs, which are incredibly sensitive to pressure, are frequently linked to pain in the neck and shoulder. In these situations, both the TPs in the painful area and the remote ipsilateral TPs must be treated.

3.8.1.1. Treatment Course and Prognosis

To interrupt the pain cycle, a local anesthetic or physiological saline injection into the TPs is frequently sufficient (Bray & Sigmond, 1941; Frost et al., 1980; Tfelt-Hansen et al., 1980).

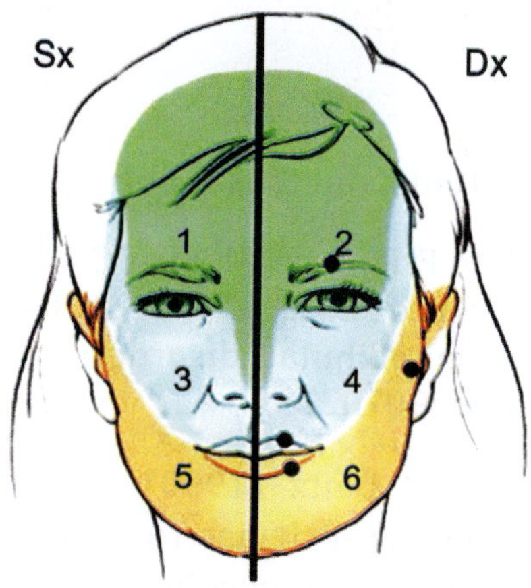

Figure 3.2. Template showing the six areas based on the trigeminus branches innervation.

Source. Caroccia F, Raimondi L, Moscagiuri F, D'Attilio M. Stimulation of myofascial trigger points in the sternocleidomastoid evokes facial thermal response correlated with the referred pain. *Applied Sciences*. 2021; 11(14):6510. https://doi.org/10.3390/app11146510.

Note: Area 1: left frontal region comprising the left nose pyramid up to the tip of it;

Area 2: right frontal region comprising the right nose pyramid up to the tip of it;

Area 3: left temporal region comprising the left hemiface cheekbone, nostril, and upper lip;

Area 4: right temporal region comprising the right hemiface cheekbone, nostril, and upper lip;

Area 5: left mandibular ramus and mandibular angle area, left hemiface, lower lip, and chin;

Area 6: right mandibular ramus and mandibular angle area, right hemiface, lower lip, and chin.

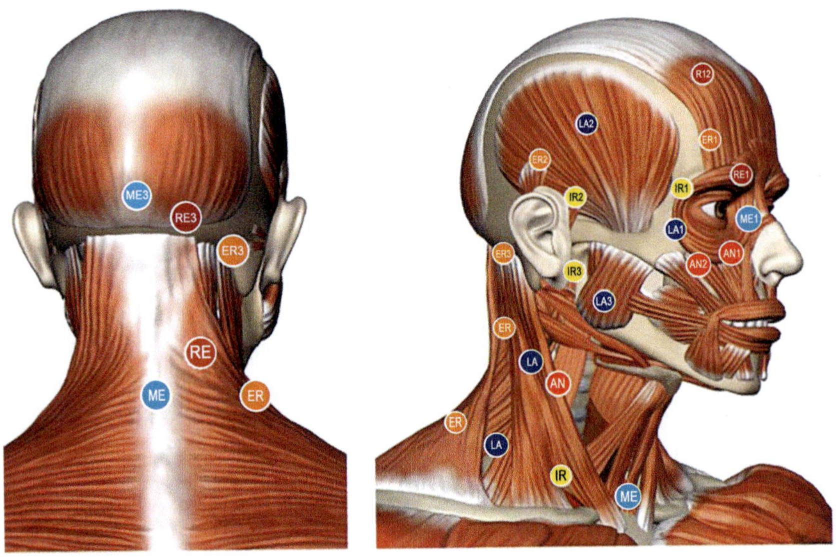

Figure 3.3. Understanding pain.

Source. Sekito F, Pintucci M, Pirri C, Ribeiro de Moraes Rego M, Cardoso M, Soares Paixão K, Ribeiro da Silva V, Stecco A. Facial pain: RCT between conventional treatment and fascial manipulation® for temporomandibular disorders. *Bioengineering*. 2022; 9(7):279. https://doi.org/10.3390/bioengineering9070279.

Travell and Daitz (1990) demonstrated the usefulness of using vasocoolants, such as fluoromethane spray. It has frequently been discovered that the insertion of thin, solid needles alone—known as "dry needling," as defined by Gunn (1989)—is just as effective as an injection, saving the patient from the additional tissue disruption that comes with using hypodermic needles with edges. Injection of a weak solution of dexamethasone (1 cc diluted in 100 cc of normal saline) is a helpful procedure when dry needling, local anesthetic, or saline injection proves inadequate (Edagawa, 1994). This therapy is based on the assumption that there are no clotting disorders or diabetes that would prevent the use of steroids. Treatment is never more than moderately effective in relieving pain when the cause is another stimulus, especially nerve root lesions or nerve compression. When the pain cycle is broken and the underlying disorder can be revealed, this procedure is helpful as a differential diagnostic tool. Additional therapies are being investigated. According to Lawrence (1978), periosteal stimulation improves the efficiency of TP injection by lowering myofascial pain.

Additionally, intriguing research is being done on the use of electromagnetic fields to reduce pain, as well as new work on the application of laser therapy.

3.8.2. Reflex Dystrophy-Like Syndromes

Among the sympathetic disorders that include reflex dystrophies are those that cause throbbing, burning, or aching pain, hyperesthesia, hyperalgesia, edema, and/or erythema. These conditions are severe, excruciating, and incapacitating. Hemiplegia, adhesive capsulitis, bicipital tendinitis, coronary ischemia, trauma, or even minor sprains or bruises can cause the onset. In a study involving 140 patients, 40% of the cases had soft tissue injury as the cause, 25% had fractures as the cause, 20% had postoperative symptoms, 12% had myocardial infarction, and 3% had a cerebrovascular accident. Furthermore, it was found that at the time of onset, 37% of these patients experienced severe emotional disturbances. Accordingly, the entire myofascial pain cycle of stressors, trigger-point activation, pain, and sympathetic involvement, as well as CNS involvement, are components of the process (Pak et al., 1970). Physical therapy and anesthetic-corticosteroid mixture injections into the impacted trigger points by a specialist are part of the immediate treatment plan. Sympathetic blocks, oral corticosteroids, and, in the worst-case scenario, sympathectomy are the only options available if this doesn't help. Breaking this cycle through early treatment of the TPs affected has shown great promise.

3.8.3. Shoulder–Hand Syndrome

- **Signs and Symptoms:** There are various stages to the illness. Onset is typically sneaky. The patient may exhibit hand and finger vasomotor abnormalities along with a burning pain in the shoulder. This stage could go on for a few months. Following this initial stage, the pain in the shoulder may subside, but trophic changes such as thickening of the palmar fascia, atrophy of the nails, demineralization, and atrophy of the muscles in the affected extremity, occur. After severe treatment, it is very difficult to stop the disease process once these trophic changes have taken place, and the final result is finger flexion deformities. Vasomotor changes are not present at this point.
- **Treatment Course and Prognosis:** Treatment for this condition must be aggressive. Generally speaking, residual damage cannot be repaired surgically; function cannot be successfully restored. Shoulder-hand syndrome patients often require narcotics for pain management due to the severe nature of their pain. Other sedatives may be used instead of phenobarbital, which is not advised. Early in the course of the disease, sympathetic blocks and corticosteroid therapy may be beneficial. It may also be beneficial to inject local anesthetics into the suprascapular nerve or other sensitive areas of the shoulder. To preserve function, an intense physical therapy program needs to be implemented in conjunction with treatment from the beginning.

3.8.4. Overuse Syndromes

A tissue may be stressed beyond its anatomical or physiological limits by excessive repetition, even though a particular action or combination of actions may be well within the body's capabilities. These factors include waste product accumulation, interference with circulation, and repeated microinjuries. The stressor can be static, as in the case of prolonged bracing or maintaining a specific posture, or dynamic, as in the case of repetitive movement. One should suspect an overuse syndrome when a patient reports that he or she:

1. performs a repetitive task
2. maintains a fixed posture for long periods of time
3. lifts above or below a mechanically strainful height
4. performs a tedious or monotonous task.

It should also raise suspicions when a large number of other employees or participants are unable to complete the same tasks. A result like this would indicate that a workplace ergonomics assessment is necessary (Sheon et al., 1987; Khalil et al., 1994). Various sports such as tennis, swimming, and baseball, as well as prolonged periods of wrist strain from cycling, are known to cause overuse injuries. Similarly, certain professions can also contribute to these types of injuries. Physical examination of patients with overuse syndrome often does not reveal inflammation, making it difficult to determine whether the affected structure is a tendon, muscle, ligament, joint capsule, or a combination of these (Sataloff et al., 1990).

3.8.5. Carpal Tunnel Syndrome

Only low back pain is more common among industrial injuries in the US than carpal tunnel syndrome. The most susceptible groups to this syndrome are those who work in jobs requiring a lot of wrist movement, such as data entry operators, grocery checkers, pipefitters, tool workers, carpenters, secretaries, and pianists. According to recent research, psychological stressors like boredom, insecurity, or the strain of other unpleasant processes may make the condition worse. Pressure on the median nerve results in carpal tunnel syndrome; this can be brought on by increased synovial hypertrophy, which can happen in gout, rheumatoid arthritis, diabetes, hypothyroidism, ganglion tumors or lipomas, pregnancy, and trauma. Research on biomechanics has demonstrated that flexor and ulnar deviation specifically increase intracarpal pressure. When diagnosing carpal tunnel syndrome, Rosenbaum and Ochoa (1993) contend that Tinel's nerve stimulation of the median nerve at the wrist is less accurate than Phalen's wrist flexion test.

- **Signs and Symptoms:** Along the median nerve into the hand and wrist, this syndrome results in paresthesias and dysesthesias. The wrist is the only possible location for the pain, but it can also retrogradely spread to the elbow or shoulder. The lymphatic or circulatory systems may be involved in a pressure gradient that is relieved by shaking or moving the hand. However, cervical radiculitis should be suspected if such shaking results in increased pain. There could be thenar atrophy.
- **Treatment Course and Prognosis:** Conservative treatment options include cortisone injections, rest, splinting, and/or activity modifications. Therapy for trigger points in the neck, forearm, shoulder, and frequently the gluteal region may help reduce pain and syndromes resembling dystrophy. To build strength and endurance in cases of complex cumulative disorders, patients should ideally start a "work-hardening" program under the guidance of certified hand, occupational, or physical therapists. Workplace ergonomic upgrades might also be necessary. Surgical release is advised when non-surgical methods prove to be successful. While 58% of surgically treated patients go back to their previous jobs, none of them return to jobs requiring vigorous repetitive motion, according to Silverstein et al. (1987).

3.8.6. Other Peripheral Entrapment Syndromes

The peripheral neuropathies are some of the most mysterious pains of the extremities. Since cervical nerve root irritation must be taken into consideration, the causes are unclear and differential diagnosis is challenging (Kopell & Thompson, 1973; Dyck et al., 1976). Evidence suggests that radiculitis makes a person more vulnerable to nerve entrapment (Bland, 1987; Upton & McComas, 1973). Some guidelines to distinguish between peripheral radiculopathy and entrapment are available in research (Dawson et al., 1983, 1990).

Table 3.4. Crude (Model 1) and Adjusted (Model 2) for Demographical and Socioeconomic Factors Association Between the Existence of Diagnosed and Surgically Treated Carpal Tunnel Syndrome (CTS), Ulnar Nerve Entrapment (UNE), or Both and Use of Psychotropic Drugs During the Follow-Up in the 5,751,152 Individuals aged 25–80 Residing in Sweden by 2010. Values are Prevalence Ratios (PR) and 95% Confidence Intervals (CI)

	Model 1	**Model 2**
	PR (95% CI)	**PR (95% CI)**
Nerve compression disorders		
• None	Ref	Ref
• CTS	1.50 (1.45–1.56)	1.06 (1.02–1.10)
• UNE	1.83 (1.64–2.05)	1.16 (1.04–1.29)
• Both	1.90 (1.45–2.49)	1.08 (0.83–1.42)
Age (years)		
• 25–34		Ref
• 35–44		1.12 (1.11–1.13)
• 45–54		1.20 (1.19–1.21)
• 55–64		1.30 (1.29–1.31)
• 65–80		1.49 (1.48–1.50)
Men		Ref
• Women		1.15 (1.15–1.16)
Income		
• Low		1.07 (1.07–1.08)
• Middle		1.07 (1.06–1.07)
• High		Ref
Native		Ref
• Immigrants		0.89 (0.89–0.90)
Occupational qualification level		
• Low		1.06 (1.05–1.07)
• Middle-low		1.04 (1.03–1.04)

	Model 1	Model 2
	PR (95% CI)	PR (95% CI)
• Middle-high		1.00 (1.00–1.01)
• High		Ref
• Missing		1.27 (1.26–1.42)
Previous psychotropic drugs use		
• Yes		15.59 (15.50–15.67)
AUC	0.501	0.885

Source: Dahlin LB, Perez R, Nyman E, Zimmerman M, Merlo J. Carpal Tunnel Syndrome and Ulnar Nerve Entrapment Are Associated with Impaired Psychological Health in Adults as Appraised by Their Increased Use of Psychotropic Medication. *Journal of Clinical Medicine*. 2022; 11(13):3871. https://doi.org/10.3390/jcm11133871.

It's important to distinguish peripheral radiculopathy from cervical spondylosis as well as other, less frequent causes of cervical root irritation, including tumors, infections, osteophytes, prolapsed discs, fractures, and epidural abscesses. It should be noted that most patients are able to discriminate between pain that originates in the neck or shoulder and travels to the hand versus pain that radiates from the hand to the shoulder. In addition to standard radiological studies, electromyography and nerve conduction studies provide the only conclusive means of diagnosing peripheral neuropathy.

Pain in the hands, forearms, and shoulders that is inconsistent in nature can result from any one of the entrapment syndromes. The muscles distal to the entrapment may or may not be involved in pain, but there is typically some local pain at the site of entrapment. A common occurrence is low-grade, sporadic pain that gets worse at night. Pain patterns resulting from compression of peripheral nerves are often distorted by myofascial disruptions and scapulocostal irritation. The most prevalent nerve compression syndrome affecting the median nerve is carpal tunnel syndrome. Pronator teres syndrome and anterior interosseous nerve syndrome are two additional conditions primarily associated with compression of the median nerve. The radial nerve is affected by the posterior interosseous syndrome and radial palsy. Guyon's canal compression and cubital tunnel syndrome are linked to ulnar nerve compression. Dorsal scapular nerve syndrome can result in pain, especially in the posterolateral aspect of the shoulder, and compression of the suprascapular nerve can cause deep, dull pain in the rhomboid area.

- **Treatment Course and Prognosis:** Both the pain and the dystrophy like syndromes can be relieved by treating trigger points in the affected and related areas, rest, splinting, cortisone injections, altering activities, and resting. The course of treatment for these syndromes is similar to that for carpal tunnel syndrome.

3.8.7. Tennis Elbow or Epicondylitis

- **Signs and Symptoms:** The patient reports having excruciating elbow pain that frequently spreads to the wrist and shoulder. Any grasping motion causes pain, and the patient could let go of objects. Most people characterize the pain as "deep." Severe pain results from applying pressure to the lateral condyles. Wrist dorsiflexion can cause pain. A history of overusing the wrist extensors and supinators in sports like tennis and golf as well as in jobs requiring similar motions like hammering is typically present with this clinical picture of pain. This lesion is much less treatable in older patients and more likely to be a chronic condition unrelated to any particular activity.

Table 3.5. The ROC Curve Shows the Capability of MRI to Diagnose Lateral Epicondylitis for Each Evaluation Method

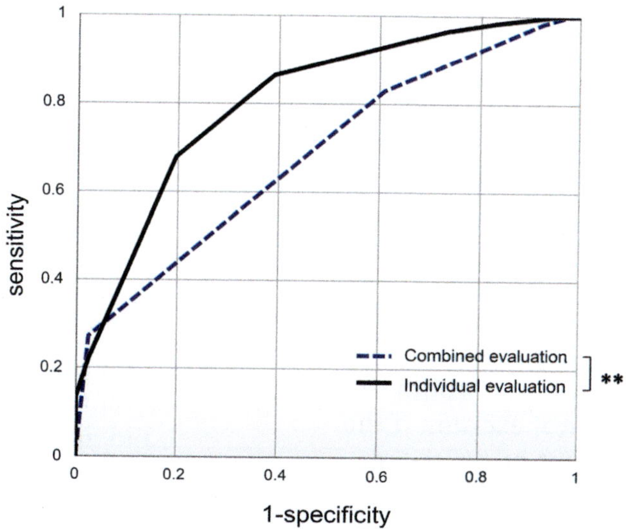

ROC curve of	Variable	AUC				Cut-off value				
		AUC	95% confidence interval	Standard error	P-value	Cut-off value	Sensitivity	specificity	PPV	NPV
Combined evaluation	MRI socre	0.69	0.60-0.78	0.046	< 0.001	3	0.83	0.40	0.66	0.62
Individual evaluation	MRI socre	0.81	0.73-0.89	0.043	< 0.001	6	0.68	0.80	0.83	0.63

Source: Ikeda K, Ogawa T, Ikumi A, Yoshii Y, Kohyama S, Ikeda R, Yamazaki M. Individual Evaluation of the Common Extensor Tendon and Lateral Collateral Ligament Improves the Severity Diagnostic Accuracy of Magnetic Resonance Imaging for Lateral Epicondylitis. *Diagnostics*. 2022; 12(8):1871. https://doi.org/10.3390/diagnostics12081871.

- **Treatment Course and Prognosis:** Treatment is contingent upon the entangled structures. Local anesthetics and steroids typically produce an effect on the common extensor and flexor tendons. A local anesthetic may be necessary when the extensor carpi radialis tendon is affected because the pain may start in the muscle instead of the epicondyle. It is unusual for the supracondylar ridge to involve muscles. Tennis elbow-like pain can be brought on by joint dysfunction at any one of the three elbow joints. They are handled through manipulation. Surgery is usually used to treat tennis elbow that is resistant to treatment. Any of the muscles surrounding the elbow joint may develop trigger points, and injection therapy is often effective in treating them. Pain in this region can often be referred to by trigger points in the scalenus anticus muscle (Zohn & Mennell, 1976).

3.8.8. Olecranon Bursa

- **Signs and Symptoms:** Injuries to the olecranon bursa, located above the bony olecranon process, are often caused by repetitive mechanical pressure. Symptoms include redness, swelling, warmth, and tenderness in the affected area. In rare cases, the bursa may become infected. Individuals with gout and rheumatoid arthritis are more susceptible to developing this condition.
- **Treatment Course and Prognosis:** Using a cushioning ring around the irritated area usually reduces pain and swelling by preventing further mechanical pressure. If the pain doesn't go away, fluid from the bursal sac can be aspirated and checked for signs of infection or to rule out other possible causes. The best course of action may be surgical excision if the condition is recurrent or persistent.

3.8.9. Ligamental Injuries

Wrist ligament injuries are frequently sustained. Localized pain and tenderness are used to make the diagnosis. The most common of these injuries is an ulnar collateral ligament sprain, which hurts when one moves their arm radially. In cases of sprains or tears in the radial ligament, ulnar deviation is painful. Another common sprain is the ulnar-capitate sprain. The dorsal aspect of the wrist hurts when the wrist is flexed.

- **Treatment Course and Prognosis:** For ligamentous injuries, local management combined with steroid injection therapy is typically successful. Surgery might be necessary to treat rips.

3.8.10. De Quervain's Disease (Constrictive Tenosynovitis)

- **Signs and Symptoms:** The patient will present with grip weakness and wrist and thumb pain. In the acute phase, wrist sprain-like symptoms could include localized swelling. Examining the area over the styloid process, tendons, abductor pollicis longus, and extensor pollicis brevis will reveal noticeable tenderness to pressure.

  The sheath around the tendons is stenotic and thickening, which is the cause of the pain. Maintaining the thumb in flexion while abducting the wrist confirms the diagnosis of De Quervain's disease. There is pain in response to this.
- **Treatment Course and Prognosis:** It is advised to immobilize the area and inject a long-acting anesthetic. Moreover, injectable steroid therapy is suitable.

3.8.11. Trigger Finger

The finger may snap in extension if a nodule formed by tiny tears in the flexor tendon prevents the tendon from gliding through the tendon sheath normally. The tendon sheath will typically hurt when palpated.

Similar to the treatment for De Quervain's disease, this involves immobilization, steroid injections, and, if required, surgery to release the patient.

3.8.12. Impingement Syndromes

Impingement syndromes are frequently seen in athletes and those who perform strenuous physical work. Positive findings on forward flexion with internal rotation and point tenderness over the anterior insertion of the supraspinatus tendon are indicative of impingement. The key test involves using a local anesthetic injected into the anterior acromial process (coracoid acromial ligament) to relieve symptoms.

Adhesive capsulitis, rotator cuff tears, and tendinitis can all be signs of a degenerative process starting at impingement. When young people have impingement syndromes, racquet sports, swimming, baseball, football, and repetitive overhead motions are nearly always linked to the condition (Moseley, 1969; Post, 1987; Nichols & Hershman, 1990).

Neer and Welsh (1977) have suggested three stages:

- Stage I is characterized by oedema and/or inflammation and usually occurs in patients between the ages of 15 and 30 years. Treatment at this stage is conservative; restriction of shoulder movement, anti-inflammatory medications, and ice packs. Occasionally steroid injections are given if these measures do not provide relief.
- Stage II is characterized by fibrosis and thickening of the rotator cuff, which further compromises subacromial mechanisms. If the patient does not respond to conservative treatment and cuff tear has been ruled out, a partial anterior acromioplasty and sectioning of the coracoid acromial ligament may be necessary.
- Stage III is usually associated with patients over the age of 40 years when further degeneration has taken place, and it may include partial tears of the rotator cuff and bony changes. Surgery may be necessary to correct the condition, particularly if tears are involved (Post, 1987). The diagnosis can be confirmed by an arthrogram.

3.8.13. Thoracic Outlet Syndrome

Most frequently, the pectoralis minor muscle, ribs, clavicle, or scalene muscles compress or irritate the inferior portion of the brachial plexus, resulting in thoracic outlet syndrome. The ulnar and occasionally the medial nerves are affected by this. Compression of the subclavian vein occurs in a small proportion of cases.

- **Signs and Symptoms:** Frequently, discomfort begins gradually and progresses to upper extremity, shoulder, arm, and lower neck pain. The pain is usually sporadic and related to movement, especially when lifting things above head height. The patient may report feeling like they have "pins and needles" in their wrists and forearms, and their fourth or fifth fingers may be weak or numb. Generally speaking, morning symptoms are worse than afternoon ones. The condition is more common in women and is observed in young adult patients with bad posture.

  Examining someone by palpation or percussion may reveal brachial plexus tenderness. The patient should be asked to sit with both arms raised to 90° abduction with external rotation as a confirmation test. The elbows are kept slightly in front of the frontal plane. The hands are slowly opened and closed as the position is maintained for three minutes. The test is positive if the patient exhibits the typical symptoms but the radial pulses are still strong.
- **Treatment course and Prognosis:** A conservative approach to treatment suggests doing mild exercise to strengthen shoulder muscles and therapy related to posture. If there is a specific activity or sleeping position that is linked to the issue, these should

be adjusted. It might be necessary to take medication to relax the muscles. All of these options, though, are limited if the disease has gotten worse to the point where decompression can only be achieved through surgery.

3.8.14. Cervical Sprain

A cervical sprain, sometimes known as a "whiplash" injury, is characterized by the neck quickly accelerating into hyperextension or flexion, followed by a rebound and reflex splint. Whiplash is most frequently linked to some trauma to the supporting muscles, tendons, and ligaments, though it can also cause damage to the spinal cord. Additionally, it could be linked to direct injury to the cervical nerve roots or functional compromise caused by the pressures of ensuing muscle spasms (Bland, 1987; Bonica, 1990; Johnson, 1996).

Cervical sprain symptoms in the short term include headaches, hoarseness or dysphagia (in anterior damage), stiffness and pain in the neck and shoulder girdle, and other symptoms similar to sympathetic dystrophy. A normal neurological examination that shows no signs of swelling or neck trauma is a good sign that there isn't any damage to the spinal cord or spinal cord. The patient needs to be closely monitored for a few days after the incident, even if the injury seems minor (Borchgrevink et al., 1998). In 4–6 weeks, ligaments and muscles heal, but intervertebral discs heal more slowly because they lack a blood supply. A transtable lateral view of the entire cervical spine must be obtained if there is any suspicion of damage to the cervical spine or cord.

After a spinal injury has been ruled out, nonsteroidal anti-inflammatory drugs, physical therapy, and the application of mild cervical traction are the first lines of treatment. For a brief period of time, a soft cervical collar might be recommended, though these haven't been proven to be very helpful. The affected muscle spasms and TPs may have an impact on nerve roots as low as T7. Lower back muscles are also frequently affected. To find painful foci and trigger points, one must carefully examine the lower torso, paying special attention to the paraspinal muscles and the gluteal muscle group. In addition to causing localized pain, trigger points in these muscles can worsen issues in the neck and shoulders, decreasing the efficacy of treatment in those areas if ignored.

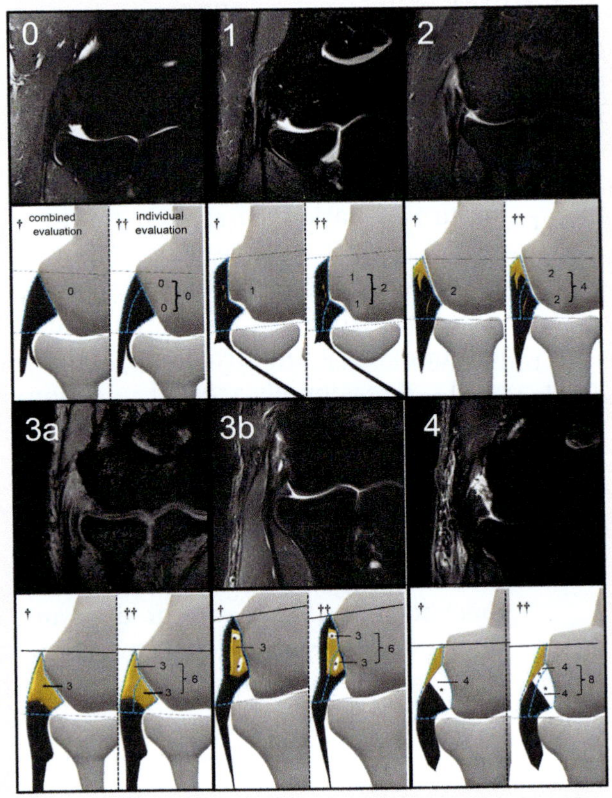

Figure 3.4. MRI examples of each score and its corresponding schema.

Source. Ikeda K, Ogawa T, Ikumi A, Yoshii Y, Kohyama S, Ikeda R, Yamazaki M. Individual evaluation of the common extensor tendon and lateral collateral ligament improves the severity diagnostic accuracy of magnetic resonance imaging for lateral epicondylitis. *Diagnostics.* 2022; 12(8):1871. https://doi.org/10.3390/diagnostics12081871.

Note: The scoring criteria are as follows: (0) (normal), dark, linear low-signal structure without changes in signal intensity; (1) (mild degeneration), thickening or mild signal change below the signal intensity of the muscle; (2) (localized degeneration), high signal change above the signal intensity of the muscle, localized below 50% of the evaluation range; (3a) (extensive degeneration), high signal change above the signal intensity of the muscle, beyond 50% of the evaluation range; (3b) (partial tear), high signal change equivalent to joint fluid, within 75% of the tendon or ligament width; (4) (extensive tear), high signal change equivalent to joint fluid, more than 75% of the tendon or ligament's width. The yellow area indicates degeneration; * tear; MRI, magnetic resonance imaging. The blue dotted line surrounds the region of interest for MRI scoring in each evaluation method. Black lines are auxiliary lines to determine the evaluation area, which runs parallel to the articular surface of the radial head. † combined evaluation; †† individual evaluation; yellow area, degeneration.

Activation of trigger points (TPs) that exist along the entire length of a muscle can cause or intensify pain felt in muscles supplied by any common nerve segment. Therefore, pain experienced along a muscle such as the semispinalis capitis can contribute to shoulder pain. Injection treatment of posterior primary rami muscles beginning at T6 is indicated if hypersensitive TPs are found in the muscles.

3.8.15. Multiple Upper Extremity Lesions

Multiple lesions may be contributing to upper extremity pain, which makes management challenging. This is especially true if the patient is elderly or middle-aged and gets hurt. When the site of injury appears to have healed satisfactorily, pain that does not go away or persists should always indicate that a cervical examination is necessary. Examining the shoulder, elbow, and wrist for joint dysfunction as well as hypersensitive TPs and tendons, bursae, rotator cuff, and joint capsule for unidentified injuries along the shock absorption pathway should be part of the further evaluation. A dystrophy-like syndrome could develop at any site of injury. Since these sequelae are typically treatable and relieve pain, it is unfortunate for the patient if the clinician ignores them.

A Closer Look

Spondylosis

Spondylosis, also known as spinal osteoarthritis, is a condition characterized by the degeneration of the spine's vertebrae and the discs between them. It is a common condition that typically develops with age, though it can also be influenced by genetic factors, lifestyle, and previous injuries. Spondylosis can occur in any part of the spine but most commonly affects the cervical (neck) and lumbar (lower back) regions.

The hallmark feature of spondylosis is the gradual deterioration of the intervertebral discs, which act as cushions between the vertebrae, and the formation of bone spurs (osteophytes) along the edges of the vertebrae. These changes can lead to various symptoms including neck or back pain, stiffness, and decreased flexibility. In some cases, spondylosis can also cause nerve compression, resulting in radiating pain, numbness, or weakness in the arms or legs.

Diagnosis of spondylosis typically involves a combination of medical history, physical examination, and imaging studies such as X-rays, MRI, or CT scans. Treatment aims to alleviate symptoms, improve mobility, and prevent further deterioration. This may include:

1. **Pain Management:** Over-the-counter or prescription medications such as nonsteroidal anti-inflammatory drugs (NSAIDs), muscle relaxants, or analgesics can help alleviate pain and inflammation.
2. **Physical Therapy:** Exercise programs, stretching, and strengthening exercises prescribed by a physical therapist can improve flexibility, strengthen supporting muscles, and reduce pain.
3. **Lifestyle Modifications:** Maintaining a healthy weight, practicing good posture, and avoiding activities that exacerbate symptoms can help manage spondylosis.
4. **Invasive Procedures:** In severe cases where conservative treatments fail to provide relief, invasive procedures such as epidural steroid injections or surgery may be considered to decompress nerves or stabilize the spine.

While spondylosis is a chronic condition that cannot be cured, proper management can significantly improve the quality of life and reduce the impact of symptoms. Regular exercise, healthy lifestyle choices, and prompt medical attention for worsening symptoms are essential for effectively managing spondylotic illness.

Summary

- The etiology of chronic back and upper extremity pain is multifactorial, often involving a combination of biomechanical, structural, neurological, and psychosocial factors.
- Back pain is usually not an early characteristic of the disease, so the diagnosis is known when back pain occurs.
- Endogeneous depression was the most common diagnosis. The psychiatrists involved with these patients separated this diagnosis from the reactive depression seen much more commonly.
- The syndrome of spinal stenosis is signified by back pain and leg pain with claudication. Patients typically present first with simple gait disturbance.
- The failed back syndrome is an imprecise term usually used to categorize a large group of patients who have undergone one or more operations on the lumbar spine without benefit.
- Intrinsic pain is most often caused by acute trauma, minor chronic trauma (overuse or strain), arthritides (osteoarthritis is fairly common, rheumatoid arthritis less so), local infection or tumor, infectious arthritis, and capsulitis in association with any condition that causes splinting.
- Cervical radiculopathy affecting the C5–T1 roots is a common neurological cause of shoulder pain; however, cervical lesions may cause multilevel nerve root irritation without radiculitis.
- Tendinitis is generally a non-traumatic lesion that occurs as the result of gradual degenerative changes in the rotator cuff.
- Bicipital tendinitis should be suspected if there is pain and tenderness to pressure over the bicipital groove.
- Adhesive capsulitis affects the glenohumeral joint. Adhesions form as a result of an inflammatory response,
- Lesions of the acromioclavicular joint are one of the most overlooked causes of shoulder and arm pain.

References

1. Ackerman, S. J., Steinberg, E. P., Bryan, R. N., BenDebba, M., & Long, D. M. (1997). Persistent low back pain in patients suspected of having herniated nucleus pulposus: Radiologic predictors of functional outcome—Implications for treatment selection. *Radiology, 203*(3), 815–822.
2. Adson, A. W. (1951). Cervical ribs: Symptoms, differential diagnosis and indications for section of the insertion of the scalenus anticus muscle. *Journal of the International College of Surgeons, 16*, 546–559.
3. Anderson, G. B. J. (1996). The epidemiology of spinal disorders. In J. W. Frymoyer (Ed.), *The Adult Spine, Principles and Practice* (2nd ed.). Lippincott.
4. Bandschuh, C. V., Stein, L., Slusser, J. H., et al. (1990). Distinguishing between scar and recurrent herniated disk in postoperative patients: Value of contrast-enhanced and MR imaging. *American Journal of Neuroradiology, 11*, 949–958.

5. Bateman, J. E. (1978). *The Shoulder and Neck* (2nd ed.). Saunders.

6. Bell, G. R., & Rothman, R. H. (1984). The conservative treatment of sciatica. *Spine, 9*, 54–56.

7. BenDebba, M., Torgerson, W. S., & Long, D. M. (1997). Personality traits, pain duration and severity, functional impairment, and psychological distress in patients with persistent low back pain. *Pain, 72*, 115–125.

8. Berman, A. T., Garbarino, J. L., Jr., Fisher, S. M., et al. (1984). The effects of epidural injection of local anesthetics and corticosteroids on patients with lumbosciatic pain. *Clinical Orthopaedics, 188*, 144–151.

9. Bigos, S. J., Bowyer, O., Braen, G., et al. (1994). Acute low back problems in adults. In *Clinical Practice Guideline No. 14 (AHCPR Publication No. 95-0642)*. US Department of Health and Human Services.

10. Bland, J. H. (1987). *Disorders of the Cervical Spine: Diagnosis and Medical Management.* Saunders.

11. Boden, S. D., Davis, D. O., Dina, T. S., et al. (1990). Abnormal magnetic resonance scans of the lumbar spine in asymptomatic subjects: A prospective investigation. *Journal of Bone and Joint Surgery, 72A*, 403–408.

12. Bogduk, N. (1991). The lumbar disc and low back pain. *Neurosurgery Clinics of North America, 2*, 791–806.

13. Bogduk, N., & Long, D. M. (1980). Percutaneous lumbar medial branch neurotomy. A modification of facet denervation. *Spine, 5*(2), 193–200.

14. Bogduk, N., Aprill, C., & Derby, R. (1995a). Discography. In A. H. White (Ed.), *Spine Care: Diagnosis and Conservative Treatment*. CV Mosby, pp. 219–238.

15. Bogduk, N., Aprill, C., & Derby, R. (1995b). Selective nerve root blocks. In D. J. Wilson (Ed.), *Interventional Radiology of The Musculoskeletal System*. Edward Arnold, pp. 121–132.

16. Bonica, J. J. (1990). *The Management of Pain* (2nd ed.). Lea & Febiger.

17. Borchgrevink, G. E., Kaasa, A., McDonagh, D., Stiles, T. C., Haraldseth, O., & Lereim, I. (1998). Acute treatment of whiplash neck sprain injuries. A randomized trial of treatment during the first 14 days after a car accident. *Spine, 23*(1), 25–31.

18. Bowman, S. J., Wedderburn, L., Whaley, A., et al. (1993). Outcome assessment after epidural corticosteroid injection for low back pain and sciatica. *Spine, 18*, 1345–1350.

19. Bray, E. A., & Sigmond, H. (1941). The local and regional injection treatment of low back pain and sciatica. *Annals of Internal Medicine, 15*, 840–852.

20. Brody, I. A., & Wilkins, R. H. (1969). Lhermitte's sign. *Archives of Neurology, 21*, 338–340.

21. Bush, K., Cowan, N., Katz, D. E., et al. (1992). The natural history of sciatica associated with disc pathology: A prospective study with clinical and independent radiologic follow-up. *Spine, 17*, 1205–1212.

22. Calliet, R. (1981). *Shoulder Pain* (2nd ed.). Davis.

23. Calvin, W. H., Devor, M., & Howe, J. F. (1982). Can neuralgias arise from minor demyelination? Spontaneous firing, mechanosensitivity and after-discharge from conducting axons. *Experimental Neurology, 75*, 755–763.

24. Cavanagh, S., Stevens, J., & Johnson, J. R. (1993). High-resolution MRI in the investigation

of recurrent pain after lumbar discectomy. *Journal of Bone and Joint Surgery, 75B*, 524–528.

25. Cholewicki, J., & McGill, S. M. (1996). Mechanical stability of the in vivo lumbar spine: Implications for injury and chronic low back pain. *Clinical Biomechanics, 11*, 1–15.
26. Choy, D. S., Case, R. B., Field, W., et al. (1987). Letter: Percutaneous laser nucleolysis of lumbar disks. *New England Journal of Medicine, 317*, 771–772.
27. Dawson, D. M., Hallet, M. L., & Millender, L. H. (1990). *Entrapment Neuropathies* (2nd ed.). Little, Brown.
28. Dawson, D. M., Hallet, M., & Millender, L. H. (1983). *Entrapment Neuropathies*. Little, Brown.
29. DePalma, A. F. (1957). *Degenerative Changes in Sternoclavicular and Acromioclavicular Joints in Various Decades*. Thomas.
30. DePalma, A. F. (1973). *Surgery of the shoulder* (2nd ed.). Lippincott.
31. Devor, M., Basbaum, A. I., Bennett, G. J., et al. (1991). Mechanisms of neuropathic pain following peripheral injury. In A. I. Basbaum & J. M. R. Besson (Eds.), *Towards a New Pharmacotherapy of Pain*. Wiley, pp. 417–440.
32. Deyo, R. A., Rainville, J., & Kent, D. L. (1992). What can the history and physical examination tell us about low back pain? *Journal of American Medical Association, 268*, 760–765.
33. Dyck, P. J., Lambert, E. H., & O'Brien, P. C. (1976). Pain in peripheral neuropathy related to rate and kind of nerve fiber degeneration. *Neurology, 26*, 466–477.
34. Edagawa, N. (1994). *Body Wall Medicine*. W4 Group.
35. Fager, C. A., & Freidberg, S. R. (1980). Analysis of failures and poor results of lumbar spine surgery. *Spine, 5*, 87–94.
36. Finnegan, W. J., Fenlin, J. M., Marvel, J. P., et al. (1979). Results of surgical intervention in the symptomatic multiply-operated back patient: Analysis of sixty-seven cases followed for three to seven years. *Journal of Bone and Joint Surgery, 61A*, 1077–1082.
37. Frost, F. A., Jeason, B., & Siggaard-Andersen, J. A. (1980). A controlled, double-blind comparison of mepivacaine injection versus saline injection for myofascial pain. *Lancet, 1*, 499–501.
38. Frymoyer, J. W., & Cats-Baril, W. L. (1991). An overview of the incidences and costs of low back pain. *Orthopaedic Clinics of North America, 22*, 263–271.
39. Frymoyer, J. W., Matteri, R. E., Hanley, E. N., et al. (1978). Failed lumbar disc surgery requiring second operation: A long-term follow-up study. *Spine, 3*, 7–11.
40. Gerhart, T. N., Dohlman, L. E., & Warfield, C. A. (1985). Clinical diagnosis of shoulder pain. *Hospital Practice, 20*(9), 134–141.
41. Gracely, R. H., Lynch, S. A., & Bennett, G. J. (1992). Painful neuropathy: Altered central processing maintained dynamically by peripheral input. *Pain, 51*, 175–194.
42. Gunn, C. C. (1989). Treating myofascial pain: Intramuscular stimulation (IMS) for myofascial pain syndromes of neuropathic origin. Health Sciences Center for Educational Resources, University of Washington, Seattle.
43. Hanley, E. N. Jr., Phillips, E. D., & Kostuik, J. P. (1991). Who should be fused? In J. W. Frymoyer, T. B. Ducker, N. M. Hadler, et al. (Eds.), *The Adult Spine: Principles and Practice, vol 2*. Raven Press, pp. 1893–1917.

44. Heliovaara, M. (1987). Body height, obesity, and risk of herniated lumbar intervertebral disc. *Spine, 12*, 469–472.
45. Heyse-Moore, G. H. (1978). A rational approach to the use of epidural medication in the treatment of sciatic pain. *Acta Orthopaedica Scandinavica, 49*, 366–370.
46. Hsieh, C. Y., Phillips, R. B., Adams, A. H., et al. (1992). Functional outcomes of low back pain: Comparison of four treatment groups in a randomized controlled trial. *Journal of Manipulative Physiological Therapeutics, 15*, 4–9.
47. Hurme, M., & Alaranta, H. (1987). Factors predicting the result of surgery for lumbar intervertebral disc herniation. *Spine, 12*, 933–938.
48. Johnson, G. (1996). Hyperextension soft tissue injuries of the cervical spine—A review. *Journal of Accident and Emergency Medicine, 13*(1), 3–8.
49. Jonsson, B., & Stromqvist, B. (1993). Symptoms and signs in degeneration of the lumbar spine: A prospective, consecutive study of 300 operated patients. *Journal of Bone and Joint Surgery, 75B*, 381–385.
50. Kambin, P. (1988). Percutaneous lumbar discectomy: Current practice. *Surgical Rounds of Orthopaedics, 2*, 31–35.
51. Kelsey, J. L. (1975). An epidemiological study of acute herniated lumbar intervertebral discs. *Rheumatological Rehabilitation, 14*, 144–159.
52. Kelsey, J. L. (1982). Idiopathic low back pain: Magnitude of the problem. In A. A. White III & S. L. Gordon (Eds.), *American Academy of Orthopaedic Surgeons Symposium on Idiopathic Low Back Pain*. CV Mosby, pp. 5–8.
53. Khalil, T., Abdel-Moty, E., Steele-Rosomoff, R., & Rosomoff, H. (1994). The role of ergonomics in the prevention and treatment of myofascial pain. In E. S. Rachlin (Ed.), *Myofascial Pain and Fibromyalgia*. Mosby, pp. 311–322.
54. Knox, B. D., & Chapman, T. M. (1993). Anterior lumbar interbody fusion for discogram concordant pain. *Journal of Spinal Disorders, 6*, 242–244.
55. Koes, B. W., Bouter, L. M., van Mameren, H., et al. (1992). The effectiveness of manual therapy, physiotherapy, and treatment by the general practitioner for nonspecific back and neck complaints: A randomized clinical trial. *Spine, 17*, 28–35.
56. Kopell, H. P., & Thompson, W. (1973). *Peripheral Entrapment Neuropathies*. Williams & Wilkins.
57. Kozak, J. A., & O'Brien, J. P. (1990). Simultaneous combined anterior and posterior fusion: An independent analysis of a treatment for the disabled low-back pain patient. *Spine, 15*, 322–328.
58. Kraft, G. H., Johnson, E. W., & LaBan, M. M. (1968). The fibrositis syndrome. *Archives of Physiological Medicine and Rehabilitation, 49*, 155–162.
59. Kraus, H. (1970). *Clinical Treatment of Back and Neck Pain*. McGraw–Hill.
60. Kuslich, S. D., Ulstrom, C. L., & Michael, C. J. (1991). The tissue origin of low back pain and sciatica: A report of pain response to tissue stimulation during operations on the lumbar spine using local anesthesia. *Orthopedic Clinics of North America, 22*, 181–187.
61. Lawrence, R. M. (1978). New approach to the treatment of chronic pain: Combination therapy. *American Journal of Acupuncture, 6*, 59–62.

62. Lippert, F. G. III, & Teitz, C. C. (1987). *Diagnosing Musculoskeletal Problems—A Practical Guide*. Williams & Wilkins.

63. Liu, S. S., Williams, K. D., Drayer, B. P., et al. (1990). Synovial cysts of the lumbosacral spine: Diagnosis by MR imaging. *American Journal of Roentgenology, 154*, 163–166.

64. Long, D. M. (1991). Failed back surgery syndrome. *Neurosurgery Clinics of North America, 2*(4), 899–919.

65. Long, D. M., & Zeidman, S. M. (1994). Outcome of low back pain therapy. In M. N. Hadley (Ed.), *Perspectives in Neurological Surgery, vol 5, no 1*. Quality Medical, pp. 41–51.

66. Long, D. M., BenDebba, M., Torgerson, W. S., et al. (1996). Persistent back pain and sciatica in the United States: Patient characteristics. *Journal of Spinal Disorders, 9*(1), 40–58.

67. Long, D. M., Erickson, D., Campbell, J., & North, R. (1981). Electrical stimulation of the spinal cord and peripheral nerves for pain control. A 10-year experience. *Applied Neurophysiology, 44*, 207–217.

68. Long, D. M., Filtzer, D. L., BenDebba, M., & Hendler, N. H. (1988). Clinical features of the failed-back syndrome. *Journal of Neurosurgery, 69*, 61–71.

69. Martins, A. N., Ramirez, A., Johnston, J., et al. (1978). Double-blind evaluation of chemonucleolysis for herniated lumbar discs: Late results. *Journal of Neurosurgery, 49*, 816–827.

70. McCombe, P. F., Fairbank, J. C., Cockersole, B. C., et al. (1989). Reproducibility of physical signs in low-back pain. *Spine, 14*, 908–918.

71. McLaughlin, H. L. (1961). The 'frozen shoulder.' *Clinical Orthopedics, 20*, 126–131.

72. Meade, T. W., Dyer, S., Browne, W., et al. (1995). Randomized comparison of chiropractic and hospital outpatient management for low back pain: Results from extended follow up. *British Medical Journal, 311*, 349–351.

73. Melzack, R., Stillwell, D. M., & Fox, E. J. (1977). Trigger points and acupuncture points for pain: Correlations and implications. *Pain, 3*, 3–23.

74. Mense, S. (1991). Considerations concerning the neurobiological basis of muscle pain. *Canadian Journal of Physiological Pharmacology, 69*, 610–616.

75. Moran, R., O'Connell, D., & Walsh, M. G. (1988). The diagnostic value of facet joint injections. *Spine, 13*, 1407–1410.

76. Moseley, H. F. (1969). *Shoulder Lesions, 3rd edn*. E & S Livingstone, pp. 75–81, 243–292.

77. Neer, C. S. II, & Welsh, R. P. (1977). The shoulder in sports. *Orthopedic Clinics of North America, 8*, 583–591.

78. Neviaser, J. S. (1975). Arthrography of the shoulder: The diagnosis and management of the lesions visualized. *CC Thomas, 63(4), 335*.

79. Nichols, J. A., & Hershman, E. B. (1990). *The Upper Extremity in Sports Medicine*. Mosby.

80. O'Connell, J. E. A. (1951). Protrusions of the lumbar intervertebral discs: A clinical review based on five hundred cases treated by excision of the protrusion. *Journal of Bone and Joint Surgery, 33B*, 8–30.

81. Onik, G., Mooney, V., Maroon, J. C., et al. (1990). Automated percutaneous discectomy: A prospective multi-institutional study. *Neurosurgery, 26*, 228–233.

82. Pak, T. J., Martin, G. M., Magnes, J. L., & Kavanaugh, G. J. (1970). Reflex sympathetic dystrophy. *Minnesota Medicine, 53*, 507–512.

83. Panjabi, M. M., Goel, V. K., & Takata, K. (1982). Physiologic strains in lumbar spinal ligaments: An in vitro biomechanical study. *Spine, 7*, 192–203.

84. Pope, M. H., Phillips, R. B., Haugh, L. D., et al. (1994). A prospective randomized three-week trial of spinal manipulation, transcutaneous muscle stimulation, massage and corset in the treatment of subacute low back pain. *Spine, 19*, 2571–2577.

85. Post, M. (1987). *Physical Examination of the Musculoskeletal System*. Year Book Medical Publishers.

86. Raugstad, T. S., Harbo, K., Oogberg, A., et al. (1982). Anterior interbody fusion of the lumbar spine. *Acta Orthopaedica Scandinavica, 53*, 561–565.

87. Revel, M., Payan, C., Vallee, C., et al. (1993). Automated percutaneous lumbar discectomy versus chemonucleolysis in the treatment of sciatica: A randomized multicenter trial. *Spine, 18*, 1–7.

88. Roberts, J. R., & Hedges, J. R. (1991). *Clinical Procedures in Emergency Medicine, 2nd ed.* Saunders, chap 64.

89. Rosenbaum, R. B., & Ochoa, J. L. (1993). *Carpal Tunnel Syndrome and Other Disorders of the Median Nerve*. Butterworth-Heinemann.

90. Saal, J. A., & Saal, J. S. (1989). Nonoperative treatment of herniated lumbar intervertebral disc with radiculopathy: An outcome study. *Spine, 14*, 431–437.

91. Saal, J. A., Saal, J. S., & Herzog, R. J. (1990). The natural history of lumbar intervertebral disc extrusions treated nonoperatively. *Spine, 15*, 683–686.

92. Saha, A. K. (1961). *Theory of Shoulder Mechanism*. Thomas.

93. Sataloff, R. T., Brandfonbrenner, A. G., & Lederman, R. J. (1990). *Textbook of Performing Arts Medicine*. Raven Press.

94. Schwarzer, A. C., Aprill, C. N., Derby, R., et al. (1995). The prevalence and clinical features of internal disc disruption in patients with chronic low back pain. *Spine, 20*, 1878–1883.

95. Sheon, R. P., Moskowitz, R. W., & Goldberg, V. M. (1987). *Soft Tissue Rheumatic Pain, 2nd ed.* Lea & Febiger.

96. Silverstein, B., Fine, L., & Stetson, D. (1987). Hand-wrist disorders among investment casting plant workers. *Journal of Hand Surgery, 12A*, 838–844.

97. Simons, D. G. (1975). Muscle pain syndromes. Part I. *American Journal of Physical Medicine, 54*, 289–311.

98. Simons, D. G. (1976). Muscle pain syndromes. Part II. *American Journal of Physical Medicine, 55*, 15–42.

99. Sola, A. E. (1981). Myofascial trigger point therapy. *Resident Staff Physicians, 27*, 38–48.

100. Sola, A. E. (1984). Treatment of myofascial pain syndromes. In C. Benedetti et al. (Eds.), *Advances in Pain Research and Therapy*. Raven Press, p. 13.

101. Sola, A. E., & Kuitert, J. H. (1955). Myofascial trigger point pain in the neck and shoulder girdle: 100 cases treated by normal saline. *Northwest Medicine, 54*, 980–984.

102. Sola, A. E., & Williams, R. L. (1956). Myofascial pain syndromes. *Neurology, 6*, 91–95.

103. Sola, A. E., Rodenberg, M. L., & Getty, B. B. (1955). Incidence of hypersensitive areas in posterior shoulder muscles. *American Journal of Physical Medicine, 34*, 585–590.

104. Spangfort, E. V. (1972). The lumbar disc herniation: A computer-aided analysis of 2,504 operations. *Acta Orthopaedica Scandinavica, 142(suppl)*, 1–95.

105. Spengler, D. M., & Freeman, C. W. (1979). Patient selection for lumbar discectomy: An objective approach. *Spine, 4*, 129–134.

106. Steindler, A. (1959). *Lectures on the Interpretation of Pain in Orthopedic Practice*. Thomas.

107. Steinmann, J. C., & Herkowitz, H. N. (1982). Pseudarthrosis of the spine. *Clinical Orthopaedics, 284*, 80–90.

108. Tfelt-Hansen, P., Olesen, J., Lous, I., et al. (1980). Lignocaine versus saline in migraine pain. *Lancet, 1*, 1140.

109. Travell, J. (1976). Myofascial trigger points. In J. J. Bonica (Ed.), *Advances in Pain Research and Therapy*. Raven Press.

110. Travell, J., & Daitz, B. (1990). *Myofascial Pain Syndromes: The Travell Trigger Point Tapes*. Williams & Wilkins Electronic Media.

111. Travell, J., & Rinzler, S. H. (1952). The myofascial genesis of pain. *Postgraduate Medicine, 11*, 425–434.

112. Travell, J., & Simons, D. G. (1983). *Myofascial Pain and Dysfunction: The Trigger Point Manual*. Williams & Wilkins.

113. Turner, J. A., Ersek, M., Herron, L., et al. (1992). Patient outcomes after lumbar spinal fusions. *Journal of American Medical Association, 268*, 907–911.

114. Waddell, G. (1987a). A new clinical model for the treatment of low back pain. *Spine, 12*, 632–644.

115. Waddell, G. (1987b). Failures of disc surgery and repeat surgery. *Acta Orthopaedica Belgica, 53*, 300–302.

116. Waddell, G., McCulloch, J. A., Kummel, E., et al. (1980). Nonorganic physical signs in low back pain. *Spine, 5*, 117–125.

117. Wall, P. D., & Gutnick, M. (1974). Ongoing activity in peripheral nerves: The physiology and pharmacology of impulses originating from a neuroma. *Experimental Neurology, 43*, 580–593.

118. Weber, H. (1983). Lumbar disc herniation: A controlled, prospective study with ten years of observation. *Spine, 8*, 131–140.

119. Weber, H. (1994). The natural history of disc herniation and the influence of intervention. *Spine, 19*, 2234–2238.

120. Wiesel, S. W., Cuckler, J. M., Deluca, F., et al. (1980). Acute low-back pain: An objective analysis of conservative therapy. *Spine, 5*, 324–330.

121. Wiesel, S. W., Tsourmas, N., Feffer, H. L., et al. (1984). A study of computer assisted tomography: I. The incidence of positive CAT scans in an asymptomatic group of patients. *Spine, 9*, 549–551.

122. Zdeblick, T. A. (1993). A prospective, randomized study of lumbar fusion: Preliminary results. *Spine, 18*, 983–991.

123. Zimmermann, M. (1979). Peripheral and central nervous mechanisms of nociception, pain

and pain therapy: Facts and hypotheses. In J. J. Bonica, J. C. Liebeskind, & D. G. Albe-Fessard (Eds.), *Advances in Pain Research and Therapy (Vol. 3,* pp. 3–32). Lippincott–Raven.

124. Zohn, D. A., & Mennell, J. M. (1976). *Musculoskeletal Pain: Diagnosis and Physical Treatment.* Little, Brown.

Chapter

FIBROMYALGIA AND ABDOMINAL PAIN

4

Contents

Introduction

Abdominal pain frequently coexists with fibromyalgia, a chronic condition marked by fatigue, tenderness, and widespread musculoskeletal pain. This complicates management and treatment for those who are affected. Although fibromyalgia mainly affects the soft tissues and muscles, it can also affect other organ systems, such as the gastrointestinal tract, in addition to the musculoskeletal system.

One of the most prevalent and incapacitating symptoms of fibromyalgia for many people is abdominal pain. Along with other gastrointestinal symptoms like diarrhea, constipation, nausea, and indigestion, it may present as cramps, bloating, discomfort, or a sharp, stabbing pain in the abdomen. The precise processes that underlie the correlation between fibromyalgia and abdominal pain are intricate and multifaceted, encompassing the interplay of neuroendocrine, immune, and psychosocial elements.

Numerous theories have been put forth to explain the connection between stomach pain and fibromyalgia. Visceral hypersensitivity and a changed perception of abdominal pain may also be caused by changes in the central sensitization mechanisms and pain processing pathways linked to fibromyalgia. An additional theory suggests that there is a dysregulation of the autonomic nervous system, which may have an impact on pain perception, visceral sensation, and gastrointestinal motility. Furthermore, comorbid illnesses like functional dyspepsia, GERD, and irritable bowel syndrome (IBS) may make abdominal symptoms worse if they are already present in fibromyalgia patients.

A thorough and multidisciplinary approach is necessary for the management of abdominal pain associated with fibromyalgia, intending to address both the gastrointestinal manifestations and the underlying symptoms of the condition. Pharmacotherapy is one possible treatment method to reduce pain, enhance gastrointestinal motility, and control related symptoms like bloating and nausea. Reducing stomach discomfort and enhancing general well-being may also benefit from dietary changes, stress reduction methods, and lifestyle therapies.

Abdominal pain and fibromyalgia often coexist and can have a substantial negative effect on an individual's quality of life. Comprehending the intricate relationship between gastrointestinal symptoms and fibromyalgia is crucial for offering all-encompassing care and formulating efficacious treatment plans customized for each patient suffering from this difficult ailment.

Orientation and Directional Terms

Term	Definition	Illustration
Abdominal pain	Abdominal pain, also known as stomach pain, can be felt anywhere from below the ribs to the pelvis.	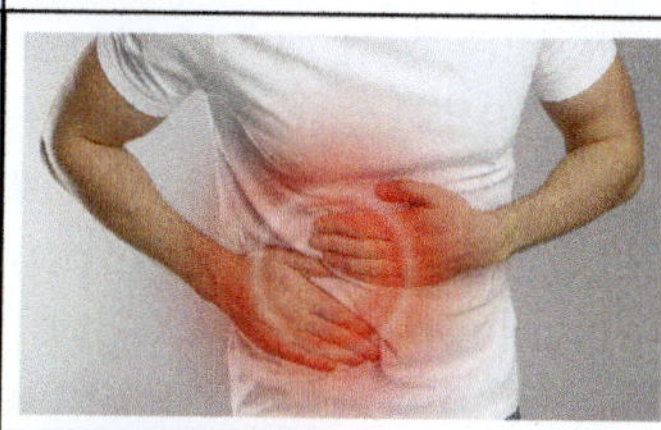
Fibromyalgia	Fibromyalgia is a disorder characterized by widespread musculoskeletal pain accompanied by fatigue, sleep, memory and mood issues.	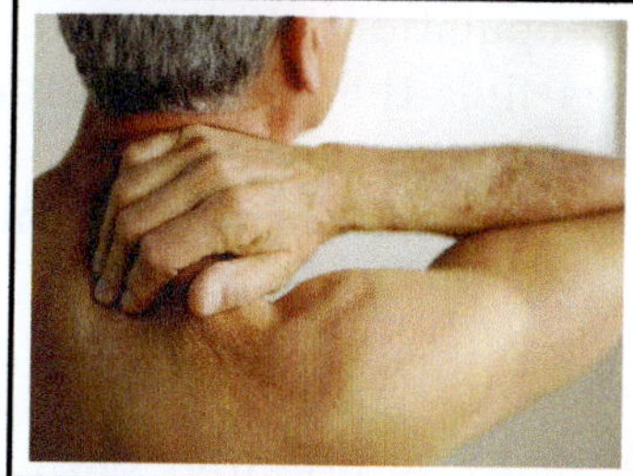
Stabbing pain	Stabbing pain in the chest that comes and goes can have various causes, from heart attacks to muscle strains.	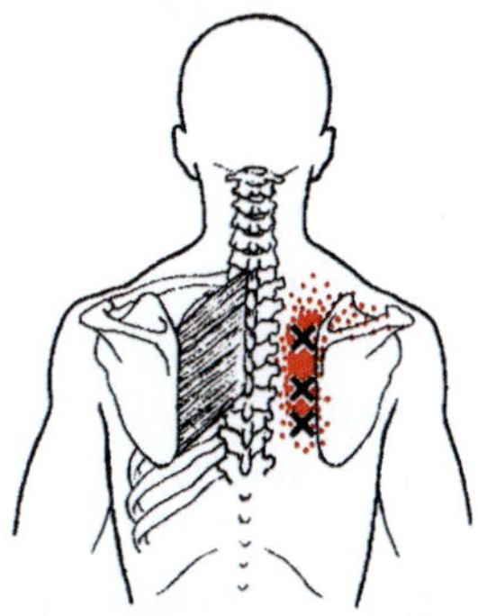
Dysautonomia	Dysautonomia, also known as autonomic failure or autonomic dysfunction, is a condition that occurs when the autonomic nervous system (ANS) malfunctions.	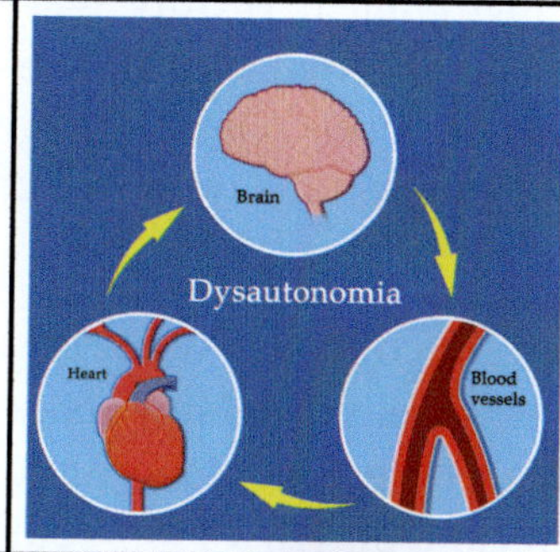
Dolorimetry	A dolorimeter is an instrument used to measure pain threshold and pain tolerance.	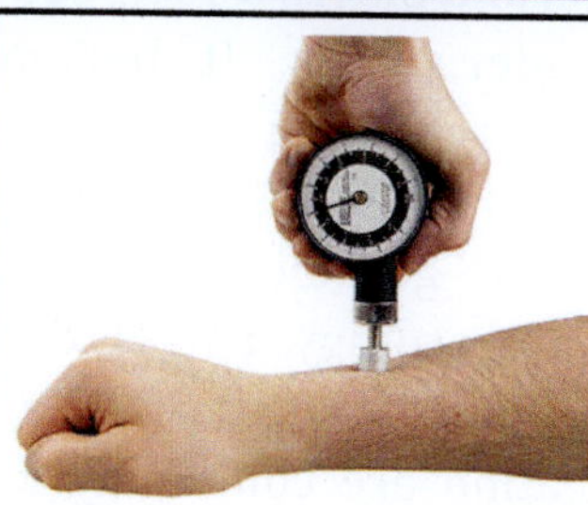

4.1: Fibromyalgia

The primary characteristic of fibromyalgia, a multisymptomatic syndrome, is chronic, widespread pain (Bennett, 1981; Yunus et al., 1981; Goldenberg, 1987). In addition to extreme exhaustion, many of these patients also have visceral hyperalgesia-related symptoms like irritable bowel and bladder. About 20% of patients in North America who consult rheumatologists belong to this population (White et al., 1995). Current studies link the symptomatology of these patients to abnormalities in sensory processing and neuroendocrine dysfunction.

4.1.1. Historical Perspective

Sir William Gowers is credited with coining the term "fibrositis" in a 1904 lecture on lumbago that was published in the British Medical Journal (Gowers, 1904). As stated in this lecture: "I believe we need to call this inflammation of the fibrous tissue—we can call it fibrositis, conveniently drawing on the analogy of "cellulitis." In 1904, Glasgow pathologist Ralph Stockman reported "myalgic nodules," which are foci of inflammation in the interstitium of muscle bundles (Stockman, 1904). These histological results were never confirmed, and for the majority of the middle third of the twentieth century, the diagnosis of "fibrositis" was synonymous with "psychogenic rheumatism."

The "fibrositis concept" was reevaluated in the 1980s as a result of Moldofsky's 1976 description of an objective sleep abnormality in these patients and Smyth's 1977 rediscovery of defined tender areas. It became clear that a sizable fraction of patients visiting rheumatologists were these individuals. To provide diagnostic guidelines, the American College of Rheumatology (ACR) decided to commission a multicenter study. The findings of this investigation are commonly known as the 1990 ACR guidelines and were published in 1990 (Wolfe et al., 1990). They changed the name from "fibrositis," which was thought to reflect a pathological idea that had been debunked, to "fibromyalgia."

4.1.2. Diagnosis

The most commonly used criteria in use today for diagnosing fibromyalgia are those from the 1990 American College of Rheumatology (Wolfe et al., 1990). They consist of one physical discovery and one historical feature. Three months or longer of widespread pain has been the historical feature.

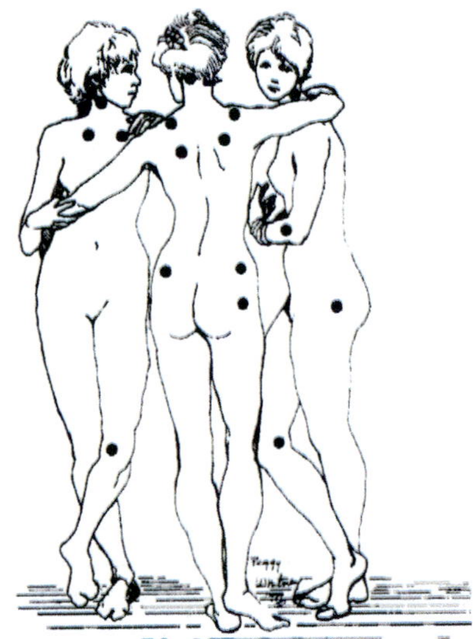

Figure 4.1. Location of the 18 tender points established as criteria for FMS diagnosis by the American College of Rheumatology (ACR).

Source. Galvez-Sánchez CM, Reyes del Paso GA. Diagnostic criteria for fibromyalgia: Critical review and future perspectives. *Journal of Clinical Medicine*. 2020; 9(4):1219. https://doi.org/10.3390/jcm9041219.

Pain in an axial distribution, as well as pain on the left and right sides of the body and above and below the waist, are all considered widespread. The presence of 11 or more of the 18 designated tender points is the physical finding. The location and the patient's experience of pain upon digital palpation with an approximate force of 4 kg (the amount of pressure required to blanch a thumbnail) are used to define a tender point.

4.1.3. Epidemiology

The general population frequently experiences chronic musculoskeletal pain. According to Croft et al. (1993), the prevalence rates of chronic widespread pain (11:2%) and regional pain (43%), respectively, were observed in the north of England. According to a Kansas study (Wolfe et al., 1995), the prevalence of chronic widespread musculoskeletal pain increased gradually from 18 to 70 years of age, peaking at 23% in the seventh decade. The prevalence was higher in women. Some subjects with regional pain syndromes seem to be more likely to develop fibromyalgia, which is characterized by widespread pain (Forseth et al., 1999a). In Kansas, the general prevalence of fibromyalgia was 2%; in women, it was 3%, and in men, it was 0%. It is believed that fibromyalgia is one end of a continuous spectrum of chronic pain, and all epidemiological studies have shown that chronic widespread pain is more common than the ACR-defined diagnosis of fibromyalgia (MacFarlane, 1999).

4.2. Clinical Features

4.2.1. Pain

Chronic, all-over pain is the primary symptom of fibromyalgia (FM) syndrome (Wolfe et al., 1990). Although many fibromyalgia patients also report joint pain, the pain is typically thought to originate from the muscles (Reilly & Littlejohn, 1992). Most FM patients experience stiffness, which is worse in the morning. When combined with the sensation of articular pain, this can further the impression of an arthritic condition. According to Moldofsky (1994), the pain and stiffness associated with fibromyalgia usually fluctuate throughout the day, reaching its lowest point between 11:00 am and 3:30 pm.

4.2.2. Fatigue

Fibromyalgia is characterized by easy fatigability to physical and mental exertion as well as psychological stressors (Yunus et al., 1981). Numerous factors are thought to contribute to the etiology of fatigue in fibromyalgia, including deconditioning, depression, dysautonomia, inadequate coping strategies, and secondary endocrine dysfunction involving the hypothalamic pituitary adrenal axis and growth hormone deficiency (Bennett et al., 1997; Pillemer et al., 1997). There are numerous parallels between FM 96 patients and those suffering from chronic fatigue syndrome (CFS) (Aaron & Buchwald, 2001). Approximately 75% of patients who satisfy the CFS diagnostic criteria also satisfy the FM diagnostic criteria (Goldenberg et al., 1990).

4.2.3. Disordered Sleep

Patients with fibromyalgia typically report having trouble sleeping (Moldofsky et al., 1975). They wake up feeling exhausted even after 8 to 10 hours of nonstop sleep. We call this kind of sleep non-restorative. The majority report being light sleepers, easily startled by quiet sounds or bothersome thoughts. An alpha-delta EEG pattern is seen in many, which could account for why they never reach the restorative stages 3 and 4 of non-REM sleep (Moldofsky, 1989). Hauri and Hawkins (1973) noted that an alpha intrusion rhythm in delta sleep is neither specific nor invariant in fibromyalgia. It has been noted that musculoskeletal pain, stiffness, and/or tenderness can be brought on by experimentally inducing alpha-delta sleep in healthy individuals (Moldofsky & Scarisbrick, 1976). The next day, fibromyalgia symptoms frequently get worse after a restless night (Affleck et al., 1996).

4.2.4. Cognitive Dysfunction

Many fibromyalgia patients self-report that cognitive dysfunction is a major problem (Park et al., 2001). Patients frequently report issues with motivation, logical reasoning, short-term memory, and focus. Research on cognitive function issues in fibromyalgia patients is expanding as these issues are becoming more widely recognized (Glass & Park, 2001). As of right now, verbal fluency, episodic memory, and working memory have been used to characterize defects. According to estimates, these declines in cognitive function are the same as 20 years of aging (Glass & Park, 2001).

4.2.5. Associated Disorders

In addition to musculoskeletal pain, a variety of other somatic complaints, including irritable bowel syndrome, restless leg syndrome, dysautonomia, chemical hypersensitivity, and irritable bladder, are frequently experienced by fibromyalgia patients (Clauw, 1995). It is now believed that the neuroendocrine effects of chronic stress and abnormal sensory processing contribute to these symptoms.

4.2.6. Psychological Distress

Patients with fibromyalgia are more likely to receive psychological diagnoses, as is the case with many chronic conditions. Compared to healthy controls, fibromyalgia patients have a higher prevalence of depression (Burckhardt et al., 1994; Yunus, 1994). Fassbender et al. (1997) noted that fibromyalgia is uncommon among patients experiencing major depression and that even depressed individuals who reported pain did not exhibit multiple tender points. Who becomes a patient with fibromyalgia may depend in part on psychological distress (Aaron et al., 1996). The idea that fibromyalgia and post-traumatic stress disorder are related is becoming more widely accepted (Amir et al., 1997). Although psychiatric disorders are more common in fibromyalgia patients than in non-patients, they appear to be a consequence of the severity of fibromyalgia symptoms rather than being inherently linked to the pathophysiology of the syndrome (Aaron et al., 1996).

4.2.7. Initiation and Maintenance of Fibromyalgia

Fibromyalgia rarely appears suddenly. The majority of patients mention acute injuries, pain from repetitive tasks, sports injuries, or other types of pain. Fibromyalgia frequently develops from a regional pain syndrome (Forseth et al., 1999b). Some people believe that toxins, stress, and infections are the causes. Low back pain, rheumatoid arthritis, SLE, Sjogren's and inflammatory bowel disease, and osteoarthritis are all frequently associated with fibromyalgia (Morand et al., 1994; Urrows et al., 1994; Lapossy et al., 1995; Bennett, 1997; Sperber et al., 1999). One year following whiplash injuries, fibromyalgia prevalence is reported to be 22% (Buskila et al., 1997). According to a report by Buskila et al. (1996), fibromyalgia is remarkably common in families. This implies that individuals who are prone to developing fibromyalgia are either genetically predisposed (nature) or have experienced events or situations in their past that support its development later on (nurture).

4.2.8. Prognosis and Impact

The symptomatology of fibromyalgia frequently lasts for years (Bengtsson et al., 1994). A patient's quality of life is frequently negatively impacted by chronic musculoskeletal pain (Burckhardt et al., 1993). Following a 7-year follow-up, an analysis of 1604 fibromyalgia patients under observation in academic centers found that pain, fatigue, sleep disturbance, functional status, anxiety, depression, and health status remained largely unaltered (Wolfe et al., 1997a). According to some research, patients with fibromyalgia who are seen in community settings as opposed to tertiary care facilities have a better prognosis (Granges et al., 1994). Pain and fatigability have an impact on motor function; people with fibromyalgia take longer to complete daily tasks, take longer to get going in the morning, and frequently need more rest breaks during the day (Henriksson, 1994). If frequent breaks aren't taken, they struggle with prolonged, repetitive motor tasks. Short-term task tolerance may be high, but prolonged task performance can lead to aggravating factors (Waylonis et al., 1994). The adjustments that people with fibromyalgia must make to reduce their pain frequently have a detrimental effect on their recreational and professional lives.

4.2.9. Disability

Many fibromyalgia patients struggle to maintain their competitiveness in the workforce, despite the condition's outward appearance of normalcy (Bennett, 1996a). According to the majority of FM patients, exhaustion and persistent pain have a detrimental influence on their quality of life and their capacity to find competitive employment (Henriksson, 1995). The degree of FM disability that is reported varies significantly between nations, most likely due to variations in political ideologies and socioeconomic conditions. 70% of fibromyalgia patients seen in academic centers said they thought of themselves as disabled in a survey. Social Security benefits (SSD) were received by 16% of the population, or 22% of the US population (Wolfe et al., 1997b).

4.3. Pathogenesis

A complex hyperalgesic pain syndrome, which is the current etiological paradigm for fibromyalgia, is caused by abnormalities in central sensory processing that interact with peripheral pain generators and neuro-endocrine pathways to produce a wide range of patient symptoms and distress. It is now believed that the expression of symptoms classified as fibromyalgia is influenced to varying degrees by both peripheral and central factors.

The majority of the 20th century saw fibrositis and fibromyalgia classified as illnesses of the muscles. It is now understood that fibromyalgia cannot be defined in terms of a particular tissue pathology due to the lack of characteristic muscle changes (Simms, 1996). This does not imply, however, that pathogenesis has nothing to do with non-pathological muscle pain issues, such as exertional muscle microtrauma. In fact, it is theorized that any peripheral pain generator—a tissue-generated source of pain—can amplify and/or prolong central pain mechanisms.

Myofascial trigger points are the focal areas of muscle pain. These are hyperalgesic zones in the muscle, which palpably feel indurated. Long-term pressure applied to these points may result in a distal referral pattern of pain, which is why they are called "trigger points" (Travell and Simons, 1992). Kellgren (1938) was the first to conduct studies with hypertonic saline to assess the correlates of painful foci within muscle. According to Graven-Nielsen (Basbaum and Fields, 1984; Graven-Nielsen et al., 1997), hypertonic saline-induced muscle pain exhibits temporal and spatial summations influenced by central facilitatory and inhibitory mechanisms. These experiments are thought to be relevant to abnormal sensory processing in fibromyalgia patients, as they emphasize the significance of focal muscle pain in eliciting a state of central sensitization (Henriksson, 1994; Bennett, 1996c).

One possible explanation for peripheral nociceptive input in fibromyalgia patients is muscle microtrauma, which is a common occurrence in healthy individuals (Bennett, 1993). Diagnosing this phenomenon is challenging because biopsying a muscle can result in trauma. NMR spectroscopy, on the other hand, can assess live, trauma-free muscle. Three NMR studies (Jubrias et al., 1994; Park et al., 2000; Sprott et al., 2000) have found that phosphodiester peaks are higher in fibromyalgia patients than in control groups. Phosphodiester peaks are associated with aging (Satrustegui et al., 1988) and musculodystrophies (Younkin et al., 1987). They are believed to be the outcome of sarcolemmal membrane proteins' lipid peroxidation. When there is muscle microtrauma, or calcium-activated muscle damage, this process takes place (Armstrong et al., 1991).

Multiple lines of evidence indicate that abnormalities in central sensory processing may contribute to the pain experienced by fibromyalgia patients.

4.3.1. Qualitative Differences in Pain

Dolorimetry provides an objective measurement of the force applied to a tender point (Campbell et al., 1983). An electronic dolorimeter was used in a study to record the subjects' pain intensity ratings, which ranged from 98 on a 0-to 10-cm visual analog scale (VAS) at different applied force levels (Bendtsen et al., 1997). Response curves that were noticeably different from those of controls and fibromyalgia patients were found. Heat and cold-related abnormalities in pain processing have also been documented in fibromyalgia patients (Kosek et al., 1996).

4.3.2. Deficient Pain Modulation in Response to Repeated Thermal Stimuli

Repeated non-noxious skin stimulation can be used to demonstrate an up-regulation of pain threshold in healthy individuals. Transcutaneous nerve stimulators (TENS) are used to treat chronic pain states on the basis of this. The physiological basis for this effect is the persistent stimulation of type A myelinated axons, which inhibits the excitability of dorsal horn neurons (Wall & Cronly-Dillon, 1960). According to Lautenbacher and Rollman (1997), fibromyalgia patients exhibit a deficiency in diffuse noxious inhibitory control (DNIC), which lends credence to the theory that their descending inhibitory pain system is malfunctioning (Mense, 2000).

4.3.3. Hyper-Responsive Somatosensory Induced Potentials

The term "somatosensory-induced potentials" describes the electrical activity in the brain that results from stimulation of peripheral senses and can be detected using electrodes in the skull. In comparison to ten matched controls, Gibson et al. found that ten FM patients had a higher late nociceptive (CO_2-laser stimulation of skin) evoked somatosensory response (Gibson et al., 1994). When compared to controls stimulated by laser stimulation of the skin, Lorenz et al. (1996) found that fibromyalgia patients had larger amplitudes of the N170 and P390 brain somatosensory potentials. They also noticed a response in both hemispheres, as opposed to controls, who only experienced a response on one side of the brain. These two studies offer objective proof that, when compared to pain-free controls, fibromyalgia patients process nociceptive stimuli differently.

4.3.4. Secondary Hyperalgesia on Electrocutaneous Stimulation

The typical experience of pain resulting from nociceptor stimulation in damaged tissue is known as primary hyperalgesia. Pain induced by uninjured tissues is referred to as secondary hyperalgesia (Magerl et al., 1998). Arroyo and Cohen (1993) observed sensory phenomena indicative of secondary hyperalgesia while trying to treat fibromyalgia patients with electrical nerve stimulation.

4.3.5. Abnormalities on SPECT Imaging

Several imaging modalities can now be used to visualize changes in brain blood flow or metabolism brought on by pain (Bradley et al., 2000). Reduced thalamic blood flow has been observed in fibromyalgia patients, according to reports (Mountz et al., 1995; Kwiatek et al., 2000). It's interesting to note that while acute pain increases thalamic blood flow, chronic pain states have been linked to decreased thalamic blood flow. A limbic network's activation as a result of the disinhibition of the medial thalamus is thought to be the cause of this discrepancy (Craig, 1998).

4.3.6. Elevated Levels of Substance P in the CSF

One significant nociceptive neurotransmitter is substance P. According to three conclusive studies (Vaeroy et al., 1988; Russell et al., 1994; Liu et al., 2000), substance P levels in the CSF of fibromyalgia patients were three times higher than in controls. Substance P has been shown to be relevant in human pain states and to be a major etiological factor in central sensitization in animal models of hyperalgesia and hypoalgesia (Abbadie et al., 1996).

4.3.7. Elevated Levels of Nerve Growth Factor

Normal sympathetic and sensory neuron development requires nerve growth factor, or NGF. When compared to healthy controls and other pain patients, Giovengo et al. found that the CSF of patients with primary fibromyalgia had four times the amount of NGF (Giovengo et al., 1999). When humans receive recombinant nerve growth factor intravenously, they experience a fibromyalgia-like muscular pain syndrome that can persist up to a week following the initial injection. It is thought that NGF stimulates protein synthesis in the central nervous system, which is the mechanism by which it causes hyperalgesia (Bennett, 2001).

4.3.8. Beneficial Response to an NMDA Receptor Antagonist

Non-nociceptive pain is primarily produced by the excitatory amino acid glutamine interacting with NMDA (N-methyl-D-aspartic acid) receptors. According to two studies, intravenous ketamine, an NMDA receptor antagonist, improves muscle endurance in FM patients while also reducing pain and raising pain threshold (Sorensen et al., 1995). Ketamine is used to lessen the effects of intramuscular experimental induction of pain summation and referral in fibromyalgia by hypertonic saline (Graven-Nielsen et al., 2000).

4.3.9. Experimentally Induced Central Hyperexcitability

There is strong experimental evidence that this neurophysiological process is a crucial step in the development of central sensitization. Temporal summation of nociceptive impulses at the spinal cord level typically happens when unmyelinated C fiber input exceeds a rate of one impulse every 2–3 s. (Koltzenburg et al., 1994). Both intramuscular electrical stimulation of muscle (Sorensen et al., 1998) and repetitive thermal stimulation of the palmar skin in fibromyalgia patients have been shown to amplify temporal summation (Staud et al., 2001).

4.4. Management

The goal of treating fibromyalgia patients is to minimize their symptoms while preserving their emotional and physical abilities. The bio-psycho-social model of disease must be thoroughly examined in order to effectively treat fibromyalgia patients. The primary management concerns that typically need to be addressed are listed in Table 4.1.

4.4.1. Diagnosis and Evaluation

The 1990 recommendations of the American College of Rheumatology classification criteria (Wolfe et al., 1990) are typically used to diagnose fibromyalgia. But it's becoming more and more clear that many patients with diffuse pain have fewer tender points than the recommended 11 out of 18. Patients who experience widespread pain and tenderness in multiple areas are unlikely to have a different neuro-physiological cause for their pain than those whose fibromyalgia is strictly defined by the American College of Radiology. It is crucial to investigate additional locations that frequently contain myofascial trigger points. This more thorough assessment is necessary for two reasons: (1) to determine whether a patient with fewer than 11 tender points has fibromyalgia, and (2) to identify relevant myofascial pain generators that may benefit from trigger point therapy (Borg-Stein & Stein, 1996).

Table 4.1. Compounds with Antioxidant and Analgesic Properties for Fibromyalgia Management

Compound	Effects
Melatonin	In an animal study, melatonin was able to improve behavioral defects, oxidative and nitrosative stress, mast cell infiltration and activation of microglia in a reserpine-induced FM model.
	In a clinical trial, the exogenous administration of 10 mg of melatonin once every 24 h increased endogenous pain inhibition, assessed on a numerical scale (0–10). The combination of amitriptyline and melatonin provided better results than amitriptyline alone, as calculated by the visual analog pain scale, in subjects with FM.
	A randomized trial found that melatonin alone or in combination with fluoxetine was beneficial for the treatment of FM. Using melatonin (3 or 5 mg/day) in combination with 20 mg/day fluoxetine caused a significant reduction in both total and individual components of the Fibromyalgia Impact Questionnaire score compared to the pretreatment values.
Coenzyme Q10	CoQ10 treatment showed effects on clinical symptoms, blood mononuclear cells and markers of mitochondrial and oxidative stress in women with FM.
	The results of this clinical study suggest that CoQ10 supplementation plays a role in the modulation of mitochondrial dysfunction and oxidative stress that induce headaches in individuals with FM.
	In a clinical study, CoQ10 supplementation was shown to provide additional benefits for relieving pain sensation in FM patients treated with pregabalin, possibly by improving mitochondrial function, reducing inflammation and decreasing brain activity.
Vitamins D and E	A clinical study found that women with FM had a lower qualitative and quantitative intake than control subjects. In particular, an association has been found between vitamin D deficiency and FM. However, its role in FM pathophysiology and the clinical relevance of its identification and treatment requires further clarification. Only vitamin E appears to be related to quality of life and pain sensation.

Palmitoylethanolamide (PEA)	PEA is a major anti-inflammatory, analgesic and neuroprotective mediator in central and peripheral organs and systems and acts on several molecular targets.
	PEA is emerging as a candidate biomarker due to its anti-inflammatory and anti-hyperalgesic effects via the downregulation of mast cell activation. Preclinical and clinical studies support the idea that PEA merits further consideration as a therapeutic approach for controlling inflammatory responses, pain, related peripheral neuropathic pain and symptoms of FM.

Source: Siracusa R, Paola RD, Cuzzocrea S, Impellizzeri D. Fibromyalgia: Pathogenesis, mechanisms, diagnosis and treatment options update. *International Journal of Molecular Sciences*, 2021; 22(8):3891. https://doi.org/10.3390/ijms22083891.

According to the 1990 ACR criteria, fibromyalgia is not a diagnosis of exclusion, so imaging studies and laboratory testing are not relevant in making the diagnosis. In terms of peripheral pain generators that can accentuate and maintain central sensitization, fibromyalgia patients may have concomitant conditions that are relevant to overall management. These concurrent issues frequently require an investigative approach to diagnosis. A crucial prerequisite for gathering information for a successful management program is a history and examination that is specifically focused on fibromyalgia. The history and physical examination will likely point out specific issues that require additional assessment in the form of specialist referrals or inquiries.

4.4.2. Education

Strong evidence suggests that a better prognosis for many chronic diseases is linked to higher educational attainment (Ramos-Remus et al., 2000). The benefits of education for fibromyalgia patients have been shown in a number of studies (Gowans et al., 1999; Mannerkorpi et al., 2000). Setting goals and reevaluating priorities are two aspects of education that are similar to cognitive behavioral techniques.

Table 4.2. Candidate Genes in the Pathogenesis of FM

Gene	Type of Study
5-HTT	Human
COMT	Human
TAAR1	Human
Opioid receptor μ1 gene A118G	Human
RGS4	Human
CNR1	Human
GRIA4	Human
SLC64A4	Human
TRPV2	Human

MYT1L	Human
NRXN3	Human
CYP450	Human
BDNF	Human
NAT15	Human
HDAC4	Human
PRKCA	Human
RTN1	Human
PRKG1	Human
SLC1A5	Human
SLC25A22	Human
GRM6	Human

Source: Siracusa R, Paola RD, Cuzzocrea S, Impellizzeri D. Fibromyalgia: Pathogenesis, mechanisms, diagnosis and treatment options update. *International Journal of Molecular Sciences.* 2021; 22(8):3891. https://doi.org/10.3390/ijms22083891.

4.4.3. Pain (Would Pain in Fibromyalgia be a Better Title?)

It makes sense to concentrate on the main areas of pain generation and processing when managing pain in FM, which include the descending pain pathway, psychological effects, dorsal horn sensitization, and peripheral pain generation.

Fibromyalgia is not associated with any particular tissue pathology, at least not in peripheral tissues (Simms, 1996). This fact does not, however, imply that peripheral nociceptive mechanisms are less significant. Peripheral pain generators will not only be felt as more painful once the central nervous system (CNS) is sensitized, but a constant onslaught of nociceptive impulses will also intensify and prolong the biochemical mechanisms causing central sensitization. NSAIDs may be helpful for certain peripheral pain generators, such as arthritic disorders, but they are typically ineffective for treating central pain. Therefore, using NSAIDs in addition to centrally acting analgesics is usually recommended. Treatments for specific pain generators might include 5-HT1D antagonists for vascular headaches and gabapentin for neuropathic pain, for example. Injections of local corticosteroids may be beneficial for certain pain generators, such as bursitis or osteoarthritis of the knees. In other situations, surgery might be necessary (e.g., endometriosis, Chiari malformation, and severe hip osteoarthritis). Myofascial trigger points are the most common source of pain for most fibromyalgia patients. Therefore, it is critical to identify and manage these trigger points effectively using pacing, stretching, improved physical conditioning, self-help techniques like acupressure and spray and stretch, and medical intervention such as procaine or botulinum toxin injections.

The majority of medications used to treat pain function at the dorsal horn level. Pharmacological factors primarily influence the modulation of "nociceptive amplification" that takes place at the first synapse (Reveille, 2000). Spinal cord sensitization is impacted by the descending pain system, which starts in the midbrain and ends at the level of dorsal horn neurons (Willis & Westlund, 1997). The action of opioids, fear-induced hypoalgesia, anticipatory hyperalgesia, the placebo effect, the advantages of cognitive behavioral therapy, and inflammation-induced hyperalgesia are all attributed to this descending system. Therefore, emotional states associated with attention, motivation, and cognition can modulate dorsal horn activity through cortical and subcortical circuits. Only medications that activate or amplify the descending pain system are currently FDA-approved to modulate dorsal horn cell reactivity; these medications include opioids, tricyclic antidepressants, and alpha-2 adrenergic agonists.

Table 4.3. ACR2010 and Modified Criteria for the Diagnosis of Fibromyalgia

Widespread Pain Index (WPI)			
Areas	**Specification**		
Number of areas in which the patient has had pain over the past week	0–19 points		
Areas to be considered	shoulder girdle, hip (buttock, trochanter), jaw, upper back, lower back, upper arm, upper leg, chest, neck, abdomen, lower arm, and lower leg (all these areas should be considered bilaterally)		
Symptom Severity Scale (SSS) Score			
Symptom	**Level of Severity**	**Symptom Level**	**Score**
Fatigue Waking unrefreshed Cognitive symptoms (e.g., working memory capacity, recognition memory, verbal knowledge, anxiety, and depression)	For each of these 3 symptoms, indicate the level of severity over the past week using the following scale: 0 = no problem 1 = slight or mild problems, generally mild or intermittent 2 = moderate; considerable problems, often present and/or at a moderate level 3 = severe; pervasive, continuous, life-disturbing problems	Considering somatic symptoms in general, indicate whether the patient has the following: 0 = no symptoms 1 = few symptoms 2 = a moderate number of symptoms 3 = a great deal of symptoms	Final score between 0 and 12
Criteria			
Specification	**Conditions**		
A patient satisfies diagnostic criteria for fibromyalgia if the following 3 conditions are met	(a)WPI ≥ 7/19 and SS scale score ≥ 5 or WPI 3–6 and SS scale score ≥ 9 (b) symptoms have been present as a similar level for at least 3 months (c) the patient does not have a disorder that would otherwise explain the pain		

Modified Criteria		
Specification	**Conditions**	**Final Score**
A patient satisfies diagnostic criteria for fibromyalgia if the following 3 conditions are met	(a)WPI (as above) (b) SS scale score (as above, but without extent of somatic symptoms) (c) presence of abdominal pain, depression, headaches (yes = 1, no = 0)	The number of pain sites (WPI), the SS scale score, and the presence of associated symptoms are summed to give a final score between 0 and 31

Source: Maffei ME. Fibromyalgia: Recent advances in diagnosis, classification, pharmacotherapy and alternative remedies. *International Journal of Molecular Sciences*. 2020; 21(21):7877. https://doi.org/10.3390/ijms21217877.

Amitriptyline, an antidepressant, has long been a staple in the management of chronic pain conditions, including fibromyalgia (Carette et al., 1986). Thirteen randomized, placebo-controlled trials were examined in a meta-analysis of antidepressant use in the treatment of fibromyalgia (O'Malley et al., 2000). With therapy, the odds ratio for improvement was 4 points. When the impact on particular symptoms was examined, antidepressants were found to improve well-being, pain, fatigue, and sleep, in that order. A single study discovered a link between the reduction of symptoms and the amelioration of depression. The long-term effectiveness of antidepressants in treating fibromyalgia pain has not been thoroughly established, despite their widespread use (Carette et al., 1994).

In the majority of acute and chronic pain conditions, opioids are useful. Despite being used fairly frequently to treat fibromyalgia (Wolfe et al., 1997a), no controlled clinical trials have been conducted on the drug. The effects on cognition decreased motivation to seek non-pharmacological treatment modalities, exacerbation of depression, and negative stigmatization by the medical community and society at large are the primary issues associated with long-term opioid use (Savage, 1996). Addiction is now known to be unfounded, occurring in only 0.5% of patients receiving opioid treatment for chronic pain (Portenoy, 1996). It is normal for all patients taking opioids to experience dependency; this is not the same as addiction, but it does mean that stopping these drugs suddenly will cause withdrawal symptoms in the patient. The unchecked use of drugs for their mind-altering effects can lead to addiction, a dysfunctional state that is frequently accompanied by medical system manipulation and obtaining drugs from sources other than pharmacies. "Pseudo-addiction" is not the same as addiction. This is a drug-seeking behavior brought on by attempts to get the right pain relief when pain is not being adequately treated (Weissman and Haddox, 1989). While opiates shouldn't be used as a first resort for fibromyalgia pain, they also shouldn't be avoided if less potent medications haven't worked.

Chronic pain conditions such as fibromyalgia are finding success with the use of Tramadol (Ultram) as a pain reliever (Roth, 1998;

Schnitzer et al., 2000). Tramadol functions by inhibiting the reuptake of serotonin and noradrenaline (norepinephrine) at the dorsal horn level in addition to its dual mechanism as a weak opioid agonist (Lewis & Han, 1997). At an average dose of 200 mg/day, a double-blind study showed its effectiveness and tolerability in the treatment of fibromyalgia pain (Russell et al., 1997). There have also been reports of benefits for fibromyalgia pain and other symptoms when tramadol and acetaminophen (Ultracet) are combined (Bennett et al., 2001).

Tizanidine (Zanaflex), an alpha-2 adrenergic agonist, has been effectively used to treat many chronic pain conditions (Fogelholm & Murros, 1992). The finding that intrathecally administered alpha-2 adrenergic agonists, but not beta-adrenergic receptor agonists, produce a potent analgesia in both experimental animals and humans provides the experimental basis for this antinociceptive action (Nabeshima et al., 1987; Coward, 1994). These medications have not been the subject of any fibromyalgia trials. Tizanidine has been shown to be helpful in treating fibromyalgia-related pain in anecdotal reports. This is because, in addition to being an antinociceptive, it also acts as an antispasmodic (Smith and Barton, 2000), which makes patients drowsy and may be beneficial if taken in the evening.

Several positive short-term trials involving 5-HT3 antagonists and fibromyalgia patients have been conducted (Farber et al., 2000; Haus et al., 2000). Only neuronal tissues, both central and peripheral, contain 5-HT3 receptors (Tecott et al., 1993). Because of the intricate biochemistry of 5-HT3 receptors, antagonists may act as nociceptive or antinociceptive depending on the situation. The 5-HT3 receptor modifies the release of neuro-active molecules like substance P, serotonin, GABA, acetylcholine, cholecystokinin, and dopamine by causing a rapid membrane depolarization and subsequent rise in cytosolic Ca++ (Wolf, 2000). Before the effectiveness of this class of medications can be thoroughly assessed, longer-term studies involving fibromyalgia patients are required.

It is less common to use medications that alter the ascending pain system. Nonetheless, ketamine-blocking NMDA receptors have been shown in experiments to reduce pain in fibromyalgia patients (Sorensen et al., 1995). Weak NMDA receptor antagonist dextromethorphan has been effectively used to treat neuropathic pain (McQuay et al., 1994); more recently, it has been used to treat fibromyalgia in conjunction with tramadol (Clark & Bennett, 2000). It makes sense that preventing substance P from releasing or from interacting with the NK-1 receptor would be advantageous. In chronic pain states, however, first-generation substance P antagonist clinical trials yielded disappointing results (Hill, 2000). NGF antagonists have not yet been employed in clinical trials involving humans.

4.4.4. Fatigue

The following are common, treatable causes of persistent fatigue in fibromyalgia patients: (1) mishandled medication dosage (TCAs, antihistamine-acting medications, benzodiazepines, etc.). 2), (3) aerobic deconditioning, (4) depression, and (5) a primary sleep disorder (e.g., apnea), (4) neurologically mediated hypotension (discussed above), (5) non-restorative sleep, and (6) growth hormone deficiency (Bennett et al., 1998). Non-pharmacological interventions are most effective in treating many of these causative factors. On the other hand, medication is a suitable treatment for endocrine dysfunction, depression, sleep issues, and other psychological stressors. Both chronic fatigue syndrome and fatigue related to fibromyalgia have been shown to benefit from recent studies employing the 5-HT3 receptor antagonist tropisetron (Spath et al., 2000). Anecdotal evidence suggests that modafinil (Provigil), a non-amphetamine medication used to treat narcolepsy and sleep deprivation, may help with non-specific fatigue (Lyons & French, 1991).

4.4.5. Sleep

The majority of people with fibromyalgia report being light sleepers who are easily startled by background sounds or bothersome thoughts. An alpha-delta EEG pattern is seen in many, which could account for why they never reach the restorative stages 3 and 4 of nonREM sleep (Drewes et al., 1995). Following the fundamental guidelines for good sleep hygiene and engaging in regular low-intensity exercise are crucial nonpharmacological components of sleep management. Low-dose tricyclic antidepressants (such as imipramine, doxepin, trazodone, and amitriptyline) are used has been the cornerstone of FM patients' sleep medication (Goldenberg, 1989; Carette et al., 1994). For many fibromyalgia patients, the level of daytime drowsiness or weight gain from TCAs is intolerable. Alprazolam (Russell et al., 1991), zolpidem (Moldofsky et al., 1996), and zopiclone (Drewes et al., 1991) are examples of benzodiazepine like drugs that have been shown in a few trials to be helpful in these patients. Some fibromyalgia patients have a primary sleep disorder that necessitates medical attention. Positive airway pressure (CPAP) or surgery is typically needed to treat sleep apnea, which affects 15% of female and 25% of male fibromyalgia patients. Restless leg syndrome, also known as periodic limb movement disorder, is by far the most prevalent sleep disorder among people with fibromyalgia. L-dopa/carbidopa (Sinemet 10/100 mg at suppertime) or clonazepam (Klonopin 0.5 or 1 mg at bedtime) are typically used as treatments (Montplaisir et al., 1992). Other dopamine agonists, including pergolide, tolixe pole, and pramixepole, have shown promise in more recent research.

4.4.6. Psychological Distress

An existential crisis-like series of emotional reactions can frequently result from having a chronic, painful disease for which there is currently no recognized cure (Chapman & Gavrin, 1999). About 60% of fibromyalgia patients have had depressive illness at some point in their lives, and 30% of them currently experience significant depression (Okifuji et al., 2000). Most people believe that treating fibromyalgia patients with depression is the same as treating patients with primary depressive illness. The topic of treating depression in patients with FM has not been the subject of any trials; nevertheless, Gruber et al. (1996) provided a helpful review of the literature on the subject. While antidepressant drugs are frequently prescribed to fibromyalgia patients for pain and sleep disorders, the dosages of these drugs are typically insufficient to treat depression. Additionally, patients with FM may be more susceptible to side effects from medication and may be taking numerous other medications that have the potential to interact negatively. Given that FM patients frequently experience stressors associated with psychosocial or economic problems, cognitive restructuring and problem-solving techniques therapy may be helpful adjuncts to medication therapy. Individuals who have trouble coping frequently have a tendency to over-dramatize negative life events that they believe they have no control over. For these patients, psychological intervention is crucial for enhancing the internal locus of control and facilitating more efficient problem-solving. Group therapy may help cognitive-behavioral therapy techniques, which seem especially well-suited to bringing about these changes (Goldenberg et al., 1994).

4.4.7. Deconditioning

The widely acknowledged modern reality that "exercise is good for fibromyalgia patients" (Clark et al., 2001) is backed by numerous studies. While there is solid scientific evidence supporting the benefits of exercise, there is also a potential risk (Mengshoel et al., 1995). The benefits and drawbacks of exercise for individuals with fibromyalgia likely depend on a variety of factors, including age, level of conditioning at the moment, rate of intensity increase, frequency of exercise, ratio of eccentric to concentric muscle use, hormonal anabolic status, and negative factors like obesity, arthritis, and concurrent muscle disease. The overtraining syndrome and the symptomatology of fibromyalgia share certain similarities. According to Urhausen et al. (1998), overtraining causes a syndrome that includes decreased performance, depression, chronic fatigue, altered hormonal stress responses, and an increased risk of infections and muscle damage. To maximize the benefits and reduce increased pain and fatigue, an individual exercise program must always be carefully planned (Clark, 1994).

4.4.8. Endocrine Dysfunction

There is insufficient evidence to conclude that an endocrine disorder is the primary cause of fibromyalgia. However, common issues like menopausal symptoms and hypothyroidism frequently exacerbate pain and fatigue, necessitating the use of appropriate replacement therapy. The hypothalamic-pituitary-adrenal (HPA) axis abnormalities in fibromyalgia patients have drawn a lot of attention (Crofford et al., 1994; Pillemer et al., 1997). Patients with fibromyalgia are generally thought to have a somewhat lower HPA responsiveness. However, it was not demonstrated that replacement therapy using 15 mg/day of Prednisone was therapeutically helpful for fibromyalgia (Clark et al., 1985). Growth hormone deficiency affects about one-third of fibromyalgia patients (Bennett et al., 1997), and replacement therapy has been shown to help these patients (Bennett et al., 1998).

4.4.9. Associated Disorders

An essential component of the overall management plan is the identification and treatment of issues that are frequently linked to fibromyalgia.

- **Chronic Fatigue:** The following are common, treatable causes of persistent fatigue in fibromyalgia patients: (1) mishandled medication dosage (TCAs, antihistamine-acting medications, benzodiazepines, etc.). 2), (3) aerobic deconditioning, (4) depression, and (5) a primary sleep disorder (e.g., sleep apnea, growth hormone deficiency, neurally mediated hypotension, non-restorative sleep), and (5) sleep apnea (Bennett et al., 1997, 1998).
- **Restless Leg Syndrome:** L-dopa/levodopa (Sinemet) in an early evening dose of 10/100 mg is a straightforward and highly effective treatment (a minority requires a higher dose or use of the long-acting preparations). Gabapentin works for certain patients. Low-dose opioid therapy frequently helps cases that are resistant to treatment.
- **Irritable Bowel Syndrome:** The treatment plan includes removing trigger foods, managing stress, following a regular bowel routine, and using medications to address specific symptoms like constipation (such as stool softeners, fiber supplements, and gentle laxatives), diarrhea (like loperamide or diphenoxylate), and antispasmodics (including dicycloverine or anticholinergic/sedative drugs like Donnatal).
- **Irritable Bladder Syndrome:** Increasing water intake, avoiding bladder irritants like fruit juices (especially cranberry), and performing pelvic floor exercises (e.g., Kegel exercises), and (4) antispasmodic drug prescriptions (e.g., hyoscyamine, flavoxate, and oxybutinin).

- **Cognitive Dysfunction:** A lot of people with fibromyalgia deal with this issue frequently. It has a negative impact on one's capacity to find competitive employment and raises the possibility of an early-stage neurodegenerative disease. Patients can feel reassured as the latter concern has never presented a problem in practice. For most patients, the distracting effects of long-term pain and mental exhaustion are the cause of memory loss and concentration issues. As a result, treating cognitive dysfunction in fibromyalgia effectively depends on managing the other symptoms as well.
- **Cold Intolerance:** Keeping warm, low-grade aerobic exercise (which enhances peripheral circulation), treating neurally mediated hypotension (see below), and prescribing vasodilators like calcium channel blockers (although these may exacerbate the condition in patients with hypotension) are the four main forms of treatment.
- **Multiple Sensitivities:** Using avoidance strategies and acknowledging that this is a fibromyalgia-related issue are part of the treatment. It's common to start taking medications at half the recommended dosage.
- **Dizziness:** There are several treatable causes of fibromyalgia: (1) deconditioning of the muscles leading to proprioceptive dysfunction; (2) myofascial trigger points in the 104 sterno-cleido-mastoids and other neck muscles; (3) neurally mediated hypotension (see below); and (4) adverse drug reactions. A correct diagnosis is necessary before beginning treatment.
- **Neurally Mediated Hypotension:** Treatment consists of three steps: (1) educating patients about the triggering factors and how to avoid them; (2) raising plasma volume (salinizing more, prescribing florinef); and (3) avoiding medications that worsen hypotension (e.g., TCAs, antihypertensives), (4) decreasing the reflex's efferent limb (α-adrenergic agonists or anticholinergic agents), and (5) preventing the reflex (β-adrenergic antagonists or disopyramide).

4.4.10. Multidisciplinary Team Therapy

The majority of management recommendations are predicated on a one-on-one doctor-patient interaction. The needs of these patients are frequently difficult to meet in the age of cost-effective medicine. Nonetheless, a group of interested medical professionals (nurses, clinical psychologists, exercise physiologists, mental health care providers, and social workers) can implement the majority of these same recommendations into a multidisciplinary treatment program (Goldenberg, 1989; Bennett, 1996b; Turk et al., 1998). In this manner, several times a month, groups of 5 to 15 patients can be seen in scheduled sessions. Patients are typically grateful to connect with others who are experiencing similar issues, and group therapy's dynamics are frequently a potent tool for helping patients change their cognitive and behavioral patterns. It is possible to foster a sense of camaraderie among these groups as they work together to solve problems. According to Bennett et al. (1996), this type of therapy has shown promise in a single 6-month program, with improvements lasting up to two years after the program ends.

4.5. Abdominal Pain

Most patients who present with abdominal pain, a common symptom that affects people of all ages, have no apparent physical cause for their pain, and most of the time the symptoms are transient. Therefore, when we categorize abdominal pain as organic or non-organic, we are really referring to the cause that led up to it. Even non-organic pain frequently has a well-defined physiological mechanism, but the presence of a pathological process that causes pain may depend on psychological factors.

Abdominal pain that starts suddenly is a very common and significant diagnostic issue. Fewer than 5% of young individuals who exhibit this symptom get hospitalized for observation, and even fewer have surgery (Stevenson, 1985). Identifying the central abdomen and the four quadrants of the abdomen, then talking about the differential diagnosis for each quadrant, is a useful diagnostic strategy.

4.5.1. Right Lower Quadrant Pain

4.5.1.1. Acute Appendicitis

Acute appendicitis is the primary differential diagnosis for right lower quadrant pain, particularly in male children (Michalowski et al., 2001). The pain, which is frequently linked to anorexia, nausea, and frequent vomiting, usually begins in the periumbilical region and spreads to the lower right quadrant after a few hours. It is also frequently accompanied by a mild fever of 39°C, either with or without frequent bowel movements or micturition. The clinical challenge lies in correctly diagnosing appendicitis to avoid needless surgery as well as in detecting it early enough to avoid complications like perforation that raise morbidity. Asking about prior similar attacks is crucial because up to 10% of patients may have recurrent appendicitis (Barber et al., 1997). Except for patients with retrocaecal appendix, who are particularly tender in the right side on rectal examination, the patient is typically extremely tender in the right lower quadrant and feels as though there is a mass there. It's unlikely that an abdominal X-ray will reveal any diagnostic information. Urinalysis reveals more white blood cells, and blood tests typically show a polymorphonuclear leucocytosis, typically >20,000/mm (Barber et al., 1997; Michalowski et al., 2001). In one study, a straightforward 24-hour observation period more than halved the >40% incidence of negative surgical explorations in uncertain cases, with over 60% of admissions finding to have an infection not requiring surgery (Wenham, 1982).

Appendiceal ultrasonography was added, and as a result, no patients had unnecessary surgeries for a normal appendix (100% specificity), but the sensitivity was only 75% (Puylaert et al., 1987). Laparoscopy has been added because the differential diagnosis in women is longer. This decreased the percentage of needless appendicectomy cases from 37 to 7% (Olsen et al., 1993).

A study conducted on 100 consecutive patients recently found that routine appendiceal computed tomography (CT) was 98% accurate. This resulted in 59 patients having their recommended management changed, including the recommendation for unnecessary surgery or admission for a 24-hour observation period (Rao et al., 1998). Although there were overall savings of $447 per patient, CT is more expensive and radiation-intensive than ultrasound. Therefore, it is important to maintain clinical skills and foster proficiency in appendiceal ultrasound (McColl, 1998).

4.5.1.2. Mesenteric Lymphadenitis

There are many different diagnoses in this case. Mesenteric lymphadenitis is a likely substitute in children and young adolescents, who present with acute appendicitis most frequently. This typically happens in the context of an upper respiratory tract virus "epidemic" or contact history. The patients' symptoms are similar to those of acute appendicitis. One useful point of differentiation in mesenteric lymphadenitis is that, although it can be unexpectedly high, the white blood count is typically normal with a relative lymphocytosis. In the hopes of lowering the number of young people with this condition who have a normal appendix removed, abdominal imaging should show lymphadenopathy along with a normal appendix.

4.5.1.3. Infective Distal Ileocaecitis

Acute appendicitis is typically associated with fewer systemic symptoms than infectious ileocaecitis. Patients who have consumed potentially contaminated water or swum in lakes frequently report having distal ileitis caused by Yersinia. It is recommended to conduct serial serological investigations for Yersinia (Attwood et al., 1987). The growing number of immunocompromised patients has resulted in a significant extension of the differential diagnosis for infective ileocaecitis.

4.5.1.4. Crohn's Disease

Individuals diagnosed with Crohn's disease typically report a history of recurrent episodes of abdominal pain, including distension, changes in bowel habits, and weight loss, either alone or in conjunction with other systemic symptoms. A mass in the lower right quadrant is the most significant differential diagnostic sign found during examination. While barium radiographs are useful for diagnosing Crohn's disease, non-invasive imaging is preferred for additional diagnostic support when a patient has an acute appendicitis differential diagnosis.

4.5.1.5. Ovarian Tubular Disorders

Ovarian tumors become more significant in young women in their third and fourth decades of life. Consequently, getting a thorough menstrual history is crucial. While a history of promiscuity would point to the possibility of acute salpingitis, a period of amenorrhea suggests the possibility of an ectopic pregnancy. But typically, this is bilateral. When a vaginal examination is performed, these conditions typically result in tenderness.

4.5.1.6. Renal and Ureteric Colic

Renal colic begins on either side of the flank and spreads to the groin and surrounding area. Usually, a ureteric calculus that causes obstruction passes from the renal pelvis into the ureter. The colicky pain, which is caused by more peristaltic contractions as the calculus is pushed farther toward the bladder, usually comes in waves and intensifies gradually, making the patient sweat and queasy. Even though there is still soreness after the pain wave passes, the patient experiences significant relief until the next one starts. The calculous is typically visible on an ultrasound or flat plate scan of the abdomen.

4.5.2. Right Upper Quadrant Pain

- **Biliary Colic and Acute Cholecystitis:** Usually originating in the upper right quadrant, biliary colic radiates to the back, sometimes accompanied by pain that is referred to the tip of the right shoulder. These individuals frequently have right upper quadrant tenderness, especially during deep inspiration. In contrast, the right upper quadrant is extremely tender and the patient experiences continuous pain when they have acute gallbladder inflammation or cholecystitis without the passage of a gallstone. Acute hepatic congestion and duodenal ulcer perforation are two additional conditions that need to be taken into account when dealing with acute right upper quadrant pain.
- **Acute Duodenal Ulcer Perforation:** Pain results from a duodenal ulcers

acute perforation. Stress frequently triggers acute ulcers. Following the abrupt onset of intense pain in the area, peritonism symptoms and signs such as "guarding" and "boardlike" rigidity of the anterior abdominal wall appear. Under the right diaphragm, a straight abdominal radiograph may reveal a gas shadow outside the duodenal lumen.

- **Acute Hepatic Congestion:** The liver, which is the main organ in the right upper quadrant, can occasionally cause acute pain that is typically accompanied by acute enlargement and stretching of the hepatic capsule. This can happen because of acute congestion brought on by acute heart failure or hepatic vein obstruction, which is known as the Budd-Chiari syndrome, or because of inflammation, as in acute viral hepatitis. Every condition causes varying degrees of jaundice as well as an abrupt release of hepatic enzymes into the bloodstream, particularly transaminases, which can range in level from less than 50 to more than 1,000 IU/L.

If there is a suspicion of acute Budd-Chiari syndrome, a liver-spleen radionuclide scan may reveal the distinct pattern of hepatic "wipe-out," along with the caudate lobe being spared or experiencing hypertrophy due to direct drainage into the inferior vena cava. Confirmation of the diagnosis requires a Doppler ultrasound of the hepatic veins and hepatic venography to visualize the blockage.

4.5.3. Central Abdomen

4.5.3.1. Colic of the Small Intestine

The most common cause of intestinal colic is acute bowel inflammation, such as acute gastroenteritis, which manifests as acute nausea with or without vomiting and crampy or colicky abdominal pain that is frequently relieved by passing loose or watery stools. The infection can be bacterial, parasitic, or viral—usually contracted during an epidemic—from tainted food or water. Stool culture and microscopic analysis for parasites, ova, and inflammatory cells may be diagnostic methods. On the other hand, depending on the location and the patient's age, intestinal obstruction may be the secondary cause of intestinal colic. Abdominal distension and partial or total constipation are linked to this. Vomiting is related to the obstruction site; the likelihood of vomiting is higher the closer the lesion is to the site.

The conditions that cause colic are best diagnosed using non-invasive methods. A non-calcified stone may be seen on ultrasonography, but a calcified stone in the ureter, gallbladder, or bile duct may be visible on a flat plate of the abdomen. When there is an intestinal blockage, both a supine and an erect film will demonstrate intestinal distension near the obstruction, while the erect film will demonstrate various air–fluid levels.

4.5.3.2. Acute Pancreatitis

Pancreatic pain is one of the rare pains that starts in the middle of the abdomen. One of the worst pains there is acute pancreatitis, which can have several causes. When none of these factors are present, idiopathic acute pancreatitis (IAP) is diagnosed. A variety of unexpected diagnoses may be found with endoscopic ultrasound. Pancreatitis causes constant central pain that typically radiates to the back. Traditionally, patients have found relief by sitting forward and cradling their knees. Deep palpation may reveal tenderness in the patient during examination. Significantly elevated pancreatic enzymes, serum amylase, and particularly lipase, confirm the diagnosis. The sensitivity and specificity of this test are

75% and 90%, respectively. More recently, it was demonstrated that a urine trypsinogen-2 dipstick test had a 95% negative predictive value, 95% sensitivity, and 95% specificity (Kemppainen et al., 1997).

4.5.3.3. Abdominal Angina

Intestinal ischemia may be the cause of central abdominal pain that is more often felt after large meals than after small ones. Only angiographic evidence of constricted coeliac or superior mesenteric vessels, along with evidence of a pressure differential across the stricture, can establish the diagnosis.

4.5.4. Left Upper Quadrant

- **Splenic Pain:** The spleen, located in the left upper quadrant, is rarely painful unless it is involved in a serositis, as in familial Mediterranean fever, or after a splenic infarct. Much more frequently, when the spleen enlarges for any reason, it hurts or feels like it's dragging.
- **Splenic Flexure of the Colon:** Although this usually happens in the transverse or descending colon, the splenic flexure of the colon may cause pain if it becomes acutely distended, as in the case of patients with toxic megacolon secondary to ulcerative colitis. Elderly patients with ischemic colitis frequently involve this site, and secondary stricture formation may happen there as well.
- **Miscellaneous:** This region may experience pain that comes from the tail of an inflamed pancreas or from distension or ulceration in the stomach.

4.5.5. Left Lower Quadrant

- **Acute Diverticulitis:** When an elderly patient has acute diverticulitis, the typical location of pain is the left lower quadrant. They typically experience pain, fever, and either constipation or bloody stools. Upon inspection, they might have an uncomfortable lump.
- **Non-specific Ulcerative Colitis:** The left lower quadrant is where ulcerative colitis patients experience pain the most frequently. The patient frequently has tenderness over the colon's descent. By observing the typical features of the colonic and rectal mucosa colonoscopy, the diagnosis is made. However, because it spreads proximally, it can affect any portion of the colon and, as a result, cause pain and tenderness over the colon's surface markings, particularly in patients who have toxic megacolon.
- **Peritonitis:** Acute peritonitis typically results from direct contact with an inflammatory organ, like the pancreas, or from a viscus perforation. Despite the possibility of beginning in the region of the perforated organ, the pain is typically widespread. The patient learns to lie very still because the pain intensifies with any movement of the abdomen. Examining the abdomen reveals that it is motionless and that breathing is not occurring in the anterior abdominal wall. When the anterior abdominal wall muscles "guard" the inflamed mucosa underneath, it feels "boardlike" to the touch. Loss of intestinal sounds occurs as a result of peritonitis because the inflammation paralyzes the intestines and causes an ileus. Large dilated loops of both large and small bowel, as well as extraluminal collections, are visible on abdominal radiographs and ultrasounds.

From a clinical perspective, the doctor has the following choices to make. Is surgery the cause? The management of a perforation, medical, infected, or noninfected inflammation depends on its cause.

4.5.6. Diagnosis of Difficult Cases of Acute Abdominal Pain

The possibility that a generalized medical condition could manifest as acute abdominal pain is something that all doctors need to be aware of. The diagnostic technique of fine catheter aspiration cytology may be used when the cause of acute abdominal pain is unclear and laparotomy is a possibility (Stewart et al., 1986). The cytosieve method was used to prepare cytological specimens, and 500 cells were counted to determine the neutrophil count. 27 patients had a successful test. In 14 patients before the test, the prelaparotomy diagnosis was accurate; in 20 patients following the test, it was not.

4.6. Chronic Abdominal Pain

4.6.1. Chronic Abdominal Wall Pain

It's critical to rule out pain coming from the anterior abdominal wall before talking about the causes of chronic visceral pain. This is primarily accomplished by taking this diagnosis into account and then searching for the typical examination findings of this pain, which include superficial tenderness that endures when the patient tenses the anterior abdominal wall. The local anesthetic should be injected directly into the tender area, and the pain and tenderness should go away afterward. The anterior cutaneous branch of the thoracoabdominal nerve being trapped and stretched is the most likely cause of this pain, which can be treated with a local anesthetic injection. It is necessary to rule out the possibility of a small ventral hernia, though.

4.6.2. Organic causes of Chronic Abdominal Pain

4.6.2.1. Atypical Gastro-Oesophageal Reflux Disorders (GERD)

A small percentage of GERD patients experience epigastric pain, despite the fact that heartburn and other thoracic symptoms characterize the great majority of cases. When any of the following tests are suspected, some or all of them is needed to make the diagnosis: endoscopy with biopsy, manometry with 24-hour monitoring for acid reflux, radionuclide technetium swallows for reflux, and serological tests for H. pylori. pylori. If it is, treating it with triple therapy—which includes using a proton pump inhibitor—to eradicate the infection could provide some relief (Klinkenberg-Knol et al., 2000).

4.6.2.2. Gastric Ulcer

Patients who have gastric ulcers often report experiencing intermittent pain in the upper abdomen spanning a considerable area. This pain is usually associated with meals and usually starts shortly after the patient eats. Antacid medications typically provide some degree of pain relief. Patients with gastric ulcers may experience mild weight loss in correlation with reduced food consumption. It is now evident that *Helicobacter pylori* infection plays a major role in the etiology of peptic ulcer disease. The cagA genotype of *Helicobacter pylori* causes inflammation and ulceration by infecting the mucosal environment. The therapy is one of several one-week courses of triple therapy (Maastricht Consensus Report, 1997) that includes two antibiotics and antacid therapy, such as a proton pump inhibitor.

4.6.2.3. Gastric Malignancy

The primary differential diagnosis in gastric ulcer treatment is the presence or absence of malignancy. Malignant ulcers typically cause unusual, continuous pain that is unrelated to meals, but they can also cause anorexia and significant weight loss. Dysphagia and regurgitation are brought on by fundic cancer, while vomiting and gastric outlet obstruction are caused by prepyloric lesions.

Up to 10% of stomach cancers are primary low-grade lymphomas of the mucosaassociated lymphoid tissue (MALT). This type of cancer is comparatively uncommon. It's evident now that H. pylori infection plays a role in the pathogenesis of lymphoma and stomach cancer, and eliminating the infection may cause the lymphoma to go away (Sackman et al., 1997).

4.6.2.4. Duodenal Ulcer

With or without radiation through to the back, patients with duodenal ulcers can frequently localize their epigastric pain with one finger. This pain is typically located to the right of the midline or very high up in the midline. Additionally, the pain is typically associated with fasting, waking the patient up in the wee hours of the morning and going away when food, liquids, or antacid medication are consumed.

These days, unusual symptoms include vomiting, nausea, and distension in the abdomen. Because they eat frequently to ease their pain, these patients may gain weight rather than lose it.

4.6.2.5. Treatment

The goal of therapy is to eradicate H pylori once the diagnosis has been made. pylori infection, using a combination of triple therapies. In addition to antacid therapy with a proton pump inhibitor, H2-receptor antagonist, or bismuth compound, these usually involve two antibiotics, such as clarithromycin, amoxicillin, tetracycline, with or without metronidazole (Wyeth et al., 1996; Maastricht Consensus, Report, 1997).

4.6.2.6. Gastroparesis

There's no denying that pain can result from gastric distension. Patients with gastroparesis, the majority of whom have diabetes, provide some of the best evidence. This was once believed to be only mildly treatable with prokinetic medications. Recently, cardiac pacing wires implanted on the serosal surface have been used in conjunction with gastric pacing. Gastric emptying and symptoms, including pain, improved when pacing entrained the stomach slow wave and transformed tachygastria into regular 3-cpm slow waves (McCallum et al., 1998). Moreover, a recent study has demonstrated that somatic pain processing-related structures are activated by symptomatic gastric distension (Ladabaum et al., 2001).

4.6.2.7. Chronic Intestinal Pseudo-Obstruction

Intestinal distension, the migrating motor complex, and peristaltic control loss are caused by disorders of the smooth muscle and myenteric plexus. The patient's symptoms may initially resemble IBS and then progress to chronic intestinal obstruction, which includes pain and distension in the abdomen, either with or without vomiting, and diarrhea brought on by bacterial overgrowth and malabsorption. Alternatively, the esophagus, stomach, or colon may be affected, resulting in constipation or gastroparesis. Drug use may run in the family or have a previous history.

As a result, to make the diagnosis, the patient will undergo a clinical history, examination, radiography, endoscopy, and surgery with an intestinal wall full-thickness biopsy. Patients with inflammatory degenerative neuropathy have recently been found to have antibodies against the enteric nervous system. The diagnosis will determine the course of treatment.

4.6.2.8. Chronic Pancreatitis and Carcinoma of the Pancreas

Less than 10% of patients experience the development of chronic pancreatitis after an episode of acute pancreatitis. Most of these patients have chronic relapsing pancreatitis, which causes recurrent episodes of pain that resemble the acute attacks linked to elevated pancreatic enzymes. Less than 20% of people have chronically persistent pain. This pain is explained by two theories. First, there is inflammatory or scar tissue that affects the pancreatic nerves; in this case, a medical nerve block is the recommended course of treatment. The second explanation is that stricture formation-related pancreatic ductular hypertension is the cause of the pain. Attempting to lower pancreatic secretion is the medical treatment for this. According to Amman and Muelhaupt (1999), patients with alcoholic chronic pancreatitis may benefit from quitting drinking, and many can anticipate their pain subsiding in 7 to 10 years.

Pancreatic cancer typically causes deep, center-abdominal pain that radiates to the back. It has nothing to do with meals; it's a typical severe pain that calls for strong analgesics. Abdominal CT is the preferred test once the diagnosis is suspected because it can reveal pancreatic enlargement. Endoscopic retrograde cholangiopancreatography (ERCP) examination can verify this. Regretfully, the percentage of these cancers that can be operated on is quite low.

4.6.2.9. Gastrointestinal Food Hypersensitivity

The recent release of the document outlining the AGA's official recommendation has provided clarification on the assessment of food allergies (Sampson et al., 2001). It is a real thing that usually consists of nuts, eggs, fish, and proteins from cow's milk and soy. Particularly in atopic infants, there is a distinct symptom complex that includes bloating, abdominal pain, and diarrhea. Adults with such allergies are rarely found to have them. Identifying the potential cause and eliminating the offending food can cause symptoms to go away, regardless of the exact mechanism.

4.6.2.10. Unusual Causes

Lastly, if a diagnosis cannot be made, the doctor needs to be aware of the numerous uncommon causes of persistent abdominal pain, which include grumbling appendicitis, which can be diagnosed with a colonoscopy if inflammation appears to be localized to the appendix's root in the caecal region (Johnson & De Cosse, 1998), leishmaniasis (Magill et al., 1993), and mesenteric panniculitis (sclerosing mesocolitis, Weber-Christian disease) (Steely & Gooden, 1986).

4.6.2.11. Carbohydrate Maldigestion and Malabsorption

Through colonic bacterial fermentation, five grams of indigestible carbohydrates can yield 1,000 milliliters of carbon dioxide, 400 milliliters of methane (in methane producers), and 200 milliliters of hydrogen (Hightower, 1977). However, recent research has demonstrated that it's critical to differentiate between bloating that occurs in irritable bowel syndrome with normal gas production and excess gas formation, as in hypolactasia (Levitt et al., 1996).

4.6.2.12. Hypolactasia

In many regions of the world, intestinal lactase deficiency is highly prevalent. As a result, lactose malabsorption happens when milk or some dairy products are consumed, which causes colonic gaseous fermentation, cramping pain in the abdomen surrounding the colon, diarrhea, and excessive flatus. The lactose hydrogen breath test (Metz et al., 1975) can confirm the diagnosis, which can also be made based on the patient's history. A lactose-free diet helped 24% of the 137 children with recurrent abdominal pain who had lactose maldigestion (Webster et al., 1995). The patient is first put on a gluten-free diet to treat any underlying pathology, such as celiac syndrome, and then they are placed on a lactose-free diet. Alternatively, dairy products and milk can be given along with synthetic lactases if the patient requires them or enjoys them.

4.6.2.13. Hyposucrasia and Multiple Sugar Malabsorptions

Other disaccharidase deficiencies are either rare or never occur due to their position further down the villi and their greater number and quantity. For instance, sucrase deficiency case reports are scarce. After consuming foods containing sucrose, the patients exhibit similar symptoms. The sucrose hydrogen breath test (Metz et al., 1976a) is used to diagnose the patients, and the removal of sucrose from the diet is the method of treatment. If symptoms do not improve, patients may present with non-ulcer dyspepsia and other sugars such as fructose and sorbitol may be involved (Mishkin et al., 1997).

4.6.2.14. Stagnant Loop Syndrome

Patients with small intestinal bacterial colonization may also experience maldigestion of carbohydrates. Bacteria are typically "swept downstream" with food after meals when the upper small intestine becomes significantly colonized. Malabsorption occurs when luminar contents in patients with specific small intestine pathologies stagnate and become colonized. Examples of this include radiation enteropathy, jejunal diverticulosis, fistulae causing a blind loop, such as Crohn's disease, systemic sclerosis of the duodenum and jejunum, and incomplete obstruction (Newman et al., 1973). These circumstances are collectively referred to as "stagnant loop syndrome," and if they occur close together, they cause monosaccharide fermentation, which raises the amount of hydrogen produced from glucose (Metz et al., 1976b). A stagnant loop can be diagnosed based on signs of vitamin B12 or bile acid malabsorption, and radiology can confirm the diagnosis by showing the lesion anatomically.

4.6.2.15. Colonic Maldigestion

Normal colonic "maldigestion" of carbohydrates happens when a diet high in indigestible carbohydrates is consumed. Gaseous abdominal pain can be brought on by an excessive amount of unabsorbed carbohydrates, such as those found in fruit, vegetables, or sorbitol in chewing gum.

4.6.2.16. Constipation

Constipated people experience cramping pain in their colons from the accumulation of gas and feces. This can happen to older people, in the absence of any colonic pathology, or in conjunction with a colon disease called diverticular disease. Clinical examination and flat plate abdominal imaging are used to make this diagnosis. Treatment entails returning bowel movements to normal while using a combination of laxatives, diet, and, if required, colonic lavage. In children, constipation is also a particularly common cause of abdominal pain; however, it is necessary to rule out several other possible causes first (Seth and Heyman, 1994).

4.6.3. Non-Organic or Psychogenic Pain

1. The location, distribution, timing, quality, and intensity of the pain do not relate to established pathophysiological patterns.
2. There is often a marked discrepancy between the severity of the pain and the patient's behavior.
3. The patient usually has or has had

multiple pains in many other parts of the body, which may have been fully investigated without any obvious abnormality being discovered. In other words, the patient is 'pain prone.'

4. The onset of pain may bear an obvious temporal relationship to stress. This is particularly the case with bereavement, where the onset may coincide with the death of a close relative or friend in whom abdominal pain may have been a major symptom.

The abdomen is the second most common site in patients with chronic pain (Merskey, 1965). Chronic abdominal pain is functional in most older children and adolescents (Daum, 1997). Further understanding of this issue and advancements in therapy should result from extensive research into the relationships between the brain and the gut (Aziz and Thompson, 1998).

4.6.4. Gaseous Distension Syndromes

4.6.4.1. Aerophagy

Acute pharyngitis and peptic esophagitis are two organic conditions that can cause pain or discomfort in the pharynx and esophagus and lead to aerophagy, or excessive air swallowing. Swallowing air causes the patient to feel some temporary relief from discomfort because it is assumed that this creates an air "cushion" between the inflammatory surfaces.

Anxiety and depression are among the non-organic, far more prevalent causes of aerophagy (Song et al., 1993). When swallowing food, anxious people often swallow more air, eat faster, and inhale excessive amounts of air. This causes food to accumulate in the stomach's fundus, which stimulates stretch receptors in the viscera's wall, causing discomfort and eventually pain throughout the gastrointestinal tract. Belching out the air will then provide the patient with momentary relief, and the process is repeated. There was a high rate of bereavement of a close relative who passed away from stomach pain in one series. Antidepressant treatment alleviated the pain in a small subset of these patients (Blendis et al., 1978).

4.6.4.2. Non-ulcer Dyspepsia

Upon examination, it is discovered that 30–60% of patients who report non-specific upper abdominal pain or dyspepsia have an *H pylori* infection. Whether this infection is the source of the symptoms is still unknown. Triple therapy may help some patients' symptoms go away, but there is no proof that it is any more effective than a placebo (Blum et al., 1998; Talley et al., 1999). However, this is still a persistent problem, and some writers continue to support triple therapy for functional dyspepsia with *H. pylori* positivity (McColl et al., 1998). Alternative therapy, such as psychodynamic-interpersonal psychotherapy, may be beneficial if symptoms continue after successful eradication (Hamilton et al., 2000). Alternatively, there might be another reason. In a referral center, for instance, delayed gastric emptying with gastric distension has been found in as many as 35% of 116 dyspeptic patients (Stanghellini et al., 1996). This syndrome tended to respond to prokinetic agents and was linked to female sex, postprandial fullness, and vomiting.

4.6.5. Irritable Bowel Syndrome

4.6.5.1. Definition

As stated at the beginning of the chapter, the majority of people experience non-organic abdominal pain occasionally, which is often linked to stress or occurs after a gastroenteritis episode. For most people, though, the symptoms eventually go away. As a result, up to 15% of children may experience irritable bowel syndrome (IBS), which is defined as symptoms that persist for more than three months (Milla,

2001). Therefore, symptoms of abdominal pain and irregular bowel movements lasting longer than 12 weeks without an organic cause can be classified as IBS. Nonetheless, given that 50% of patients may experience symptom changes from one category to another over a one-year period, classifying patients as having non-ulcer dyspepsia or IBS may be artificial (Agreus et al., 1995).

4.6.5.2. Incidence

Studies conducted recently in the United States suggest that 20–30% of people have IBS symptoms. Females are affected by IBS more frequently than males; ratios in published series range from 1:5:1. According to a published study, there may be a history of physical and/or sexual abuse in up to 44% of women who present with IBS (Drossman et al., 1990). The third decade is the peak age of onset. Nonetheless, according to Hahn et al. (1997), up to 70% of people with the same IBS symptoms choose not to seek medical assistance.

4.6.5.3. Clinical Features

In children, abdominal pain is primarily periumbilical (Milla et al., 2001), but in adults, it typically occurs over the colon's surface markings, with the left lower quadrant being the most common site and the right or left upper quadrant over the hepatic or splenic flexures being less common. It rarely keeps the patient awake at night, but it can range in intensity from a dull ache to severe attacks that last for minutes, hours, or even the entire day. "Air trapping," which results in the segmental accumulation of gas, is the cause of "meteorism."

Up to 90% of patients experience constipation, diarrhea, or altered bowel habits. Defecation relieves pain and eating aggravates it in about half of the patients. But since the patient's appetite is rarely impacted, a history of notable weight loss (i.e., more than 3.5 kg – I think it is important to state in what time length does the weight loss need to happen to be out of the ordinary) is out of the ordinary and should prompt consideration of a different diagnosis.

IBS symptoms can start after a gastroenteritis attack. IBS pain is linked to nausea without vomiting, dyspepsia, urinary symptoms, particularly dysuria, gynecological symptoms, particularly dysmenorrhea, and headaches (Gwee et al., 1999). Compared to 32% of age-matched controls, 60% of women visiting gynecological clinics, 40% undergoing elective hysterectomy, and 60% undergoing dilatation and curettage for dysmenorrhea, may have had pelvic pain due to IBS (Crowell et al., 1994). They frequently had an appendectomy for "chronic appendicitis" in the past. Another common observation with these patients is their fear of cancer.

The Rome II Criteria were recently refined at a second IBS conference held in Rome. Although the Rome II Criteria are great for bringing discipline and standardization to the field of therapeutic trials, their extreme rigidity creates artificial constraints that will need to be reviewed in the future (Camilleri, 1998). Examining the patient reveals that, although appearing well, there is typically a discrepancy between the severity of their symptoms and their physical state. A particular region of the colon, usually the descending colon, will cause the patient to become tender. A rectal examination reveals that some patients are extremely tender. Sigmoidoscopic examination is typically normal, but because of pain and spasms, it is very difficult to go past the rectosigmoid junction. Using a sigmoidoscope, the patients may also exhibit mucosal hyperalgesia to light touch. Sedimentation rate is one of the routine blood tests that should be normal.

4.6.5.4. Psyche

There is a lot of historical data supporting affective disorders. Although insomnia may also be an issue, persistent fatigue is nearly universal, with some patients reporting tiredness even after getting a full night's sleep. On the other hand, they might experience depression and often feel like crying. Even in patients who had acute gastroenteritis prior to developing IBS, the patients' formal testing results showed higher scores for anxiety, neuroticism, and introversion compared to either normal controls or patients with ulcerative colitis. Their neurosis score fell between normal and frank neurosis. (Gwee et al., 1999). However, according to Kumar et al. (1990), the psychological abnormalities associated with IBS may not be the primary cause of the disorder but rather be a determinant of the patient's decision to seek medical attention (Smith et al., 1990).

4.6.5.5. Investigations

Any indication of leucocytosis, anemia, etc., should be looked into more to rule out other illnesses like inflammatory bowel disease. A barium enema or colonoscopy is eventually performed on most of these patients, which is normal aside from varying degrees of spasm, even though it's important psychologically not to overinvestigate them. According to Bohmer and Tuynman (1996), up to 25% of patients may be lactose intolerant or have another type of dietary intolerance (Nanda et al., 1989). Eliminating the problematic food may cause a noticeable improvement in symptoms.

4.6.5.6. Motility Studies

Although studies on the motility of the small intestine, upper gastrointestinal tract, and even the esophagus have revealed abnormalities linked to hypersensitivity of lumbar splanchnic afferents, colon motility has often been demonstrated to be abnormal in IBS patients (Lembo et al., 1994; Accarino et al., 1995). According to van Ginkel et al. (2001), distension of the relevant intestinal region, particularly the distal colon and rectum, in adults and particularly in children, replicated the pain, with pain thresholds lower than those of normal volunteers—a phenomenon now known as hypersensitivity (Mayer and Gebhart, 1994).

Clinically, patients were separated into constipated and diarrheal types. The former had decreased colonic activity and was linked to a cholinergic disorder, while the latter had increased and disordered colonic motor activity and was linked to an adrenergic abnormality (Aggarwal et al., 1994).

4.6.5.7. Treatment

A compassionate, understanding, and sometimes creative doctor who is willing to spend time talking with the patient about their symptoms and the etiology of IBS is essential to the treatment of IBS. Though it is not generally accepted, a high-fiber diet utilizing soluble, cereal fiber, like natural bran, has been suggested as the foundation of therapy in an effort to normalize intestinal transit. Since lactose, fructose, or sorbitol consumption frequently triggers abdominal symptoms in IBS patients, it is worthwhile to try eliminating each of these carbohydrates from the diet one at a time. In addition, constipated patients may benefit from using stool-softening medications like diocyte sodium 100 mg twice a day. Patients with cramps and bloating have been treated with antispasmodic drugs, either with or without sedatives, with varying degrees of success (Jailwala et al., 2000). Since serotonin reuptake antagonists and tricyclic antidepressants have neuromodulatory and analgesic effects at lower dosages, they have been recommended for patients who experience severe pain regularly (Jackson et al., 2000). Despite placebo response rates of more than 50%, they are successful in randomized controlled trials (Drossman et al.,

1997). Whether tricyclics specifically act as an antidepressant in IBS remains to be determined (Jackson et al., 2000). Brain-gut function is modulated in large part by serotonin. In patients with diarrhea-predominant IBS, the use of 5-HT3 receptor inhibitors, such as ondanstron, improved stool consistency and decreased frequency. Alosetron improved pain both directly by increasing compliance to distension and indirectly by inhibiting the activation of spinal cord neurons by colonic distension. Alosetron primarily inhibited diarrhea by slowing left colonic transit. One such randomized controlled trial involved 1 mg of alosetron. I. d. caused a noticeable three-month improvement in pain and bowel function over a 12-week period, but it also increased constipation when compared to a placebo (Camilleri et al., 2000). Regretfully, there have been numerous reports of serious side effects, such as complete constipation with fecal impaction and ischemic colitis, since the FDA approved this extremely promising therapy (Friedel et al., 2001). Tegaserod, a 2 mg b (i. d) partial agonist of the 5-HT4 receptor. was demonstrated to be more effective than a placebo in reducing abdominal bloating, discomfort, and constipation (Pandolfino et al., 2000) and to dramatically accelerate proximal colonic filling, a measure of orocaecal transit, at 6 h (Prather et al., 2000). Nonetheless, anotherreview found that there was still a great deal of doubt regarding the effectiveness and, consequently, the outcomes of controlled trials in IBS (Klein, 1998).

4.6.5.8. Prognosis

It is thought that irritable bowel syndrome is a chronic pain condition that can last for many years. Nonetheless, nearly 70% of patients in a study on the vigorous use of bulking agents and high-fiber diets were said to be pain-free after five years (Harvey et al., 1987). Significant advancements in the treatment of IBS have recently resulted from and will continue to result from our growing understanding of the gut-brain axis and the psychopathology of the condition.

A Closer Look

Dysautonomia

Dysautonomia encompasses a spectrum of disorders stemming from dysfunction within the autonomic nervous system (ANS), the body's automatic control center governing vital functions like heart rate, blood pressure, digestion, and temperature regulation. This intricate system relies on a network of nerves and neurotransmitters to maintain balance, and when disrupted, it can manifest in a multitude of symptoms spanning various organ systems. Among the most prevalent types is Postural Orthostatic Tachycardia Syndrome (POTS), where individuals experience an abnormal surge in heart rate upon standing, often leading to dizziness, fatigue, and fainting. Neurocardiogenic Syncope (NCS) presents as sudden drops in blood pressure and heart rate, culminating in fainting episodes typically triggered by stress or prolonged standing. Additionally, conditions like Multiple System Atrophy (MSA) and Pure Autonomic Failure (PAF) underscore the more severe end of the dysautonomia spectrum, with MSA being a progressive neurodegenerative disorder affecting multiple bodily systems, including autonomic functions, and PAF characterized by a broad failure in autonomic regulation. Diagnosis involves a comprehensive evaluation encompassing medical history, physical examinations, and specialized tests gauging autonomic function, such as tilt table tests and sweat tests. Treatment primarily targets symptom management and enhanced quality of life, employing strategies like lifestyle adjustments, medication to regulate blood pressure and heart rate, physical therapy, and ongoing medical support. Despite its challenges, individuals with dysautonomia can often lead fulfilling lives by leveraging tailored management plans and accessing support networks to mitigate the impact of their condition on daily functioning.

Summary

- Fibromyalgia, a chronic condition characterized by widespread musculoskeletal pain, tenderness, and fatigue, often coexists with abdominal pain, further complicating the management and treatment of affected individuals.
- Abdominal pain is a common and debilitating symptom experienced by many individuals with fibromyalgia.
- Fibromyalgia is a multisymptomatic syndrome defined by the core feature of chronic widespread pain.
- Fibromyalgia patients usually report disturbed sleep. Even if they sleep continuously for 8 to 10 h they awake feeling tired.
- The contemporary etiological paradigm for fibromyalgia is that of a complex hyperalgesic pain syndrome, in which abnormalities of central sensory processing interact with peripheral pain generators and neuro-endocrine pathways to generate a wide spectrum of patient symptomatology and distress.
- Primary hyperalgesia is the normal perception of pain from nociceptor stimulation in an injured tissue.
- The management of fibromyalgia patients is an exercise in symptom palliation and maintenance of physical and emotional functionality.
- Pain in the right lower quadrant is common, and the main differential diagnosis is that of acute appendicitis, especially in a male child.
- Infectious ileocaecitis is usually associated with more systemic symptoms than acute appendicitis. Patients with distal ileitis due to Yersinia very often have a history of swimming in a lake or drinking possibly contaminated water.
- Renal colic starts in either flank and radiates around and down into the groin. It is usually due to a ureteric calculus passing from the renal pelvis into the ureter causing obstruction.
- Patients with gastric ulcers complain of periodic upper abdominal pain over a fairly large area, which is frequently related to meals and occurs soon after the patient starts eating.

References

1. Aaron, L. A., et al. (1996). Psychiatric diagnoses in patients with fibromyalgia are related to health care-seeking behavior rather than to illness. *Arthritis and Rheumatism, 39*(3), 436–445.
2. Aaron, L. A., & Buchwald, D. (2001). A review of the evidence for overlap among unexplained clinical conditions. *Annals of Internal Medicine, 134*(9 Pt 2), 868–881.
3. Abbadie, C., et al. (1996). Spinal cord substance P receptor immunoreactivity increases in both inflammatory and nerve injury models of persistent pain. *Neuroscience, 70*(1), 201–209.
4. Accarino, A. M., Azpiroz, F., & Malagelada, J.-R. (1995). Selective dysfunction of mechanosensitive intestinal afferents in irritable bowel syndrome. *Gastroenterology, 108*(2), 636–643.
5. Affleck, G., et al. (1996). Sequential daily relations of sleep, pain intensity, and attention to pain among women with fibromyalgia. *Pain, 68*(3), 363–368.

6. Aggarwal, A., et al. (1994). Predominant symptoms in irritable bowel syndrome correlate with specific autonomic nervous system abnormalities. *Gastroenterology, 106*(4), 945–950.

7. Agreus, L., et al. (1995). Irritable bowel syndrome and dyspepsia in the general population: Overlap and lack of stability. *Gastroenterology, 109*(2), 671–680.

8. Amir, M., et al. (1997). Posttraumatic stress disorder, tenderness and fibromyalgia. *Journal of Psychosomatic Research, 42*(6), 607–613.

9. Amman, R. W., & Muelhaupt, B. (1999). The natural history of pain in alcoholic chronic pancreatitis. *Gastroenterology, 116*(5), 1132–1140.

10. Armstrong, R. B., Warren, G. L., & Warren, J. A. (1991). Mechanisms of exercise-induced muscle fiber injury. *Sports Medicine, 12*(3), 184–207.

11. Arroyo, J. F., & Cohen, M. L. (1993). Abnormal responses to electro cutaneous stimulation in fibromyalgia. *Journal of Rheumatology, 20*(11), 1925–1931.

12. Attwood, S. E. A., et al. (1987). Yersinia infection and acute abdominal pain. *Lancet, 1*(8524), 529–533.

13. Aziz, Q., & Thompson, D. G. (1998). Brain–Gut axis in health and disease. *Gastroenterology, 114*(3), 559–578.

14. Babior, B. M., & Matzner, Y. (1997). The familial Mediterranean fever gene cloned at last. *New England Journal of Medicine, 337*(21), 1548–1549.

15. Barber, M. D., McLaren, J., & Rainey, J. B. (1997). Recurrent appendicitis. *British Journal of Surgery, 84*(1), 110–112.

16. Basbaum, A. I., & Fields, H. L. (1984). Endogenous pain control systems: Brainstem spinal pathways and endorphin circuitry. *Annual Review of Neuroscience, 7*, 309–338.

17. Bendtsen, L., et al. (1997). Evidence of qualitatively altered nociception in patients with fibromyalgia. *Arthritis and Rheumatism, 40*(1), 98–102.

18. Bengtsson, A., et al. (1994). Long term follow-up of fibromyalgia patients: Clinical symptoms, muscular function, laboratory tests—An eight-year comparison study. *Journal of Musculoskeletal Pain, 2*(2), 67–80.

19. Bennett, D. L. (2001). Neurotrophic factors: Important regulators of nociceptive function. *Neuroscientist, 7*(1), 13–17.

20. Bennett, R. (1997). The concurrence of lupus and fibromyalgia: Implications for diagnosis and management. *Lupus, 6*(5), 494–499.

21. Bennett, R. M. (1993). The origin of myopia: An integrated hypothesis of focal muscle changes and sleep disturbance in patients with the fibromyalgia syndrome. *Journal of Musculoskeletal Pain, 1*(3–4), 95–112.

22. Bennett, R. M. (1996a). Fibromyalgia and the disability dilemma. A new era in understanding a complex, multidimensional pain syndrome. *Arthritis and Rheumatism, 39*(10), 1627–1634.

23. Bennett, R. M. (1996b). Multidisciplinary group programs to treat fibromyalgia patients. *Rheumatic Disease Clinics of North America, 22*(2), 351–367.

24. Bennett, R. M. (1996c). The contribution of muscle to the generation of fibromyalgia symptomatology. *Journal of Musculoskeletal Pain, 4*(3), 35–59.

25. Bennett, R. M., et al. (1996). Group treatment of fibromyalgia: A 6-month outpatient program. *Journal of Rheumatology, 23*(3), 521–528.

26. Bennett, R. M., et al. (1997). Hypothalamic-pituitary-insulin-like growth factor-I axis dysfunction in patients with fibromyalgia. *Journal of Rheumatology, 24*(7), 1384–1389.

27. Bennett, R. M., et al. (2001). Efficacy and safety of a tramadol/acetaminophen combination (Ultracet) in the management of fibromyalgia-related pain: A multicenter, outpatient, randomized, double-blind, placebo-controlled study. *Arthritis & Rheumatology, 44*(9), S67–S67

28. Bennett, R. M., Clark, S. R., & Walczyk, J. (1998). A randomized, double-blind, placebo-controlled study of growth hormone in the treatment of fibromyalgia. *American Journal of Medicine, 104*(3), 227–231.

29. Blendis, L. M., Hill, O. W., & Merskey, H. (1978). Abdominal pain and the emotions. *Pain, 5*(2), 179–191.

30. Blum, A. L., et al. (1998). Lack of effect of treating Helicobacter pylori positive functional dyspepsia in patients with nonulcer dyspepsia. *New England Journal of Medicine, 339*(26), 1875–1881.

31. Bohmer, C. J. M., & Tuynman, H. (1996). The clinical relevance of lactose malabsorption in irritable bowel syndrome. *European Journal of Gastroenterology and Hepatology, 8*(10), 1013–1016.

32. Borg-Stein, J., & Stein, J. (1996). Trigger points and tender points: One and the same? Does injection treatment help? *Rheumatic Disease Clinics of North America, 22*(2), 305–322.

33. Bradley, L. A., et al. (2000). Use of neuroimaging to understand abnormal pain sensitivity in fibromyalgia. *Current Rheumatology Reports, 2*(2), 141–148.

34. Burckhardt, C. S., et al. (1994). Assessing depression in fibromyalgia patients. *Arthritis Care Research, 7*(1), 35–39.

35. Burckhardt, C. S., Clark, S. R., & Bennett, R. M. (1993). Fibromyalgia and quality of life: A comparative analysis. *Journal of Rheumatology, 20*(3), 475–479.

36. Buskila, D., et al. (1997). Increased rates of fibromyalgia following cervical spine injury. A controlled study of 161 cases of traumatic injury. *Arthritis and Rheumatism, 40*(3), 446–452.

37. Buskila, D., et al. (1996). Familial aggregation in the fibromyalgia syndrome. *Seminars in Arthritis and Rheumatism, 26*(6), 605–611.

38. Camilleri, M. (1998). What's in a name? Roll on Rome II. *Gastroenterology, 114*(2), 237.

39. Camilleri, M. (2001). Management of irritable bowel syndrome. *Gastroenterology, 120*(3), 652–668.

40. Camilleri, M., et al. (2000). Efficacy and safety of alosetron in women with irritable bowel syndrome: A randomized, placebo-controlled trial. *Lancet, 355*(9209), 1035–1040.

41. Campbell, S. M., et al. (1983). Clinical characteristics of fibrositis. I. A 'blinded' controlled study of symptoms and tender points. *Arthritis and Rheumatism, 26*(6), 817–824.

42. Carette, S., et al. (1986). Evaluation of amitriptyline in primary fibrositis. A double-blind, placebo-controlled study. *Arthritis and Rheumatism, 29*(5), 655–659.

43. Carette, S., et al. (1994). Comparison of amitriptyline, cyclobenzaprine, and placebo in the treatment of fibromyalgia. *Arthritis and Rheumatism, 37*(1), 32–40.

44. Chapman, C. R., & Gavrin, J. (1999). Suffering: The contributions of persistent pain. *Lancet, 353*(9164), 2233–2237.

45. Clark, S., Tindall, E., & Bennett, R. M. (1985). A double-blind crossover trial of prednisone versus placebo in the treatment of fibrositis. *Journal of Rheumatology, 12*(5), 980–983.

46. Clark, S. R. (1994). Prescribing exercise for fibromyalgia patients. *Arthritis Care Research, 7*(4), 221–225.

47. Clark, S. R., et al. (2001). Exercise for patients with fibromyalgia: Risks versus benefits. *Current Rheumatology Reports, 3*(2), 135–140.

48. Clark, S. R., & Bennett, R. M. (2000). Supplemental dextromethorphan in the treatment of fibromyalgia: A double-blind, placebo-controlled study of efficacy and side-effects. *Arthritis and Rheumatism, 43*(9S), S333.

49. Clauw, D. J. (1995). Fibromyalgia: More than just a musculoskeletal disease. *American Family Physician, 52*, 843–851, 853–854.

50. Coward, D. M. (1994). Tizanidine: Neuropharmacology and mechanism of action. *Neurology, 44*(10 Suppl 6), S6–10.

51. Craig, A. D. (1998). A new version of the thalamic disinhibition hypothesis of central pain. *Pain Forum, 7*(1), 1–14.

52. Crofford, L. J., et al. (1994). Hypothalamic–pituitary–adrenal axis perturbations in patients with fibromyalgia. *Arthritis and Rheumatism, 37*(11), 1583–1592.

53. Croft, P., et al. (1993). The prevalence of chronic widespread pain in the general population. *Journal of Rheumatology, 20*(4), 710–713.

54. Crowell, M. D., Dubin, N. H., Robinson, J. C., et al. (1994). Functional bowel disorders in women with dysmenorrhea. *American Journal of Gastroenterology, 89*(11), 1973–1977.

55. Daum, F. (1997). Functional abdominal pain in older children and adolescents. *Gastrointestinal Diseases Today, 6*, 7–12.

56. Drewes, A. M., et al. (1991). Zopiclone in the treatment of sleep abnormalities in fibromyalgia. *Journal of Rheumatology, 20*(2), 288–293.

57. Drewes, A. M., et al. (1995). Clustering of sleep electroencephalographic patterns in patients with the fibromyalgia syndrome. *British Journal of Rheumatology, 34*(12), 1151–1156.

58. Drossman, D. A., Leserman, J., Nachman, G., et al. (1990). Sexual and physical abuse in women with functional gastrointestinal disorders. *Annals of Internal Medicine, 113*(11), 808–833.

59. Drossman, D. A., Whitehead, W. E., & Camilleri, M. (1997). Irritable bowel syndrome. *Gastroenterology, 112*(6), 2118–2137.

60. Farber, L., et al. (2000). Efficacy and tolerability of tropisetron in primary fibromyalgia—A highly selective and competitive 5-HT3 receptor antagonist. *German Fibromyalgia Study Group*, 113, 49–54.

61. Fassbender, K., et al. (1997). Tender points, depressive and functional symptoms: Comparison between fibromyalgia and major depression. *Clinical Rheumatology, 16*(1), 76–79.

62. Fishbain, D. (2000). Evidence-based data on pain relief with antidepressants. *Annals of Medicine, 32*(5), 305–316.

63. Fogelholm, R., & Murros, K. (1992). Tizanidine in chronic tension-type headache: A placebo controlled double-blind cross-over study. *Headache, 32*(9), 509–513.

64. Forseth, K. O., et al. (1999b). Prognostic factors for the development of fibromyalgia in women with self-reported musculoskeletal pain. A prospective study. *Journal of Rheumatology, 26*(11), 2458–2467.

65. Forseth, K. O., Forre, O., & Gran, J. T. (1999a). A 5.5-year prospective study of self-reported musculoskeletal pain and of fibromyalgia in a female population: Significance and natural history. *Clinical Rheumatology, 18*(2), 114–121.

66. Friedel, D., Thomas, R., & Fisher, R. S. (2001). Ischemic colitis during treatment with alosetron. *Gastroenterology, 120*(3), 557–560.

67. Gibson, S. J., et al. (1994). Altered heat pain thresholds and cerebral event-related potentials following painful CO_2 laser stimulation in subjects with fibromyalgia syndrome. *Pain, 58*(2), 185–193.

68. Giovengo, S. L., Russell, I. J., & Larson, A. A. (1999). Increased concentrations of nerve growth factor in cerebrospinal fluid of patients with fibromyalgia. *Journal of Rheumatology, 26*(7), 1564–1569.

69. Glaser, J. P., & Engel, G. L. (1977). Psychodynamics, psychophysiology and gastrointestinal symptomatology. *Clinics in Gastroenterology, 6*(3), 507–531.

70. Glass, J. M., & Park, D. C. (2001). Cognitive dysfunction in fibromyalgia. *Current Rheumatology Reports, 3*(2), 123–127.

71. Goldenberg, D. L. (1987). Fibromyalgia syndrome: An emerging but controversial condition. *Journal of the American Medical Association, 257*(20), 2782–2787.

72. Goldenberg, D. L. (1989). A review of the role of tricyclic medications in the treatment of fibromyalgia syndrome. *Journal of Rheumatology, 19*(Suppl), 137–139.

73. Goldenberg, D. L., et al. (1990). High frequency of fibromyalgia in patients with chronic fatigue seen in a primary care practice. *Arthritis and Rheumatism, 33*(3), 381–387.

74. Goldenberg, D. L., et al. (1994). A controlled study of a stress-reduction, cognitive-behavioral treatment program in fibromyalgia. *Journal of Musculoskeletal Pain, 2*(4), 53–66.

75. Gowans, S. E., et al. (1999). A randomized, controlled trial of exercise and education for individuals with fibromyalgia. *British Medical Journal, 12*, 120–128.

76. Gowers, W. R. (1904). Lumbago: Its lessons and analogues. *British Medical Journal, 1*, 117–121.

77. Granges, G., Zilko, P., & Littlejohn, G. O. (1994). Fibromyalgia syndrome: Assessment of the severity of the condition 2 years after diagnosis. *Journal of Rheumatology, 21*(3), 523–529.

78. Graven-Nielsen, T., et al. (1997). Quantification of local and referred muscle pain in humans after sequential i.m. injections of hypertonic saline. *Pain, 69*(1–2), 111–117.

79. Graven-Nielsen, T., et al. (2000). Ketamine reduces muscle pain, temporal summation, and referred pain in fibromyalgia patients. *Pain, 85*(3), 483–491.

80. Gruber, A. J., Hudson, J. I., & Pope, H. G., Jr. (1996). The management of treatment-resistant depression in disorders on the interface of psychiatry and medicine. Fibromyalgia, chronic fatigue syndrome, migraine, irritable bowel syndrome, atypical facial pain, and premenstrual dysphoric disorder. *Psychiatric Clinics of North America, 19*(2), 351–369.

81. Gwee, K. A., Leong, Y. L., Graham, C., et al. (1999). The role of psychological and biological factors in post-infective gut dysfunction. *Gut, 44*(3), 400–440.

82. Hahn, B. A., Saunders, W. B., & Maier, W. C. (1997). Differences between individuals with self-reportable irritable bowel syndrome (IBS) and IBS-like symptoms. *Digestive Diseases and Sciences, 42*(12), 2585–2590.

83. Hamilton, J., Guthrie, E., Creed, F., et al. (2000). A randomized controlled trial of psychotherapy in patients with chronic functional dyspepsia. *Gastroenterology, 119*(3), 661–669.

84. Harvey, R. F., Mauad, E. C., & Brown, A. M. (1987). Prognosis in the irritable bowel syndrome: A 5-year prospective study. *Lancet, 1*(8535), 963–965.

85. Hauri, P., & Hawkins, D. R. (1973). Alpha-delta sleep. *Electroencephalography and Clinical Neurophysiology, 34*(2), 233–237.

86. Haus, U., et al. (2000). Oral treatment of fibromyalgia with tropisetron given over 28 days: Influence on functional and vegetative symptoms, psychometric parameters and pain. *Scandinavian Journal of Rheumatology, 113*, 55–58.

87. Henriksson, C. M. (1994). Longterm effects of fibromyalgia on everyday life. A study of 56 patients. *Scandinavian Journal of Rheumatology, 23*(1), 36–41.

88. Henriksson, C. M. (1995). Living with continuous muscular pain—Patient perspectives. Part I: Encounters and consequences. *Journal of the Caring Sciences, 9*(1), 67–76.

89. Henriksson, K. G. (1994). Chronic muscular pain: An etiology and pathogenesis. *Baillière's Clinical Rheumatology, 8*(3), 703–719.

90. Hightower, N. C. (1977). Intestinal gas and gaseousness. *Clinics in Gastroenterology, 6*(3), 597–606.

91. Hill, R. (2000). NK1 (substance P) receptor antagonists—Why are they not analgesic in humans? *Trends in Pharmacological Sciences, 21*(7), 244–246.

92. Horwitz, B. J., & Fisher, R. S. (2001). The irritable bowel syndrome. *New England Journal of Medicine, 344*(24), 1846–1850.

93. Jackson, J. L., O'Malley, P. G., Tomkins, G., et al. (2000). Treatment of functional gastrointestinal disorders with antidepressant medications: A meta-analysis. *American Journal of Medicine, 108*(1), 65–72.

94. Jailwala, J., Imperiale, T. F., & Kroenke, K. (2000). Pharmacological treatment of the irritable bowel syndrome: A systematic review of randomized, controlled trials. *Annals of Internal Medicine, 133*(2), 136–147.

95. Jennette, J. C., & Falk, R. J. (1997). Small-vessel vasculitis. *New England Journal of Medicine, 337*(21), 1512–1523.

96. Johnson, T. R., & De Cosse, J. J. (1998). Colonoscopy diagnosis of grumbling appendicitis. *Lancet, 351*(9110), 495–496.

97. Jubrias, S. A., Bennett, R. M., & Klug, G. A. (1994). Increased incidence of a resonance in the phosphodiester region of 31P nuclear magnetic resonance spectra in the skeletal muscle of fibromyalgia patients. *Arthritis and Rheumatism, 37*(6), 801–807.

98. Kauppinen, R., & Mustajoki, P. (1992). Prognosis of acute porphyria. *Medicine, 71*, 1–12.

99. Kellgren, J. H. (1938). Observations on referred pain arising from muscle. *Clinical Science, 3*(4), 175–190.

100. Kemppainen, E. A., Hedstrom, J. I., Puolakkainen, P. A., et al. (1997). Rapid measurement of urinary trypsinogen-2 as a screening test for acute pancreatitis. *New England Journal of Medicine, 336*(25), 1788–1793.

101. Klein, K. B. (1998). Controlled treatment trials in the irritable bowel syndrome: A critique. *Gastroenterology, 95*(1), 232–241.

102. Klinkenberg-Knol, E. C., Nelis, F., Dent, J., et al. (2000). Long-term omeprazole treatment in resistant gastroesophageal reflux disease. *Gastroenterology, 118*(4), 661–669.

103. Koltzenburg, M., Torebjork, H. E., & Wahren, L. K. (1994). Nociceptor modulated central sensitization causes mechanical hyperalgesia in acute chemogenic and chronic neuropathic pain. *Brain, 117*(3), 579–591.

104. Kosek, E., Ekholm, J., & Hansson, P. (1996). Sensory dysfunction in fibromyalgia patients with implications for pathogenic mechanisms. *Pain, 68*(3), 375–383.

105. Kumar, D., Pfeffer, J., & Wingate, D. L. S. (1990). Role of psychological factors in the irritable bowel syndrome. *Digestion, 45*(2), 80–85.

106. Kwiatek, R., et al. (2000). Regional cerebral blood flow in fibromyalgia: Single-photon-emission computed tomography evidence of reduction in the pontine tegmentum and thalami. *Arthritis and Rheumatism, 43*(12), 2823–2833.

107. Ladabaum, U., Minoshima, S., Hasler, W. L., et al. (2001). Gastric distension correlates with activation of multiple cortical and subcortical regions. *Gastroenterology, 120*(2), 369–376.

108. Lapossy, E., et al. (1995). The frequency of transition of chronic low back pain to fibromyalgia. *Scandinavian Journal of Rheumatology, 24*(1), 29–33.

109. Lautenbacher, S., & Rollman, G. B. (1997). Possible deficiencies of pain modulation in fibromyalgia. *Clinical Journal of Pain, 13*(3), 189–196.

110. Lembo, T., Munakata, J., Mertz, H., et al. (1994). Evidence for the hypersensitivity of lumbar splanchnic afferents in irritable bowel syndrome. *Gastroenterology, 107*(6), 1686–1696.

111. Levitt, M. D., Furne, J., & Olsson, S. (1996). The relation of passage of gas and abdominal bloating to colonic gas production. *Annals of Internal Medicine, 124*(4), 422–424.

112. Lewis, K. S., & Han, N. H. (1997). Tramadol: A new centrally acting analgesic. *American Journal of Health-System Pharmacy, 54*(6), 643–652.

113. Liu, Z., et al. (2000). A high-recovery extraction procedure for quantitative analysis of substance P and opioid peptides in human cerebrospinal fluid. *Peptides, 21*(6–7), 853–860.

114. Lorenz, J., Grasedyck, K., & Bromm, B. (1996). Middle and long latency somatosensory evoked potentials after painful laser stimulation in patients with fibromyalgia syndrome. *Clinical Neurophysiology, 100*(2), 165–168.

115. Lyons, T. J., & French, J. (1991). Modafinil: The unique properties of a new stimulant. *Aviation Space and Environmental Medicine, 62*(5), 432–435.

116. Maastricht Consensus Report. (1997). The management of *H. pylori* infection. *Gut, 41*(1), 8–13.

117. MacFarlane, G. J. (1999). Generalized pain, fibromyalgia and regional pain: An epidemiological view. *Bailliere's Best Practice in Clinical Rheumatology, 13*(3), 403–414.

118. Magerl, W., Wilk, S. H., & Treede, R. D. (1998). Secondary hyperalgesia and perceptual wind-up following intradermal injection of capsaicin in humans. *Pain, 74*(2–3), 257–268.

119. Magill, A. J., Grogl, M., Gasser, R. A., et al. (1993). Visceral infection caused by leishmania tropica in veterans of Operation Desert Storm. *New England Journal of Medicine, 328*(19), 1383–1387.

120. Mannerkorpi, K., et al. (2000). Pool exercise combined with an education program for patients with fibromyalgia syndrome: A prospective, randomized study. *Journal of Rheumatology, 27*(10), 2473–2481.

121. Mayer, E. A., & Gebhart, G. F. (1994). Basic and clinical aspects of visceral hyperalgesia. *Gastroenterology, 107*(1), 271–293.

122. McCallum, R. W., Chen, J. de Z., Lin, Z., et al. (1998). Gastric pacing improves emptying and symptoms in patients with gastroparesis. *Gastroenterology, 114*(3), 456–461.

123. McColl, I. (1998). More precision in diagnosing appendicitis. *New England Journal of Medicine, 338*(3), 190–191.

124. McColl, K., Murray, L., El-Omar, E., et al. (1998). Symptomatic benefit from eradicating Helicobacter pylori infection in patients with nonulcer dyspepsia. *New England Journal of Medicine, 339*(26), 1869–1874.

125. McQuay, H. J., et al. (1994). Dextromethorphan for the treatment of neuropathic pain: A double-blind randomized controlled crossover trial with integral n-of-1 design. *Pain, 59*(1), 127–133.

126. Mengshoel, A. M., Vollestad, N. K., & Forre, O. (1995). Pain and fatigue induced by exercise in fibromyalgia patients and sedentary healthy subjects. *Clinical and Experimental Rheumatology, 13*(4), 477–482.

127. Mense, S. (2000). Neurobiological concepts of fibromyalgia—The possible role of descending spinal tracts. *Scandinavian Journal of Rheumatology, 113*(Suppl.), 24–29.

128. Merskey, H. (1965). Psychiatric patients with persistent pain. *Journal of Psychosomatic Research, 9*(3), 299–309.

129. Metz, G., Gassull, M. A., Draser, B. S., et al. (1976b). Breath hydrogen test for small intestinal bacterial colonization. *Lancet, 1*(7965), 668–669.

130. Metz, G., Jenkins, D. J. A., Peters, T. J., et al. (1975). Breath hydrogen as a diagnostic method for hypolactasia. *Lancet, 1*(7911), 1155–1157.

131. Metz, G., Jenkins, D. J. A., Peters, T. J., et al. (1976a). Breath hydrogen in hyposucrasia. *Lancet, 1*(7966), 119–120.

132. Michalowski, W., Rubin, S., Slowinski, R., et al. (2001). Triage of the child with abdominal pain. *Paediatrics and Child Health, 6*(1), 23–28.

133. Milla, P. (2001). Irritable bowel syndrome in childhood. *Gastroenterology, 120*(2), 287–307.

134. Mishkin, D., Sablauskas, L., Yalovsky, M., et al. (1997). Fructose and sorbitol malabsorption in ambulatory patients with functional dyspepsia. *Digestive Diseases and Sciences, 42*(12), 2591–2598.

135. Moldofsky, H. (1989). Sleep and fibrositis syndrome. *Rheumatic Diseases Clinics of North America, 15*(1), 91–103.

136. Moldofsky, H. (1994). Chronobiological influences on fibromyalgia syndrome: Theoretical and therapeutic implications. *Baillière's Clinical Rheumatology, 8*(4), 801–810.

137. Moldofsky, H., et al. (1975). Musculosketal symptoms and non-REM sleep disturbance in patients with 'fibrositis syndrome' and healthy subjects. *Psychosomatic Medicine, 37*(4), 341–351.

138. Moldofsky, H., Scarisbrick, P., England, R., et al. (1996). The effect of zolpidem in patients with fibromyalgia: A dose ranging, double blind, placebo controlled, modified crossover study. *Journal of Rheumatology, 23*(3), 529–533.

139. Moldofsky, H., & Scarisbrick, P. (1976). Induction of neurasthenic musculoskeletal pain syndrome by selective sleep stage deprivation. *Psychosomatic Medicine, 38*(1), 35–44.

140. Montplaisir, J., et al. (1992). The treatment of the restless leg syndrome with or without periodic leg movements in sleep. *Sleep, 15*(5), 391–395.

141. Morand, E. F., et al. (1994). Fibromyalgia syndrome and disease activity in systemic lupus erythematosus. *Lupus, 3*, 187–191.

142. Mountz, J. M., et al. (1995). Fibromyalgia in women. Abnormalities of regional cerebral blood flow in the thalamus and the caudate nucleus are associated with low pain threshold levels. *Arthritis and Rheumatism, 38*, 926–938.

143. Nabeshima, T., et al. (1987). Antinociceptive activity induced by tizanidine and alpha-2 adrenoreceptors. *Neuropharmacology, 26*, 1453–1455.

144. Nanda, R., James, R., Smith, H., et al. (1989). Food intolerance and the irritable bowel syndrome. *Gut, 30*, 1099–1104.

145. Newman, A., Katsaris, J., Blendis, L. M., et al. (1973). Small intestinal injury in women who received pelvic radiotherapy. *Lancet, 2*, 1471–1473.

146. O'Malley, P. G., et al. (2000). Treatment of fibromyalgia with antidepressants: A meta-analysis. *Journal of General Internal Medicine, 15*, 659–666.

147. Okifuji, A., Turk, D. C., Sherman, J. J. (2000). Evaluation of the relationship between depression and fibromyalgia syndrome: Why aren't all patients depressed? *Journal of Rheumatology, 27*, 212–219.

148. Olsen, J. B., Myren, C. I., Haahr, P. E. (1993). Randomized study of the value of laparoscopy before appendectomy. *British Journal of Surgery, 80*, 922–923.

149. Pandolfino, J. E., Howden, C. W., Kahrilas, P. J. (2000). Motility-modifying agents and management of disorders of gastrointestinal motility. *Gastroenterology, 118*, S32–S47.

150. Park, D. C., et al. (2001). Cognitive function in fibromyalgia patients. *Arthritis and Rheumatology, 44*, 2125–2133.

151. Park, J. H., Niermann, K. J., Olsen, N. (2000). Evidence for metabolic abnormalities in the muscles of patients with fibromyalgia. *Current Rheumatology Reports, 2*, 131–140.

152. Pillemer, S. R., et al. (1997). The neuroscience and endocrinology of fibromyalgia. *Arthritis and Rheumatism, 40*, 1928–1939.

153. Portenoy, R. K. (1996). Opioid therapy for chronic nonmalignant pain: A review of the critical issues. *Journal of Pain and Symptom Management, 11*, 203–217.

154. Prather, C. M., Camilleri, M., Zinsmeister, A. R., et al. (2000). Tegaserod accelerates orocecal

transit in patients with constipation-predominant irritable bowel syndrome. *Gastroenterology, 118*, 463–468.

155. Puylaert, J. B., Rutgers, P. H., Lalisang, R. I., et al. (1987). A prospective study of ultrasonography in the diagnosis of appendicitis. *New England Journal of Medicine, 317*, 666–670.
156. Ramos-Remus, C., et al. (2000). How important is patient education? *Bailliere's Best Practice in Clinical Rheumatology, 14*, 689–703.
157. Rao, P. M., Rhea, J. T., Novelline, R. A., Mostafavi, A. A., McCabe, C. J. (1998). Effect of computerized tomography of the appendix on treatment of patients and use of hospital resources. *New England Journal of Medicine, 338*, 141–146.
158. Reilly, P. A., Littlejohn, G. O. (1992). Peripheral arthralgia presentation of fibrositis/fibromyalgia syndrome. *Journal of Rheumatology, 19*, 281–283.
159. Reveille, J. D. (2000). The changing spectrum of rheumatic disease in human immunodeficiency virus infection. *Seminars in Arthritis and Rheumatology, 30*, 147–166.
160. Roth, S. H. (1998). Efficacy and safety of tramadol HCl in breakthrough musculoskeletal pain attributed to osteoarthritis. *Journal of Rheumatology, 25*, 1358–1363.
161. Russell, I. J., et al. (1991). Treatment of primary fibrositis/fibromyalgia syndrome with ibuprofen and alprazolam: A double-blind, placebo-controlled study. *Arthritis and Rheumatism, 34*, 552–560.
162. Russell, I. J., et al. (1994). Elevated cerebrospinal fluid levels of substance P in patients with the fibromyalgia syndrome. *Arthritis and Rheumatism, 37*, 1593–1601.
163. Russell, I. J., et al. (1997). Efficacy of Ultram™ [Tramadol HCL] treatment of fibromyalgia syndrome: Preliminary analysis of a multicenter, randomized, placebo-controlled study. *Arthritis and Rheumatism, 40*, S214.
164. Sackman, M., Morgner, A., Rudolph, B., et al. (1997). Regression of gastric MALT lymphoma after eradication of *H. pylori* is predicted by endosonographic staging. *Gastroenterology, 113*, 1087–1090.
165. Sampson, H. A., Sicherer, S. H., Birnbaum, A. H. (2001). AGA technical review on the evaluation of food allergy in gastrointestinal disorders. *Gastroenterology, 120*, 1026–1040.
166. Satrustegui, J., et al. (1988). An in vivo phosphorus nuclear magnetic resonance study of the variations with age in the phosphodiers content of human muscle. *Mechanisms of Aging and Development, 42*, 105–114.
167. Savage, S. R. (1996). Long-term opioid therapy: Assessment of consequences and risks. *Journal of Pain and Symptom Management, 11*, 274–286.
168. Schnitzer, T. J., et al. (2000). Efficacy of tramadol in treatment of chronic low back pain. *Journal of Rheumatology, 27*, 772–778.
169. Seth, R., Heyman, M. B. (1994). Management of constipation and encopresis in infants and children. *Gastroenterology Clinics of North America, 23*, 621–636.
170. Simms, R. W. (1996). Is there muscle pathology in fibromyalgia syndrome? *Rheumatic Disease Clinics of North America, 22*, 245–266.
171. Smith, H. S., Barton, A. E. (2000). Tizanidine in the management of spasticity and

musculoskeletal complaints in the palliative care population. *American Journal of Hospice and Palliative Care, 17*, 50–58.

172. Smith, R. C., Greenbaum, D. S., Vancouver, J. B., et al. (1990). Psychosocial factors are associated with health care seeking rather than diagnosis in irritable bowel syndrome. *Gastroenterology, 98*, 293–301.
173. Song, J. Y., Merskey, H., Sullivan, S., et al. (1993). Anxiety and depression in patients with abdominal bloating. *Canadian Journal of Psychology, 38*, 475–479.
174. Sorensen, J., et al. (1995). Pain analysis in patients with fibromyalgia: Effects of intravenous morphine, lidocaine and ketamine. *Scandinavian Journal of Rheumatology, 24*, 360–365.
175. Sorensen, J., et al. (1998). Hyperexcitability in fibromyalgia. *Journal of Rheumatology, 25*, 152–155.
176. Spath, M., Welzel, D., Farber, L. (2000). Treatment of chronic fatigue syndrome with 5-HT3 receptor antagonists—Preliminary results. *Scandinavian Journal of Rheumatology, 113*, 72–77.
177. Sperber, A. D., et al. (1999). Fibromyalgia in the irritable bowel syndrome: Studies of prevalence and clinical implications. *American Journal of Gastroenterology, 94*, 3541–3546.
178. Sprott, H., et al. (2000). 31P magnetic resonance spectroscopy in fibromyalgia muscle. *Rheumatology (Oxford), 39*, 1121–1125.
179. Stanghellini, V., Tosetti, C., Paternico, A., et al. (1996). Risk indicators of delayed gastric emptying of solids in patients with functional dyspepsia. *Gastroenterology, 110*, 1036–1042.
180. Starnes, H. F., Moore, F. D., Mentzer, S., et al. (1986). Abdominal pain in neutropenic cancer patients. *Cancer, 57*, 616–619.
181. Staud, R., et al. (2001). Abnormal sensitization and temporal summation of second pain (wind-up) in patients with fibromyalgia syndrome. *Pain, 91*, 165–175.
182. Steely, W. M., Gooden, S. M. (1986). Sclerosing mesocolitis. *Diseases of the Colon and Rectum, 29*, 266–268.
183. Stevenson, R. J. (1985). Abdominal pain unrelated to trauma. *Surgical Clinics of North America, 65*, 1181–1215.
184. Stewart, R. J., Gupta, R. K., Purdie, G. L., et al. (1986). Fine catheter aspiration cytology of peritoneal cavity in difficult cases of acute abdominal pain. *Lancet, 2*, 1414–1415.
185. Stockman, R. (1904). The causes, pathology and treatment of chronic rheumatism. *Edinburgh Medical Journal, 15*, 107–116.
186. Talley, N. J., Vakil, N., Ballard, D., et al. (1999). Absence of benefit of eradicating Helicobacter pylori in patients with nonulcer dyspepsia. *New England Journal of Medicine, 341*, 1106–1111.
187. Tecott, L. H., Maricq, A. V., Julius, D. (1993). Nervous system distribution of the serotonin 5-HT3 receptor mRNA. *Proceedings of the National Academy of Sciences of the USA, 90*, 1430–1434.
188. Travell, J. G., Simons, D. G. (1992). *Myofascial Pain and Dysfunction: The Trigger Point Manual, vol. 2.* Williams & Wilkins, Baltimore.
189. Turk, D. C., et al. (1998). Interdisciplinary treatment for fibromyalgia syndrome: Clinical and statistical significance. *Pain, 11*, 186–195.
190. Urhausen, A., Gabriel, H. H., Kindermann, W. (1998). Impaired pituitary hormonal response

to exhaustive exercise in overtrained endurance athletes. *Medicine and Science in Sports and Exercise, 30*, 407–414.

191. Urrows, S., et al. (1994). Unique clinical and psychological correlates of fibromyalgia tender points and joint tenderness in rheumatoid arthritis. *Arthritis and Rheumatism, 37*, 1513–1520.
192. Vaeroy, H., et al. (1988). Elevated CSF levels of substance P and high incidence of Raynaud phenomenon in patients with fibromyalgia: New features for diagnosis. *Pain, 32*, 21–26.
193. van Ginkel, R., Voskuul, W. P., Benninga, M. A., et al. (2001). Alterations in rectal sensitivity and motility in childhood irritable bowel syndrome. *Gastroenterology, 120*, 31–38.
194. Wall, P. D., Cronly-Dillon, J. R. (1960). Pain, itch and vibration. *Journal of Neurology, Neurosurgery, and Psychiatry, 23*, 365–375.
195. Waylonis, G. W., Ronan, P. G., Gordon, C. (1994). A profile of fibromyalgia in occupational environments. *American Journal of Physical Medicine and Rehabilitation, 73*, 112–115.
196. Webster, R. B., Di Palma, J. A., Gremse, D. A. (1995). Lactose maldigestion and recurrent abdominal pain in children. *Digestive Diseases and Sciences, 40*, 1506–1510.
197. Weissman, D. E., Haddox, J. D. (1989). Opioid pseudo-addiction: An iatrogenic syndrome. *Pain, 36*, 363–364.
198. Wenham, P. W. (1982). Viral and bacterial associations of acute abdominal pain in children. *British Journal of Clinical Practice, 36*, 321–326.
199. White, K. P., et al. (1995). Fibromyalgia in rheumatology practice: A survey of Canadian rheumatologists. *Journal of Rheumatology, 22*, 722–726.
200. Willis, W. D., Westlund, K. N. (1997). Neuroanatomy of the pain system and of the pathways that modulate pain. *Journal of Clinical Neurophysiology, 14*, 2–31.
201. Wolf, H. (2000). Preclinical and clinical pharmacology of the 5-HT3 receptor antagonists. *Scandinavian Journal of Rheumatology, 113*, 37–45.
202. Wolfe, F., et al. (1990). The American College of Rheumatology 1990 Criteria for the classification of fibromyalgia: Report of the Multicenter Criteria Committee. *Arthritis and Rheumatism, 33*, 160–172.
203. Wolfe, F., et al. (1995). The prevalence and characteristics of fibromyalgia in the general population. *Arthritis and Rheumatism, 38*, 19–28.
204. Wolfe, F., et al. (1997a). Health status and disease severity in fibromyalgia: Results of a six-center longitudinal study [see comments]. *Arthritis and Rheumatism, 40*, 1571–1579.
205. Wolfe, F., et al. (1997b). Work and disability status of persons with fibromyalgia. *Journal of Rheumatology, 24*, 1171–1178.
206. Wood, J. D., Alpers, D. H., Andrews, P. L. R. (1999). Fundamentals of neurogastroenterology. *Gut, 45*, 1–44.
207. Wyeth, J. W., Pounder, R. E., Duggan, A. E., et al. (1996). The safety and efficiency of ranitidine bismuth citrate in combination with antibiotics for the eradication of Helicobacter pylori. *Alimentary Pharmacology and Therapeutics, 10*, 623–630.
208. Younkin, D. P., et al. (1987). 31P NMR studies in Duchenne muscular dystrophy: Age-related metabolic changes. *Neurology, 37*, 165–169.

209. Yunus, M., et al. (1981). Primary fibromyalgia (fibrositis): Clinical study of 50 patients with matched normal controls. *Arthritis and Rheumatism, 11*, 151–171.

210. Yunus, M. B. (1994). Psychological aspects of fibromyalgia syndrome: A component of the dysfunctional spectrum syndrome. *Baillière's Clinical Rheumatology, 8*, 811–837.

Chapter 5

CHRONIC PELVIC AND OBSTETRIC PAIN

Contents

Introduction

A range of disorders affecting the pelvic region—the lower abdomen, pelvis, and reproductive organs—combine to form the complex and frequently incapacitating medical challenge known as chronic pelvic and obstetric pain (CPOP). It includes a wide range of symptoms, from chronic pelvic pain to excruciating pain that severely lowers quality of life. Numerous conditions, such as endometriosis, adenomyosis, pelvic inflammatory disease, prior childbirth trauma, and nerve entrapment syndromes, can cause CPOP. Furthermore, psychological variables might make pain worse for this group of people.

One of the unique characteristics of CPOP is its complex etiology, which includes both psychological and physical elements. As a result, managing the condition requires an all-encompassing, multidisciplinary approach. Making a diagnosis can be difficult since it frequently calls for a comprehensive medical history, a physical examination, and a range of imaging and diagnostic procedures. Moreover, CPOP has an impact on relationships, everyday functioning, mental health, and more in addition to physical discomfort. A multimodal treatment approach that includes medication, physical therapy, psychological support, and occasionally surgical intervention is usually necessary for the effective management of CPOP. However, because CPOP is heterogeneous and each patient experiences pain differently, treatment strategies need to be customized to meet the unique needs and circumstances of each patient. All things considered, treating the complexities of CPOP calls for cooperation between medical professionals and a comprehensive strategy that takes into account both the psychological and physiological aspects of pain management.

Orientation and Directional Terms

Term	Definition	Illustration
Pelvic pain	Pelvic pain can have many causes, including infections, conditions affecting pelvic organs, and problems with the female reproductive system.	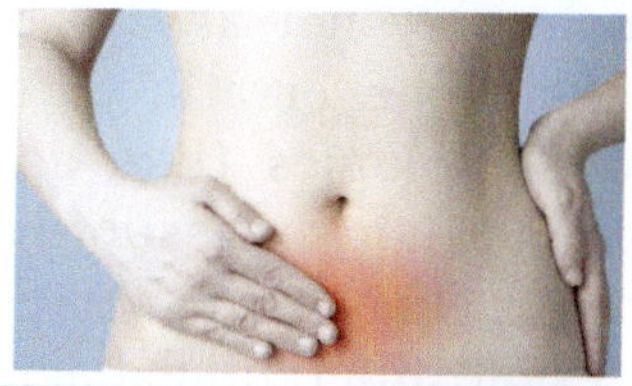
Obstetric pain	Obstetric pain is acute pain that can occur during pregnancy, labor, delivery, and after delivery.	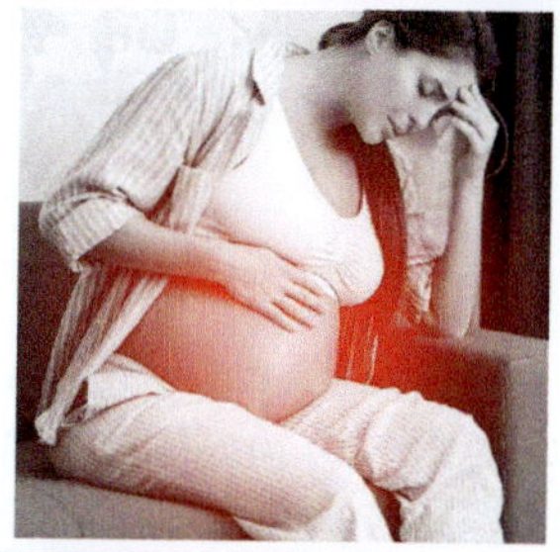
Adhesiolysis	Adhesiolysis is a surgical procedure that cuts and releases adhesions, which are fibrous tissue connections between organs or tissues.	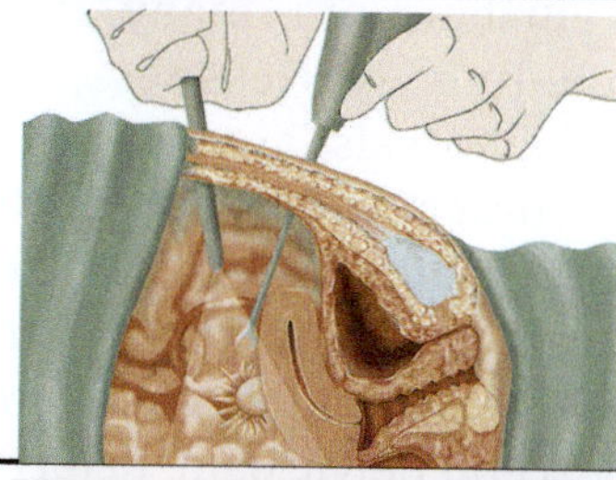
Rectovaginal septum	The rectovaginal fascia (often called rectovaginal septum or sometimes fascia of Otto) is a thin structure separating the vagina and the rectum.	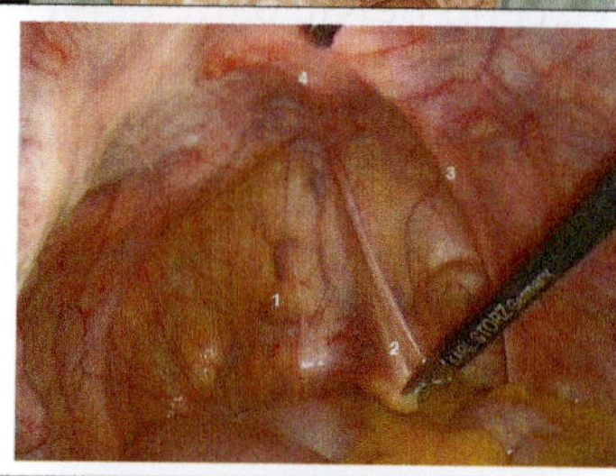
Haematuria	Hematuria is blood in the urine. When the urine is red or pink this could be linked to blood in the urine and is called "gross" or "visible" hematuria.	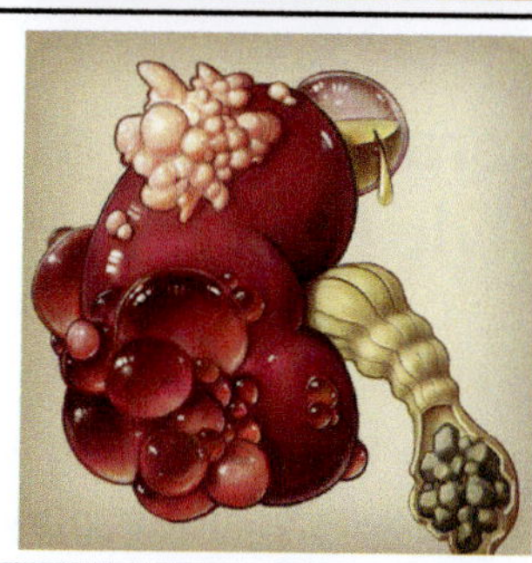

5.1. Chronic Pelvic Pain

Any pelvic pain that lasts longer than six months is classified as chronic pelvic pain (CPP). The cause of the pain may not always be clear-cut, and there may be erratic correlations between some pathologies (like adhesions, endometriosis, and pelvic congestion) and pain even after a comprehensive evaluation. This chapter discusses the differential diagnosis and treatment of persistent pelvic pain in addition to outlining the pertinent anatomy.

5.1.1. Biological Considerations

Unlike somatic pain, visceral pain is typically deep and challenging to localize (Kumazawa, 1986; Cervero & Tattersall, 1986; Wesselmann & Lai, 1997). Furthermore, many autonomic reactions, including restlessness, nausea, vomiting, and diaphoresis, are linked to acute visceral pain (Procacci et al., 1986). Referred pain, which is superficial, well-localized, and thought to originate from the dermatome receiving the visceral stimulus, is a significant component of visceral pelvic pain. Referred pain to the dermatomes associated with pelvic organ innervation characterizes a variety of acute and chronic gynecologic pain conditions, i.e., the dorsal rami of L1–L2 (lower back) and T10–L2 (anterior thighs and abdominal wall) (Slocumb, 1984; Giamberardino et al., 1995; Wesselmann & Lai, 1997).

5.2. Peripheral Causes of Chronic Pelvic Pain

5.2.1. Adhesions

Many viewpoints have been expressed regarding the role that pelvic adhesions play in the development of pelvic pain. 16–44% of patients undergoing laparoscopy for persistent pelvic pain had adhesions discovered (Kresch et al., 1984; Rapkin, 1986; Hughes, 1990). Nevertheless, the comparison group chosen will determine the prevalence of adhesions in the control group (i.e., either infertility or sterilization). Adhesions were observed by Kresch in 14% of women undergoing sterilization and 51% of CPP patients (Kresch et al., 1984). On the other hand, according to Rapkin (1986), adhesions were present in 26% of CPP patients and 39% of asymptomatic infertility patients. Moreover, there were no differences in the location or density of adhesions between the groups (Rapkin, 1986). Koninckx et al. (1991), who laparoscoped 227 patients and observed a similar prevalence and distribution of adhesions between CPP patients and asymptomatic infertility patients, corroborated the latter findings.

Table 5.1. Summary of the Pathogenesis of Pelvic Pain in the Context of Chron's Disease

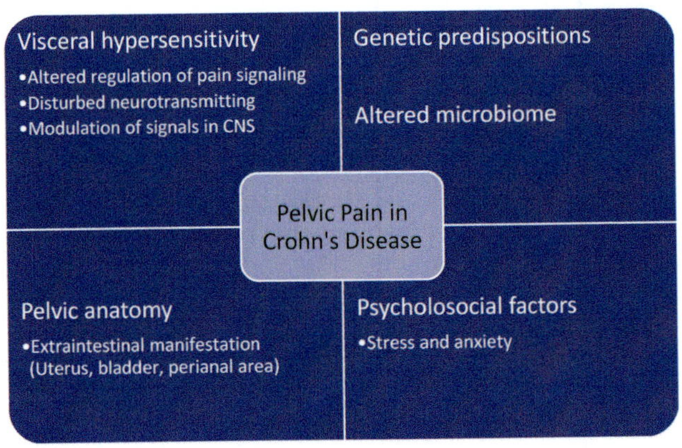

Source. Włodarczyk J, Burzyński J, Czerwiński B, Prusisz M, Socała K, Poleszak E, Fichna J, Maryńczak K, Włodarczyk M, Dziki Ł. Management of Pelvic Pain in Patients with Crohn's Disease—Current Overview. *Journal of Clinical Medicine*. 2023; 12(2):526. https://doi.org/10.3390/jcm12020526.

Table 5.2. Summary of Chronic Pelvic Pain

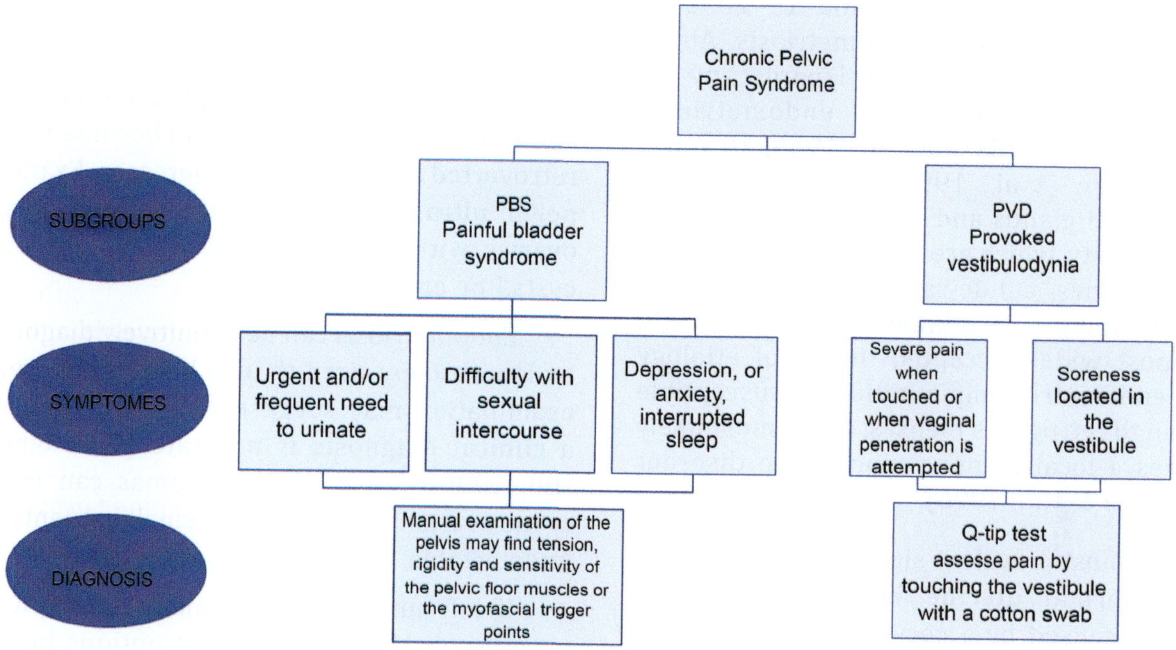

Source. Grinberg K, Sela Y, Nissanholtz-Gannot R. New Insights about Chronic Pelvic Pain Syndrome (CPPS). *International Journal of Environmental Research and Public Health*. 2020; 17(9):3005. https://doi.org/10.3390/ijerph17093005.

While it is true that women with CPP are more likely than women having sterilization to experience adhesions, these findings cannot be interpreted as causal or even strongly associated. Adhesiolysis should reduce pain if adhesions are the source of it. In women with CPP, there is only one randomized controlled trial of adhesion lysis (Peters et al., 1992). Patients with CPP who had laparoscopically diagnosed stage III to IV adhesions were either expected to be managed or had laparotomy adhesiolysis. A follow-up pain assessment conducted 16 months after surgery revealed no discernible advantage of adhesiolysis over expectant management. At an 8-month follow-up, a prospective nonrandomized adhesiolysis study also revealed no improvement in pain (Steege & Scott, 1991). With adhesiolysis, however, there was a notable improvement in pain relief for the subgroup of women without "CPP syndrome." Women who displayed four or more of the following symptoms were considered to have CPP syndrome: (1) pain lasting longer than six months; (2) inadequate relief from prior treatments; (3) reduced physical functioning due to pain; (4) vegetative signs of depression; and (5) changed roles within the family. Steege came to the conclusion that while adhesion lysis may be beneficial in certain cases, it is not recommended for women who have "CPP syndrome" (Steege & Scott, 1991).

Future research on laparoscopy performed under local anesthesia might enable "pain mapping," which would identify the tissues or adhesions most likely to be the source of the pain. Studies on pain symptoms following procedures guided by pain mapping techniques have not yet been conducted (Howard et al., 2000).

5.2.2. Endometriosis

About 1–2% of all women and 15–20–25% of infertile women have endometriosis. About 28–74% of patients having a laparoscopy for persistent pelvic pain have endometriosis (Kresch et al., 1984; Rapkin, 1986; Howard, 1993; Reese et al., 1996). The presence of endometrial glands and stroma outside of the uterine cavity, which are most frequently found in the ovaries, cul-de-sac, pelvic visceral and parietal peritoneum, is known as endometriosis. The most widely accepted theory of etiology links endometrial implantation in susceptible women to retrograde menses, and it most likely involves a local immune modulation disorder (D'Hooghe & Hill, 1996).

The most prevalent signs of endometriosis are abnormal uterine bleeding, which is typically caused by a secretory endometrium, dysmenorrhea, dyspareunia, and infertility. Endometriosis can cause pelvic pain in women at any point during the menstrual cycle, although the most common symptom is dysmenorrhea. Dysmenorrhea can start 7 to10 days before the menstrual cycle starts and last long after the bleeding stops. The patient frequently reports experiencing sharp or pressure-like pain in the rectum, lower abdomen, and back that radiates to the perineum, thighs, or vagina. When the disease affects the uterosacral ligaments, the rectovaginal septum, or the cul-de-sac (pouch of Douglas), dyspareunia or dyschezia (pain with bowel movements) is common. While many patients have inflammation of the intestinal serosa, mucosa is rarely affected, which can result in cyclic hemochromateemia. Urinary tract involvement can also be linked to frequency, urgency, and infrequently, haematuria. Patients may very rarely experience ureteral or colon blockage. Women who are postmenopausal and taking estrogen replacement therapy may still have endometriosis symptoms. In the absence of estrogen replacement, the diagnosis is quite controversial. Endometriosis patients frequently exhibit focal tenderness and nodularity on rectovaginal examination of the posterior cul-de-sac, uterosacral or broad ligaments. The cul-de-sac will become completely obliterated and fibrotic, and the uterus will become fixedly retroverted as the disease progresses. Exams or pelvic ultrasounds frequently reveal enlarged ovaries with reduced mobility and "chocolate cysts," or endometriomas.

Endometriosis can be definitively diagnosed by laparoscopy, even though history and pelvic examination may suggest it. 50% of the time, a clinical diagnosis is accurate (D'Hooghe & Hill, 1996). Since endometriomas can mimic cystic ovarian neoplasms and small implants are undetectable, ultrasound is not a diagnostic tool.

If left untreated, endometriosis typically progresses. Medical treatment options include gonadotropin-releasing hormone analogs, high-dose oral or depo progestins, androgenic hormones (Danocrine), continuous or cyclic oral contraceptive pills, and Prentice et al. (2000), Olive and Pritts (2001). In cases of severe endometriosis or endometriomas, laparoscopic electro-dessication, laser vaporization, or laparotomy with disease resection is typically advised. Individuals who do not wish to become fertile may have a total abdominal hysterectomy, which includes the removal of any remaining GI, GU, or peritoneal disease, as well as bilateral salpingo-oophorectomy and appendectomy. Multidisciplinary pain management or adjunctive acupuncture are beneficial for certain women (Rapkin & Kames, 1987).

Endometriosis may not be the primary cause of chronic pelvic pain in many women, or it may only be a contributing factor. Upon repeat laparoscopy, at least 30% of patients who experienced recurrent pain following endometriosis treatment showed no evidence of residual implants. With the exception of higher-stage diseases, which are typically linked to higher prevalence and more intense pain, there is no discernible relationship between the severity of the disease and the level of pain. Moreover, there is no connection between the site of endometriotic lesions and the location of pain (Fukaya et al., 1993). Careful reevaluation is necessary if pain does not improve with appropriate medical or surgical management of endometriosis.

5.2.3. Tumors and Cysts of the Reproductive Organs

Acute pain may result from degeneration, torsion of the leiomyomata, or adnexal torsion in the majority of reproductive organ cysts and tumors. Ultrasonography is needed to diagnose pelvic tumors, such as leiomyomata or ovarian neoplasms, which can cause persistent lower abdominal fullness and discomfort.

Leiomyomata are the most prevalent type of pelvic neoplasm. Myomata typically cause mild pelvic discomfort when the masses press against the bladder or rectum. When uterine size exceeds 14 cm, abnormal bleeding or discomfort are usually warranted for surgery, either a myomectomy or a hysterectomy.

5.2.4. Pelvic Congestion

The origin of chronic pelvic pain has been the subject of interest for the past 40 years, with some linking it to "pelvic congestion" or varicosities in the uterine and ovarian veins. Clinical manifestations of the syndrome include menorrhagia, dysmenorrhea, dyspareunia, and low back and abdominal pain. Usually bilateral, the pain is distributed lower pelvic and is made worse by the menstrual cycle and the luteal phase. Exam findings include uterine tenderness, parametria, particularly in the uterosacral ligaments, and frequently polycystic ovaries (Beard et al., 1988).

Until recently, the only diagnosis for pelvic congestion was a clinical one. Transuterine venography is a diagnostic test, but in 21% of cases, it is either technically impractical or not readable (Beard et al., 1988). A few small research have looked at pelvic ultrasound combined with Doppler or MRI to diagnose pelvic congestion (Stones et al., 1990).

Pelvic congestion has been treated with hormonal suppression that creates a hypo-estrogenic environment (Farquhar et al., 1989; Gangar et al., 1993). In a randomized, placebo-controlled treatment trial, 30 mg of medroxyprogesterone acetate (MPA) was given daily for three months. The patients who received MPA experienced a 50% reduction in pain score, while those who received a placebo experienced a 33% reduction (Beard et al., 1991). But while the pain did not return in the placebo group, it did in the MPA group following treatment cessation. 33 of the 36 patients who were followed for a year after a total abdominal hysterectomy with bilateral salpingo-oophorectomy reported no pain (Beard et al., 1991). Pelvic vein transcatheter embolization has been tried on a small number of patients with encouraging results, but the long-term risks and advantages are still unknown (Sichlau et al., 1994).

5.2.5. Salphingo-Oophoritis

Although patients typically experience symptoms and signs of acute or subacute infection before the pain becomes chronic, salpingo-oophoritis can cause persistent pelvic pain. Patients may have been diagnosed with pelvic inflammatory disease and may have experienced multiple episodes of pain accompanied by fever. The patient might not even have salpingitis, though. 50% of cases result in a clinical diagnosis that is incorrect (Westrom & Eschenbach, 1999). Diagnostic methods include peritoneal fluid cultures and laparoscopic visualization of the pelvic organs. Intravenous antibiotics are the standard treatment for salpingo-oophoritis. Hysterectomy and salpingo-oophorectomy are only infrequently necessary, usually in cases of tuboovarian abscesses.

5.2.6. Ovarian Remnant Syndrome

The ovarian remnant syndrome, in which residual ovarian cortical tissue is left in situ, can arise from a hysterectomy and bilateral salpingo-oophorectomy carried out in the context of severe anatomic distortion, such as with severe endometriosis or pelvic inflammatory disease (Siddal-Allum et al., 1994). Pain related to ovarian remnants is uncommon, despite the fact that their incidence is unknown but thought to be high.

A history, physical examination, and hormonal evaluation are used to diagnose ovarian remnant syndrome (Price et al., 1990). After surgery, flank pain, urinary tract infection, and intermittent partial bowel obstruction may occur two to five years later along with periodic pain. A sore mass in the lateral pelvis may be discovered during a pelvic exam. A mass with sonographic features of ovarian tissue is typically confirmed by ultrasound after ovarian stimulation with clomiphene. Follicle stimulating hormone (FSH) and estradiol levels in a patient who has undergone bilateral salpingo-oophorectomy and is not receiving hormonal replacement therapy show a typical premenopausal picture, though occasionally the remaining ovarian tissue may not be active enough to suppress FSH levels. Treatment requires laparotomy to remove residual ovarian tissue (Price et al., 1990). However, complications are common and can include bleeding, ureteral, bladder, and bowel injury, postoperative ileus, and recurrent remnants in 15% of cases. An acceptable substitute could be GnRH agonist treatment along with estrogen and progestin addback therapy (Carey & Slack, 1996).

5.2.7. Cyclic Pelvic Pain

Pelvic cyclic pain refers to pain that has a particular connection to the menstrual cycle. Primary and secondary dysmenorrhea are included, along with atypical cyclic pain, such as pain that starts two weeks before menstruation. An alternative form of secondary dysmenorrhea is atypical cyclic pain. An examination of a daily pain and menstrual journal is frequently necessary for the diagnosis of cyclic pain.

Up to 50% of women who menstruate experience dysmenorrhea, also known as "painful monthly flow," a common gynecologic disorder (Rapkin et al., 1997). When there is no pelvic pathology, menstrual pain is referred to as primary dysmenorrhea; when there is, it is referred to as secondary dysmenorrhea. Primary dysmenorrhea typically manifests one to two years following menarche, coinciding with the onset of ovulatory cycles, though it can last well into the forties. Suprapubic cramps that radiate down the anterior thighs and into the lumbosacral region are the source of the pain, which is frequently accompanied by nausea, vomiting, and diarrhea. The pain lasts for 48–72 hours and happens before or shortly after the start of the menstrual cycle.

Years after menarche is typically when secondary dysmenorrhea first appears, and it may coincide with anovulatory cycles. Endometriosis and adenomyosis, a disorder in which the endometrial glands penetrate the myometrium, are the most frequent causes of secondary dysmenorrhea. Table 5.2 lists uterine, fallopian tube, vaginal, cervical, adnexal, and peritoneal pathologies as additional common causes. A comprehensive history regarding the onset and duration of the pain, a pain diary, and a careful pelvic examination—focusing on the uterus's size, shape, mobility, and tenderness as well as adnexal structures and the nodularity of the uterosacral ligaments and rectovaginal septum—are necessary to distinguish between primary and secondary dysmenorrhea and chronic pelvic pain. A transvaginal ultrasound, a complete blood count with an elevated white blood cell count (ESR), and genital studies for chlamydia and gonorrhea are recommended. In the event that no anomalies are discovered and the discomfort is periodic, primary dysmenorrhea may be the tentative diagnosis.

Prostaglandin synthetase inhibitors should be started premenstrually, or at least before the pain starts, or before it gets severe, as they are effective in treating primary dysmenorrhea in up to 80% of cases (Deligeoroglou, 2000). The birth control pill is the second choice for a patient with primary dysmenorrhea who is not contraindicated for oral contraceptives. Oral contraceptive control pills provide relief for over 90% of women suffering from primary dysmenorrhea (Chan & Dawood, 1980). Pain management can be achieved with the use of narcotic analgesics. Organic pathology should be ruled out before adding narcotic medication. This is usually done with a laparoscopy and, if necessary, a hysteroscopy. Gonadotropin-releasing hormone agonists combined with continuous low-dosage (menopausal) hormone addback, continuous oral contraceptive pill administration, and high-dose progestins (oral or depo intramuscular injection) are additional methods of hormonal menstrual suppression. Potential side effects of these regimens include breakthrough bleeding and related pain. Transcutaneous electrical nerve stimulation and acupuncture may be effective (Wilson et al., 2000). Laparoscopy is necessary to rule out endometriosis and other potential causes of secondary dysmenorrhea if treatment fails. Laparoscopic uterosacral ligament ablation, presacral neurectomy, and, in certain instances of secondary dysmenorrhea, hysterectomy are among the surgical techniques for treating dysmenorrhea (Malinak, 1980).

5.2.8. Gastroenterologic Causes of Chronic Pelvic Pain

Gastroenterologic (GI) pathology is the real cause of many patients with chronic pelvic pain who are referred to gynecologists (Reiter, 1990; Walker et al., 1996). It is frequently challenging to distinguish between lower abdominal pain that is enterocolic or gynecologic because the cervix, uterus, adnexa, lower ileum, sigmoid colon, and rectum share the same visceral innervation, with pain signals traveling via the sympathetic nerves to spinal cord segments T10–L1 (Mayer & Gebhart, 1993). Additionally, pain from the GI tract is frequently diffuse and poorly localized, as is the case with other forms of visceral pain.

As many as 7 to 60% of referrals to a gynecologist for chronic pelvic pain can be attributed to irritable bowel syndrome (IBS), one of the more prevalent causes of lower abdominal pain (Reiter, 1990). The most common sign of irritable bowel syndrome is cramping, sporadic stomach pain, usually located in the lower left quadrant. Table 5.3 lists the Rome II criteria for the diagnosis of IBS. The premenstrual and menstrual phases of the cycle, as well as moments of stress, tension, anxiety, or depression, are generally associated with worsening symptoms.

IBS is diagnosed based on the patient's medical history and the rule out of other illnesses. Blood in the stool, recent antibiotic use, nocturnal awakenings, weight loss, family history of colon cancer, and abnormal pelvic or abdominal exam are examples of red flags that should not be used to rule out pathology but rather call for a colonoscopy or CAT scan. Dietary changes, bulk-forming agents, a high-fiber diet, assurance, education, stress management, and medications like anxiolytics, anticholinergics, low-dose tricyclic antidepressants, or other antispasmodics are all part of the treatment plan for IBS (Ringel et al., 2001).

Colonic diverticular disease is another factor contributing to persistent enterocolic pain. Diverticulosis affects 5 to 40% of people over 40, though most patients never get diverticulitis. Diverticulitis causes severe, acute pain in the left lower quadrant along with fever, a tender mass, and leukocytosis, whereas diverticulosis is typically asymptomatic.

Table 5.3. The Rome II Criteria for Diagnosing Irritable Bowel Syndrome

Abdominal pain or discomfort, for at least 12 weeks out of the previous 12 months, which need not necessarily be consecutive (and cannot be explained by structural or biochemical changes), and has 2 of these 3 features:	
a.	relieved by defecation
b.	onset associated with a change in frequency
c.	consistency of stool

Similar to Crohn's disease, ulcerative colitis, and granulomatous disease, inflammatory bowel diseases (IBD) typically manifest more acutely with symptoms like vomiting, fever, diarrhea, and anorexia rather than as chronic pelvic pain. An IBD diagnosis is made with a barium study or colonoscopy.

Prolonged lower abdominal pain may be caused by gastrointestinal tract tumors. Changes in bowel habits (74% of patients) and abdominal pain (65% of patients) are the most common and early symptoms of bowel carcinomas. Weight loss and rectal bleeding could indicate an advanced stage of the illness. During a rectal examination, the majority of rectal tumors are palpable. Diagnostic procedures include endoscopy, barium enema, and CAT scan with contrast.

5.2.9. Hernia

One differential diagnosis for lower abdominal pain is a hernia. Inguinal hernias in females are comparatively uncommon. Women who have anterior or posterior perineal hernias may experience lower pressure-like abdominal or perineal pain. These hernias are typically restricted to cystocele, rectocele, or enterocele. Usually, a pessary is used to treat this kind of pain, followed by surgery. A Spigelian hernia, which arises from transversalis fascia weakness and causes lower abdominal pain between the semilunar line and the lateral border of the rectus muscle, is another reason why women experience abdominal pain. This was first reported by Spagen in 1984. Ultrasound, clinical examination, and increased pain with Valsalva maneuver are useful in the diagnosis process. Surgery is required in order to repair.

5.2.10. Urologic Causes of Chronic Pelvic Pain

The anatomy and development of the urinary and genital tracts are so close that pelvic pain can be a presenting symptom of chronic pain of urologic origin. The embryonic urogenital sinus is the source of the urethra, bladder, vagina, and vestibule. About 5% of women with chronic pelvic pain present with pelvic pain due to a variety of ureteral causes, including endometriosis, ureteral obstructions, urolithiasis, recurrent cystoureteritis, urethral syndrome, urethral diverticulae, urgency, frequency syndrome, interstitial cystitis, infiltrating bladder tumors, and ectopic pelvic kidney (Reiter, 1990; Spangen, 1984). Inquire about symptoms like urgency, frequency, hesitancy, incontinence, nocturia, dyspareunia, and previous history of urinary tract treatment in the medical history. In addition to pyuria and a positive urine culture, the patient with infectious cystitis complains of suprapubic pain, dysuria, frequency, and urgency. Usually, the symptoms go away with appropriate antibiotic treatment. History, urinalysis, and culture can all be used to diagnose relapses and reinfection. In some cases, if the patient has recurrent cystoureteritis, antibiotics may need to be given post-coitally or for an extended length of time. The antibiotic and therapy duration may also need to be modified. About 25% of female cases of pyuria and urethritis are caused by chlamydial infections (Summit, 1993).

According to Bergman et al. (1989), the urethral syndrome can manifest as persistent pelvic pain or irritative symptoms of the lower urinary tract, including dysuria, urinary frequency, and dyspareunia. This is an exclusionary diagnosis. Negative results on urinalysis, low or negative colony counts (e.g., less than 104 colon/mL) on a urine culture, a negative chlamydia test, and vulvovaginitis assessment will raise the possibility of urethral syndrome diagnosis. Although urethral spasticity with periurethral muscle fatigue or chronic inflammation of the periurethral glands have been proposed as possible causes, the exact cause of the syndrome is unknown. Reeducating voiding habits through pelvic floor muscle biofeedback (Bergman et al., 1989) is one method of treatment. Another is chronic suppression with a low-dose course of broad spectrum antibiotics for three to six months, or, if chlamydia is suspected, tetracycline for two to three weeks. Urethral dilatation has been tried, if unsuccessful. For women going through menopause and beyond, vaginal estrogen is crucial (Karram, 1993). Muscle relaxants, psychotherapy, and pelvic floor muscle biofeedback should all be taken into account.

Urge/frequency syndrome and interstitial cystitis (IC) are both compatible with symptoms of suprapubic pain, nocturia, urgency, and frequency of urination along with negative laboratory results. At least two of the following symptoms must be present in order for the diagnosis of IC to be made by consensus: glomerulations on endoscopy, decreased compliance on cystometrogram, pain in the suprapubic, pelvic, urethral, vaginal, or perineal regions, or pain relieved by emptying the bladder (Kream & Carr, 1999). Urgency/frequency syndrome is the term used to describe symptoms that do not fit the criteria of the IC. The cause of interstitial cystitis is unknown, although theories include autoimmune disease, abnormalities in the bladder mucosa's glycosaminoglycan layer, and activated bladder sensory neuropeptides (Sant, 1998). Patients exhibiting the aforementioned symptoms should be evaluated with a cystoscopy performed under anesthesia, hydrodistension, and possibly a biopsy. A bladder diet, intravesical hydrodistension, transcutaneous electrical nerve stimulation (TENS), instillation of dimethylsulfoxide or glycosaminoglycan analogs, physical therapy, biofeedback to the pelvic floor muscles, or repeated anesthetic blocks are among the treatment options (hypogastric plexus). The condition is still treated empirically, with some success being achieved with less-than-ideal oral pharmacologic agents such as narcotics, anticholinergics, antispasmodics, non-steroidal anti-inflammatory drugs, and tricyclic antidepressants (Sant, 1998).

5.2.11. Nerve Entrapment or Injury

In the differential diagnosis of persistent lower abdominal pain, abdominal cutaneous nerve injury or entrapment should be taken into account, particularly in cases where no visceral etiology is evident. The syndrome can also follow trauma, car accidents, or exercise.

It most frequently develops months to years after Pfannenstiel skin or other lower abdominal incisions, including laparoscopic procedures (Sippo et al., 1987). The genitofemoral (L1, L2), ilioinguinal (T12, L1), and iliohypogastric (T12, L1) nerves are frequently affected.

Pain is one of the signs of nerve entrapment; it is usually brought on by exercise and goes away with bed rest. The rectus margin's lateral edge is the site of a stabbing, colicky pain that is frequently accompanied by a burning or aching pain that radiates to the hip or sacroiliac region. The pain is made worse by bloating, menstruation, nausea, and a full bladder or bowel.

A fingertip examination can be used to pinpoint the location of the pain (McDonald, 1993). The neuromuscular foramen at the rectus margin medial and inferior to the anterior iliac spine, or the site of exit from the aponeurosis of the other thoracic/abdominal cutaneous nerves in the event of spontaneous nerve entrapment, is the maximal point of tenderness. Asking the patient to elevate their shoulders or raise and extend their lower limbs in a straight leg raising maneuver is one maneuver that aids in the diagnosis.

Next, apply pressure with a single finger to the outer side of the rectus abdominis muscle. If there is pain in the abdominal wall, it will get worse (Thomson & Francis, 1977). A diagnostic nerve block consisting of an injection of 2–3 mL of 0.25% Bupivocaine is used to confirm the tentative diagnosis (Slocumb, 1990; McDonald, 1993). Most patients report feeling better right away, and many need up to five injections every two weeks. Surgery to remove the affected nerves should only be considered as a last resort (Hahn, 1989). Acupuncture, anticonvulsants, and tricyclic antidepressants are among the medications that are helpful in managing pain. To strengthen additional muscles and prevent reinjury, physical therapy or a change in lifestyle may be required.

5.2.12. Musculoskeletal Causes of Chronic Pain

Gynecologic pathology is rarely the cause of lower back pain in women who do not also complain of pelvic pain, though low back pain can coexist with pelvic pathology. Gynecologic, vascular, neurologic, psychogenic, or spondylogenic pathologies (relating to the axial skeleton and its structures) can all result in back pain (Baker, 1993). Chronic pelvic pain symptoms are frequently attributed to abnormalities of the musculoskeletal system. Treatment effectiveness should be increased by a physical therapist who is skilled in assessing joint range of motion, muscle strength and length, and posture.

5.2.13. Myofascial Pain

There are differing reports on the frequency of myofascial pain as a reason for pelvic pain. Myofascial syndrome was discovered by Reiter and Gambone in 15% of their patients with somatic pathology. Reiter (1990) states that 47% of all patients referred to their pelvic pain clinic had identifiable somatic pathology. Slocumb (1984, 1990) observed that 89% of women presenting with chronic pelvic pain had "trigger points," regardless of the underlying pelvic pathology.

Activity in the afflicted area and deeper visceral structures that have similar dermatomal innervation—bladder or colon activity or pathology, menses, and cervical motion and intercourse—both intensify myofascial pain (Travell, 1976; Slocumb, 1984, 1990). Any muscle or structure with T12–L4 innervation can refer pain to the lower abdomen (i.e., muscles like the rectus, illiopsoas, quadratus lumborum, piriformis, and obturators, ligaments, discs, and vertebrae). Applying pressure to the trigger point on the back, vaginal, or abdominal dermatomes causes both local and referred pain when examined digitally. The above-described straight leg raising maneuver makes pain worse. In addition to physical therapy and treatment of associated psychological factors like depression, anxiety, and learned behavior patterns that may accompany and exacerbate the condition, treatment for myofascial trigger points involves injecting the trigger points with a local anesthetic (Travell, 1976; Slocumb, 1984, 1990). Anticonvulsants and tricyclic antidepressants are two examples of medications that may be helpful.

5.3. Psychological Factors in Chronic Pelvic Pain

From a psychological standpoint, a number of things could encourage pain to become chronic. Research on women who experience persistent pelvic pain has revealed a significant degree of psychological distress (Reiter, 1990).

Compared to women with chronic pelvic pain and pathology as determined by laparoscopy, women with chronic pelvic pain without pathology were found to have higher depression scores and family histories of affective disorder (Magni et al., 1984). The prevalence of major depression, dysthymic disorder, panic disorders, somatization disorder, and sexual abuse was significantly higher in the pelvic pain group of women compared to the pain-free control group and those with pelvic pain of unknown etiology. Although no prospective studies have been conducted, depression frequently occurred before the onset of pain (Magni et al., 1984; Mayer & Gebhart, 1993).

Research has also looked at the relationship between sexual abuse and chronic pelvic pain. Women with chronic pelvic pain have been found to be highly prevalent (90%) victims of both physical and sexual abuse (Rapkin et al., 1990). The subsequent persistence of pelvic pain is strongly correlated with a history of depression and childhood sexual abuse (Harrop-Griffiths et al., 1988). Toomey reiterated the significance of finding out about past histories of physical and sexual abuse in patients with persistent pelvic pain (Toomey et al., 1993).

For patients without somatic pathology, the diagnosis of "chronic pelvic pain without obvious pathology" has been proposed (Renaer, 1980). These patients have frequently been diagnosed with psychogenic pain. It is important to recognize that neurophysiologic processes in the brain and spinal cord contribute to the persistence of chronic pain (Rapkin, 1995). In all painful conditions, Wall (1988) suggests that it is "necessary to consider the lability of central transmission pathways as well as seeking peripheral pathology."

5.4. Diagnosis and Management of Chronic Pelvic Pain

Like other chronic pain conditions, pelvic pain requires a meticulous yet compassionate multidisciplinary approach for successful diagnosis and treatment. A complete medical history must be acquired. It is important to inquire about the type of pain, its location and radiation, factors that aggravate or relieve it, the timing of the menstrual cycle, the impact of exercise, work, stress, sexual activity, and orgasm. Determine the circumstances surrounding the onset and continuation of the pain, such as prior pain episodes, the inability to carry out a family role or work, litigation, or worker's compensation. Other somatic symptoms to be noted include those related to the genital tract (abnormal vaginal bleeding, discharge, mittelschmerz, dysmenorrhea, dyspareunia, infertility), the musculoskeletal system (predominantly low back distribution, pain radiation, association with injury, fatigue, postural changes), and the urinary system (dysuria, urgency, frequency, suprapelvic pain). It is necessary to ask historical questions particular to each of the peripheral pathologies listed in Table 5.1. It is important to record past medical, surgical, gynecologic, obstetric, and sexual histories as well as medication intake and previous pain evaluations. If the patient has undergone surgery, the operational and pathology reports are crucial.

It is important to inquire about both recent and previous psychological histories, including psychosocial factors, histories of physical, sexual, and/or emotional abuse in the past or present, hospitalization histories, suicide attempts, and chemical (drug or alcohol) dependency. It is important to talk about the patient's and her family's perspective on the pain, how they have responded to it, and any recent changes in the patient's life. After building a rapport with the patient, it might be necessary to obtain the portion of the history that deals with delicate subjects again.

The possibility of an acute condition requiring immediate medical or surgical intervention should be raised by symptoms such as fever, anorexia, nausea, emesis, significant diarrhea, recurrent constipation, ascites, uterine bleeding, pregnancy, or a recent abortion, especially if they are accompanied by orthostasis, peritoneal signs, pelvic or abdominal mass, abnormal CBC, positive genital or urinary tract cultures, or a positive pregnancy test.

A thorough physical examination should be conducted, paying special attention to the examination of the pelvic floor muscles, urethrovesical junction?, abdominal, back, bimanual, and rectovaginal. In order to identify the sources of pain in the abdominal wall, the examination should involve an evaluation of the abdomen using a straight leg raising maneuver. With the aforementioned maneuvers, visceral pain is reduced and abdominal wall pain is increased (Slocumb, 1990; McDonald, 1993). The patient should be checked while standing for pelvic (cystocele, enterocele), abdominal (inguinal, femoral, and Spigelian), and hernias. Using fingertip palpation, an attempt should be made to identify the tissues (lower back, external genital, pelvic, and abdominal) that replicate the patient's pain. It is important to assess the rectum, urethra, and bladder for appearance, support, and tenderness. The examination of the S3–S5 and L2–L4 nerve roots can be facilitated by a neurologic examination of the lower limbs and the perineum. Visualizing the vaginal epithelium is important for determining vaginal estrogenization.

If laboratory tests haven't been done already, they include CBC, ESR, urinalysis and culture, pap smear, wet mount of vaginal secretions, cervical and urethral cultures (gonorrhea and chlamydia), stool guaiac, and stool culture if diarrhea is present. An ultrasound or MRI examination is recommended if the results of the pelvic or abdominal examination are insufficient or suggestive of a mass. Fiberoptic or other suitable imaging studies of other organ systems should be taken into consideration if symptoms and signs point to the involvement of other systems.

It is recommended to keep a daily pain journal to record the occurrence, severity, and mood of pain. Menstrual cycles, medication intake, and aggravating and mitigating factors ought to be documented in the diary. An analog visual scale ranging from 1 (no pain) to 10 (the most severe pain ever) is used in simple diaries. It is recommended to keep the diary for a minimum of two months.

It is best to have a psychologist with experience managing chronic pain assess the patient. Preferably, the psychologist should work out of the same clinic suite. Psychological referral completes the evaluation process and provides access to behavioral, relaxation, and stress-reduction therapies. The evaluation of the pain complaint, its influence on life circumstances, controlling factors, and coping mechanisms should be the main goals of the assessment.

Sexual functioning is likely to be impacted by pelvic pain, which could have further effects on mood, the quality of relationships, and self-esteem. To determine whether the sexual issues developed later on or before the pain, a thorough medical history is required. It is important to assess any past or present trauma, sexual abuse, or physical abuse. It is important to ascertain how the pain affects daily functioning. Standardized psychological testing is beneficial in establishing a baseline against which to measure response to treatment and directing treatment strategies in addition to determining the presence of affective disturbance.

If a particular pathology is verified, management needs to move forward. Patients should be assessed for primary or secondary dysmenorrhea and treated if their pain diary indicates cyclic or atypical cyclic pain. Diagnosing pelvic pain, particularly cyclic pain, may necessitate a laparoscopy. Treatment can start on the basis of clinical suspicion, but if pelvic congestion is suspected, imaging tests such as transuterine venography, MRI, or pelvic ultrasound may be recommended. If trigger points were injected and the pain persisted, the injection should be repeated weekly or biweekly for a maximum of five injections. A physical therapy consultation should also be considered, particularly if activity exacerbates the pain or if the low back pain is noticeable. The pharmacologic treatment of CPP is similar to that of general chronic pain. Patients with pelvic pain have responded well to the use of tricyclic antidepressants and anticonvulsants, despite the paucity of controlled studies in this area. Pelvic pain can be effectively managed with narcotics when they are used appropriately and in conjunction with a narcotic contract. Prescription selective serotonin reuptake inhibitors are used to treat depression. The patient should keep up with their regularly scheduled appointments with the gynecologist.

5.4.1. Surgical Management of Chronic Pelvic Pain

A randomized controlled trial is only found in a small number of studies on the surgical management of CPP. The average length of postoperative follow-up is less than six months, and pain assessment tools are typically insufficient.

5.4.2. Diagnostic Laparoscopy

The laparoscope has been controversial in its application to the treatment of chronic pelvic pain, despite its great utility in diagnosing and treating acute pelvic pain. Two-thirds of patients have adhesion findings, which may or may not be related to their pain, and between 14 and 77% of patients have no discernible pathology (Rapkin, 1986; Steege & Scott, 1991; Stout et al., 1991). Furthermore, regardless of the existence of "pathology," non-surgical management of chronic pelvic pain is effective in 65 to 90% of patients (Rapkin & Kames, 1987; Reiter et al., 1991; Peters et al., 1991). According to Peters et al. (1991), women with chronic pelvic pain were randomized to one of two treatment groups: the standard approach group, which underwent routine laparoscopy and had results guided by the findings; or the integrated approach group, which focused on somatic, psychological, dietary, and physiotherapeutic factors but did not routinely perform laparoscopy. Of the 49 patients in the standard group, 5% had endometriosis, 18% had adhesions, and the remaining patients had pelvic varices, ovarian cysts, or myomata. Of the patients, 65% had no abnormality. According to Peters et al. (1991), the integrated approach was substantially more successful in reducing pelvic pain (75% vs. 41%; $p < 0.01$).

5.4.3. Hysterectomy

According to Howard (1993), the only reason why 19% of hysterectomies are performed is to treat chronic pelvic pain. That being said, 30% of patients who come into pelvic pain clinics have already had hysterectomy without any pain relief. Hysterectomy is still a viable option for carefully chosen patients experiencing pain of "uterine" origin in cases of cyclic pain or dysfunctional uterine bleeding, particularly if hormonal suppression relieves their symptoms (Hillis et al., 1995).

5.4.4. Presacral Neurectomy

The initial description of presacral neurectomy, also known as sympathectomy (PSN), was given for the indication of dysmenorrhea. The major afferent supply of the presacral nerve, or superior hypogastric plexus, comes from the uterus, proximal fallopian tubes, and the cervix. Because sympathetic fibers from adnexal structures travel with the spinal cord at T9–T10, PSN cannot relieve lateralizing pain with a visceral origin.

PSN has been reported to be effective in treating central pelvic pain in the context of non-cyclic pain as well as cyclic pain (dysmenorrhea) (Vercellini et al., 1991; Candiani et al., 1992). The suprapubic, midline component of menstrual pain can be lessened with PSN (Vercellini et al., 1991). Laparoscopic surgery is technically challenging to perform (Chen & Soong, 1997). There has only been one randomized controlled trial conducted on the laparoscopic transection of the uterosacral ligaments (LUNA), and consequently uterine afferents (Lichten & Bombard, 1987). 81% of the 10 subjects experienced relief with LUNA, but only 45% showed a significant improvement at the one-year follow-up. Still, not a single control got better (Lichten & Bombard, 1987).

5.4.5. Multidisciplinary Pain Management

Chronic pelvic pain can be effectively managed through a multidisciplinary approach, which typically involves a team consisting of a gynecologist, internist, psychologist, physical therapist, anaesthesiologist, and dietitian. Treatment may include non-steroidal anti-inflammatory drugs, narcotics, tricyclic antidepressants, anticonvulsants, as well as trigger point injections and nerve blocks targeting specific areas such as the pudendal, ilioinguinal, iliohypogastric, genitofemoral and occasionally hypogastric nerves.

In 85% of the subjects, a program that included tricyclic antidepressants, acupuncture, and cognitive behavioral therapy was effective in reducing pain by at least 50% (Rapkin & Kames, 1987; Kames al, 1990). A multidisciplinary team may be able to achieve comparable outcomes, according to other research (Wood et al., 1990; Reiter et al., 1991; Peters et al., 1991; Milburn et al., 1993). The multidisciplinary approach combining traditional gynecologic treatment with input from psychological, dietary, and physical therapy was found to be more effective than traditional gynecologic (medical and surgical) management or cure in a prospective randomized, controlled study (Peters et al., 1991).

5.5. Obstetric Pain

According to the current theory of pain management during labor and delivery, pain must be effectively relieved because chronic, intense pain and the stress it causes can have negative effects on the mother and possibly the fetus. Strong clinical evidence (Shnider & Levinson, 1987; Gabbe & Steven, 1991; Bonica & McDonald, 1995) indicates that analgesia administered appropriately lowers maternal and perinatal mortality and morbidity. Obstetricians of today have a conservative view of the drugs that mothers take. The potential for medication given to mothers to have depressant effects on fetuses and neonates is well known. Moreover, mothers are far more grateful for a clear and cogent involvement in the birthing process (Lamaze & Vellay, 1952; Atlee, 1956). The obstetric scenario is extremely stable and successful; patients receive careful consideration and management during the intrapartum period in addition to antepartum evaluation and consultation. A sensitive measure of the effectiveness of this kind of care is the perinatal death rate, which is currently at an all-time low in US history. Before the administration of analgesic therapy, approximately 65–68% of primiparas and multiparas rated their labor pain as severe or very severe, and 23% of primiparas and 11% of multiparas rated their pain as "horrible," according to a systematic study using the McGill Pain Questionnaire (Melzack, 1984). Rich nations now understand the advantages of contemporary analgesia and fully anticipate pain management during childbirth.

5.5.1. Mechanisms and Pathways of the Pain of Childbirth

The logical application of pain relief during labor is based on the neural mechanisms underlying childbirth pain. The uterus, lower uterine segment, cervix, vagina, and perineum are the five general areas that make up the innervation of the reproductive organs.

Afferents with cell bodies in the dorsal root ganglia of the T10, T11, T12, and L1 segments innervate the uterus and lower uterine segments. The sympathetic nerves that comprise the cervical and pelvic plexuses are paralleled by afferent pathways. These afferents from the four segments pass via the inferior, medial, and superior hypogastric pelvic Plexi before entering the posterior roots and connecting with dorsal horn interneurons synaptically. The pain resulting from contractions of the uterus is referred to the dermatomes supplied by the same spinal cord segments that receive input from the uterus and cervix, as is typical of pain arising from the viscera. The T10–T12 pathways also innervate the cervix (Bonica, 1969).

On the other hand, the sacral nerve roots innervate the perineum, and the pudendal nerves carry the input directly to the spinal dorsal horn.

In the vagina, there are some areas of mixed overlap. Approximately 70% of the afferents from the uterine-cervical area connect to the inferior hypogastric plexus of nerves on either side of the cervix, and the remaining afferents from the lower genital tract and vagina connect to the pudendal nerve. The sympathetic nerves supply distinct innervation to the uterine horns (Kawatani & de Groat, 1991). The reproductive tract's small myelinated and unmyelinated fiber types are consistent with the innervation of other visceral organs.

Thus, the pudendal nerve and other smaller nerves derived from S2, S3, and S4 innervate the vagina and the perineum, which are innervated by the same neural pathways as the second and third stages of labor. The unusual pain that is felt in the thigh and upper legs due to pressure on the intrapelvic structures typically involves fibers as high as L2 and as low as S3.

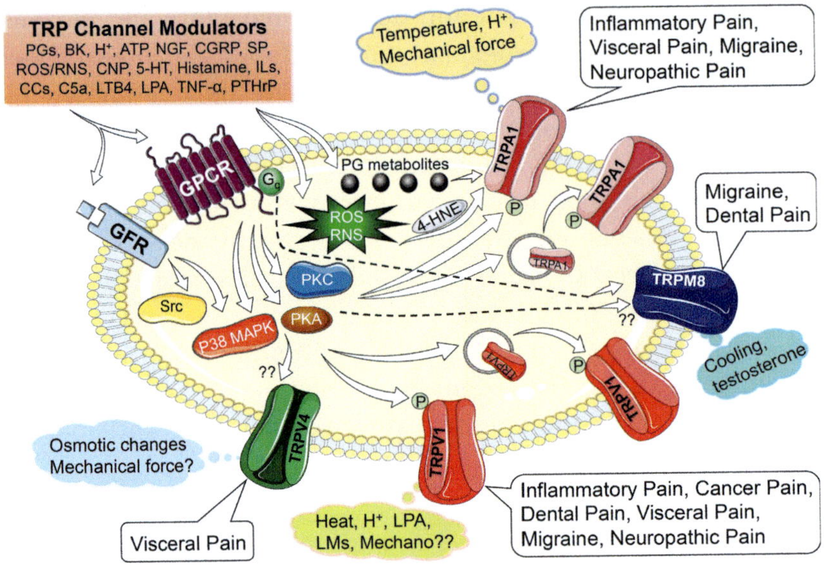

Figure 5.1. Scheme depicting specific activators and modulators of various nociceptive transient receptor potential (TRP) channels on mammalian sensory neurons. Involvement of individual TRP channels in specific pain-related pathologies are indicated/listed within call-out boxes.

Source: Mickle AD, Shepherd AJ, Mohapatra DP. Nociceptive TRP Channels: Sensory Detectors and Transducers in Multiple Pain Pathologies. *Pharmaceuticals*. 2016; 9(4):72. https://doi.org/10.3390/ph9040072.

Note: Abbreviations: 5-HT, serotonin; ATP, adenosine triphosphate; BK, bradykinin; CCs, chemokines; CGRP, calcitonin gene-related peptide; CNP, C-type natriuretic peptide; GFR, growth factor receptor; GPCR, G protein-coupled receptor; H^+, protons; ILs, interleukins; LMs, lipid mediators; LPA, lysophosphatidic acid; LTB4; leukotriene B4; NGF, nerve growth factor; p38 MAPK, p38 mitogen-activated protein kinase; PGs, prostaglandins; PKA, cAMP-dependent protein kinase; PKC, protein kinase C; PTHrP, parathyroid hormone-related peptide; ROS, reactive oxygen species; RNS, reactive nitrogen species; SP, substance P or neurokinin; Src; src-type protein kinase; TRPA1, transient receptor potential sub-family ankyrin, member-1; TRPM8, transient receptor potential sub-family melastatin, member-8; TRPV1, transient receptor potential sub-family vanilloid, member-1; TRPV4, transient receptor potential sub-family vanilloid, member-4.

5.5.2. Labor Pain

Cervical dilation and uterine contractions are the causes of the first stage of labor pain. This keeps happening during the first phase until total dilatation is attained.

Uterine contractions continue even in the face of strong resistance when the cervix has fully dilated. As the fetus descends toward the vaginal outlet, the vaginal canal continues to dilate, causing pain to develop in this second stage. The fetus descends during the second stage, reaching the anatomical level of the ischial spines, where the fetal head starts to negotiate the mid-pelvis. Distension and stretching of the mid- and lower vaginal tissues, distension of the outlet, and eventual dilatation occur as a result of the fetal head eventually passing through the mid-pelvis to allow the passage of the largest part of the fetus—the head. The dorsal root ganglia of the at the S2-S4 levels receive the greatest amount of stimulation for these anatomical changes through the nociceptive pathways of the pudendal nerves. Additionally, there is a substantial sensory spillover via the perianal, upper thigh, and lower sacrum regions to other nearby pathways. The pain in the perineal region is sharp and localized, akin to that experienced when superficial somatic structures are stimulated. By blocking the sensory nerves, this pain can be removed (Klink, 1953; Bonica, 1967).

When complete dilatation takes place, the pain might be excruciating, and it might be challenging to push against the tightness in the perineal muscles until an epidural block involving the sacral nerves or a caudal injection is used to achieve analgesia. A number of parturients experience aching, burning, or cramping discomfort in their thighs and, less frequently, in their legs during the second and late stages of labor. The stimulation of pain-sensitive structures within the pelvic cavity may be the cause of this. These structures may include the pelvic peritoneum, the bladder, urethra, and rectum; the ligaments, fascia, and muscles within the pelvic cavity; and abnormal pressure on the lumbosacral plexus roots. As previously mentioned, the pudendal nerve and other smaller branches that originate from S2, S3, and S4 are involved in the neural pathways for the second and third stages of labor.

5.6. Physiological and Psychological Effects of Labor Pain

5.6.1. Changes in Ventilation

One of the strongest respiratory stimulants during labor and delivery is the pain. Tidal volume, minute ventilation, and alveolar ventilation all noticeably rise as a result of this. Due to this physiological shift, PaCO2 drops from 32 mmHg during pregnancy to as low as 16–20 mmHg, and on rare occasions as low as 10–15 mmHg. pH rises to 7.5–7.6 as a result (Bonica, 1973; Huch et al., 1977; Peabody, 1979). The mother oxygen dissociation curve shifts to the left and cerebral and uterine blood flow decreases as a result of this respiratory alkalosis, which happens at the peak of each uterine contraction. Pain no longer stimulates breathing at the start of the relaxation phase, resulting in a brief period of hypoventilation due to the hypocapnia, which lowers the mother's $PaCO_2$ by 10–50%, with a mean of 25–30% (Huch et al., 1977; Peabody, 1979). When moms are prescribed opioids for pain management, the depressant effects of respiratory alkalosis are compounded by the opioids' own action. Fetal $PaCO_2$ decreases with late decelerations when the mother's $PaCO_2$ drops below 70 mmHg, which has a major impact on the fetus (Myers, 1975).

5.6.2. Neuroendocrine Effects

In the animal model, some of the previously reported alterations—such as decreased carbon dioxide levels—combined with the 20–40% rise in catecholamine levels brought on by noxious stimulation to result in a net decrease in uterine blood flow (Jouppila, 1977; Morishima et al., 1978; Shnider & Levinson, 1987; Berkley & Wood, 1989).

The main effect is an increase in noradrenaline (NA) levels accompanied by a 35–70% decrease in uterine blood flow. According to data from studies conducted on humans, experiencing extreme pain and anxiety during active labor can raise levels of adrenaline (epinephrine) (A) by 300–600%, noradrenaline (norepinephrine) (NA) by 200–400%, cortisol by 200–300%, and corticosteroid and ACTH by significant amounts. All of these peak at delivery or shortly thereafter (Lederman et al., 1977, 1978; Ohno et al., 1986). According to Lederman's research, there was a 200% increase in cortisol, a 150% increase in NA, and a nearly 300% increase in adrenaline (epinephrine). The correlation between elevated A and cortisol levels and pain and anxiety was very intriguing. More recent studies found a nearly two-fold increase in dopamine levels, a three-fold increase in A levels, a two-fold increase in NA levels, and a slight increase in cyclic adenosine monophosphate (cAMP) levels during labor and after delivery. These studies examined catecholamines and cyclic nucleotides extensively. Ohno et al. (1986) observed a correlation between NA and cAMP levels during labor, as well as a positive relationship between the A level and heart rate and systolic blood pressure.

5.6.3. Cardiovascular Changes

Cardiac output rises above prelabor levels during labor. When the parturient was in the supine position as opposed to the lateral position, there was a greater percentage increase in cardiac output. When the parturient was in the supine position, between contractions, her cardiac output was approximately 15% higher in the early first stage, 30% higher in the late first stage, 45% higher in the second stage, and 65–80% higher in the immediate postpartum period than in the prelabor period (Hendricks & Quilligan, 1956; Adams & Alexander, 1958; Hansen & Ueland, 1966). There was even a further increase in cardiac output of 15–20% during painful uterine contractions.

The extrusion of 250–300 ml of blood from the uterus and increased venous return from the pelvis and lower limbs into the maternal circulation are thought to be responsible for nearly half of the increase of cardiac output? during contractions. The remaining portion results from an increase in sympathetic activity brought on by labor's physical exertion, pain, anxiety, and apprehension, all of which increase cardiac output as labor progresses. When there is no analgesic, uterine contractions also result in systolic and diastolic blood pressure increases of 20 to 30 mmHg. An increase in systolic blood pressure and cardiac output causes a notable rise in left ventricular work. While healthy parturients can tolerate this, it may be harmful if the parturients have pulmonary hypertension, essential hypertension, heart disease, or pre-eclampsia (Hendricks & Quilligan, 1956; Hansen & Ueland, 1966; Robson et al., 1987).

5.6.4. Metabolic Effects

The basal metabolic rate and oxygen consumption should rise gradually during pregnancy and reach a significant 20% above normal at term (Bonica, 1967, 1969, 1980; Bonica & McDonald, 1995). The metabolism and oxygen consumption increase even more during parturition (Bonica & McDonald, 1990). Free fatty acids and lactate levels are thought to rise dramatically during labor due to sympathetic-induced lipolytic metabolism and pain-induced catecholamine release (Bonica & McDonald, 1990). This is supported by the observation that only modest increases in maternal free fatty acid, lactate levels, and acidosis are seen upon total blockade of nociceptive afferent and efferent pathways with epidural analgesia (Marx & Greene, 1964). Maternal acidosis can happen if there is inadequate analgesia during the second stage of labor. The physical strain and maternal pain brought on by the constant, active bearing-down attempts are to blame for this. As previously mentioned, labor pain and anxiety also raise the sympathetic nervous system, which in turn raises metabolic rate and oxygen consumption. Labor-related increases in oxygen consumption, combined with the kidney's loss of bicarbonate to compensate for pain-induced respiratory alkalosis, cause a progressive metabolic acidosis in the mother that is passed on to the fetus (Marx & Greene, 1964; Buchan, 1980; Bonica & McDonald, 1990). Along with a greater increase in lactate, the mother's pyruvate level rises.

Eventually, excess lactate accumulates and is reflected in a progressive offset increase in base excess (Marx & Greene, 1964; Buchan, 1980; Bonica & McDonald, 1990).

5.6.5. Gastrointestinal and Urinary Function

The gastrointestinal and urinary tracts are also impacted by labor pain and the resulting rise in sympathetic activity. According to Marx and Greene (1964), pain during labor stimulates the release of gastrin and increases the secretion of gastric acid. Furthermore, there are delays in gastric and urinary bladder function due to segmental and suprasegmental reflex inhibition of gastrointestinal and urinary motility caused by pain, anxiety, and emotional stress. Opioids, depressants, and recumbent postures all exacerbate these reflex effects of nociception (Marx & Greene, 1964; Pearson & Davies, 1973, 1974; Buchan, 1980). Therefore, food and liquids other than water may be retained for up to 36 hours or longer due to the combined effects of painkillers and depressants. During this time, gastric juices and swallowed air build up gradually, and the pH of the stomach gradually drops below the crucial level of 2.5. Therefore, especially during the induction of general anesthesia, delayed gastric emptying of the acidic gastric contents increases the risk of regurgitation and pulmonary aspiration. Due to general anesthesia, this risk has long been and continues to be one of the most frequent causes of maternal death and morbidity (Hayes et al., 1972).

5.6.6. Effects on Uterine Activity and Labor

Uterine contractility, which naturally affects the length of labor, can either increase or decrease due to the same increased secretion of catecholamines and cortisol brought on by pain and emotional stress. According to Nimmo et al. (1975), cortisol and adrenaline reduce uterine activity, while noradrenaline (norepinephrine) increases it. Nociceptive stimulation was shown in an early animal study to increase uterine activity by approximately 60%. This increase was linked to a decrease in fetal oxygen tension and fetal heart rate, which was marked by concerning signs of late decelerations (Holdsworth, 1978). Lederman and colleagues (Lederman et al., 1977, 1978) observed that in certain parturients, extreme pain and anxiety raised cortisol and adrenaline levels to such an extent that labor was prolonged and uterine activity was reduced. A tiny proportion of parturients experienced "incoordinate uterine contractions," which are characterized by ineffective labor patterns, an increase in frequency and uterine tone, and a decrease in intensity (Moir & Willocks, 1967; Holdsworth, 1978; Tomkinson et al., 1982).

5.6.7. Psychological Effects

Without a doubt, psychological factors influence the patient's mental state and attitude during labor as well as the frequency and severity of parturition pain. Anxiety, fear, and trepidation all serve to intensify the experience of pain and the behavior associated with it (Moir & Willocks, 1967; Bonica & Hunter, 1969; Brown et al., 1972; Morishima et al., 1980; Tomkinson et al., 1982). The classic source of a parturient's fear and anxiety is ignorance or misinformation. An uninformed patient, particularly one who is primipara, may experience anxiety related to pain, complications, the unknown, or even death. She might also worry that her unborn child might suffer harm (Myers, 1975; Tomkinson et al., 1982; Reading & Cox, 1985). Research has shown that patients who experience ambivalence or negative reactions to gestation, or who have an unintended or illegitimate pregnancy, report more pain during labor and delivery (Reading & Cox, 1985).

The parturient's degree of pain is also significantly influenced by her relationship with her spouse or partner. In 1984, Melzack observed that when a husband was present in the labor room as opposed to when he wasn't, the effective pain scores were higher. In any case, the finding was not erroneous, he suggested, though it might represent true higher effective pain scores or result from a purposeful selection of descriptors to impress the husband or vent frustration at him. Wallach discovered a comparable effect in a separate investigation in 1982. On the other hand, Nettelbladt et al. (1976), Norr et al. (1977), and Fridh et al. (1988) discovered that the expectant father's positive attitudes toward the pregnancy appeared to play a significant role in lowering the mother's feelings of anxiety during her pregnancy. Pregnant women felt less pain during parturition when their partners received a lot of support from their expectant fathers during pregnancy and labor.

The modulation of sensory transmissions and the effective and behavioral aspects of pain can both be influenced by other emotional factors, such as intense motivation and cultural influences. While producing distraction and dissociation from pain reduces pain behavior, cognitive intervention, such as providing the parturient with preparatory information about labor, reduces uncertainty. Lowe (1989) found that the most significant predictor of all components of pain during active labor was confidence in one's ability to handle labor in a study involving 134 low-risk parturients at term. In other words, the parturient felt less pain the more confident she was, and vice versa.

According to Marx and Greene (1964), intense labor pain can result in significant, long-lasting emotional disturbances that may harm a parturient's mental health, have a detrimental effect on her relationship with her baby during the first few critical days of life, and create anxiety about getting pregnant in the future, which may have an impact on her sexual relationship with her husband. According to Melzack et al. (1981), Gaston-Johansson et al. (1988), and Stewart (1982), a considerable proportion of women who underwent natural childbirth experienced pain during childbirth without analgesia, which led to the development or exacerbation of prelabor depression or other negative emotional reactions in the postpartum period. Melzack also mentioned that some women had to resort to using analgesics when faced with extreme pain because they were expecting "a natural painless childbirth," which added a burden of guilt, anger, and failure. Stewart stated that these patients lost interest in having sex and turned miserable, depressed, and even suicidal. Some wives who expected "natural" childbirth had to have their husbands undergo psychotherapy for severe reactions, such as feelings of guilt and subsequent impotence and phobias, after witnessing their wives go through such excruciating pain.

5.7. Current Methods to Relieve Childbirth Pain

Regional analgesia is by far the most popular technique available today in centers with access to anesthesia coverage. The safest method of treating pain during the first stage of labor was a topic of discussion in the past. The use of the lumbar epidural (LE) technique for regional analgesia has been closely examined. It is evident that the mother, the nurse, the anesthetist, and even the obstetrician prefer the tried-and-true LE method. Since different countries have different standards for anesthesia, we will quickly go over some alternative forms of labor analgesia. The focus of this chapter is on regional anesthetic methods. There are numerous medications and methods available today to relieve the pain associated with childbirth. These can all be arbitrarily divided into four groups: inhalation analgesia/anesthesia, simple pharmacological analgesia techniques, psychological analgesia, and regional analgesia/anesthesia.

There have been substantial advancements in the techniques for reducing labor pain during the last 20 years. This is supported by two surveys that included current practice in the UK, Scandinavia, and several other countries throughout the world, as well as four significant surveys of obstetric analgesia/anesthesia performed in the USA over the previous three decades (Marx & Green, 1964; Bonica & McDonald, 1995). These surveys show a trend toward a decrease in the use of inhalation and regional analgesia and an increase in the use of continuous lumbar epidural block with a diluted solution of local anesthetics and opioids in major hospitals with well-organized obstetric services and an obstetric anesthesia service available.

While 20–30% of parturients in the USA choose psychological analgesia, two-thirds eventually receive lumbar epidurals or other types of regional analgesia. Additionally, there has been a widespread trend away from inhalation anesthesia during childbirth and labor. Nonetheless, 20–50% of parturients in the UK and Scandinavia continue to use inhalation analgesia, either on their own or in conjunction with systemic opioids. Nonetheless, the UK has seen a consistent rise in the use of continuous lumbar epidural blocks for the first stage of labor as opposed to inhalation analgesia.

As expected, there are still a lot of issues in developing nations due to inadequate equipment and support systems, a lack of regional anesthesia specialists, and other factors. According to Marx & Green, 1964 and Bonica & McDonald, 1995, the majority of parturients either receive no analgesia at all or only basic inhalation and local anesthesia techniques. Based on these findings, a brief discussion of psychological analgesia, basic inhalation techniques, and regional anesthesia is provided below. The use of continuous lumbar epidural analgesia/anesthesia is adequately emphasized (Brownridge, 1991).

5.7.1. Psychological Analgesia

- **Natural Childbirth:** At a time when there were few other options available for pain relief, Dick-Read (1953) popularized natural childbirth, and for that he should be honored. At first, he gave the mother all of the attention. It was essential that she be in peak physical shape to handle the demands of labor. As a result, early on in the technique's development, conditioning played a significant role. Later on, the psychological aspects were added, but Dick-Read did not place all of the emphasis on conditioning—he also emphasized the importance of patient control over the labor process. The collaboration of an approachable and supportive nurse who would serve as a coach and facilitator for the patient during trying times considerably improved this approach.
- **Psychoprophylactic Method:** Around the same time that regional anesthesia was being reintroduced, Lamaze (1956) of France successfully brought the method to the United States, popularizing it. At this point, different ventilation exercises were included, and it was recognized that managing this aspect of breathing could be beneficial to the perception of pain. This happened in the middle of the 1970s, when there weren't many doctors practicing obstetric anesthesia. Each of these techniques required the obstetrician, teachers, nurses, and patient to work closely together and communicate. The parturient's confidence and optimism were fostered by the medical team, and

this was crucial to her having a positive and satisfying birthing experience.

- **Hypnotic Method:** Both the obstetric patient and the obstetrician must fully cooperate for the hypnotic approach to be effective. Frequently, the obstetrician serves as the hypnosis sessions' instructor. Naturally, learning hypnosis from an obstetrician is highly effective because of the strong and positive relationship that typically exists between the patient and her doctor. Sustaining enthusiasm for this approach necessitates patience, focus, commitment to picking up a new skill, and faith in the patient's inner fortitude.

5.7.2. Simple Techniques of Pharmacological Analgesia

5.7.2.1. Systemic Analgesics

The main medications used to relieve pain during labor that are not controlled by regional analgesic techniques are narcotics, or more accurately, opioids. These agents are easily administered intramuscularly by a labor nurse, who is essentially the primary healthcare provider in charge of making decisions regarding the patient's comfort. As a result, the nurse would interact with the patient during routine rounds and only get in touch with the patient's doctor when required. After good active labor was established, meperidine (Demerol) was frequently ordered initially. Other opioid medications were used, including fentanyl, morphine, alphaprodine, and nalbuphine. These drugs are now administered in tiny intravenous doses to reduce the overall amount required for labor pain and, consequently, the amount available to affect the fetus, even though they were originally administered intramuscularly in the past.

For a very long time, morphine was arguably the most traditional and widely used opioid among obstetricians. It had a potent analgesic effect when combined with scopolamine to induce twilight sleep. Both this and the depressing effect on the mother and the newborn were striking. A small amount of morphine was tried as an intravenous bolus to try and lessen the depressant effect. There might have been some fetal protective effect when given right before uterine contractions (Gerdin et al., 1990).

An opioid of the agonist and antagonist types is nalbuphine, also known as nubain. It has a similar respiratory depressant effect to morphine. One benefit of nalbuphine is that it has a ceiling effect on its depressant properties. Stated differently, a dosage that produces the greatest amount of depression can be increased without the neonate exhibiting additional signs of increased depression. This opioid has 80% of the potency of morphine. For the treatment of labor pain, the onset that occurred 2–3 minutes after intravenous injection was appealing.

100 times more potent than morphine, fentanyl is a synthetic opioid that is highly lipid soluble. Its rapid analgesic effect was its main use, but it also had the benefit of producing active metabolites that could function as respiratory depressants. While small intravenous doses of 50 μg were successfully used in the first stage of labor, there was little to no benefit over morphine, which had a much longer analgesic effect. It also crossed the placenta and quickly emerged in the fetal circulation due to its high lipid solubility (Rosaeg et al., 1992).

After managing the initial phase of labor, it's time to think about a dependable, full-pain relief second-stage method. Opioids are necessary when the moderate pain of the second stage starts. 70 to 80% of parturients report adequate relief from moderate pain, and 30 to

60% report adequate relief from severe pain (Bonica, 1967, 1969). While small doses can cause some neonatal depression, they do not cause significant respiratory depression in mothers. Nitrous oxide inhalation analgesia can be administered intermittently or continuously using a mask that is connected to an anesthesia machine. With the fetal head crowning to cause maximum dilatation of the perineum, this technique can be helpful immediately after delivery (Marx & Katsnelson, 1992). A bilateral pudendal nerve block or perineal infiltration can provide comparable pain relief during fetal delivery as an alternative analgesic technique.

Many parts of the world still do not recognize labor pain, which makes it a significant issue for pain management today. The quality of care varies greatly between third-world countries, where there is no pain relief at all, and modern centers, where 90% of patients benefit from regional analgesic techniques.

Even classes are offered in contemporary facilities to calm patients' anxieties and reassure them that their comfort and the safety of the unborn child is given the highest priority. Conversations such as these underscore the significance of the nurse in assisting the obstetrician and the anesthetist by supporting the patient during a difficult time.

5.7.3. Inhalational Analgesia/ Anesthesia

Inhalation analgesia is the logical progression from systemic analgesia. It still works well today to relieve labor pain because it doesn't result in unconsciousness or severe depression in the mother or newborn, and it quickly provides somewhat effective pain relief when it's most needed. Sevoflurane or desflurane in oxygen can be used, as can common agents such as 40–50% nitrous oxide in oxygen (Swart et al., 1991). The anesthetist's assistant or the anesthetist themselves may give nitrous oxide intermittently during uterine contractions (Carstoniu et al., 1994). In some regions of the world, premixed cylinders containing 50% nitrous oxide and 50% oxygen are used specifically for this purpose; however, most of the time, an anesthetic machine in an operating room or delivery room setting administers it for safety reasons. Anesthesiologist-trained personnel should administer the drug inhalation following safety and optimal analgesia guidelines. 10 to 15 seconds should pass between each contraction's painful phase and the inhalation. When administered appropriately, inhalational analgesia gives one-third of parturients good analgesia and another one-third partial relief (Norman et al., 1992).

Because inhalational anesthesia can be quickly induced, provides maximum control over the depth and duration of action, and can be quickly eliminated at the end of the procedure, it is still used for very brief periods of time as well as for actual delivery. However, general anesthesia is extremely risky and increases the possibility of maternal death from asphyxia brought on by a difficult endotracheal intubation (Glassenberg, 1991).

In the USA and Britain, these are the two main causes of anesthesia-related maternal death, along with regurgitation and pulmonary aspiration. Because of this, general anesthesia should be avoided; however, if it is required, it should only be administered by a qualified anesthetist who has first secured the airway through endotracheal intubation. Since there is currently insufficient data to conclude the mother's safety when using the laryngeal mask airway in obstetrics, this is a contentious topic. In addition, this is among the most challenging obstetric anesthesia areas. This method should only be used by experts in its application and then only in certain situations until further experience is obtained.

5.7.4. Regional Analgesia/ Anesthesia

Since the 1970s, the use of epidurals, a type of regional analgesia, for labor and delivery has grown significantly in popularity. Without causing any depression of the central nervous system, regional analgesia provides good pain relief. To put it another way, the mother can fully appreciate the beauty of the experience of a lifetime while maintaining total control over her entire range of abilities. There are very few, if any, complications for the mother or the fetus with the current delivery and selection of local anesthetics, and there is little to no negative impact on the length or pattern of labor. By using regional techniques, aspiration complications during delivery are prevented, as is the use of general anesthesia for operative delivery, which prevents the mother and baby from being negatively affected by depressant medications during labor.

In order to compensate for the increased vascular capacitance experienced after sympathetic block, maternal hypotension is lessened by infusing fluids prior to inducing spinal, epidural, or caudal block. The parturient is also positioned in the lateral decubitus position during labor to prevent the aortocaval compression inherent in the supine position. Preventing systemic toxic reactions can be achieved by avoiding overdosing or unintentionally injecting therapeutic doses intravenously, as well as by administering small amounts of local anesthetic doses repeatedly over short intervals of time. Furthermore, it was discovered that the use of tiny doses of adrenaline, or epinephrine, decreased the amount of time that mothers and fetuses were exposed to the local anesthetic used for the epidural (McLintic et al., 1991). Using the test dose and closely monitoring the 154 mother heart rate from injection for three minutes can sometimes identify this complication. For a brief while, the adrenaline in the test dose will cause an acute rise in heart rate.

An accidental subarachnoid injection of a local anesthetic dose meant for extradural block may cause very high or complete spinal anesthesia. If the local anesthetic dosage is large in comparison to what would be given in the subarachnoid space, it has a profound effect on the sympathetic nervous system, which is in charge of maintaining tone in the capacitance vessels. If this effect is not recognized and treated promptly, the patient may experience progressive hypotension and eventually shock. By trying to aspirate blood or cerebrospinal fluid and injecting a test dose of 2–3 ml of a solution containing 5–7.6 mg of bupivacaine and 15 mg of adrenaline, the latter two complications can be essentially avoided. A low (T10–S5) spinal anesthesia will develop in the parturient if the injection is inadvertently subarachnoid. As previously indicated, an intravenous injection of adrenaline (epinephrine) will cause moderate tachycardia and hypertension within 20 to 30 seconds, with symptoms lasting between 30 and 60 seconds (Moore & Batra, 1981). Large therapeutic doses should only be injected when neither happens.

5.7.4.1. Paracervical and Pudendal Block

Excellent first- and second-stage analgesia can be obtained by combining paracervical and pudendal block techniques, provided that the practitioner is knowledgeable about the anatomy of those particular nerve areas. Only diluted local anesthetic concentrations are currently used in some centers when performing the paracervical block. But in many cases, this wonderful regional block has been abandoned due to issues with bradycardia in the fetus following the mother's drug administration. Obstetricians in institutions without access to obstetric anesthesia services may still use bilateral pudendal block.

5.7.4.2. Epidural Analgesia

Epidural analgesia has gained popularity over the past few de cades for both cesarean sections and labor and vaginal delivery. Many changes have been made to the technique since the 1960s. The initial protocol involved injecting 12–15 ml of lignocaine, or 1%–5% lidocaine, or equianesthetic concentrations of another local anesthetic on an intermittent basis. This usually produced analgesia from T9–T10 to S5. The use of such a relatively high dose of local anesthetic increased the risk of systemic toxic reactions from an accidental intravenous injection or total spinal anesthesia from an accidental subarachnoid injection, even though it is typically effective in relieving pain during labor and delivery.

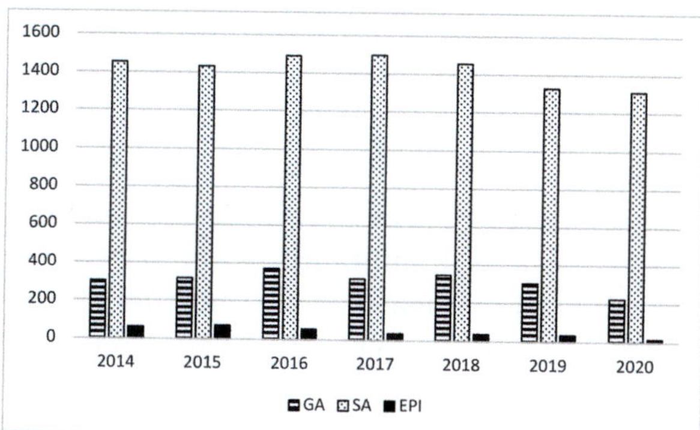

Figure 5.2. Anesthesia for cesarean sections in a retrospective analysis of anesthesia provided to obstetric patients in the tertiary care center between 1 January 2014 and 31 December 2020.

Source: Krawczyk P, Jaśkiewicz R, Huras H, Kołak M. Obstetric Anesthesia Practice in the Tertiary Care Center: A 7-Year Retrospective Study and the Impact of the COVID-19 Pandemic on Obstetric Anesthesia Practice. *Journal of Clinical Medicine*. 2022; 11(11):3183. https://doi.org/10.3390/jcm11113183.

Note: GA—general anesthesia; SA—spinal anesthesia; EPI—epidural anesthesia.

Every local anesthetic injection caused a temporary decrease in uterine activity as well as weakness or even paralysis in the perineal muscles and lower limbs in many parturients. Due to the patient's loss of control over their lower limbs, they experienced discomfort and inconvenience. Resistance forces necessary for internal rotation of the presenting part were reduced by paralysis or weakness of the perineal muscles. The reflex urge to bear down was also removed from the afferent limb by sacral anesthesia. The second stage is prolonged as a result of all these effects, and instrumental delivery is frequently required (Bonica, 1967, 1969, 1980; Bonica & McDonald, 1995).

Numerous changes resulted from these and other worries (Bonica & McDonald, 1995). First, analgesia was restricted to T10–T11 in the initial stage before being expanded to the sacral segments. An excellent method of anesthesia and analgesia during pregnancy is provided by continuous epidural block (Eddleston et al., 1992). Compared to the other epidural block techniques previously mentioned, this technique has the advantage of requiring less medication. There is no early perineal muscle weakness or numbness in the lower limbs as a result of it. As such, there's no interference with internal rotation or flexion. For parturients who request epidural analgesia, continuous epidural analgesia or its discontinuous counterpart, patient-controlled epidural infusion, are now commonly used. The double catheter technique was also used in the 1980s for parturients who needed analgesia at obstetric centers where the anesthetists had extensive experience with both lumbar epidural blocks and caudal blocks (Bonica & McDonald, 1995). These days, it's standard practice to use infusion pumps that allow for more precise administration of the analgesic solution and to add opioids (typically fentanyl) to the infusion to increase the analgesic efficacy of the local anesthetics. In many institutions where anesthetists provide an obstetric anesthesia service, it has replaced all other regional techniques for labor and vaginal delivery because it has been shown to:

1. Produce more stable levels of analgesia.
2. Lead to a smaller incidence of maternal hypotension.
3. Decrease the risk of systemic toxic reaction or accidental total spinal anesthesia.
4. Decrease and, in some instances, eliminate the incidence of unintended motor block, thus obviating the problems mentioned above (Bonica & McDonald, 1995).

Modified methods of attempting to reduce the amount of drug the fetus would be exposed to gained popularity in the early 1970s. In the beginning, attempts were made to obtain only a T10–T12 block for early labor and a T10–L2 block for later labor by using smaller volumes of 8–10 ml of local anesthetic. This approach was effective and initiated the use of different agents and dosages, a trend that has persisted. The patient will receive a very tiny injection of 0–10 ml of bupivacaine today, and she will receive a continuous dosage for the duration of her labor. A diluted local anesthetic (0.0625% bupivacaine and adrenaline (epinephrine)) and a diluted concentration of either fentanyl or sufentanil are part of the continuous infusion dosage (Bonica & McDonald, 1995). Throughout labor, the patient receives the combination via a pump until they are ready to give birth.

When it came to labor pain relief, the caudal epidural block gained more traction than the lumbar epidural block. While the caudal block works well for second-stage analgesia, it is not the best option for first-stage pain management because it requires a significant amount of local anesthetic to achieve analgesia at the T10 level, which is where the catheter tip is located at S4 or S2. To achieve first-stage pain relief, up to a 20–25 ml volume has been used in certain cases. Naturally, all of the intermediate segments are also blocked, resulting in a complete sympathetic block and all of its consequences for the patient. However, it is mentioned because it was the cornerstone of obstetric anesthesia for a very long time and is a very effective way to relieve labor pain. Several texts provide more thorough instructions on implementing caudal analgesia (Bonica, 1973; Shnider & Levinson, 1987).

5.7.4.3. Technique of Continuous Epidural Infusion

A detailed description of the technique for achieving lumbar epidural analgesia is beyond the scope of this book.

The majority of medical professionals use a single catheter inserted into the upper lumbar epidural space (Gieraerts et al., 1992). Some prefer to use the paramedian technique with a Touhy needle to introduce the catheter (Bonica, 1980). Three milliliters of 0.025% bupivacaine and 1 millionth of an adrenaline (epinephrine) are used as an anesthetic after the catheter is firmly in place and all monitoring and resuscitation equipment is ready for use right away.

As an alternative, 10 milliliters of 0.125% bupivacaine combined with 12.5 micrograms of adrenaline (epinephrine) can be utilized (Williams et al., 1990). A single bolus of 5 ml of 0.025% bupivacaine is injected as a priming dose if no indications of an intravenous or subarachnoid injection appear within 5 minutes. Typically, this results in analgesia that reaches from T9–T10 to L1–L2. As soon as this is accomplished, a continuous infusion of a solution containing 0–12% ml/h of fentanyl (2 μg/ml) and 0–0625% bupivacaine is started. This is then adjusted to maintain analgesia with the upper level at T10. Typically, 120 milliliters of solution are made.

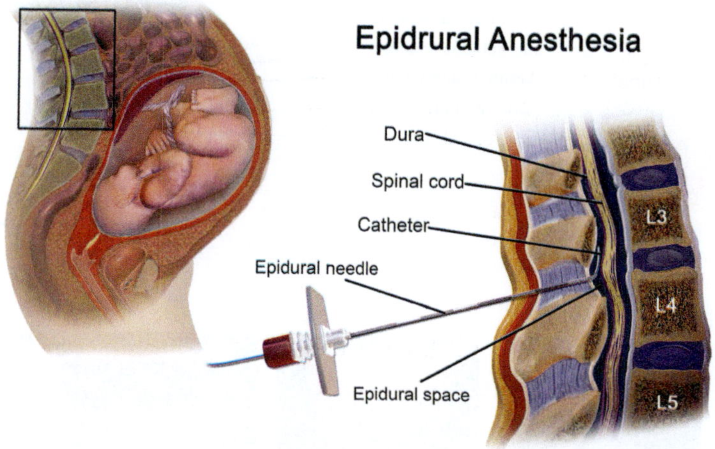

Figure 5.3. Techniques of lumbar epidural block for labor and vaginal delivery.

Source: Althobaiti M, Ali S, Hariri NG, Hameed K, Alagl Y, Alzahrani N, Alzahrani S, Al-Naib I. Recent advances in smart epidural spinal needles. *Sensors*. 2023; 23(13):6065. https://doi.org/10.3390/s23136065.

Some medical professionals mix 30 milliliters of bupivacaine (0–25%), 60 micrograms of sufentanyl, and 200 micrograms of adrenaline (epinephrine) in a 120 milliliter volume (McIntosh & Rayburn, 1991). It is simple to administer exact dosages of medication by using a pump. Because the pumps are compact and lightweight, walking around during the first stages of labor is possible. Because they think it facilitates labor, some obstetricians favor maternal ambulation in the early stages of the procedure. Having a self-contained medication cassette with a minimum capacity of 100 ml of solution, the pump eliminates the need for a separate suspended medication bottle, which is a unique benefit associated with portability. There is a large selection of suitable pumps available.

If the patient would rather lie in bed during labor and delivery, she can be placed in either the left or right lateral position, with the upper body raised between 15° and 20°. The degree of the caudal level of analgesia tends to increase with every hour, while the cephalad level stays relatively constant at T10. All of the lumbar and sacral segments are typically involved in analgesia by the third or fourth hour. About 50–60% of parturients find that sacral analgesia is adequate for providing perineal analgesia. Prior to delivery, the patient is examined. If sacral analgesia is not achieved, 10 milliliters of either 2% chloroprocaine or 1% lidocaine are administered while the patient is sitting. For the actual delivery, this typically results in adequate analgesia and perineal relaxation.

The patient-controlled epidural analgesic delivery system is an expansion of continuous epidural infusion. Research has compared these two methods and found no discernible differences in patient preferences for one over the other, as well as comparable benefits for the patients (Bonica, 1980; Gambling et al., 1990; Ferrante et al., 1991).

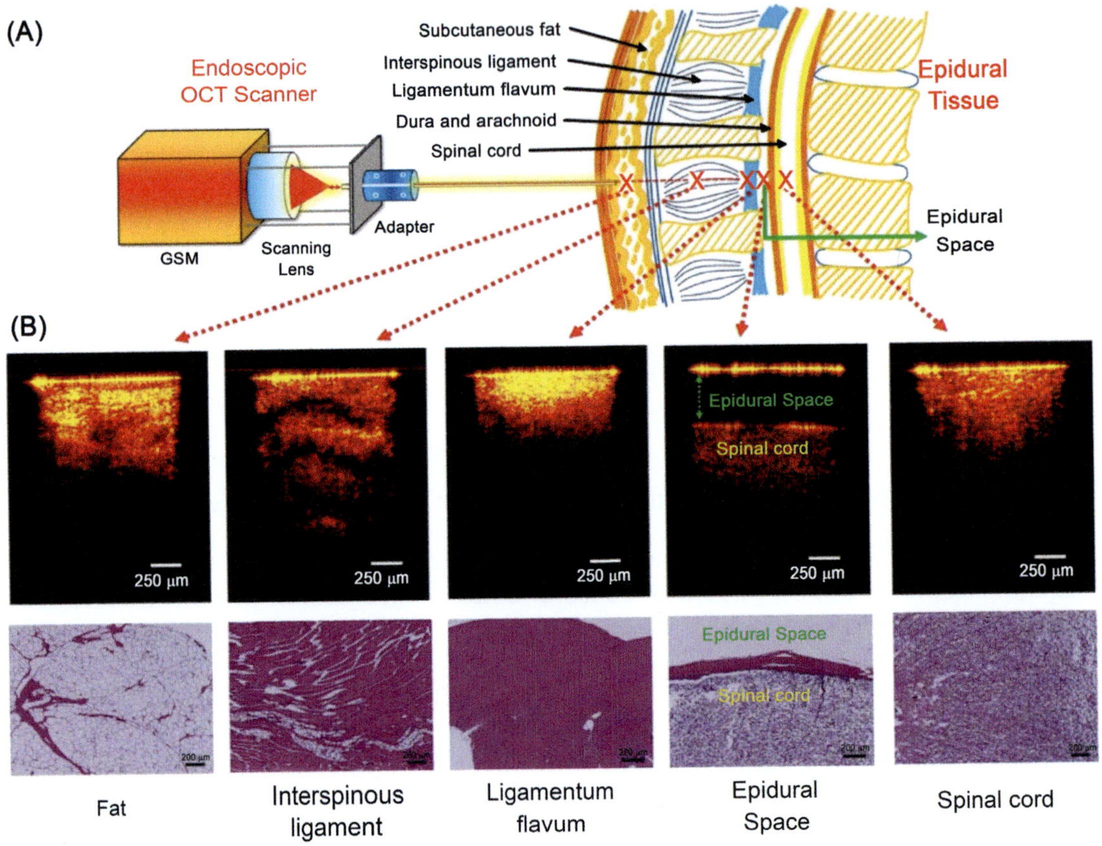

Figure 5.4. Schematic illustration showing technique of continuous epidural analgesia and the extent and intensity of analgesia during the first and second stages of labor and for delivery.

Source. Althobaiti M, Ali S, Hariri NG, Hameed K, Alagl Y, Alzahrani N, Alzahrani S, Al-Naib I. Recent advances in smart epidural spinal needles. *Sensors*. 2023; 23(13):6065. https://doi.org/10.3390/s23136065.

Note: (A) The epidural needle and catheter in place. After removing the needle, the catheter is taped to the patient's back and a test dose of local anesthetic given. (B) If after 5 min there is no sign of accidental intravenous or subarachnoid injection, a bolus of 5 ml of local anesthetic is injected while the patient is in the lateral position. (C) After signs of epidural analgesia of T9–T10 to L1–L2 are noted, the catheter is connected to the continuous infusion system and the solution is administered at a rate of 10–12 ml/h with the patient in a 15°–20° head-up position, lying on her side. (D) Extent of analgesia after 1.5–2 h of infusion. (E) Extent of analgesia in the early and mid second stage. (F) After internal rotation has occurred, injection of a bolus of 10 ml of local anesthetic solution (e.g., 1% lidocaine) produces an increase in the intensity of analgesia indicated by the more heavily shaded area involving the lower sacral segments. (G) The patient is ready for delivery. Note the wedge under the right hip and lower region to help displace the uterus to the left.

5.7.4.4. Technique of Spinal–Epidural

Finally, a method that has gained popularity recently is the spinal-epidural combination technique, which involves passing an 18-gauge thin-walled epidural needle through a 27-gauge spinal needle to deliver a small amount of subarachnoid opioid. Prior to making the customary entry into the epidural space, the lumbar epidural needle is inserted. Subsequently, the epidural needle is punctured with a small-gauge spinal needle until the dura is reached. A tiny amount of opioid is injected following the spinal needle's contact with the dura to provide analgesia without significantly impairing sympathetic nervous system function or causing severe lower limb motor paralysis. This technique is sometimes referred to as the "walking epidural" because the patient retains full motor control over her legs and experiences minimal motor loss despite the opioid's first-stage pain relief in the subarachnoid space (Norris et al., 1998). Being able to walk around is particularly crucial in the second stage because it reduces the likelihood that the presenting part will not rotate and allows the mother to actively use her expulsive forces to supplement labor in order to achieve a spontaneous delivery.

A Closer Look

Laparoscopy

Laparoscopy, also known as minimally invasive surgery or keyhole surgery, is a surgical technique that allows for the examination and treatment of abdominal and pelvic organs through small incisions using specialized instruments and a camera called a laparoscope. This approach offers several advantages over traditional open surgery, including shorter recovery times, reduced postoperative pain, smaller scars, and a lower risk of complications.

During a laparoscopic procedure, the surgeon makes several small incisions in the abdomen, typically ranging from 0.5 to 1.5 centimeters in length. Carbon dioxide gas is then pumped into the abdominal cavity to create space and improve visibility. Next, a laparoscope, a thin, flexible tube equipped with a camera and light source, is inserted through one of the incisions, allowing the surgeon to visualize the internal organs on a monitor in real-time. Additional instruments are inserted through the remaining incisions to manipulate tissues, perform procedures, and address any identified issues.

Laparoscopy is used for a variety of diagnostic and therapeutic purposes across numerous medical specialties. In gynecology, it is commonly employed for diagnosing and treating conditions such as endometriosis, ovarian cysts, fibroids, and infertility issues. In general surgery, laparoscopy is used for procedures including gallbladder removal (cholecystectomy), hernia repair, appendectomy, and bariatric surgery for weight loss. Additionally, laparoscopic techniques are utilized in urology, gastroenterology, and other fields to address a wide range of conditions.

Advances in technology have led to the development of even more specialized forms of laparoscopy, such as robotic-assisted laparoscopic surgery, which offers enhanced precision and dexterity to the surgeon. However, laparoscopy may not be suitable for all patients or conditions, and in some cases, open surgery may be necessary.

Overall, laparoscopy represents a significant advancement in surgical care, offering patients a less invasive option with faster recovery times and improved outcomes compared to traditional open surgery. Its versatility and effectiveness have made it a cornerstone of modern surgical practice across various medical disciplines.

Summary

- Chronic pelvic and obstetric pain (CPOP) presents a complex and often debilitating medical challenge, encompassing a spectrum of conditions affecting the pelvic region, including the lower abdomen, pelvis, and reproductive organs.
- Chronic pelvic pain (CPP) is defined as pain that persists for more than 6 months.
- The role of pelvic adhesions in the genesis of pelvic pain has been debated from various perspectives. Adhesions were found in 16–44% of the patients undergoing laparoscopy for chronic pelvic pain.
- Endometriosis affects about 1–2% of all women and 15–25% of infertile women. Endometriosis is found in approximately 28–74% of the patients undergoing laparoscopy for chronic pelvic pain.
- Salpingo-oophoritis can cause chronic pelvic pain, though patients usually present with symptoms and signs of acute or subacute infection before the pain becomes chronic.
- Cyclic pelvic pain implies pain occurring with a specific relationship to the menstrual cycle. It consists of primary and secondary dysmenorrhea but also includes atypical cyclic pain, such as pain beginning two weeks prior to menses.
- Patients with cyclic or atypical cyclic pain based on the evaluation of the pain diary should be evaluated and treated for primary or secondary dysmenorrhea.
- Multidisciplinary pain management is an excellent approach to chronic pelvic pain. The team usually includes a gynecologist or internist as pain manager, psychologist, and often a physical therapist, anesthesiologist, and dietitian.

References

1. Atlee, H. B. (1956). *Natural Childbirth.* Thomas, Springfield, IL.
2. Baker, P. K. (1993). Musculoskeletal origins of chronic pelvic pain. In F. W. Ling (Ed.), *Obstetrics and Gynecology Clinics of North America: Contemporary Management of Chronic Pain* (pp. 719–742). Saunders.
3. Beard, R. W., Kennedy, R. G., Gangar, K. F., Stones, R. W., Rogers, V., Reginald, P. W., & Anderson, M. (1991). Bilateral oophorectomy and hysterectomy in the treatment of intractable pelvic pain associated with pelvic congestion. *British Journal of Obstetrics and Gynecology, 98*, 988–992.
4. Beard, R. W., Reginald, P. W., & Wadsworth, J. (1988). Clinical features of women with chronic lower abdominal pain and pelvic congestion. *British Journal of Obstetrics and Gynecology, 95*, 153–161.
5. Bergman, A., Karram, M., & Bhatia, N. N. (1989). Urethral syndrome: A comparison of different treatment modalities. *Journal of Reproductive Medicine, 34*, 157–160.
6. Berkley, K. J., & Wood, E. (1989). Responses to varying intensities of vaginal distension in the awake rat. *Society of Neuroscience Abstracts, 15*, 979.
7. Bland, R. W. (1989). A randomized controlled trial of medroxyprogesterone acetate and psychotherapy for the treatment of pelvic congestion. *British Journal of Obstetrics and Gynecology, 96*, 1153–1162.

8. Bonica, J. J. (1967). *Principles and Practice of Obstetric Analgesia and Anesthesia, vol. 1*. Davis, Philadelphia.

9. Bonica, J. J. (1969). *Principles and Practice of Obstetric Analgesia and Anesthesia, vols. 1, 2*. Davis, Philadelphia.

10. Bonica, J. J. (1973). Maternal respiratory changes during pregnancy and parturition. In G. F. Marx (Ed.), *Parturition and Perinatology*. Davis, Philadelphia.

11. Bonica, J. J. (1980). *Obstetric Analgesia and Anesthesia, 2nd edn*. World Federation of Societies of Anesthesiologists/University of Washington Press.

12. Bonica, J. J., & Hunter Jr, C. A. (1969). Management in dysfunction of the forces of labor. In J. J. Bonica (Ed.), *Principles and Practice of Obstetric Analgesia and Anesthesia, vol. 2*. Davis, Philadelphia.

13. Bonica, J. J., & McDonald, J. S. (1990). The pain of childbirth. In J. J. Bonica (Ed.), *The Management of Pain, 2nd edn* (pp. 1313–1343). Lea & Febiger.

14. Bonica, J. J., & McDonald, J. S. (1995). *Principles and Practice of Obstetric Analgesia and Anesthesia, 2nd edn*. Williams & Wilkins.

15. Brown, W. A., Manning, T., & Grodin, J. (1972). The relationship of antenatal and perinatal variables to the use of drugs in labor. *Psychosomatic Medicine, 34*, 119–127.

16. Brownridge, P. (1991). Treatment options for the relief of pain during childbirth. *Drugs, 41*, 69–80.

17. Buchan, P. C. (1980). Emotional stress in childbirth and its modification by variations in obstetric management—Epidural analgesia and stress in labor. *Acta Obstetricia et Gynecologica Scandinavica, 59*, 319–321.

18. Candiani, G. B., Fedele, L., Vercellini, P., Bianchi, S., & Di Nola, G. (1992). Presacral neurectomy for the treatment of pelvic pain associated with endometriosis: A controlled study. *American Journal of Obstetrics and Gynecology, 167*, 100–103.

19. Candido, K. D., & Winnie, A. P. (1992). A dual-chambered syringe that allows identification of the epidural space using the loss of resistance technique with air and with saline. *Regional Anesthesia, 17*, 163–165.

20. Carey, M. P., & Slack, M. C. (1996). GnRH analogue in assessing chronic pelvic pain in women with residual ovaries. *British Journal of Obstetrics and Gynecology, 103*, 150–153.

21. Cervero, F., & Tattersall, J. E. H. (1986). Somatic and visceral sensory integration in the thoracic spinal cord. In F. Cervero & J. Morrison (Eds.), *Visceral Sensation* (pp. 189–205). Elsevier.

22. Chan, W. Y., & Dawood, M. Y. (1980). Prostaglandin levels in menstrual fluid of non-dysmenorrhea and of dysmenorrhea subjects with and without oral contraceptive or ibuprofen therapy. *Advances in Prostaglandin, Thromboxane and Leukotriene Research, 8*, 1443–1447.

23. Chen, F.-P., & Soong, Y.-K. (1997). The efficacy and complications of laparoscopic presacral neurectomy in pelvic pain. *Obstetrics and Gynecology, 90*, 974–977.

24. D'Hooghe, T. M., & Hill, J. A. (1996). Endometriosis. In J. S. Berek, E. Y. Adashi, & P. A. Hillard (Eds.), *Novak's Gynecology, 12th edn.* (pp. 887–914). Williams & Wilkins.

25. Deligeoroglou, E. (2000). Dysmenorrhea. *Annals of the New York Academy of Science, 900*, 237–244.

26. Dick-Read, G. (1953). *Childbirth Without Fear*. Harper.

27. Eddleston, J. M., Maresh, M., Horsman, E. L., & Young, H. (1992). Comparison of maternal and fetal effects associated with intermittent or continuous infusion or extradural analgesia. *British Journal of Anesthesia, 69*, 154–158.

28. Farquhar, C. M., Rogers, V., Franks, S., Pearce, S., & Wadsworth, J. Beard RW, A randomized controlled trial of medroxyprogesterone acetate and psychotherapy for the treatment of pelvic congestion. Br J Obstet Gynaecol. 1989;96(10):1153.

29. Ferrante, F. M., Lu, L., Jamison, S. B., & Datta, S. (1991). Patient-controlled epidural analgesia: Demand dosing. *Anesthesia and Analgesia, 73*, 547–552.

30. Fridh, G., Kopare, T., Gaston-Johansson, F., & Norvell, K. T. (1988). Factors associated with more intense labor pain. *Research in Nursing and Health, 11*, 117–124.

31. Fukaya, T., Hoshiai, H., & Yajima, A. (1993). Is pelvic endometriosis always associated with chronic pain? A retrospective study of 618 cases diagnosed by laparoscopy. *American Journal of Obstetrics and Gynecology, 169*, 719–722.

32. Gabbe, S. G. (1991). *Obstetrics—Normal and Problem Pregnancies (2nd edn.)* Churchill Livingstone.

33. Gambling, D. R., McMorland, G. H., Yu, P., & Laszlo, C. (1990). Comparison of patient-controlled epidural analgesia and conventional intermittent 'top-up' injections during labor. *Anesthesia and Analgesia, 70*, 256–261.

34. Gangar, K. V., Stones, R. W., Saunders, D., Rogers, V., Rae, T., Cooper, S., & Beard, R. W. (1993). An alternative to hysterectomy? GnRH analogue combined with hormone replacement therapy. *British Journal of Obstetrics and Gynecology, 100*, 360–364.

35. Gaston-Johansson, F., Fridh, G., & Turner-Norvell, K. (1988). Progression of labor pain in primiparas and multiparas. *Nursing Research, 37*, 86–90.

36. Gaylard, D. (1990). Epidural analgesia by continuous infusion. In F. Reynolds (Ed.), *Epidural and Spinal Blockade in Obstetrics* (pp. 49–58). Bailliere Tindall.

37. Gerdin, A., Salmonson, T., Lindberg, B., & Rane, A. (1990). Maternal kinetics of morphine during labor. *Journal of Perinatal Medicine, 18*, 479–487.

38. Giamberardino, M. A., Berkley, K. J., Iezzi, S., di Bigotina, P., & Vecchiet, L. (1995). Changes in skin and muscle sensitivity in dysmenorrhea vs. normal women as a function of body site and monthly cycle. *Society of Neuroscience Abstracts, 1638*.

39. Gieraerts, R., Van Zundert, A., De Wolf, A., & Vaes, L. (1992). Ten ml bupivacaine 0.125% with 12.5μ epinephrine is a reliable epidural test dose to detect inadvertent intravascular injection in obstetric patients. A double-blind study. *Acta Anaesthesiologica Scandinavica, 36*, 656–659.

40. Glassenberg, R. (1991). General anesthesia and maternal mortality. *Seminars in Perinatology, 15*, 386–396.

41. Hahn, L. (1989). Clinical findings and results of operative treatment in ilioinguinal nerve entrapment syndrome. *British Journal of Obstetrics and Gynecology, 96*, 1080–1083.

42. Hansen, J. M., & Ueland, K. (1966). The influence of caudal analgesia on cardiovascular dynamics during normal labor and delivery. *Acta Anaesthesiologica Scandinavica, 23*(suppl 10), 449–452.

43. Harrop-Griffiths, J., Katon, W., Walker, E., Helm, L., Russo, J., & Hickok, C. (1988). The association between chronic pelvic pain, psychiatric diagnoses and childhood sexual abuse. *Obstetrics and Gynecology, 71*, 589–594.
44. Hayes, J. R., Ardill, J., Kennedy, T. L., Shanks, R. G., & Buchanan, K. D. (1972). Stimulation of gastrin release by catecholamines. *Lancet, 1*, 819–821.
45. Hendricks, C. H., & Quilligan, E. J. (1956). Cardiac output during labor. *American Journal of Obstetrics and Gynecology, 71*, 953–972.
46. Hillis, S. D., Marchbanks, P. A., & Peterson, H. B. (1995). The effectiveness of hysterectomy for chronic pelvic pain. *Obstetrics and Gynecology, 86*, 941–945.
47. Holdsworth, J. D. (1978). Relationships between stomach contents and analgesia in labor. *British Journal of Anesthesia, 50*, 1145–1148.
48. Howard, F. M. (1993). The role of laparoscopy in chronic pelvic pain: Promise and pitfalls. *Obstetrical and Gynecological Survey, 48*, 357–387.
49. Howard, F. M., El-Minawi, A. M., & Sanchez, R. A. (2000). Conscious pain mapping by laparoscopy in women with chronic pelvic pain. *Obstetrics and Gynecology, 96*, 934–944.
50. Huch, A., Huch, R., Schneider, H., & Rooth, G. (1977). Continuous transcutaneous monitoring of fetal oxygen tension during labor. *British Journal of Obstetrics and Gynecology, 84*(suppl 1), 1–39.
51. Hughes, J. M. (1990). Psychological aspects of pelvic pain. In I. Rocker (Ed.), *Pelvic pain in women: Diagnosis and Management* (pp. 13–20). Springer-Verlag.
52. Jouppila, R. (1977). The effect of segmental epidural analgesia on hormonal and metabolic changes during labor. *Acta Universitatis Ouluensis, Series D, Medica No 16, Anaesthesiologica No 2*.
53. Kames, L. D., Rapkin, A. J., Naliboff, B. D., Afifi, S., & Ferrer-Brechner, T. (1990). Effectiveness of an interdisciplinary pain management program for the treatment of chronic pelvic pain. *Pain, 41*, 41–46.
54. Karram, M. M. (1993). Frequency, urgency, and painful bladder syndrome. In M. D. Walters & M. M. Karram (Eds.), *Clinical Urogynecology* (pp. 285–298). Mosby.
55. Kawatani, M., & de Groat, W. C. (1991). A large proportion of afferent neurons innervating the uterine cervix of the cat contain VIP and other neuropeptides. *Cell and Tissue Research, 266*, 191–196.
56. Klink, E. W. (1953). Perineal nerve block: An anatomic and clinical study in the female. *Obstetrics and Gynecology, 1*, 137–146.
57. Koninckx, P. R., Meuleman, C., Demeyere, S., Lesaffre, E., & Cornillie, F. J. (1991). Suggestive evidence that pelvic endometriosis is a progressive disease, whereas deeply infiltrating endometriosis is associated with pelvic pain. *Fertility and Sterility, 55*, 759–770.
58. Kream, R. M., & Carr, D. B. (1999). Interstitial cystitis. *Pain Forum, 8*, 139–145.
59. Kresch, A. J., Seifer, D. B., Sachs, L. B., & Barrese, I. (1984). Laparoscopy in 100 women with chronic pelvic pain. *Obstetrics and Gynecology, 64*, 672–674.
60. Kumazawa, T. (1986). Sensory innervation of reproductive organs. In F. Cervero & J. Morrison (Eds.), *Visceral Sensation* (pp. 115–131). Elsevier.

61. Lederman, R. P., Lederman, E., Work, B. A. Jr., & McCann, D. S. (1978). The relationship of maternal anxiety, plasma catecholamines, and plasma cortisol to progress in labor. *American Journal of Obstetrics and Gynecology, 132*, 495–500.

62. Lederman, R. P., McCann, D. S., Work, B., & Huber, M. J. (1977). Endogenous plasma epinephrine and norepinephrine in last-trimester pregnancy and labor. *American Journal of Obstetrics and Gynecology, 129*, 5–8.

63. Lichten, E. M., & Bombard, J. (1987). Surgical treatment of primary dysmenorrhea with laparoscopic uterine nerve ablation. *Journal of Reproductive Medicine, 32*, 37–41.

64. Lowe, N. K. (1989). Explaining the pain of active labor: The importance in maternal confidence. *Research in Nursing and Health, 12*, 237–245.

65. Magni, G., Salmi, A., deLeo, D., & Ceola, A. (1984). Chronic pelvic pain and depression. *Psychopathology, 17*, 132–136.

66. Malinak, L. R. (1980). Operative management of pelvic pain. *Clinical Obstetrics and Gynecology, 23*, 191–199.

67. Marx, G. F., & Greene, N. M. (1964). Maternal lactate, pyruvate and excess lactate production during labor and delivery. *American Journal of Obstetrics and Gynecology, 90*, 786–793.

68. Marx, G. F., & Katsnelson, T. (1992). The introduction of nitrous oxide into obstetrics. *Obstetrics and Gynecology, 80*, 715–718.

69. Mayer, E. A., & Gebhart, G. F. (1993). Functional bowel disorders and the visceral hyperalgesia hypothesis. In E. A. Mayer & H. E. Raybould (Eds.), *Pain Research and Clinical Management, vol 9* (pp. 3–28). Elsevier.

70. McDonald, J. S. (1993). Management of chronic pain. In F. W. Ling (Ed.), *Obstetrics and Gynecology Clinics of North America: Contemporary Management of Chronic Pain* (pp. 817–839). Saunders.

71. McIntosh, D. G., & Rayburn, W. F. (1991). Patient-controlled analgesia in obstetrics and gynecology. *Obstetrics and Gynecology, 70*, 202–204.

72. McLintic, A. J., Danskin, S. H., Reid, J. A., & Thorburn, J. (1991). Effects of adrenaline on extradural anesthesia, plasma lignocaine concentrations and feto-placental unit during elective cesarean section. *British Journal of Anesthesia, 67*, 683–689.

73. Melzack, R. (1984). The myth of painless childbirth. The John J. Bonica Lecture. *Pain, 19*, 321.

74. Melzack, R., Taenzer, P., Feldman, P., & Kinch, R. A. (1981). Labour is still painful after prepared childbirth training. *Canadian Medical Association Journal, 125*, 357–363.

75. Milburn, A., Reiter, R. C., & Rhomberg, A. T. (1993). Multidisciplinary approach to chronic pelvic pain. In F. W. Ling (Ed.), *Obstetrics and Gynecology Clinics of North America: Contemporary Management of Chronic Pelvic Pain* (pp. 643–661). Saunders.

76. Moir, D. D., & Willocks, J. (1967). Management of incoordinate uterine action under continuous epidural analgesia. *British Medical Journal, 3*, 396–400.

77. Moore, D. C., & Batra, M. S. (1981). The components of an effective test dose prior to epidural block. *Anesthesiology, 55*, 693–696.

78. Morishima, H. O., Pedersen, H., & Finster, M. (1978). The influence of maternal psychological stress on the fetus. *American Journal of Obstetrics and Gynecology, 131*, 286–290.

79. Morishima, H. O., Pedersen, H., & Finster, M. (1980). Effects of pain on mother, labor and fetus. In G. F. Marx & G. M. Bassel (Eds.), *Obstetric Analgesia and Anesthesia* (pp. 197–210). Elsevier/North Holland.

80. Myers, R. E. (1975). Maternal psychological stress and fetal asphyxia: A study in the monkey. *American Journal of Obstetrics and Gynecology, 122*, 47–59.

81. Nettelbladt, P., Fagerstrom, C. F., & Uddenberg, N. (1976). The significance of reported childbirth pain. *Journal of Psychosomatic Research, 20*, 215–221.

82. Nimmo, W. S., Wilson, J., & Prescott, L. F. (1975). Narcotic analgesics and delayed gastric emptying during labor. *Lancet, 1*, 890.

83. Norman, P. H., Kavanagh, B., Daley, M. D., et al. (1992). Nitrous oxide analgesia in labor (abstract). *Anesthesia and Analgesia, 74*, S222.

84. Norr, K. L., Block, C. R., Charles, A., Meyering, S., & Meyers, E. (1977). Explaining pain and enjoyment in childbirth. *Journal of Health and Social Behavior, 18*, 260–275.

85. Norris, M. C., Fogel, S. T., & Holtmann, B. (1998). Intrathecal sufentanil (5 vs. 10 microg) for labor analgesia: Efficacy and side effects. *Regional Anesthesia and Pain Medicine, 23*, 252–257.

86. Ohno, H., Yamashita, K., Yahata, et al. (1986). Maternal plasma concentrations of catecholamines and cyclic nucleotides during labor and following delivery. *Research Communications in Chemical Pathology and Pharmacology, 51*, 183–194.

87. Olive, D. L., & Pritts, E. A. (2001). Treatment of endometriosis. *New England Journal of Medicine, 345*, 266–275.

88. Peabody, J. L. (1979). Transcutaneous oxygen measurement to evaluate drug effect. *Clinical Perinatology, 6*, 109–121.

89. Pearson, J. F., & Davies, P. (1973). The effect of continuous epidural analgesia on the acid-base status of maternal arterial blood during the first stage of labor. *Journal of Obstetrics and Gynecology of the British Commonwealth, 80*, 218–224.

90. Pearson, J. F., & Davies, P. (1974). The effect of continuous lumbar epidural analgesia on the acid-base status of maternal arterial blood during the first stage of labor. *Journal of Obstetrics and Gynecology of the British Commonwealth, 81*, 975–979.

91. Peters, A. A. W., Trimbos-Kemper, G. C. M., Admiraal, C., & Trimbos, J. B. (1992). A randomized clinical trial on the benefit of adhesiolysis in patients with intraperitoneal adhesions and chronic pelvic pain. *British Journal of Obstetrics and Gynecology, 99*, 59–62.

92. Peters, A. A., Van Dorst, E., Jellis, B., Van Zuuren, E., Hermans, J., & Trimbos, J. B. (1991). A randomized clinical trial to compare two different approaches in women with chronic pelvic pain. *Obstetrics and Gynecology, 77*, 740–744.

93. Prentice, A., Deary, A. J., Goldbeck-Wood, S., Farquhar, C., & Smith, S. K. (2000). Gonadotrophin-releasing hormone analogues for pain associated with endometriosis (Cochrane Review). *The Cochrane Library, issue 4*. Update Software.

94. Price, F. V., Edwards, R., & Buchsbaum, H. J. (1990). Ovarian remnant syndrome: Difficulties in diagnosis and management. *Obstetrical and Gynecological Surgery, 45*, 151–156.

95. Procacci, P., Zoppi, M., & Maresen, M. (1986). Clinical approach to visceral sensation. In F. Cervero & J. Morrison (Eds.), *Visceral Sensation* (pp. 21–36). Elsevier.

96. Rapkin, A. J. (1986). Adhesions and pelvic pain: A retrospective study. *Obstetrics and Gynecology, 68*, 13–15.

97. Rapkin, A. J. (1995). Gynecological pain in the clinic: Is there a link with the basic research? In G. F. Gebhart (Ed.), *Visceral Pain: Progress in Pain Research and Management* (pp. 469–488). IASP Press.

98. Rapkin, A. J., & Kames, L. D. (1987). The pain management approach to chronic pelvic pain. *Journal of Reproductive Medicine, 32*, 323–327.

99. Rapkin, A. J., Kames, L. D., & Darke, L. L. (1990). History of physical and sexual abuse in women with chronic pelvic pain. *Obstetrics and Gynecology, 76*, 90–96.

100. Rapkin, A. J., Rasgon, N. L., & Berkley, K. J. (1997). Dysmenorrhea. In T. L. Yaksh et al. (Eds.), *Anesthesia. Biologic foundations* (pp. 785–793). Lippincott-Raven.

101. Reading, A. E., & Cox, D. N. (1985). Psychosocial predictors of labor pain. *Pain, 22*, 309–315.

102. Reese, K. A., Reddy, S., & Rock, J. A. (1996). Endometriosis in an adolescent population: The Emory experience. *Journal of Pediatric and Adolescent Gynecology, 9*, 125–128.

103. Reiter, R. C. (1990). Occult somatic pathology in women with chronic pelvic pain. *Clinical Obstetrics and Gynecology, 33*, 154–160.

104. Reiter, R. C., Gambone, J. C., & Johnson, S. R. (1991). Availability of a multidisciplinary pelvic pain clinic and frequency of hysterectomy for pelvic pain. *Journal of Psychosomatic Obstetrics and Gynecology, 12*(suppl), 109.

105. Renaer, M. (1980). Chronic pelvic pain without obvious pathology in women: Personal observation and a review of the problem. *European Journal of Obstetrics and Gynecology, 10*, 415–463.

106. Ringel, Y., Sperber, A. D., & Drossman, D. A. (2001). Irritable bowel syndrome. *Annual Review of Medicine, 52*, 319–338.

107. Robson, S. C., Dunlop, W., Boys, R. J., & Hunter, S. (1987). Cardiac output during labor. *British Medical Journal, 295*, 1169–1172.

108. Rosaeg, O. P., Kitts, J. B., Koren, G., & Byford, L. L. (1992). Maternal and fetal effects of intravenous patient-controlled fentanyl analgesia during labor in a thrombocytopenic parturient. *Canadian Journal of Anesthesia, 39*, 277–281.

109. Sant, G. R. (1998). Interstitial cystitis—A urogynecology perspective. *Contemporary OB/GYN, June*, 119–130.

110. Shnider, S. M., & Levinson, G. (1987). *Anesthesia for Obstetrics, 3rd edn.* Williams & Wilkins.

111. Sichlau, M. J., Yao, J. S. T., & Vogelzang, R. L. (1994). Transcatheter embolotherapy for the treatment of pelvic congestion syndrome. *Obstetrics and Gynecology, 83*, 892–896.

112. Siddall-Allum, J., Rae, T., Rogers, V., Witherow, R., Flanagan, A., & Beard, R. W. (1994). Chronic pain caused by residual ovaries and ovarian remnants. *British Journal of Obstetrics and Gynecology, 101*, 979–985.

113. Sippo, W. C., Burghardt, A., & Gomez, A. C. (1987). Nerve entrapment after Pfannensteil incision. *American Journal of Obstetrics and Gynecology, 157*, 420–421.

114. Slocumb, J. C. (1984). Neurological factors in chronic pelvic pain: Trigger points and the abdominal pelvic pain syndrome. *American Journal of Obstetrics and Gynecology, 149*, 536–543.

115. Slocumb, J. C. (1990). Chronic somatic myofascial and neurogenic abdominal pelvic pain. In R. P. Porreco & R. C. Reiter (Eds.), *Clinical Obstetrics and Gynecology* (pp. 145–153). Lippincott.

116. Spangen, L. (1984). Spigelian hernia. *Surgical Clinics of North America, 64*, 351–366.

117. Steege, J. F., & Scott, A. L. (1991). Resolution of chronic pelvic pain after laparoscopic lysis of adhesions. *American Journal of Obstetrics and Gynecology, 165*, 278–283.

118. Stewart, D. E. (1982). Psychiatric symptoms following attempted natural childbirth. *Canadian Medical Association Journal, 127*, 713–716.

119. Stones, R. W., Rae, T., Rogers, V., Fry, R., & Beard, R. W. (1990). Pelvic congestion in women: Evaluation with transvaginal ultrasound and observation of venous pharmacology. *British Journal of Radiology, 63*, 710–711.

120. Stout, A. L., Steege, J. F., Dodson, W. C., & Hughes, C. L. (1991). Relationship of laparoscopic findings to self-report of pelvic pain. *American Journal of Obstetrics and Gynecology, 164*, 73–79.

121. Summit, R. L. (1993). Urogynecology causes of chronic pelvic pain. In F. W. Ling (Ed.), *Obstetrics and Gynecology Clinics of North America: Contemporary Management of Chronic Pain* (pp. 685–698). Saunders.

122. Swart, F., Abboud, T. K., Zhu, J., et al. (1991). Desflurane analgesia in obstetrics: Maternal and neonatal effects (abstract). *Anesthesiology, 75*, A844.

123. Thomson, H., & Francis, D. M. A. (1977). Abdominal-wall tenderness: A useful sign in the acute abdomen. *Lancet, 2*, 1053–1055.

124. Tomkinson, J., et al. (1982). Report on confidential inquiries into maternal death in England and Wales 1976–1978. Report on Health and Social Subjects No. 16. HMSO.

125. Toomey, T. C., Hernandez, J. T., Gittelman, D. F., & Hulka, J. F. (1993). Relationship of sexual and physical abuse to pain and psychological assessment variables in chronic pelvic pain patients. *Pain, 53*, 105–109.

126. Travell, J. (1976). Myofascial trigger points: Clinical view. *Advances in Pain Research and Therapy, 1*, 919–926.

127. Vercellini, P., Fedele, L., Bianchi, S., & Candiani, G. B. (1991). Pelvic denervation for chronic pain associated with endometriosis: Fact or fancy? *American Journal of Obstetrics and Gynecology, 165*, 745–749.

128. Walker, E. A., Gelfand, A. N., Gelfand, M. D., Green, C., & Katon, W. J. (1996). Chronic pelvic pain and gynecological symptoms in women with irritable bowel syndrome. *Journal of Psychosomatic Obstetrics and Gynecology, 17*, 39–46.

129. Wall, P. D. (1988). The John J. Bonica distinguished lecture. Stability and instability of central pain mechanisms. In R. Dubner (Ed.), *Proceedings of the Fifth World Congress on Pain* (pp. 13–24). Elsevier.

130. Wesselmann, U., & Lai, J. (1997). Mechanisms of referred visceral pain: Uterine inflammation in the adult virgin rat results in neurogenic plasma extravasation in the skin. *Pain, 73*, 209–317.

131. Westrom, L., & Eschenbach, D. (1999). Pelvic inflammatory disease. In K. K. Holmes et al. (Eds.), *Sexually Transmitted Diseases, Third edn.* (pp. 783–809). McGraw-Hill.

132. Williams, B., Kwan, K., Chen, B., & Wu, Y. (1990). Comparison of 0.0312% bupivacaine plus

sufentanil and 0.0625% bupivacaine plus sufentanil for epidural anesthesia during labor and delivery. *Anesthesiology, 73*, A950.

133. Wilson, M., Farquhar, C., Kennedy, S., & Jin, X. (2000). Transcutaneous electrical nerve stimulation and acupuncture for primary dysmenorrhea (Protocol for a Cochrane Review). *The Cochrane Library, Issue 4*. Update Software.

134. Wood, D. P., Weisner, M. G., & Reiter, R. C. (1990). Psychogenic chronic pelvic pain. *Clinical Obstetrics and Gynecology, 33*, 179–195.

135. Zarzur, E., & Gonzalves, J. J. (1992). The resistance of the human dura mater to needle penetration. *Regional Anesthesia, 17*, 216–218.

Chapter 6

OROFACIAL PAIN MANAGEMENT

Contents

Introduction

A wide range of disorders affecting the mouth, jaws, face, and related structures are included in orofacial pain management; these disorders frequently present difficult diagnostic and therapeutic challenges. It includes a wide range of conditions, such as headaches, neuropathic pain syndromes, dental pain, trigeminal neuralgia, and temporomandibular joint disorders (TMD). Numerous factors, such as dental pathology, trauma, inflammation, muscle dysfunction, nerve injury, or systemic diseases, can lead to these conditions.

The multifactorial nature of orofacial pain, which frequently involves interactions between biological, psychological, and social factors, is one of its unique features. As a result, comprehensive and interdisciplinary approaches combining knowledge from different medical specialties like neurology, otolaryngology, dentistry, and pain management are usually necessary for effective management.

The diagnosis of orofacial pain disorders is primarily based on a comprehensive clinical assessment, which is frequently augmented by specialized diagnostic tests and imaging studies. The goals of orofacial pain treatment are to reduce symptoms, increase function, and improve quality of life. Pharmaceutical treatments, dental therapies, physical modalities, behavioral therapies, and occasionally surgical procedures are some examples of these.

Treatment regimens must be customized to take into account the various underlying causes of orofacial pain disorders as well as the individual needs of each patient. In order to effectively manage the complexities of orofacial pain and optimize outcomes, collaboration between patients and healthcare providers is imperative.

Orientation and Directional Terms

Term	Definition	Illustration
Orofacial pain	Orofacial pain (OFP) is a common dental specialty that deals with pain in the face, mouth, jaw, head, and neck.	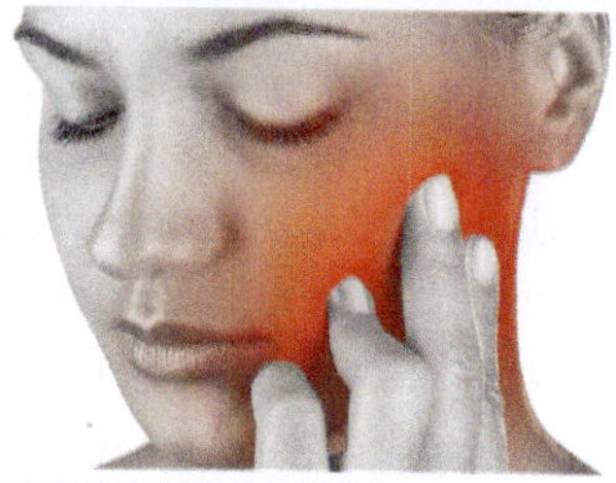
Temporomandibular disorders	Temporomandibular disorders (TMDs) are a group of conditions that cause pain and dysfunction in the jaw joint and muscles that control jaw movement.	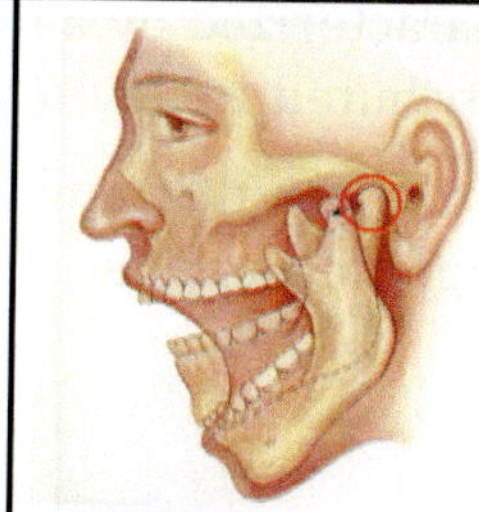
Muscle dysfunction	Muscle dysfunction, also known as a muscle disorder or myopathy, can cause weakness, pain, or paralysis in your muscles.	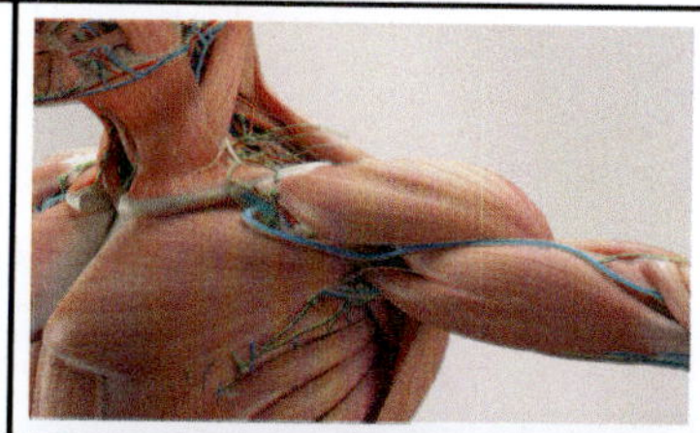
Retrodiscitis	Retrodiscitis is an inflammatory condition of the retrodiscal tissues in the temporomandibular joint (TMJ).	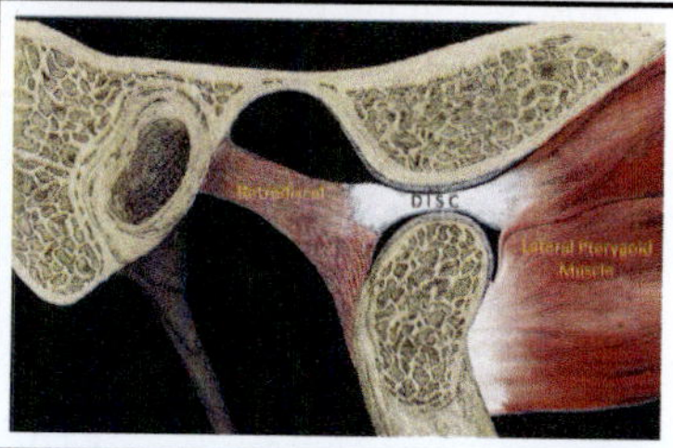
Cyclobenzaprine	Cyclobenzaprine is used with rest, physical therapy, and other measures to relax muscles and relieve pain and discomfort caused by strains, sprains, and other muscle injuries.	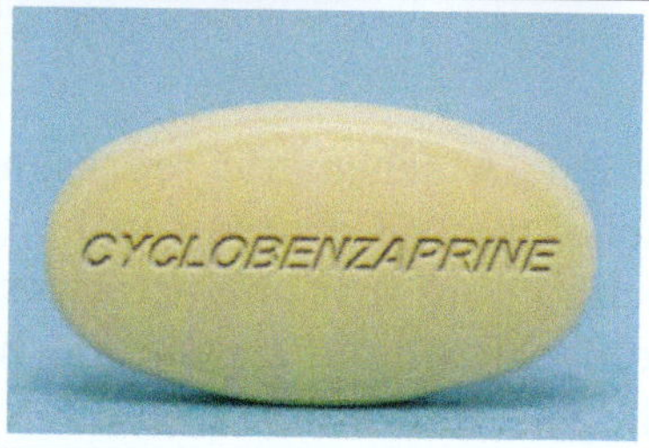

6.1. Orofacial Pain

Orofacial pain is among the most common health issues that have a detrimental impact on day-to-day activities. When looking at the entire orofacial district, a significant portion of patients report pain that is primarily localized at the oral/dental site; in fact, the most common cause of orofacial pain is dental disease. We can therefore classify it as odontogenic pain.

Tooth decay and dental caries are generally the most common causes of dental pain. Furthermore, if left untreated, even a straightforward dental caries can develop into a more widespread oral problem, which can result in pulpitis, a general inflammation of the dental pulp that is most frequently linked to dental and orofacial pain. Dentine hypersensitivity is a common odontogenic pain condition characterized by a brief, sharp pain that is triggered by different exogenous stimuli and cannot be attributed to any other organic cause.

It's feasible to argue that any external stimulus could hurt if it was aimed at the tooth with pulpitis or the exposed dentine.

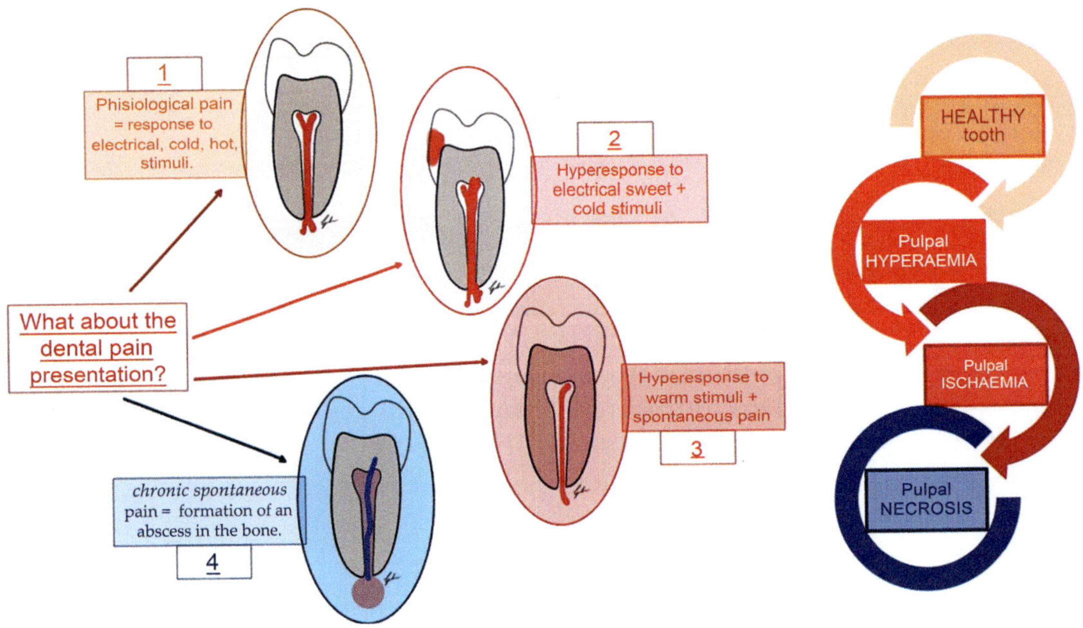

Figure 6.1. A schematic representation of the many guises of dental pain. In dental pain and toothache, many features can be described. Among them, the most common are represented by the elicited pain that characterizes the form of reversible pulpitis, in which the response to touch and cold can mimic trigeminal neuralgia, post-traumatic neuropathies, trigeminal autonomic cephalalgias, and other secondary neuropathies. In the end, the episodic intense throbbing pain associated with irreversible pulpitis can mimic myofascial pain and migraine.

Source: Labanca M, Gianò M, Franco C, Rezzani R. Orofacial pain and dentistry management: guidelines for a more comprehensive evidence-based approach. *Diagnostics*, 2023; 13(17):2854. https://doi.org/10.3390/diagnostics13172854.

Above all, though, we must take into account how special and intricate the sensory system and innervation are in the tooth and throughout the orofacial region. Consequently, the transduction of the nociceptive signal and, thus, the treatment, differ even though many dental conditions are well-known and well-defined. In actuality, some of these underlying mechanisms are still unknown, which may result in the oral pain being undertreated, being overtreated even when avoidable, or, in the end, receiving the wrong kind of care.

6.1.1. Orofacial Pain Disorders

Orofacial pain disorders are extremely common, severely incapacitating conditions that affect the neck, face, and head. Because pain can originate from multiple sources in the orofacial region due to its complexity, these conditions pose a challenge to clinicians. For an accurate diagnosis, the clinician must possess a thorough understanding of the pain conditions resulting from these structures. It is highly recommended that a multidisciplinary approach to management be employed.

According to Okeson, there are two categories for orofacial pain: physical (Axis 1) and psychological (Axis 2) conditions. Physical conditions include neuropathic pains, which include episodic (e.g., trigeminal neuralgia [TN]) and continuous (e.g., peripheral/centralized mediated) pains, as well as neurovascular disorders (e.g., migraine). Temporomandibular disorders (TMD) include disorders of the temporomandibular joint (TMJ) and disorders of the musculoskeletal structures (e.g., masticatory muscles and cervical spine). Anxiety and mood disorders are examples of psychological disorders. This review will only address TMD, neuropathic pain, and headaches, with an emphasis on current viewpoints in orofacial pain management. For a more thorough explanation of the pathophysiology and diagnosis of the conditions shown in this classification as well as other painful conditions affecting the head, face, and neck.

6.2. TMD

A variety of clinical issues involving the TMJ, related structures, and the masticatory musculature are categorized as "TMD." Among musculoskeletal disorders, TMD is thought to be a subclassification and is the most common ailment for which patients seek medical attention. To properly form a differential diagnosis, these facial structures must be carefully evaluated in conjunction with clinical symptoms. The patient's complaint could be as minor as general facial fullness or pressure, but it could also include jaw pain, ear pain, toothache, facial pain, and/or headache. A number of factors, such as the primary complaint, medical history, presenting symptoms, examination, and diagnosis, influence treatment planning. Although TMD cases were once thought to be challenging to diagnose and treat, current research in orofacial pain and pain management has made this possible for clinicians to offer patients a variety of treatment options with higher success rates by using a more standardized classification system and improved diagnostic and therapeutic techniques (Okeson JP. Bell's Orofacial Pains).

6.2.1. Natural History and Epidemiology of TMD

The majority of epidemiological studies unequivocally show that women experience TMD symptoms more frequently than men do, and that many symptoms appear to start in adolescence or the early twenties and may last intermittently well into middle age. Despite these facts, TMD symptomatology does improve over time, which supports a conservative approach to treatment. In a research by Solberg et al., 26% of participants between the ages of 18 and 25 had at least one symptom and 76% of participants had one or more signs of TMD.

Merely 10% of this cohort exhibited symptoms deemed severe enough by the participants to warrant medical attention. According to Rasmussen's research, the majority of TMJ clicking cases did not progress to an open or closed locking state. Rasmussen reported that the majority of painful and incapacitating symptoms eventually subsided, even though joint noises usually persisted throughout the natural course of internal derangement. Acute TMD symptoms also lasted an average of 50.5 years. Könönen et al. followed 128 adult Finns for nine years, and their findings were similar in that clicking frequency rose with age. But none of the patients experienced locking. In a more recent study, patients with a mean age range of 52 years showed a prevalence of crepitus, whereas patients with a mean age range of 38 years did not. The presence of degenerative joint disorders was found to be the discriminating factor in two different age subgroups.

6.2.2. Disorders of the TMJ

TMJ disorders arise from disc–condyle incoordination, which affects the biomechanics of the TMJ. These conditions include internal derangements, such as disc displacements with or without reduction, or disc interference disorders. The latter can be asymptomatic or symptomatic as a result of inflammation (capsulitis/synovitis, for example).

Reduction in disc displacements can cause a click that is either painful or not. Disk displacements that are not reduced could cause excruciating limitations when they open. When the pain is caused by inflammation originating from the retrodiscal tissues, capsulitis, or synovitis processes, retrodiscitis and TMJ subluxation may manifest symptomatology. When an aggressive systemic disease influences osteoarthritic changes, as in the case of polyarthritis, the changes can start in the articular surfaces of the TMJ.

6.2.3. Muscular Disorders

Myalgia from a strained or injured muscle typically manifests as a dull aching pain. Although it is frequently observed in acute forms, it can also manifest for longer periods of time if muscle tension persists. Muscle relaxants, hot or cold compresses, stretching exercises, and rest are some possible treatments. Another way that myofascial pain (MFP) manifests itself is as a dull, constant aching pain with fluctuating intensity. According to Simons et al.'s mapping, MFP causes pain upon palpation that is localized and may refer to other sites. MFP is typically observed in cases of more persistent muscle pain, characterized by constant tension. In MFP, trigger points are frequently observed and can be restricted to a tense muscle band. Furthermore, trigger points are linked to shortened muscles and can cause a local twitch response when activated. The diagnosis should be confirmed by palpating the trigger points in the same way that the patient complains of pain. A conclusive diagnosis may also be obtained by obstructing the masseter muscle, which is the source of the pain, with a vapocoolant spray or local anesthetic injection.

Myositis is a temporary, localized swelling of the face and muscles. Localized tenderness and increased pain with mandibular movement are common, usually after an injury or infection.

6.2.4. Patient Evaluation

An evaluation of the TMJs, an assessment of the mandibular range of motion (ROM), a thorough intraoral examination, a general examination of the head and neck, and an examination of the masticatory muscles should all be part of the TMD assessment process.

6.2.4.1. Evaluation of the TMJs and Mandibular ROM

A TMJ evaluation involves looking for any indications of dysfunction or pain symptomatology. When the mandible is closed and at rest, light pressure is applied with the fingertips to the lateral and posterior aspects of the TMJs to open them. Symptoms that appear in reaction to pressure placed on the lateral aspect of the TMJs could indicate capsulitis or synovitis. Retrodiscitis or posterior capsulitis could be the cause of symptoms that are reported in response to force applied to the posterior aspect of the condyle.

Joint sounds, which can manifest as pops, clicks, or crepitus, should be recognized by the clinician. 1 A stethoscope inserted into the TMJ region or, occasionally, palpation are used to assess these sounds. Pops and clicks are frequently connected to disc displacements with reduction, and crepitation is frequently linked to osteoarthritic alterations in the TMJ's articular surfaces. TMJ imaging could be helpful during the examination. Furthermore, determining any TMJ restrictions is crucial. To identify any mandibular deviations, the clinician should observe the patient's opening and closing patterns. Using a millimeter ruler, measure comfort opening, active opening, passive opening, protrusion, and left and right lateral excursions while recording the location and degree of pain felt when moving the jaw. This is how mandibular range of motion is evaluated. This is especially useful for telling the difference between pain in the muscles and joints. The patient defines comfort opening as wide as they can open without experiencing any pain, active opening as wide as they can open while experiencing pain, and passive opening as far as the clinician is concerned, which is when they gently stretch the patient past active opening and note whether the end feels soft or hard. Approximately 40 mm, or roughly the width of three of the patient's fingers, is considered a reasonably normal interincisal distance. If the patient is properly questioned, they will typically disclose any recent limitations in range of motion. During the initial examination, it's important to record any instances of TMJ clicking, crepitus, or jaw opening interferences, whether or not they cause pain. These baseline results will serve as a reference for future changes in TMD symptoms and will help establish the differential diagnosis and available treatments.

6.2.4.2. Evaluation of the Muscles of Mastication

With 2–3 pounds of pressure, or the amount required to cause the fingernail to blanch, the muscles of mastication should be palpated bilaterally for firmness and tenderness. When palpating the patient's muscles, it is important to find out how much of the primary complaint is replicated, whether the pain is localized to one site or multiple, and how severe the tenderness is. Before performing a palpation, it might be useful to inquire about the patient's use of analgesics to help explain any decreased symptoms found during the examination.

6.2.5. Management of TMD

The majority of the time, patients will see the clinician when they experience pain or dysfunction. Examples of these symptoms include headaches, joint locking episodes (open lock/TMJ subluxation), pain associated with mandibular function (chewing), and limitations in opening.

Reducing pain, regaining normal range of motion, and regaining normal jaw and masticatory function are the objectives of TMD treatment. Numerous TMDs have the potential to be self-limiting and cyclical, with intervals of total symptom remission.

Research on disc-condyle incoordinations indicates that some patients may experience self-limiting symptoms with no significant disability, despite the possibility that they may progress (e.g., from a disc displacement with reduction to a disc displacement without reduction). It is crucial to stress that patients who receive conservative, reversible treatments do not experience a recurrence of their symptoms; therefore, conservative treatment is the modality that should always be used. Thus, the emphasis of initial treatment should be on a conservative and reversible strategy. The three main forms of treatment are medical (non-surgical care), surgical, and home care/self-care programs.

6.2.5.1. Patient Education: Home Care Program

Generally, the first course of action should be home care, if not as part of a more comprehensive treatment plan. It has been demonstrated that using a home care program is beneficial for managing TMD. Research indicates that following their first patient education/counseling visit, patients have reported feeling less pain right away. This could be due to an instant decrease in stress/tension-related parafunctional activity. Patient education is one of the most subtle, underappreciated, and successful treatments for TMD, and it is an essential component of home care. Thus, providing the patient with information and reassurance about their condition and symptoms may significantly reduce anxiety and enhance the effectiveness of treatment.

A good home care program will emphasize a soft diet, parafunctional habit modification, moist heat and/or ice therapy, and resting the masticatory muscles by limiting jaw movements. Muscle rest may entail minimizing jaw movements (such as chewing, yawning, and talking) during the course of treatment and possibly even after symptoms have subsided. When the condition is acute, patients with disc displacement without reduction should be told not to try to open their mouths too widely. Instead, they should be told that with the right care, their range of motion will improve and return to normal. Limiting the range of motion in the mandible would help promote healing and stop additional damage. This could be achieved by eating only soft foods, abstaining from chewing gum and hard foods, closing your mouth when you yawn, and practicing habit awareness by not biting, clenching, or bruxing. To reduce prolonged masticatory muscle contractions, patients may have diurnal (daytime) parafunctional habits (clenching, grinding, posturing) that are frequently unconscious. These habits should be addressed. Reducing and eventually stopping the daytime activity that contributes to the progression of TMD requires patient education and understanding of the physiological rest position (lips together, teeth apart). Many patients will return for follow-up after being asked to monitor their jaw position over time, realizing that they are, in fact, doing something with their jaws that exacerbates their symptoms. Furthermore, offering cues for habit control could be useful in reminding the patient to check their bite position throughout the day. Saying the letter "N," for instance, a few times a day can serve as a reminder to the patient to relax or stop grinding their teeth. For the purpose of managing muscle and TMJ pain and preventing worsening of the condition while receiving treatment, a soft diet is also essential. Lastly, it may be suggested to try applying moist heat or ice therapy to the sore spots on the head, neck, and face. When treating muscle pain or tension, moist heat works better because it promotes circulation and relaxes the affected muscles. For TMJ capsulitis, ice works better because it lessens inflammation.

6.2.6. Medical Care (Non-Surgical)

6.2.6.1. Physical Therapy

It has been demonstrated that giving the patient instructions to apply moist heat or cold compresses, or to alternate between the two modalities, is beneficial because it promotes analgesia and relaxation and may facilitate better movement.

Physical therapy helps to reduce inflammation, promote strength and repair, and restore normal function to the TMJ, masticatory muscles, and cervical muscles. Physical therapy for TMJ disorders can be administered by a licensed clinician or by a skilled physical therapist with experience. Stretching tired, chronically contracted muscles, increasing range of motion, and lowering the activity of trigger points in the muscles are the main objectives of the physical therapy portion of the treatment plan. N-stretch, which involves stretching the jaw by placing the tip of the tongue on the roof of the mouth, chin to chest, which involves gently pulling the head forward and bringing the chin toward the chest, and head tilt, which involves turning the head to one side and then tilting it posteriorly, are a few of the exercises that are frequently used to treat muscle disorders related to the TMJ. For best results, perform these exercises four to six times a day. Before stretching the muscles, the patient should also apply moist heat for 10 to 15 minutes and then ethyl chloride spray. With the help of vaporcoolant spray, muscles can be temporarily sedated to facilitate more intense stretches without experiencing pain. Throughout the day, at least three of the six exercise sessions should be conducted with the heat and cooling spray. If patients combine transcutaneous electrical nerve stimulation with a rigorous stretching regimen and biofeedback training as a cognitive behavioral procedure to teach them to maintain reduced muscular tension and pain, they can expect an even higher likelihood of treatment success.

6.2.6.2. Pharmacotherapy

To effectively manage the symptomatology of intracapsular disorders, medications can be added. Analgesics, nonsteroidal anti-inflammatory drugs (NSAIDs), local anesthetics, injectable and oral corticosteroids, sodium hyaluronate injections, muscle relaxants, injections of botulinum toxin, and antidepressants are among the pharmacological agents that are frequently used to treat TMJ disorders. Tricyclic antidepressants are typically used more for chronic TMD pain in conjunction with tension-type headaches; analgesics and corticosteroids are indicated for acute TMD pain; NSAIDs, local anesthetics, and muscle relaxants are used for both acute and chronic conditions. There is a dearth of research on the effectiveness of botulinum toxin in treating muscular disorders associated with traumatic musculoskeletal disorders (TMD), but there is some evidence in favor of administering high injection volumes and low concentrations of the toxin to various muscle sites.

6.2.6.3. NSAIDs

For mild-to-moderate acute inflammatory conditions, NSAIDs are recommended. NSAIDs that are frequently used include naproxen and ibuprofen. The patient should take NSAIDs for at least two weeks, and their dosage should be time-contingent rather than based on the patient's level of pain. As long as the activity causing the inflammatory process can be decreased, long-term NSAID use is not advised. Long-term use of NSAIDs, such as COX-2 inhibitors like celecoxib, may be considered in some cases of chronic arthritis; however, it is important to consider potential side effects, such as gastrointestinal upset.

6.2.6.4. Local Anesthetics

Myofascial trigger points are the main situation in which local anesthetics are used. Myofascial trigger points can be found in many different muscles, including the splenius capitis and upper trapezius, but they are typically identified in the mastication muscles. Although 1% or 2% lidocaine is also frequently used, 1% procaine (1 cc) is advised due to its low toxicity to muscles. The trigger point, which is typically located in a taut band of muscle, is located using the trigger point injection technique, and the area is needled.

The patient should be informed that while there may be some soreness in the muscles for the first 48 hours following the injection, these should start to feel better. The effectiveness of trigger point injections varies greatly and is primarily reliant on the patient adhering to a rigorous physical therapy program in addition to the injections. To confirm a diagnosis, local anesthetics can also be used to block the most likely source of pain.

6.2.6.5. TMJ Injections

Corticosteroid injections intracapsularly significantly lessen pain in the TMJ. When the joint is still acutely inflamed, as in the case of polyarthritic disorders and acute disc displacements without reduction, it is indicated for treating acute and painful arthritic TMJ that has not responded to other treatment modalities. TMJ injections typically involve the use of triamcinolone or dexamethasone along with 2% lidocaine without epinephrine.

A TMJ tomography or other radiographic examination is necessary before administering an injection into the joint space. Animal research has revealed that steroid injections might boost osteoclastic activity. There is no proof that a single steroid injection harms the body; however, several injections may, so the number of injections should be carefully considered because there is a chance that the injection site may resorb bone (Okeson JP. Bell's Orofacial Pains).

Table 6.1. Different Types of Pain, Different Treatment Strategies.

Orofacial Pain Management	
Type of Pain	**Main Drugs**
Inflammatory pain	1. Anti-inflammatory drugs; 2. Pain reliever drugs (e.g., paracetamol) H D, Wellish, & Gilden, (2003)
Post-surgery pain	1. Anti-inflammatory drugs; 2. Pain reliever drugs (e.g., paracetamol) H D, Wellish, & Gilden, (2003)
Temporomandibular joint-associated pain	1. Anti-inflammatory drugs; 2. Pain reliever drugs (e.g., paracetamol) H D, Wellish, & Gilden, (2003)
Neuropathic pain	1. Opioids; 2. Tricyclic antidepressants; 3. Serotonin noradrenaline reuptake inhibitors.

Source: Labanca M, Gianò M, Franco C, Rezzani R. Orofacial pain and dentistry management: Guidelines for a more comprehensive evidence-based approach. *Diagnostics*. 2023; 13(17):2854. https://doi.org/10.3390/diagnostics13172854.

*Pain in the Orofacial Region can be associated with several different causes, and it can be characterized by many different features and patterns of presentation. Consequently, it is not possible to think of a single therapeutic strategy; instead, targeted therapies with specific actions are needed, depending on the mechanism that is causing the pain itself.

Sodium hyaluronate injections have been shown to alleviate symptoms in patients with osteoarthritis of the knee; however, results for the treatment of TMD have been equivocal, and further research is necessary.

6.2.6.6. Muscle Relaxants

When TMJ disorders are linked to acute muscle tension, physicians may prescribe muscle relaxants. These are typically taken in the evening before going to bed because of the potential for drowsiness. Therefore, in addition to their ability to prevent muscle pain, these medications are especially useful in treating insomnia in patients with irregular sleep patterns. Cyclobenzaprine is a frequently used and efficient muscle relaxant. It is recommended to start with lower dosages (5–10 mg) and to take it 1–2 hours before bed.

6.2.6.7. Antidepressants

For more persistent MFP, tricyclic antidepressants such as nortriptyline and amitriptyline may be used. They may also be recommended for TMD patients who experience depression, insomnia, poor appetite, or tension-type headaches (TTH). It is crucial to let the patient know that when these drugs are prescribed to treat headaches and/or muscle pain, the dosages are typically too high to produce antidepressant effects. The recommended dosages of amitriptyline (10–25 mg) and nortriptyline (10–30 mg) should be gradually increased until the desired therapeutic effect is obtained or side effects, such as sleepiness, dry mouth, or weight gain, appear. Tricyclic antidepressants keep the patient in deeper sleep stages and also have anti-nociceptive effects. Patients with concomitant heart conditions, concurrent psychotropic use, and/or psychiatric illness, such as bipolar disorder, should use caution.

6.2.6.8. Occlusal Appliance Therapy

Oral appliances (OAs) are processed acrylic devices with various designs that have been used for years to treat TMD. Research has shown a decrease in TMD symptoms, or at least enough data to support their use in treating masticatory system myalgia and arthralgia. An in-depth analysis of OA use and TMD management came to the conclusion that OAs are still thought to be a helpful adjunct therapy in certain TMD cases.

The goals of stabilization appliances, such as flat plane splints, are to lessen the strain on the masticatory muscles, distribute parafunctional forces in the jaw equally, and shield the occlusal surfaces of the teeth from persistent nighttime bruxing. OAs will shield teeth from excessive tooth wear in cases of nocturnal bruxism, but they might not completely eliminate parafunctional habits. They might, however, lessen their frequency, duration, and intensity. As long as parafunctional activity is managed during the day with education and bite relation awareness, teaching the patient to be aware of when they are clenching their teeth during the day, the patient is typically only required to wear the splint at night. All maxillary or mandibular teeth should be covered by the splint, which should have minimal to no anterior contacts and bilateral posterior contacts. When the stabilization appliance is first fitted, it should feel comfortable to the patient. A week later, the patient should have another assessment. Because chronic bruxism may cause changes in the shape and function of the splint, adjustments should be made every three to six months.

Clinicians prescribe different anterior repositioning splints for different patients, but they are typically used for patients who have chronic intermittent closed-locking. Short-term (6-week) use of this appliance is highly advised in addition to close monitoring, as long-term use of repositioning appliances may result in permanent occlusal and bite changes. The patient should be advised to stop using the splint if bite abnormalities begin, and the splint may need to be changed into a stabilizing non-repositioning appliance. Some patients may find that wearing a splint makes their pain worse. In this instance, it is advised to stop using the splint if the pain doesn't go away and to reevaluate both the splint and the original diagnosis.

When compared to the use of no appliance, soft stabilization appliances, anterior bite appliances, and non-occluding appliances, well-adjusted hard stabilization appliances are more effective in treating joint and muscle pain, according to a systematic review and meta-analysis of randomized controlled trials. These OAs showed some promise in easing joint and muscular pain, but there was also a greater chance of unfavorable outcomes (such as occlusal abnormalities).

6.2.6.9. Occlusal Adjustment

The effectiveness of occlusal adjustments in the treatment or prevention of TMD is not well-established. Occlusal adjustments are an irreversible treatment option for TMD, and conservative measures should be taken in its management.

6.2.7. Surgical Care

TMJ surgery is not recommended as a preventive measure or in patients who are asymptomatic or only mildly symptomatic; rather, it should only be performed when non-surgical therapy has failed. In addition to moderate-to-severe pain and incapacitating dysfunction, surgical recommendations, such as arthrocentesis and arthroscopy, rely on the degree of internal derangement and the history of prior TMJ treatment. Discouragement of surgical procedures is crucial in cases where pharmacological management, physical medicine, and splint therapy have not been tried. When treating this specific patient group, it is best to collaborate closely with an oral and maxillofacial surgeon skilled in TMJ surgery.

A conservative treatment called arthrocentesis is helpful when there are intra-articular movement restrictions, such as disc displacement without reduction. It entails intra-articular lavage with or without the deposit of corticosteroids. Patients with joint restrictions and those who have developed an acute or chronic closed lock are advised to undergo this procedure, which is frequently combined with mandibular manipulation.

Arthroscopy is a closed surgical technique that is helpful in cases of fibrosis and hypomobility brought on by joint derangement because it permits direct observation and sampling of joint tissue. It is primarily used for lysis and lavage, but it can also be used for biopsy and adhesion ablation. It is mostly done in the upper joint space.

Arthrotomy is an open surgical procedure that modifies the anatomy of the joint. It is necessary for patients with advanced TMD who meet the surgical criteria and have not responded to other modalities. This procedure can involve total or partial joint reconstruction or replacement. It is applied to cases of severe chronic arthritis, severe chronic dislocations, neoplasia, and bony or fibrous ankylosis. It is crucial to collaborate closely with a skilled TMJ surgeon to determine whether this procedure is required if more conservative measures have failed to yield positive outcomes.

6.2.8. Acupuncture and TMD

For a variety of orofacial pain disorders, primarily musculoskeletal in nature, acupuncture has been investigated as a complementary and alternative medicine treatment modality. To stimulate the energy flow that is thought to be blocked, acupuncture points are stimulated. This is one type of Traditional Chinese Medicine (TCM) known as acupuncture. It's been suggested that the lack of conclusive research on acupuncture's effectiveness in treating pain stems from the fact that studies on the subject frequently overlook complementary therapies like Qigong and herbal remedies. In a study on TMD, individuals receiving traditional acupuncture treatment reported less pain and, more significantly, less need for NSAIDs. In a subsequent study, TCM with acupuncture was compared to specialty care that included patient education, physical therapy, occlusal splint therapy, self-care, and psychosocial counseling. It was discovered that the TCM arm significantly reduced pain and factors that were associated with psychosocial problems. Furthermore, research has demonstrated that MFP, when considered independently of TMD, benefits from acupuncture in comparison to a sham acupuncture procedure. Because the two procedures are similar, it is important to explain to MFP patients the differences between acupuncture and traditional trigger point injection therapy. In addition to conventional therapies, acupuncture seems to be a helpful treatment for TMD. It could also be used as a backup if pharmaceutical treatment is not appropriate.

Table 6.2. Nociceptive Pain Treatment. Schematic Summary of the Main Drugs and Therapeutic Strategies that Can be Used in the Management of Nociceptive Pain

Nociceptive Pain Management	
Step	Main drugs
1—mild pain	Non-opioid analgesics: 1. Acetaminophen; 2. Aspirin; 3. Other non-steroidal anti-inflammatory drugs.
2—moderate pain	**Moderate opioids:** 1. Tramadol; 2. Codeine; 3. Oxycodone; (Associated with other non-opioid adjuvants).
3—severe pain	**Strong opioids:** 1. Morphine; 2. Levorphanol; 3. Oxycodone.

Source: Labanca M, Gianò M, Franco C, Rezzani R. Orofacial pain and dentistry management: guidelines for a more comprehensive evidence-based approach. *Diagnostics*. 2023; 13(17):2854. https://doi.org/10.3390/diagnostics13172854.

6.3. Neuropathic Pain

Neuroplastic alterations affecting the peripheral and central nervous systems along with immune mechanisms are implicated in the development and maintenance of chronic neuropathic pain, according to basic and clinical research. According to estimates, 5 to 10 cases of chronic orofacial neuropathic pain occur for every 100,000 individuals. Neuropathic pain conditions in the orofacial region are commonly classified into two categories: continuous pain disorders, which often arise from deafferentation following injury in the peripheral and central nervous system, as in the case of neuromas and idiopathic trigeminal neuropathic pains, such as atypical odontalgia (AO), and episodic pain disorders, such as trigeminal neuralgia (TN) and glossopharyngeal neuralgia. The frequency, etiology, and course of treatment for these disorders vary widely. You can find more thorough reviews of the pathophysiology, etiology, and classification of neuropathic pain elsewhere.

Treatment information for trigeminal neuropathic pain is still scarce. The evidence supporting the treatment of pain in other body regions serves as the foundation for this one. The reference books by Dworkin et al. and Zakrzewska are excellent.

When it comes to treating neuralgic pain, anticonvulsant drugs are the first line of treatment because of their demonstrated efficacy in treating trigeminal neuropathic pain. For more persistent pain, such as idiopathic trigeminal neuropathic pain in AO, topical drugs like capsaicin and lidocaine, as well as tricyclic antidepressants and serotonin noradrenaline reuptake inhibitors, are used.

6.3.1. Trigeminal Neuralgia

One person with TN experiences severe, lancinating, electric-like pain that is unilateral in nature. TN is a chronic paroxysmal neuropathic pain condition. It is most frequently localized to the trigeminal nerve's second and third distributions (V2 and V3), both intraorally and extraorally, and it can manifest simultaneously in both distributions. The trigeminal distribution typically contains a trigger zone that, when activated, can cause an unbearably painful attack. Pain episodes can occur frequently throughout the day, lasting anywhere from a few seconds to several minutes. Pain in TN frequently goes into remission, sometimes lasting for several months or even longer.

Vascular compression, which has the potential to cause focal demyelination, is frequently linked to the genesis of TN. Attacks of trigeminal neural pain have been linked to compression of the superior cerebellar artery on the trigeminal root; however, nonvascular compression caused by a cerebellopontine angle tumor, such as acoustic neuromas, meningiomas, cholesteatomas, and neurofibromas, has also been implicated in TN pain. An examination of the cranial nerve can reveal additional neural deficits that might be brought on by a mass pressing on the trigeminal root. Thus, to rule out any intracranial pathology, brain computed tomography (CT) and magnetic resonance imaging (MRI) should be requested. Moreover, it has been demonstrated that myelin loss resulting from multiple sclerosis is a causal disorder associated with the paroxysmal pain firing of TN attacks.

The preferred medications for treating TN are antiepileptic ones. Gabapentin, oxcarbazepine, and carbamazepine are frequently prescribed as first-line drugs. A systematic review that assessed the medication found that carbamazepine was the most successful course of action. Second-line medications like baclofen and lamotrigine may be added to treat pain attacks if these medications are ineffective or if side effects prevent the therapeutic range from being reached. Doses should be decreased in these situations. If necessary, it is best to completely stop the pain attacks by taking multiple medications. Once the patient is pain-free and has been monitored for pain episodes for at least three to six months, a gradual taper off of medication will show whether TN has entered remission. Pharmacologic management should be resumed right away if pain attacks return. Microvascular decompression or gamma knife radiosurgery are two neurosurgical options that may be explored if medication is no longer effective or if uncontrollable side effects occur.

6.3.2. Glossopharyngeal Neuralgia

A rare disorder called glossopharyngeal neuralgia is characterized by pain in the glossopharyngeal nerve's supply area. The tonsil, larynx, ear, throat, posterior portion of the tongue, and nasopharynx are among the painful locations. When stimulation of the oropharyngeal region is applied, this disorder manifests as shooting paroxysms of pain that can happen several times a day. Common triggers can include chewing, swallowing, coughing, talking, and moving the head. They can also involve mechanical stimulation of the trigger zone. The excruciating episodes might recur for months before ending on their own. Glossopharyngeal neuralgia may coexist with a cardiac dysrhythmia such as bradycardia, asystole, or syncope because of the close proximity of the vagal sensory nerves. By using topical or local anesthetics to block the tonsillar and pharyngeal region, the diagnosis can be verified. Imaging tests, including a brain MRI and a CT scan of the head, should be performed to rule out pathology associated with the compression of the nerve and potential oropharyngeal carcinoma. Similar to treatment for TN, glossopharyngeal neuralgia can be treated pharmacologically with antiepileptic drugs. Surgery such as radiofrequency thermocoagulation, gamma knife radiosurgery, rhizotomy, or microvascular decompression to relieve pressure on the glossopharyngeal nerve may be considered if medication management is unsuccessful.

6.3.3. Peripheral Trigeminal Neuropathic Pain

Traumatic nerve injuries can cause peripheral neuropathic pain, which manifests as persistent, burning pain at the site of the injury. A traumatic neuroma is the result of a transected nerve occasionally attempting to heal itself through axonal sprouting after injury. Tapping (Tinel's sign) or lightly pressing on the suspected neuroma site can be used to make the diagnosis. Additionally, the region of the nerve injury or the area next to it will frequently exhibit allodynia and hyperalgesia. It is advised to do a somatic block using a local anesthetic (such as an injection of lidocaine) after performing a diagnostic block of the painful site with a topical anesthetic (such as benzocaine). Topical creams or ointments can be used to treat the pain if either of these blocks reduces or eliminates it. One useful strategy to lessen the possibility of systemic side effects when treating neuropathic pain is the application of topical medications. Usually applied in cream or gel form, capsaicin is a commonly used locally acting pharmacologic agent. Its concentration ranges from 0–5%. It can also be mixed with 20% benzocaine and applied using a neurosensory stent to cover the affected area. In the US and Europe, 8% capsaicin has recently been approved for topical application and has shown promise in pain relief. Furthermore, analgesics/sedatives like ketamine, NSAIDs like diclofenac, anticonvulsants like gabapentin and carbamazepine, and tricyclic antidepressants like nortriptyline and amitriptyline can all be combined to create a cream by compounding pharmacies.

6.3.4. Centralized Trigeminal Neuropathic Pain

Extended activation of peripheral nociceptors may ultimately result in alterations to the central nervous system. In these cases, hyperalgesia and allodynia are present, and the pain is characterized as persistent, aching, and burning. Centrally acting systemic medications are used as a form of treatment for centralized neuropathic pain because diagnostic local anesthetic blocking of the affected site typically does not relieve the pain. Tricyclic antidepressants like amitriptyline, when combined with antiepileptic medications like gabapentin and valproic acid, may lessen pain, although treating this condition is frequently challenging.

6.3.5. Atypical Odontalgia

AO is a trigeminal neuropathy that is often centralized and localized in a tooth or tooth area. It is frequently misdiagnosed, leading to unnecessary dental treatments in an effort to relieve the pain. AO is a persistent idiopathic pain that does not meet the diagnostic criteria for cranial neuralgias and is not associated with another disorder. The pain can be described as throbbing and burning in nature. The pharmacological management of AO may involve both topical and systemic medications. If the pain is localized to a peripheral origin and a diagnostic block gives an unclear response but leads to a decrease in pain, a topical medication can be used and a neurosensory stent can be created. Systemic treatments, such as tricyclic antidepressants, calcium channel blockers (pregabalin and gabapentin), sodium channel blockers (carbamazepine), and antiepileptics like topiramate, may be utilized for managing AO. Managing AO is a challenging task that requires a multidisciplinary approach. Orofacial pain specialists and neurologists, as well as psychiatric and psychological evaluations, should be involved to identify any comorbidities with depression and anxiety (Okeson JP. *Bell's Orofacial Pains)*.

6.4. Headache

An additional cause of non-odontogenic toothaches and orofacial pains could be a trigeminovascular system disruption. Migraine headaches are typically thought of as unilateral headaches that hurt behind the eyes, neck, and skull; however, they can also occur in the lower face, especially in the teeth. The possibility of this localization, in addition to the clinical characteristics of a migraine, must be known by the orofacial pain clinician in order to prevent misdiagnosis as an odontogenic toothache or another form of orofacial pain, which could result in inappropriate management.

The trigeminal system is also responsible for primary headaches, which include migraine and TTH. These conditions can be chronic and incapacitating, impacting more than 15% of the US population at any given time and costing the country's economy more than $19 trillion annually. Meningeal blood vessel dilatation caused by neurological events leads to migraine, a primary brain disorder that is further explained as a neurovascular disorder involving further nociceptive activation of the trigeminovascular system. Although the exact cause of migraines is still unknown, important peripheral and central anatomical structures are known to be involved. The ophthalmic branch (V1) of the trigeminal nerve and its afferent connection to the trigeminal nucleus caudalis (TNC) in the central nervous system, as well as a reflex connection from the trigeminal nucleus to the parasympathetic outflow to the cranial vasculature through the superior salivatory nucleus, comprise the trigeminovascular system. The dura mater, which envelops the meninges and spinal cord, the dural meningeal blood vessels (cranial vasculature), and the innervations of these structures are furnished by the trigeminovascular system.

The TNC, brainstem, and higher processing centers receive information from these structures about nociceptive pain. Cervical inputs are also received by the TNC. The C2 and C3 regions are also stimulated by dura mater stimulation, which is referred to as the trigeminocervical complex (TCC). This anatomical relationship could help to explain why the neck region can occasionally experience a migraine headache.

The trigeminovascular system, specifically the afferent meningeal nociceptor projections to the ophthalmic division of the trigeminal nerve, is thought to be activated and sensitized in primary headaches, specifically migraine. This activation and sensitization is thought to cause the release of vasoactive neuropeptides, such as substance P (SP), neurokinin A (NKA), and calcitonin gene-related peptide (CGRP), which is elevated during a chronic migraine attack. Although the exact cause of trigeminovascular activation is still unknown, it has been suggested that malfunctions in the brainstem and diencephalon nuclei may activate this system and transmit nociceptive information to other central structures. It is well known that CGRP released from the trigeminal nerve contributes to neurogenic inflammation, which in turn facilitates the transmission of pain and causes allodynia and hyperalgesia. These nociceptive mediators will cause the trigeminovascular system to become more sensitized, edematous, and activate mast cells.

6.4.1. Facial Migraine

Facial migraine is described as a subset of patients who present with the typical migraine headache, but localized in the face rather than as a subtype, ("Migraine without aura") of the new International Classification of Headache Disorders, Third Edition (ICHD-3 beta version). A facial migraine may be diagnosed using the same criteria as migraine without aura (ICHD-3 1.1), which are as follows: unilateral, recurrent, moderate-to-severe headache with pulsating quality that lasts for 4–72 hours, aggravated by routine physical activity, and associated with nausea, phonophobia, and photophobia. Since most cranial structures are innervated by the ophthalmic division of the trigeminal nerve, this may help to explain why the majority of migraine sufferers experience pain in the periorbital area and behind their eyes. On the other hand, a facial migraine only affects the lower portion of the face. There have been reports of migraines that are restricted to the maxillary branch distribution (V2) region. The localization of the pain in the maxillary region may be explained by the nervus meningeus medius, which is produced by V2 and innervates the dura mater of the anterior floor of the middle fossa. There have also been reports of migraine symptomatology that is restricted to the V3 territory. This could be explained by the well-known fact that stimulation of the dura mater causes pain in any of the three divisions of the trigeminal nerve in humans undergoing neurosurgery and in animals participating in electrophysiological experiments. You can find other comprehensive reviews of migraine pathophysiology.

6.4.1.1. Management

Both pharmaceutical and nonpharmacological methods are used to treat migraines. A thorough medical examination by a neurologist is an essential part of any migraine treatment plan in order to rule out any secondary causes of the headache, such as tumors, systemic diseases, or abnormalities of the cerebrovascular system.

6.4.1.1.1. Nonpharmacological Approaches

Patients must receive education regarding the pain they are feeling. Patients experiencing facial migraines, which are localized to the lower face, teeth, or gums, should be reassured that, despite the pain being intense and throbbing, they are not suffering from a toothache or other dental issue. This is critical because it will stop needless dental procedures from being performed because of incorrect diagnoses of orofacial pain or odontogenic toothaches.

The management protocol for facial migraine is the same as that for other migraine headaches, as stated in the ICDH-3 (beta version), despite having a different localization. It is advised to ask the patient to list any potential triggers for a migraine attack. Using a pain diary, where the patient records the features of their headache episodes and the circumstances leading up to them, is a useful way for the patient to provide this information. The patient is advised to avoid or address the triggers as soon as they are recognized, for example, by making dietary changes, practicing good sleep hygiene, or managing their stress. This is a fantastic chance for the patient to understand how much lifestyle modifications can affect their headaches and, as a result, feel more in control of the condition.

Additional non-pharmacological approaches such as biofeedback, relaxation techniques, hypnosis, and psychological therapies have shown promise in treating migraine and TTH.

6.4.1.1.2. Pharmacological Approaches

As previously mentioned, the TNC is an essential anatomical relay center for sending sensory data, primarily nociceptive, from the head and its cranial vasculature, the orofacial region, and higher pain processing centers in the brain. It also sends and receives projections from the superior salivatory nucleus and descending inhibitory system structures, including the rostral ventromedial medulla and ventrolateral periaqueductal gray. Because of these anatomical relationships, the TNC is now a viable therapeutic target with the ability to reduce or prevent trigeminovascular nociceptive activation and subsequent sensitization.

Since facial migraine has a different headache location (the face), but the same disorder and pathophysiology, the same medications used for managing migraines are also used to treat it. A medication for abortive migraine attacks should be taken into consideration if they happen less frequently than twice a month. Preventive medicine is the best course of action if the migraine attack occurs more frequently.

6.4.1.1.3. Abortive Medications

When treating a migraine acutely, drugs intended to cause abortions are the first line of treatment. It has been demonstrated that taking NSAIDs, such as ibuprofen and naproxen sodium, can likely relieve a headache attack. Nevertheless, patients who take NSAIDs frequently run the risk of aggravating their pre-existing headaches and developing medication overuse headaches.

For years, moderate-to-severe migraines have been treated with ergotamine derivatives, such as dihydroergotamine (DHE). However, triptans have largely replaced ergotamine derivatives due to their superior tolerability and pharmacological specificity. In addition to acting at other receptors, DHE is an agonist for both 5-HT1B and 5-HT1D, and it can be helpful for patients who have not responded to triptan therapy. DHE comes in injectable and intranasal forms; the latter is particularly well-liked for use as an abortive agent in emergency rooms.

Sumatriptan is one of the more recent and well-established serotonin 5-HT1B/1D receptor agonists (triptans) used for the acute treatment of migraines. According to studies, they act in the thalamus and ventrolateral periaqueductal gray, as well as on neuronal activation, preventing the presynaptic release of CGRP at the TCC. 5-HT1B/1D receptors are found in humans and rodents at the level of the TNC and on the trigeminal ganglion. Human intracranial arteries are the site of 5-HT1B receptor localization. It has been demonstrated that sumatriptan inhibits TCC neurons' central sensitization but does not reverse it. This could account for the effectiveness of triptans when taken as soon as a migraine appears.

Subcutaneous and intranasal formulations provide a quick onset of action and are a good alternative for patients experiencing gastrointestinal side effects, in addition to oral dosing formulations. When selecting the right triptan for a patient, it is important to take into account the variations in their pharmacokinetic properties.

New combination preparations, like sumatriptan with naproxen sodium, have demonstrated good tolerability in the acute management of migraine as well as additive effects in improving pain relief and migraine-associated symptoms, like phonophobia, photophobia, and nausea, when compared with monotherapy.

Triptans are contraindicated in patients with disorders of the cardiovascular and cerebrovascular systems due to their vasoconstrictor properties, which can cause these effects. On the other hand, brand-new drugs under development, such CGRP receptor antagonists like oral telcagepant, have demonstrated to be effective migraine preventives without having any negative vascular effects. Research indicates that the 5-HT1F receptor is a potentially effective new target for the treatment of migraines. Double-blind placebo-controlled trials have demonstrated the clinical efficacy of lasmiditan, a 5-HT1F receptor agonist, in treating acute migraines.

6.4.1.1.4. Preventives

Preventive therapy can help patients who experience frequent migraine attacks, such as 15 headache days per month. However, little is known about the current preventive medications' mode of action. Certain medications have shown to be helpful: tricyclic antidepressants like amitriptyline; beta adrenergic blockers like propranolol and atenolol; calcium channel blockers like verapamil and flunarizine; serotonin antagonists like methysergide; and antiepileptics like topiramate and valproate.

Evidence suggests that more recent therapeutic approaches hold promise. It has been demonstrated that using injections of botulinum toxin for the prevention of migraines, as well as the treatment of chronic migraine and TTH, is safe and well-tolerated. Furthermore, it has been demonstrated that neuromodulative techniques, such as occipital nerve stimulation methods, are useful in treating refractory headaches, like cluster headaches and chronic migraines, so that weeks without pain are possible. You can find other, more thorough evaluations of migraine prevention strategies elsewhere (Graff-Radford, 2004).

6.4.2. Tension Type Headache

The most prevalent primary headache condition in the general public is the Tension Type Headache or TTH. Although the exact pathophysiology is unknown, both central and peripheral mechanisms probably play a role. TTH may arise from a model that posits a relationship between the limbic system, the descending inhibitory system, and peripheral inputs like intracranial vasculature and myofascial inputs.

The patient may describe the headache as dull and non-pulsating, like a tight headband compressing their head. Regular physical activity won't make the bilateral, mild-to-moderately intense headache worse. Although it can start out as sporadic episodes, it can develop into a more chronic condition. Pericranial tenderness and headaches can occasionally be related. The temporalis muscle and cervical muscles, such as the splenius, sternocleidomastoid, and upper trapezius muscles, are palpably tender. Myofascial trigger point-related headaches may fit the criteria for both episodic and chronic

TTH. This is crucial to remember during the examination because the goal of treatment should be to address the MFP condition. Injection therapy for trigger points and physical therapy are helpful.

As with migraine, TTH is managed with both pharmacological and nonpharmacological methods. It has been demonstrated that modifying one's lifestyle to include better sleep hygiene, keeping a pain journal to identify triggers, managing stress, and practicing relaxation are beneficial. Pharmacological methods, like administering injections of botulinum toxin in addition to NSAIDs and tricyclic antidepressants, have shown promise.

6.4.2.1. Headache and TMD

Headache and orofacial pain disorders, including TMD, are well-known to affect a large portion of the general population. There appears to be a clinical comorbidity between TMD and primary headaches.

Table 6.3. Diagnostic Criteria of Tension-Type Headache Subtypes

<table>
<tr><th>Infrequent Episodic TTH</th><th>Frequent Episodic TTH</th><th>Chronic TTH</th></tr>
<tr><td>A. At least 10 episodes of headache occurring on <1 day per month on average (<12 days per year) and fulfilling criteria B–D</td><td>A. At least 10 episodes of headache occurring on 1–14 days per month on average for >3 months
(12 and <180 days per year) and fulfilling criteria B–D</td><td>A. Headache occurring on 15 days per month on average for >3 months (180 days per year), fulfilling criteria B–D</td></tr>
<tr><td colspan="2">B. Lasting from 30 min to 7 days</td><td>B. Lasting hours to days, or unremitting</td></tr>
<tr><td colspan="3">C. At least two of the following four characteristics:
1. Bilateral location;
2. Pressing or tightening (non-pulsating) quality;
3. Mild or moderate intensity;
4. Not aggravated by routine physical activity such as walking or climbing stairs.</td></tr>
<tr><td colspan="2">D. Both of the following:
1. No nausea or vomiting;
2. No more than one of photophobia or phonophobia.</td><td>D. Both of the following:
1. No more than one of photophobia, phonophobia or mild nausea;
2. Neither moderate or severe nausea nor vomiting.</td></tr>
<tr><td colspan="3">E. Not better accounted for by another ICHD-3 diagnosis.</td></tr>
</table>

Source: Baglioni V, Orecchio S, Esposito D, Faedda N, Natalucci G, Guidetti V. Tension-Type Headache in Children and Adolescents. *Life*. 2023; 13(3):825. https://doi.org/10.3390/life13030825.

Epidemiological research has demonstrated that patients with primary headaches, such as migraine, episodic tension headache, and chronic daily headache, are more likely to experience TMD symptomatology. Patients with TMD also had higher rates of primary headache prevalence, particularly migraine. Furthermore, there is a higher impact on disability in patients with musculoskeletal headache and orofacial pain disorders. Since these nociceptive inputs convey in TNC where intracranial inputs do not, it is possible that extracranial trigeminal nociceptive inputs originating from the craniofacial structures as a result of a TMD could affect the activation of the trigeminovascular system. Therefore, a headache disorder may influence and/or exacerbate an existing TMD condition, and a TMD condition may exacerbate a headache disorder. Therefore, it is critical that such comorbidity be addressed during treatment. Establishing a relationship between the orofacial pain specialist and the neurologist (headache specialist) is necessary because the management of both conditions should be prioritized due to their significant correlation in terms of headache and TMD prevalence (Bendtsen & Jensen, 2011).

6.4.3. Trigeminal Autonomic Cephalalgias (TACs)

Severe headaches that are less common than migraine but are known for their infamous parasympathetic autonomic symptoms include cluster headache, paroxysmal hemicranias, and short-lasting unilateral neuralgiform headache attacks with conjunctival injection and tearing. Although they can occur anywhere in the orofacial region, including the mandible, TMJ, and dental areas, these headaches usually occur in the orbital, temporal, or supraorbital regions. It is crucial to make an appropriate differential diagnosis in order to prevent unnecessary dental treatments or misdiagnosis as other types of orofacial pains with non-neurological etiologies. These headaches require neurological evaluation and management. You can find other comprehensive reviews of trigeminal autonomic cephalalgias and their management (Graff-Radford, 2004).

A Closer Look

Odontogenic Pain

Odontogenic pain refers to pain originating from the teeth or surrounding structures, often resulting from dental conditions such as tooth decay, infection, trauma, or gum disease. This type of pain can vary in intensity, duration, and location, and may present as sharp, throbbing, or constant discomfort. Understanding the underlying causes of odontogenic pain is crucial for appropriate diagnosis and management.

One of the most common causes of odontogenic pain is dental caries, commonly known as tooth decay. When bacteria in the mouth produce acids that erode tooth enamel, it can lead to the formation of cavities, exposing the sensitive inner layers of the tooth to stimuli such as heat, cold, or pressure, resulting in pain. Untreated dental caries can progress to involve the dental pulp, where the tooth's nerve and blood vessels reside, leading to more severe and persistent pain.

Dental infections, such as periapical or periodontal abscesses, can also cause significant odontogenic pain. These infections typically occur when bacteria invade the pulp or surrounding tissues, leading to inflammation, swelling, and the formation of pus. The pressure buildup from an abscess can cause excruciating pain and may be accompanied by fever, swelling of the face or gums, and general malaise.

Trauma to the teeth or surrounding structures, such as fractures, dislocations, or injuries to the temporomandibular joint (TMJ), can also result in odontogenic pain. Additionally, conditions like gum disease (periodontitis) or dental procedures such as tooth extractions or root canal treatment may cause temporary discomfort or exacerbate pre-existing pain.

Diagnosis of odontogenic pain typically involves a comprehensive dental examination, including visual inspection, dental X-rays, and sometimes additional tests such as pulp vitality testing or imaging studies. Treatment options vary depending on the underlying cause but may include dental restorations (fillings, crowns), root canal therapy, extraction of the affected tooth, antibiotic therapy for infections, or referral to specialists such as endodontists or oral surgeons.

Prevention of odontogenic pain involves maintaining good oral hygiene practices, such as regular brushing and flossing, routine dental check-ups, and timely treatment of dental issues to prevent their progression. Early intervention is key to preventing complications and minimizing the impact of odontogenic pain on oral health and overall well-being.

Summary

- Orofacial pain management encompasses a diverse array of conditions affecting the mouth, jaws, face, and associated structures, often presenting complex challenges in diagnosis and treatment.
- Orofacial pain represents one of the most widespread health problems that negatively affects daily living activities.
- Orofacial pain disorders are highly prevalent and debilitating conditions involving the head, face, and neck. These conditions represent a challenge to the clinician since the orofacial region is complex and therefore, pain can arise from many sources.
- "TMD" defines a number of clinical problems that involve the masticatory musculature, the TMJ, and associated structures. TMD is considered to be a subclassification of musculoskeletal disorders and is the most prevalent condition for which patients seek treatment.
- Myalgia usually presents as a dull aching pain due to muscle injury or strain. It is commonly seen in acute forms, though, with continued muscle tension, can present for longer periods of time.
- NSAIDs are indicated for mild-to-moderate acute inflammatory conditions. Commonly used NSAIDs include ibuprofen and naproxen.
- Antiepileptic medications are the drugs of choice for the management of TN. Carbamazepine, oxcarbazepine, and gabapentin are commonly used as first-line medications.
- Peripheral neuropathic pain can arise as a result of a traumatic nerve injury resulting in chronic aching, continuous burning-like pain at the site of the injury.
- Ergotamine derivatives, such as dihydroergotamine (DHE), have been used for years for the treatment of moderate to severe migraine; however, triptans, because of their better tolerability and pharmacological specificity, have replaced ergotamine derivatives in the majority of cases.

References

1. Akerman, S., & Romero-Reyes, M. (2013). Insights into the pharmacological targeting of the trigeminocervical complex in the context of treatments of migraine. *Expert Review of Neurotherapeutics, 13*(9), 1041–1059.
2. Akerman, S., Holland, P. R., & Goadsby, P. J. (2011). Diencephalic and brainstem mechanisms in migraine. *Nature Reviews Neuroscience, 12*(10), 570–584.
3. Anand, P., & Bley, K. (2011). Topical capsaicin for pain management: Therapeutic potential and mechanisms of action of the new high-concentration capsaicin 8% patch. *British Journal of Anaesthesia, 107*(4), 490–502.
4. Andreou, A. P., Summ, O., Charbit, A. R., Romero-Reyes, M., & Goadsby, P. J. (2010). Animal models of headache: From bedside to bench and back to bedside. *Expert Review of Neurotherapeutics, 10*(3), 389–411.
5. Aurora, S. K., Gawel, M., Brandes, J. L., Pokta, S., Vandenburgh, A. M., & BOTOX North American Episodic Migraine Study Group. (2007). Botulinum toxin type A prophylactic treatment of episodic migraine: A randomized, double-blind, placebo-controlled exploratory study. *Headache, 47*(4), 486–499.

6. Baad-Hansen, L. (2008). Atypical odontalgia–Pathophysiology and clinical management. *Journal of Oral Rehabilitation, 35*(1), 1–11.

7. Bakshi, R., Lerner, A., Fritz, J. V., & Sambuchi, G. D. (2001). Vascular compression in trigeminal neuralgia shown by magnetic resonance imaging and magnetic resonance angiography image registration. *Archives of Neurology, 58*(8), 1290–1291.

8. Bartsch, T., & Goadsby, P. J. (2003). The trigeminocervical complex and migraine: Current concepts and synthesis. *Current Pain and Headache Reports, 7*(5), 371–376.

9. Bendtsen, L., & Fernández-de-la-Peñas, C. (2011). The role of muscles in tension-type headache. *Current Pain and Headache Reports, 15*(6), 451–458.

10. Bendtsen, L., & Jensen, R. (2011). Treating tension-type headache–An expert opinion. *Expert Opinion on Pharmacotherapy, 12*(7), 1099–1109.

11. Bendtsen, L., Evers, S., Linde, M., Mitsikostas, D. D., Sandrini, G., & Schoenen, J.; EFNS. (2010). EFNS guideline on the treatment of tension-type headache–Report of an EFNS task force. *European Journal of Neurology, 17*(11), 1318–1325.

12. Benoliel, R., Elishoov, H., & Sharav, Y. (1997). Orofacial pain with vascular-type features. *Oral Surgery, Oral Medicine, Oral Pathology, Oral Radiology, and Endodontology, 84*(5), 506–512.

13. Bernstein, C., & Burstein, R. (2012). Sensitization of the trigeminovascular pathway: Perspective and implications to migraine pathophysiology. *Journal of Clinical Neurology, 8*(2), 89–99.

14. Bezuur, J. N., Habets, L. L., Jimenez Lopez, V., Naeije, M., & Hansson, T. L. (1988). The recognition of craniomandibular disorders–A comparison between clinical and radiographic findings in eighty-nine subjects. *Journal of Oral Rehabilitation, 15*(3), 215–221.

15. Blaustein, D., & Heffez, L. (1988). Diagnostic arthroscopy of the temporomandibular joint. Part II. Arthroscopic findings of arthrographically diagnosed disk displacements. *Oral Surgery, Oral Medicine, Oral Pathology, 65*(2), 135–141.

16. Bramwell, B. L. (2010). Topical orofacial medications for neuropathic pain. *International Journal of Pharmaceutical Compounding, 14*(3), 200–203.

17. Buckley, M. J., Merrill, R. G., & Braun, T. W. (1993). Surgical management of internal derangement of the temporomandibular joint. *Journal of Oral and Maxillofacial Surgery, 51*(1 Suppl 1), 20–27.

18. Burstein, R., & Jakubowski, M. (2004). Analgesic triptan action in an animal model of intracranial pain: A race against the development of central sensitization. *Annals of Neurology, 55*(1), 27–36.

19. Burstein, R., Levy, D., & Jakubowski, M. (2005). Effects of sensitization of trigeminovascular neurons to triptan therapy during migraine. *Revue Neurologique (Paris), 161*(6–7), 658–660.

20. Buzzi, M. G., & Moskowitz, M. A. (1991). Evidence for 5-HT1B/1D receptors mediating the antimigraine effect of sumatriptan and dihydroergotamine. *Cephalalgia, 11*(4), 165–168.

21. Carleton, S. C., Shesser, R. F., Pietrzak, M. P., et al. (1998). Double-blind, multicenter trial to compare the efficacy of intramuscular dihydroergotamine plus hydroxyzine versus intramuscular meperidine plus hydroxyzine for the emergency department treatment of acute migraine headache. *Annals of Emergency Medicine, 32*(2), 129–138. https://doi.org/10.1016/S0196-0644(98)70175-9.

22. Carlson, C. R., Okeson, J. P., Falace, D. A., Nitz, A. J., & Anderson, D. (1991). Stretch-based relaxation and the reduction of EMG activity among masticatory muscle pain patients. *Journal of Craniomandibular Disorders, 5*(3), 205–212.

23. Castro, M. E., Pascual, J., Romón, T., del Arco, C., del Olmo, E., & Pazos, A. (1997). Differential distribution of [3H] sumatriptan binding sites (5-HT1B, 5-HT1D and 5-HT1F receptors) in human brain: Focus on brainstem and spinal cord. *Neuropharmacology, 36*(4–5), 535–542. https://doi.org/10.1016/S0028-3908(97)00032-5.

24. Clark, G. T. (1984). A critical evaluation of orthopedic interocclusal appliance therapy: Effectiveness for specific symptoms. *Journal of the American Dental Association, 108*(3), 364–368.

25. Clark, G. T. (1984). A critical evaluation of orthopedic interocclusal appliance therapy: Design, theory, and overall effectiveness. *Journal of the American Dental Association, 108*(3), 359–364.

26. Clark, G. T., Adachi, N. Y., & Dornan, M. R. (1990). Physical medicine procedures affect temporomandibular disorders: A review. *Journal of the American Dental Association, 121*(1), 151–162.

27. Clark, G. T., Beemsterboer, P. L., Solberg, W. K., & Rugh, J. D. (1979). Nocturnal electromyographic evaluation of myofascial pain dysfunction in patients undergoing occlusal splint therapy. *Journal of the American Dental Association, 99*(4), 607–611.

28. Clark, G. T., Seligman, D. A., Solberg, W. K., & Pullinger, A. C. (1989). Guidelines for the examination and diagnosis of temporomandibular disorders. *Journal of Craniomandibular Disorders, 3*(1), 7–14.

29. Danzig, W. N., & Van Dyke, A. R. (1983). Physical therapy as an adjunct to temporomandibular joint therapy. *Journal of Prosthetic Dentistry, 49*(1), 96–99.

30. Daudia, A. T., & Jones, N. S. (2002). Facial migraine in a rheological setting. *Clinical Otolaryngology and Allied Sciences, 27*(6), 521–525. https://doi.org/10.1046/j.1365-2273.2002.00624.x.

31. de Leeuw, R. (2008). Temporomandibular disorders. In R. de Leeuw (Ed.), *Orofacial Pain: Guidelines for Assessment, Diagnosis, and Management* (4th ed., pp. 158–176). Quintessence Publishing Co, Inc. (The American Academy of Orofacial Pain).

32. Derry, S., Sven-Rice, A., Cole, P., Tan, T., & Moore, R. A. (2013). Topical capsaicin (high concentration) for chronic neuropathic pain in adults. *Cochrane Database of Systematic Reviews, 2*, CD007393. https://doi.org/10.1002/14651858.CD007393.pub3.

33. Dimitroulis, G., Dolwick, M. F., & Martinez, A. (1995). Temporomandibular joint arthrocentesis and lavage for the treatment of closed lock: A follow-up study. *British Journal of Oral and Maxillofacial Surgery, 33*(1), 23–27. https://doi.org/10.1016/0266-4356(95)90081-4.

34. Divine, J. G., Zazulak, B. T., & Hewett, T. E. (2007). Viscosupplementation for knee osteoarthritis: A systematic review. *Clinical Orthopaedics and Related Research, 455*, 113–122. https://doi.org/10.1097/BLO.0b013e31802c9b09.

35. Dodick, D. W., Turkel, C. C., DeGryse, R. E., et al. (2010). PREEMPT Chronic Migraine Study Group Onabotulinumtoxin A for treatment of chronic migraine: Pooled results from the double-blind, randomized, placebo-controlled phases of the PREEMPT clinical program. *Headache, 50*(6), 921–936. https://doi.org/10.1111/j.1526-4610.2010.01678.x.

36. Dodick, D., Lipton, R. B., Martin, V., et al. (2004). Triptan Cardiovascular Safety Expert Panel Consensus statement: Cardiovascular safety profile of triptans (5-HT agonists) in the acute treatment of migraine. *Headache, 44*(5), 414–425. https://doi.org/10.1111/j.1526-4610.2004.04079.x.

37. Dube, C., Rompre, P. H., Manzini, C., Guitard, F., de Grandmont, P., & Lavigne, G. J. (2004). Quantitative polygraphic controlled study on efficacy and safety of oral splint devices in tooth-grinding subjects. *Journal of Dental Research, 83*(5), 398–403. https://doi.org/10.1177/154405910408300509.

38. Durham, P. L. (2006). Calcitonin gene-related peptide (CGRP) and migraine. *Headache, 46*(Suppl 1), S3–S8. https://doi.org/10.1111/j.1526-4610.2006.00449.x.

39. Dworkin, R. H., O'Connor, A. B., Audette, J., et al. (2010). Recommendations for the pharmacological management of neuropathic pain: An overview and literature update. *Mayo Clinic Proceedings, 85*(Suppl 3), S3–S14. https://doi.org/10.4065/mcp.2009.0649.

40. Dworkin, S. F. (2011). Temporomandibular disorder (TMD) pain-related disability found related to depression, nonspecific physical symptoms, and pain duration at 3 international sites. *Journal of Evidence-Based Dental Practice, 11*(3), 143–144. https://doi.org/10.1016/j.jebdp.2011.03.015.

41. Dworkin, S. F., Huggins, K. H., LeResche, L., et al. (1990). Epidemiology of signs and symptoms in temporomandibular disorders: Clinical signs in cases and controls. *Journal of the American Dental Association, 120*(3), 273–281.

42. Elder, C., Ritenbaugh, C., Aickin, M., et al. (2012). Reductions in pain medication use associated with traditional Chinese medicine for chronic pain. *The Permanente Journal, 16*(3), 18–23. https://doi.org/10.7812/TPP/12-006.

43. El-Hakim, I. E., Abdel-Hamid, I. S., & Bader, A. (2005). Tempromandibular joint (TMJ) response to intra-articular dexamethasone injection following mechanical arthropathy: A histological study in rats. *International Journal of Oral and Maxillofacial Surgery, 34*(3), 305–310. https://doi.org/10.1016/j.ijom.2004.07.015.

44. Ernberg, M., Hedenberg-Magnusson, B., List, T., & Svensson, P. (2011). Efficacy of botulinum toxin type A for treatment of persistent myofascial TMD pain: A randomized, controlled, double-blind multicenter study. *Pain, 152*(9), 1988–1996. https://doi.org/10.1016/j.pain.2011.04.024.

45. Färkkilä, M., Diener, H. C., Géraud, G., et al. (2012). Efficacy and tolerability of Lasmiditan, an oral 5-HT(1F) receptor agonist, for the acute treatment of migraine: A phase 2 randomized, placebo-controlled, parallel-group, dose-ranging study. *The Lancet Neurology, 11*(5), 405–413. https://doi.org/10.1016/S1474-4422(12)70056-6.

46. Feinerman, D. M., & Goldberg, M. H. (1994). Acoustic neuroma appearing as trigeminal neuralgia. *Journal of the American Dental Association, 125*(8), 1122–1125.

47. Fernández-de-Las-Peñas, C., Alonso-Blanco, C., Cuadrado, M. L., & Pareja, J. A. (2006). Myofascial trigger points in the suboccipital muscles in episodic tension-type headache. *Manual Therapy, 11*(3), 225–230. https://doi.org/10.1016/j.math.2006.05.002.

48. Fernández-de-las-Peñas, C., Alonso-Blanco, C., Cuadrado, M. L., Gerwin, R. D., & Pareja, J. A. (2006). Myofascial trigger points and their relationship to headache clinical parameters in chronic tension-type headache. *Headache, 46*(8), 1264–1272. https://doi.org/10.1111/j.1526-4610.2006.00565.x.

49. Ferrari, M. D., Färkkilä, M., Reuter, U., et al. (2010). European COL-144 Investigators. Acute treatment of migraine with the selective 5-HT1F receptor agonist Lasmiditan–A randomized proof-of-concept trial. *Cephalalgia, 30*(10), 1170–1178. https://doi.org/10.1177/0333102410365101.

50. Franco, A. L., Gonçalves, D. A., Castanharo, S. M., Speciali, J. G., Bigal, M. E., & Camparis, C. M. (2010). Migraine is the most prevalent primary headache in individuals with temporomandibular disorders. *Journal of Orofacial Pain, 24*(3), 287–292.

51. Fricton, J. (2007). Myogenous temporomandibular disorders: Diagnostic and management considerations. *Dental Clinics of North America, 51*(1), 61–83. https://doi.org/10.1016/j.cden.2006.09.003.

52. Fricton, J., Look, J. O., Wright, E., et al. (2010). Systematic review and meta-analysis of randomized controlled trials evaluating intraoral orthopedic appliances for temporomandibular disorders. *Journal of Orofacial Pain, 24*(3), 237–254.

53. Fromm, G. H., Terrence, C. F., & Chattha, A. S. (1984). Baclofen in the treatment of trigeminal neuralgia: Double-blind study and long-term follow-up. *Annals of Neurology, 15*(3), 240–244. https://doi.org/10.1002/ana.410150306.

54. Gady, J., & Ferneini, E. M. (2013). Botulinum toxin A and headache treatment. *Connecticut Medicine, 77*(3), 165–166.

55. Gangarosa, L., & Mahan, P. E. (1982). Pharmacologic management of TMD-MPDS. *Ear, Nose, and Throat Journal, 61*, 670–678.

56. Goadsby, P. J. (2005). Migraine, allodynia, sensitization and all of that. *European Neurology, 53*(Suppl 1), 10–16. https://doi.org/10.1159/000085706.

57. Goadsby, P. J., Cohen, A. S., & Matharu, M. S. (2007). Trigeminal autonomic cephalalgias: Diagnosis and treatment. *Current Neurology and Neuroscience Reports, 7*(2), 117–125.

58. Goadsby, P. J., Edvinsson, L., & Ekman, R. (1990). Vasoactive peptide release in the extracerebral circulation of humans during migraine headache. *Annals of Neurology, 28*(2), 183–187. https://doi.org/10.1002/ana.410280213.

59. Goadsby, P. J., Lipton, R. B., & Ferrari, M. D. (2002). Migraine–Current understanding and treatment. *New England Journal of Medicine, 346*(4), 257–270. https://doi.org/10.1056/NEJMra010917.

60. Gonçalves, D. A., Bigal, M. E., Jales, L. C., Camparis, C. M., & Speciali, J. G. (2010). Headache and symptoms of temporomandibular disorder: An epidemiological study. *Headache, 50*(2), 231–241. https://doi.org/10.1111/j.1526-4610.2009.01542.x.

61. Graff-Radford, S. B. (2001). Regional myofascial pain syndrome and headache: Principles of diagnosis and management. *Current Pain and Headache Reports, 5*(4), 376–381. https://doi.org/10.1007/s11916-001-0075-7.

62. Graff-Radford, S. B. (2004). Myofascial pain: Diagnosis and management. *Current Pain and Headache Reports, 8*(6), 463–467. https://doi.org/10.1007/s11916-004-0075-4.

63. Gregg, J. M., & Rugh, J. D. (1983). Pharmacological therapy. In N. D. Mohl, A. George, G. E. Carlsson, & J. D. Rugh (Eds.), *A Textbook of Occlusion* (pp. 351–375). Quintessence.

64. Guarda-Nardini, L., Piccotti, F., Mogno, G., Favero, L., & Manfredini, D. (2012). Age-related

differences in temporomandibular disorder diagnoses. *Cranio, 30*(2), 103–109. https://doi.org/10.1179/crn.2012.014.

65. Guarda-Nardini, L., Stecco, A., Stecco, C., Masiero, S., & Manfredini, D. (2012). Myofascial pain of the jaw muscles: Comparison of short-term effectiveness of botulinum toxin injections and fascial manipulation technique. *Cranio, 30*(2), 95–102. https://doi.org/10.1179/crn.2012.013.
66. H D, Wellish, M., & Gilden, D. (2003). Topical ketamine treatment of postherpetic neuralgia. *Neurology, 60*(8), 1391. https://doi.org/10.1212/01.WNL.0000058901.81396.1A.
67. Headache Classification Committee of the International Headache Society (IHS). (2013). The international classification of headache disorders (3rd ed., beta version). *Cephalalgia, 33*(9), 629–808. https://doi.org/10.1177/0333102413485658.
68. Herman, C. R., Schiffman, E. L., Look, J. O., & Rindal, D. B. (2002). The effectiveness of adding pharmacologic treatment with clonazepam or cyclobenzaprine to patient education and self-care for the treatment of jaw pain upon awakening: A randomized clinical trial. *Journal of Orofacial Pain, 16*(1), 64–70.
69. Ho, T., Ferrari, M., Dodick, D., et al. (2008). Efficacy and tolerability of MK-0974 (telcagepant), a new oral antagonist of calcitonin gene-related peptide receptor, compared with zolmitriptan for acute migraine: A randomized, placebo-controlled, parallel-treatment trial. *The Lancet, 372*, 2115–2123. https://doi.org/10.1016/S0140-6736(08)61626-8.
70. Holland, S., Silberstein, S. D., Freitag, F., Dodick, D. W., Argoff, C., Ashman, E., & Quality Standards Subcommittee of the American Academy of Neurology and the American Headache Society. (2012). Evidence-based guideline update: NSAIDs and other complementary treatments for episodic migraine prevention in adults: Report of the Quality Standards Subcommittee of the American Academy of Neurology and the American Headache Society. *Neurology, 78*(17), 1346–1353. https://doi.org/10.1212/WNL.0b013e3182535d0c.
71. Humphrey, P. P., & Feniuk, W. (1991). Mode of action of the anti-migraine drug sumatriptan. *Trends in Pharmacological Sciences, 12*(12), 444–446. https://doi.org/10.1016/0165-6147(91)90637-F.
72. International Association for the Study of Pain, Subcommittee on Taxonomy. (1986). Classification of chronic pain. Descriptions of chronic pain syndromes and definitions of pain terms. *Pain Supplement, 3*, S1–S226.
73. Jannetta, P. J. (1967). Arterial compression of the trigeminal nerve at the pons in patients with trigeminal neuralgia. *Journal of Neurosurgery, 26*(1), 159–162.
74. Jensen, R., Rasmussen, B. K., Pedersen, B., & Olesen, J. (1993). Muscle tenderness and pressure pain thresholds in headache: A population study. *Pain, 52*(2), 193–199. https://doi.org/10.1016/0304-3959(93)90100-V.
75. Jensen, T. S., Rasmussen, P., & Reske-Nielsen, E. (1982). Association of trigeminal neuralgia with multiple sclerosis: Clinical and pathological features. *Acta Neurologica Scandinavica, 65*(3), 182–189. https://doi.org/10.1111/j.1600-0404.1982.tb03018.x.
76. Kaniecki, R. G. (2012). Tension-type headache. *Continuum (Minneapolis, Minn.), 18*(4), 823–834. https://doi.org/10.1212/01.CON.0000421621.41183.06.
77. Katusic, S., Williams, D. B., Beard, C. M., Bergstralh, E. J., & Kurland, L. T. (1991). Epidemiology and clinical features of idiopathic trigeminal neuralgia and glossopharyngeal neuralgia:

Similarities and differences, Rochester, Minnesota, 1945–1984. *Neuroepidemiology, 10*(5–6), 276–281. https://doi.org/10.1159/000110260.

78. Kirk, W. S., Jr., & Calabrese, D. K. (1989). Clinical evaluation of physical therapy in the management of internal derangement of the temporomandibular joint. *Journal of Oral and Maxillofacial Surgery, 47*(2), 113–119. https://doi.org/10.1016/0278-2391(89)90309-1.

79. Kitt, C. A., Gruber, K., Davis, M., Woolf, C. J., & Levine, J. D. (2000). Trigeminal neuralgia: Opportunities for research and treatment. *Pain, 85*(1), 3–7. https://doi.org/10.1016/S0304-3959(99)00252-0.

80. Klasser, G. D., & Greene, C. S. (2009). Oral appliances in the management of temporomandibular disorders. *Oral Surgery, Oral Medicine, Oral Pathology, Oral Radiology, and Endodontology, 107*(2), 212–223. https://doi.org/10.1016/j.tripleo.2008.09.026.

81. Koh, H., & Robinson, P. G. (2003). Occlusal adjustment for treating and preventing temporomandibular joint disorders. *Cochrane Database of Systematic Reviews*, (1), CD003812. https://doi.org/10.1002/14651858.CD003812.

82. Könönen, M., Waltimo, A., & Nyström, M. (1996). Does clicking in adolescence lead to painful temporomandibular joint locking? *The Lancet, 347*(9008), 1080–1081. https://doi.org/10.1016/S0140-6736(96)90647-8.

83. Kopp, S., Akerman, S., & Nilner, M. (1991). Short-term effects of intra-articular sodium hyaluronate, glucocorticoid, and saline injections on rheumatoid arthritis of the temporomandibular joint. *Journal of Craniomandibular Disorders, 5*(4), 231–238.

84. Kreiner, M., Betancor, E., & Clark, G. T. (2001). Occlusal stabilization appliances. Evidence of their efficacy. *Journal of the American Dental Association, 132*(6), 770–777. https://doi.org/10.14219/jada.archive.2001.0271.

85. Lance, J. W., & Goadsby, P. J. (Eds.). (2005). *Mechanism and Management of Headache* (7th ed.). Elsevier Butterworth Heinemann.

86. Latremoliere, A., & Woolf, C. J. (2009). Central sensitization: A generator of pain hypersensitivity by central neural plasticity. *The Journal of Pain, 10*(9), 895–926. https://doi.org/10.1016/j.jpain.2009.06.012.

87. Lee, E. J., Calcaterra, T. C., & Zuckerbraun, L. (1998). Traumatic neuromas of the head and neck. *Ear, Nose, & Throat Journal, 77*(8), 670–674.

88. Leone, M., & Bussone, G. (2009). Pathophysiology of trigeminal autonomic cephalalgias. *The Lancet Neurology, 8*(8), 755–764. https://doi.org/10.1016/S1474-4422(09)70134-6.

89. LeResche, L. (1997). Epidemiology of temporomandibular disorders: Implications for the investigation of etiologic factors. *Critical Reviews in Oral Biology & Medicine, 8*(3), 291–305. https://doi.org/10.1177/10454411970080030501.

90. Levy, D., Jakubowski, M., & Burstein, R. (2004). Disruption of communication between peripheral and central trigeminovascular neurons mediates the antimigraine action of 5HT 1B/1D receptor agonists. *Proceedings of the National Academy of Sciences of the United States of America, 101*(12), 4274–4279. https://doi.org/10.1073/pnas.0306147101.

91. Li, X. D., Shi, Z. D., & Tian, W. D. (2004). An outcome analysis of two methods of intra-capsular injection of sodium hyaluronate for temporomandibular disorders. *Hua Xi Kou Qiang Yi Xue Za Zhi, 22*(2), 135–137. [Article in Chinese]

92. Lipton, J. A., Ship, J. A., & Larach-Robinson, D. (1993). Estimated prevalence and distribution of reported orofacial pain in the United States. *Journal of the American Dental Association, 124*(10), 115–121. https://doi.org/10.14219/jada.archive.1993.0396.

93. Lipton, R. B., Bigal, M. E., Diamond, M., Freitag, F., Reed, M. L., & Stewart, W. F. (2007). Migraine prevalence, disease burden, and the need for preventive therapy. *Neurology, 68*(5), 343–349. https://doi.org/10.1212/01.wnl.0000252808.97649.21.

94. Longmore, J., Shaw, D., Smith, D., et al. (1997). Differential distribution of 5HT1D- and 5HT1B-immunoreactivity within the human trigemino-cerebrovascular system: Implications for the discovery of new anti-migraine drugs. *Cephalalgia, 17*(8), 833–842. https://doi.org/10.1046/j.1468-2982.1997.1708833.x.

95. Lutz, J., Linn, J., Mehrkens, J. H., et al. (2011). Trigeminal neuralgia due to neurovascular compression: High-spatial-resolution diffusion tensor imaging reveals microstructural neural changes. *Radiology, 258*(2), 524–530. https://doi.org/10.1148/radiol.10101259.

96. Ma, Q. P. (2001). Co-localization of 5-HT(1B/1D/1F) receptors and glutamate in trigeminal ganglia in rats. *Neuroreport, 12*(8), 1589–1591. https://doi.org/10.1097/00001756-200106130-00035.

97. Ma, Q. P., Hill, R., & Sirinathsinghji, D. (2001). Colocalization of CGRP with 5-HT1B/1D receptors and substance P in trigeminal ganglion neurons in rats. *European Journal of Neuroscience, 13*(11), 2099–2104. https://doi.org/10.1046/j.0953-816x.2001.01581.x.

98. Manfredini, D., Piccotti, F., & Guarda-Nardini, L. (2010). Hyaluronic acid in the treatment of TMJ disorders: A systematic review of the literature. *Cranio, 28*(3), 166–176. https://doi.org/10.1179/crn.2010.025.

99. Marbach, J. J. (1999). Medically unexplained chronic orofacial pain. Temporomandibular pain and dysfunction syndrome, orofacial phantom pain, burning mouth syndrome, and trigeminal neuralgia. *Medical Clinics of North America, 83*(3), 691–710.

100. Marks, P. V., & Purchas, S. H. (1992). Life-threatening glossopharyngeal neuralgia. *Australian and New Zealand Journal of Surgery, 62*(8), 660–661.

101. Martin, W. J., & Forouzanfar, T. (2011). The efficacy of anticonvulsants on orofacial pain: A systematic review. *Oral Surgery, Oral Medicine, Oral Pathology, Oral Radiology, and Endodontology, 111*(5), 627–633. https://doi.org/10.1016/j.tripleo.2010.11.005.

102. Mathew, N. T., Frishberg, B. M., Gawel, M., Dimitrova, R., Gibson, J., Turkel, C., & BOTOX CDH Study Group. (2005). Botulinum toxin type A (BOTOX) for the prophylactic treatment of chronic daily headache: A randomized, double-blind, placebo-controlled trial. *Headache, 45*(4), 293–307. https://doi.org/10.1111/j.1526-4610.2005.05067.x.

103. Mathew, N. T., Landy, S., Stark, S., et al. (2009). Fixed-dose sumatriptan and naproxen in poor responders to triptans with a short half-life. *Headache, 49*(7), 971–982. https://doi.org/10.1111/j.1526-4610.2009.01428.x.

104. Mathews, G. J. O. J. (1972). Painful traumatic neuroma. *Surgical Clinics of North America, 52*(5), 1313–1324.

105. Matsuka, Y., Fort, E. T., & Merrill, R. L. (2000). Trigeminal neuralgia due to an acoustic neuroma in the cerebellopontine angle. *Journal of Orofacial Pain, 14*(2), 147–151.

106. May, A. (2006). Update on the diagnosis and management of trigemino-autonomic headaches. *Journal of Neurology, 253*(12), 1525–1532. https://doi.org/10.1007/s00415-006-0309-9.

107. May, A., & Goadsby, P. J. (1999). The trigeminovascular system in humans: Pathophysiologic implications for primary headache syndromes of the neural influences on the cerebral circulation. *Journal of Cerebral Blood Flow & Metabolism, 19*(2), 115–127. https://doi.org/10.1097/00004647-199902000-00001.

108. McNaughton, F. L., & Feindel, W. (1977). Innervation of intracranial structures: A reappraisal. In F. C. Rose (Ed.), *Physiological Aspects of Clinical Neurology* (pp. 279–293). Oxford: Blackwell Scientific.

109. McNeill, C. (1993). *Temporomandibular Disorders: Guidelines for Classification, Assessment, and Management* (2nd ed.). Chicago, IL: Quintessence Publishing Co, Inc.

110. Mejersjö, C., & Carlsson, G. E. (1983). Long-term results of treatment for temporomandibular joint pain-dysfunction. *Journal of Prosthetic Dentistry, 49*(6), 809–815.

111. Mejersjö, C., & Carlsson, G. E. (1984). Analysis of factors influencing the long-term effect of treatment of TMJ-pain dysfunction. *Journal of Oral Rehabilitation, 11*(3), 289–297.

112. Merrill, R. L. (1997). Head and neck pain. *Seminars in Anesthesia, Perioperative Medicine, and Pain, 16*(4), 280–291.

113. Merrill, R. L. (1997). Orofacial pain mechanisms and their clinical application. *Dental Clinics of North America, 41*(2), 167–188.

114. Merrill, R. L., & Graff-Radford, S. B. (1992). Trigeminal neuralgia: How to rule out the wrong treatment. *Journal of the American Dental Association, 123*(2), 63–68.

115. Mitrirattanakul, S., & Merrill, R. L. (2006). Headache impact in patients with orofacial pain. *Journal of the American Dental Association, 137*(9), 1267–1274. https://doi.org/10.14219/jada.archive.2006.0064.

116. Mueller, O., Diener, H. C., Dammann, P., et al. (2013). Occipital nerve stimulation for intractable chronic cluster headache or migraine: A critical analysis of direct treatment costs and complications. *Cephalalgia*. Advance online publication. https://doi.org/10.1177/0333102413491323.

117. Nicholson, R., Buse, D. C., Andrasik, F., & Lipton, R. B. (2011). Nonpharmacologic treatments for migraine and tension-type headache: How to choose and when to use. *Current Treatment Options in Neurology, 13*(1), 28–40. https://doi.org/10.1007/s11940-010-0103-6.

118. Nickerson, J. W., & Boering, G. (1989). Natural course of osteoarthrosis as it relates to internal derangement of the temporomandibular joint. *Oral and Maxillofacial Surgery Clinics of North America, 1*, 27–45.

119. Nitzan, D. W., Dolwick, M. F., & Martinez, G. A. (1991). Temporomandibular joint arthrocentesis: A simplified treatment for severe, limited mouth opening. *Journal of Oral and Maxillofacial Surgery, 49*(11), 1163–1167. https://doi.org/10.1016/0278-2391(91)90438-K.

120. Obermann, M. (2010). Treatment options in trigeminal neuralgia. *Therapeutic Advances in Neurological Disorders, 3*(2), 107–115. https://doi.org/10.1177/1756285610366108.

121. Obermann, M., Mueller, D., Yoon, M. S., Pageler, L., Diener, H., & Katsarava, Z. (2007). Migraine with isolated facial pain: A diagnostic challenge. *Cephalalgia, 27*(11), 1278–1282. https://doi.org/10.1111/j.1468-2982.2007.01425.x.

122. Ohrbach, R., & Gale, E. N. (1989). Pressure pain thresholds, clinical assessment, and differential diagnosis: Reliability and validity in patients with myogenic pain. *Pain, 39*(2), 157–169. https://doi.org/10.1016/0304-3959(89)90224-8.

123. Okeson, J. P. (2008). The classification of orofacial pains. *Oral and Maxillofacial Surgery Clinics of North America, 20*(2), 133–144. https://doi.org/10.1016/j.coms.2007.11.002.

124. Okeson, J. P. (Ed.). (2005). *Bell's Orofacial Pains: The Clinical Management of Orofacial Pain* (6th ed.). Carol Stream, IL: Quintessence Publishing Co, Inc.

125. Olds, M. J., Woods, C. I., & Winfield, J. A. (1995). Microvascular decompression in glossopharyngeal neuralgia. *American Journal of Otology, 16*(3), 326–330.

126. Olesen, J. (1991). Clinical and pathophysiological observations in migraine and tension-type headache explained by integration of vascular, supraspinal and myofascial inputs. *Pain, 46*(2), 125–132. https://doi.org/10.1016/0304-3959(91)90043-5.

127. Oshinsky, M. L. (2006). Insights from experimental studies into allodynia and its treatment. *Current Pain and Headache Reports, 10*(3), 225–230. https://doi.org/10.1007/s11916-006-0039-8.

128. Patel, S. B., Boros, A. L., & Kumar, S. K. (2012). Atypical odontalgia – An update. *Journal of the California Dental Association, 40*(9), 739–747.

129. Peñarrocha, M., Bandrés, A., Peñarrocha, M., & Bagán, J. V. (2004). Lower-half facial migraine: A report of 11 cases. *Journal of Oral and Maxillofacial Surgery, 62*(12), 1453–1456. https://doi.org/10.1016/j.joms.2004.03.023.

130. Pistoia, F., Sacco, S., & Carolei, A. (2012). Behavioral therapy for chronic migraine. *Current Pain and Headache Reports, 17*(1), 1–8. https://doi.org/10.1007/s11916-012-0246-3.

131. Randolph, C. S., Greene, C. S., Moretti, R., Forbes, D., & Perry, H. T. (1990). Conservative management of temporomandibular disorders: A posttreatment comparison between patients from a university clinic and from private practice. *American Journal of Orthodontics and Dentofacial Orthopedics, 98*(1), 77–82. https://doi.org/10.1016/0889-5406(90)70031-V.

132. Rapoport, A., & Winner, P. (2006). Nasal delivery of antimigraine drugs: Clinical rationale and evidence base. *Headache, 46*(Suppl), S192–S201. https://doi.org/10.1111/j.1526-4610.2006.00603.x.

133. Rasmussen, B. K. (1993). Migraine and tension-type headache in a general population: Precipitating factors, female hormones, sleep pattern and relation to lifestyle. *Pain, 53*(1), 65–72. https://doi.org/10.1016/0304-3959(93)90057-V.

134. Rasmussen, O. C. (1981). Description of population and progress of symptoms in a longitudinal study of temporomandibular arthropathy. *Scandinavian Journal of Dental Research, 89*(2), 196–203. https://doi.org/10.1111/j.1600-0722.1981.tb00986.x.

135. Reeves, J. L. (1976). EMG-biofeedback reduction of tension headache: A cognitive skills-training approach. *Biofeedback and Self-Regulation, 1*(2), 217–225. https://doi.org/10.1007/BF00998941.

136. Reisner, L., & Pettengill, C. A. (2001). The use of anticonvulsants in orofacial pain. *Oral Surgery, Oral Medicine, Oral Pathology, Oral Radiology, and Endodontology, 91*(1), 2–7. https://doi.org/10.1067/moe.2001.109284.

137. Riley, J. L., 3rd, Myers, C. D., Currie, T. P., et al. (2007). Self-care behaviors associated with

myofascial temporomandibular disorder pain. *Journal of Orofacial Pain, 21*(3), 194–202.

138. Ritenbaugh, C., Hammerschlag, R., Calabrese, C., et al. (2008). A pilot whole systems clinical trial of traditional Chinese medicine and naturopathic medicine for the treatment of temporomandibular disorders. *Journal of Alternative and Complementary Medicine, 14*(5), 475–487. https://doi.org/10.1089/acm.2007.0643.
139. Rodrigues, D., Siriani, A. O., & Bérzin, F. (2004). Effect of conventional TENS on pain and electromyographic activity of masticatory muscles in TMD patients. *Brazilian Oral Research, 18*(4), 290–295. https://doi.org/10.1590/S1806-83242004000400005.
140. Romero-Reyes, M., & Graff-Radford, S. (2007). Is there hope for chronic pain and headache? *Headache, 47*(8), 1262–1271. https://doi.org/10.1111/j.1526-4610.2007.00814.x.
141. Samiee, A., Sabzerou, D., Edalatpajouh, F., Clark, G. T., & Ram, S. (2011). Temporomandibular joint injection with corticosteroid and local anesthetic for limited mouth opening. *Journal of Oral Science, 53*(3), 321–325. https://doi.org/10.2334/josnusd.53.321.
142. Sanitá, P. V., & de Alencar Júnior, F. G. P. (2009). Myofascial pain syndrome as a contributing factor in patients with chronic headaches. *Journal of Musculoskeletal Pain, 17*(1), 15–25. https://doi.org/10.1080/10582450902766710.
143. Sarlani, E., Balciunas, B. A., & Grace, E. G. (2005). Orofacial pain–Part I: Assessment and management of musculoskeletal and neuropathic causes. *AACN Clinical Issues, 16*(3), 333–346. https://doi.org/10.1016/j.ccell.2005.03.001.
144. Sarlani, E., Balciunas, B. A., & Grace, E. G. (2005). Orofacial pain – Part II: Assessment and management of vascular, neurovascular, idiopathic, secondary, and psychogenic causes. *AACN Clinical Issues, 16*(3), 347–358. https://doi.org/10.1016/j.ccell.2005.03.002.
145. Schurks, M., Diener, H. C., & Goadsby, P. (2008). Update on the prophylaxis of migraine. *Current Treatment Options in Neurology, 10*(1), 20–29. https://doi.org/10.1007/s11940-008-0015-0.
146. Shen, Y. F., Younger, J., Goddard, G., & Mackey, S. (2009). Randomized clinical trial of acupuncture for myofascial pain of the jaw muscles. *Journal of Orofacial Pain, 23*(4), 353–359.
147. Shields, K. G., & Goadsby, P. J. (2006). Serotonin receptors modulate trigeminovascular responses in ventroposteromedial nucleus of thalamus: A migraine target? *Neurobiology of Disease, 23*(3), 491–501. https://doi.org/10.1016/j.nbd.2006.04.012.
148. Silberstein, S. D. (2009). Preventive migraine treatment. *Neurologic Clinics, 27*(2), 429–443. https://doi.org/10.1016/j.ncl.2008.11.007.
149. Silberstein, S. D., Dodick, D. W., Saper, J., et al. (2012). Safety and efficacy of peripheral nerve stimulation of the occipital nerves for the management of chronic migraine: Results from a randomized, multicenter, double-blinded, controlled study. *Cephalalgia, 32*(16), 1165–1179. https://doi.org/10.1177/0333102412459283.
150. Silberstein, S. D., Lipton, R. B., & Dalessio, D. J. (Eds.). (2001). *Wolff's Headache and Other Head Pain* (7th ed., pp. 478–479). New York: Oxford University Press.
151. Silberstein, S., & Kori, S. (2013). Dihydroergotamine: A review of formulation approaches for the acute treatment of migraine. *CNS Drugs, 27*(5), 385–394. https://doi.org/10.1007/s40263-013-0051-2.
152. Simons, D. G., Travel, J. G., & Simons, L. S. (1998). *Myofascial Pain and Dysfunction: The Trigger Point Manual. Upper Half of Body* (2nd ed., p. 1). Atlanta, GA: Lippincott Williams & Wilkins.

153. Singh, P. M., Kaur, M., & Trikha, A. (2013). An uncommonly common: Glossopharyngeal neuralgia. *Annals of Indian Academy of Neurology, 16*(1), 1–8. https://doi.org/10.4103/0972-2327.107680.

154. Smith, D., Hill, R. G., Edvinsson, L., & Longmore, J. (2002). An immunocytochemical investigation of human trigeminal nucleus caudalis: CGRP, substance P and 5-HT1D-receptor immunoreactivities are expressed by trigeminal sensory fibers. *Cephalalgia, 22*(6), 424–431. https://doi.org/10.1046/j.1468-2982.2002.00420.x.

155. Smith, D., Shaw, D., Hopkins, R., et al. (1998). Development and characterization of human 5-HT1B- or 5-HT1D-receptor specific antibodies as unique research tools. *Journal of Neuroscience Methods, 80*(2), 155–161. https://doi.org/10.1016/S0165-0270(98)00047-2.

156. Smith, T. R., Sunshine, A., Stark, S. R., Littlefield, D. E., Spruill, S. E., & Alexander, W. J. (2005). Sumatriptan and naproxen sodium for the acute treatment of migraine. *Headache, 45*(8), 983–991. https://doi.org/10.1111/j.1526-4610.2005.05169.x.

157. Solberg, W., Woo, M., & Houston, J. (1979). Prevalence of mandibular dysfunction in young adults. *Journal of the American Dental Association, 98*(1), 25–34. https://doi.org/10.14219/jada.archive.1979.0054.

158. Song, P. C., Schwartz, J., & Blitzer, A. (2007). The emerging role of botulinum toxin in the treatment of temporomandibular disorders. *Oral Diseases, 13*(3), 253–260. https://doi.org/10.1111/j.1601-0825.2007.01353.x.

159. Sprenger, T., & Goadsby, P. (2009). Migraine pathogenesis and state of pharmacological treatment options. *BMC Medicine, 7*, 71. https://doi.org/10.1186/1741-7015-7-71.

160. Stewart, W. F., Ricci, J. A., Chee, E., & Morganstein, D. (2003). Lost productive work time costs from health conditions in the United States: Results from the American productivity audit. *Journal of Occupational and Environmental Medicine, 45*(12), 1234–1246. https://doi.org/10.1097/01.jom.0000100000.17063.03.

161. Stoll, M. L., Good, J., Sharpe, T., et al. (2012). Intra-articular corticosteroid injections to the temporomandibular joints are safe and appear to be effective therapy in children with juvenile idiopathic arthritis. *Journal of Oral and Maxillofacial Surgery, 70*(8), 1802–1807. https://doi.org/10.1016/j.joms.2011.12.038.

162. Subcutaneous Sumatriptan International Study Group. (1991). Treatment of migraine attacks with sumatriptan. *New England Journal of Medicine, 325*(5), 316–321. https://doi.org/10.1056/NEJM199108013250503.

163. Toller, P. A. (1977). Use and misuse of intra-articular corticosteroids in treatment of temporomandibular joint pain. *Proceedings of the Royal Society of Medicine, 70*(7), 461–463. [PMC free article] https://www.ncbi.nlm.nih.gov/pmc/articles/PMC1543216/ (accessed on 26 June 2024).

164. Tsuga, K., Akagawa, Y., Sakaguchi, R., & Tsuru, H. (1989). A short-term evaluation of the effectiveness of stabilization-type occlusal splint therapy for specific symptoms of temporomandibular joint dysfunction syndrome. *Journal of Prosthetic Dentistry, 61*(5), 610–613. https://doi.org/10.1016/0022-3913(89)90310-5.

165. Wenneberg, B., Kopp, S., & Gröndahl, H. G. (1991). Long-term effect of intra-articular injections of a glucocorticosteroid into the TMJ: A clinical and radiographic 8-year follow-up. *Journal of Craniomandibular Disorders, 5*(1), 11–18.

166. Zakrzewska, J. M. (2010). Medical management of trigeminal neuropathic pains. *Expert Opinion on Pharmacotherapy, 11*(8), 1239–1254. https://doi.org/10.1517/14656561003702713.

167. Zakrzewska, J. M., Chaudhry, Z., Nurmikko, T. J., Patton, D. W., & Mullens, E. L. (1997). Lamotrigine (Lamictal) in refractory trigeminal neuralgia: Results from a double-blind placebo-controlled crossover trial. *Pain, 73*(2), 223–230. https://doi.org/10.1016/S0304-3959(97)00110-8.

Chapter 7

HEART, VASCULAR, AND HEMOPATHIC PAIN

Contents

Introduction

Together, the terms "heart," "vascular," and "hemopathic pain" describe a range of pain experiences that stem from blood-related illnesses and the cardiovascular system. These illnesses may present with a variety of symptoms, ranging from minor discomfort to excruciating pain, and they can have a serious negative effect on a person's general health and quality of life. It is crucial to comprehend the underlying causes, mechanisms, and management techniques of these kinds of pain to treat patients with cardiovascular and hematologic conditions efficiently.

Cardiac pain, or pain that originates in the heart, usually results from ischemia, inflammation, or other pathological processes that impact the heart muscle or coronary arteries. Coronary artery disease, which reduces blood flow to the heart muscle and can cause angina or myocardial infarction (heart attack), is the most common cause of cardiac pain. A common description of cardiac pain is pressure, tightness, or squeezing in the chest. It can also refer to the arms, shoulders, neck, jaw, or back. Pain from blood vessels, such as arteries, veins, and capillaries, is referred to as vascular pain. Vasculitis, varicose veins, deep vein thrombosis, and peripheral artery disease are a few conditions that can cause vascular pain. Vascular pain can manifest as aching, throbbing, or cramping in the afflicted limbs or other areas of the body, depending on the underlying cause. Vascular pain can occasionally be severe enough to cause accompanying symptoms like skin ulcers, discoloration, or swelling.

Hemopathic pain refers to pain that is caused by blood disorders, including leukemia, hemophilia, sickle cell disease, and thrombocytopenia. These illnesses can result in different degrees of pain and discomfort due to bone marrow expansion, joint inflammation, and nerve compression. Depending on the particular hematologic disorder and its complications, hemopathic pain can present as headaches, muscle, joint, or bone pain.

A comprehensive approach that addresses the underlying cause, relieves symptoms, and enhances the patient's overall cardiovascular and hematologic health is necessary for the effective management of heart, vascular, and hemopathic pain. Medication, lifestyle changes, physical therapy, interventional procedures, and, in certain situations, surgical interventions are some examples of treatment strategies. To further improve outcomes and quality of life for patients with hematologic and cardiovascular conditions, healthcare providers must collaborate, educate, and support their patients.

Orientation and Directional Terms

Term	Definition	Illustration
Stable angina	Stable angina is a type of chest pain that's usually caused by poor blood flow to the heart's coronary arteries.	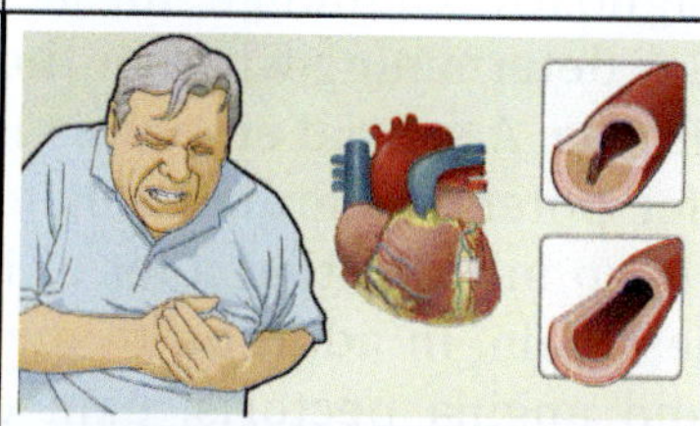
Ischemia	Ischemia is a serious condition that occurs when blood flow to a part of the body is restricted, which can deprive tissues, muscles, or organs of oxygen and nutrients.	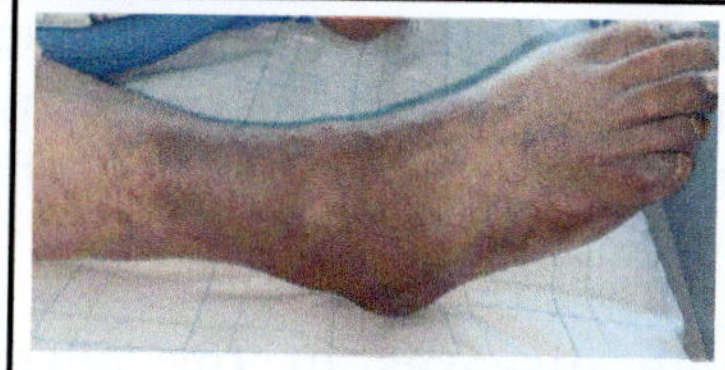
Myocardial infarction	Myocardial infarction (MI), also known as a heart attack, occurs when blood flow to the heart muscle is blocked, preventing the heart from getting enough oxygen and causing heart cells to die.	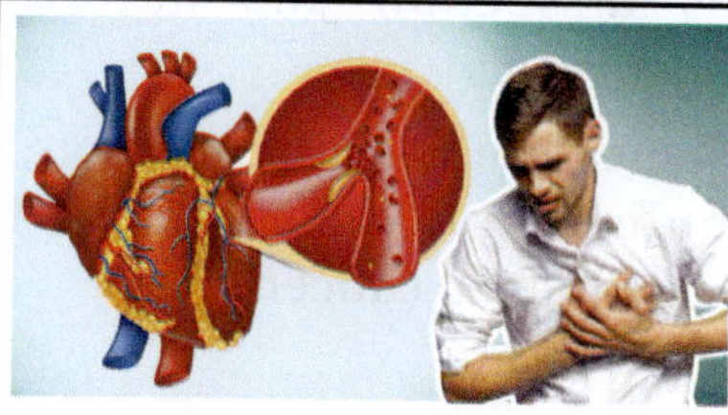
Vasculitis	Vasculitis is a rare group of conditions that cause inflammation and swelling of blood vessels.	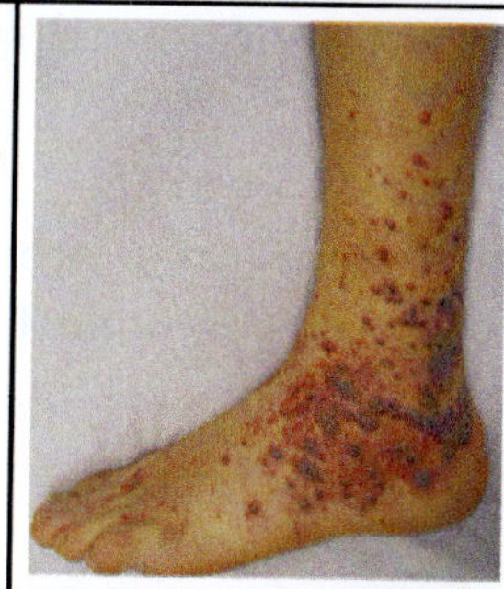
Pleuritis	Pleuritis, also known as pleurisy, is inflammation of the pleura, the two thin layers of tissue that line the chest cavity and surround the lungs.	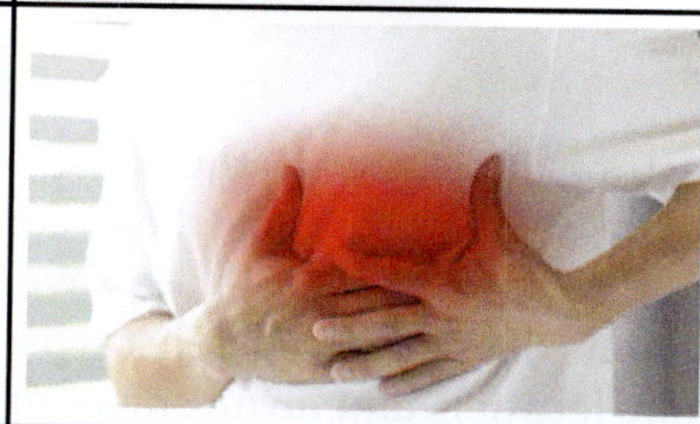

7.1. Heart Pain

When a patient presents with chest pain, the primary diagnostic challenge for a medical professional is determining whether the patient has heart disease. A special emphasis is placed on looking for potential cardiac ischemia. Still, we have to keep in mind that a lot of illnesses result in chest pain. In addition to myocardial infarction and angina pectoris, pain can also occur in pericarditis and certain valvular heart diseases. Many thoracic diseases may cause chest pain that often resembles pain from the heart, including:

1. some diseases of the aorta, such as dissection and atherosclerotic aneurysms
2. some diseases of the lungs, such as pulmonary embolism, infarction, pneumonia, cancer
3. pleuritis
4. diseases of the esophagus, such as alterations of motility and inflammation.

Additionally, chest injuries, Tietze's syndrome, or herpes zoster may precede or follow chest wall pain i.e., discomfort that is restricted to palpably painful swelling in the costochondral and costosternal joints.

7.1.1. General Considerations on Pain from Ischemic Heart Disease

Every doctor is familiar with the pain associated with ischemic heart disease because it is a commonly observed symptom. However, due to varying points of reference, distinct types of pain in the same location, and involvement of regions distant from the heart, descriptions found in textbooks and everyday experience convey the impression of a broad range of symptoms. That being said, this pain doesn't seem to follow any rules. We think that's why doctors focus more on laboratory and instrumental investigations rather than making a precise observation of the patient's pain.

It is only when we look closely at the different kinds of pain that the patient experiences that we can see that there are no rules for cardiac pain. In fact, identifying the location of pain is not sufficient; additional steps include differentiating between genuine visceral pain and referred pain as well as figuring out whether the pain is referred to deep or superficial parietal structures. We can only obtain such information by conducting a thorough and sufficient investigation into the patient. As a result, a brief overview of the clinical features of visceral pain should come before any discussion of cardiac pain.

7.1.2. Clinical Characteristics of Visceral Pain

True visceral pain has distinct characteristics from deep pain or cutaneous pain. Visceral pain is not well localized and can be dull, aching, or boring. It is always accompanied by a feeling of unwellness and malaise. Strong autonomic reactions, including vasomotor reactions, changes in heart rate and blood pressure, and diffuse sweating, are linked to it, as well as a strong alarm response.

Pain is gradually felt in more superficial structures, sometimes even far from the site of origin, when an algogenic process affecting a viscus recurs frequently or intensifies and lasts longer. In English, this phenomenon is typically referred to as "referred pain," but German writers refer to it more appropriately—transferred pain, in our opinion—using a less common term. Autonomic reflexes may accompany referred pain. Zones of tenderness in the muscles and cutaneous hyperalgesia are frequently observed. When experiencing unpleasant visceral sensations, patients frequently choose to use terms other than pain, such as pressure, tightness, discomfort, or squeezing. There is a range of unpleasantness and intensity between the absence of sensory symptoms and the actual pain.

7.1.3. Pain in Myocardial Infarction

This pain can strike out of nowhere during stressful activities, right after a big meal, or while you're sleeping or resting. Sometimes it's preceded by unpleasant stomach sensations like indigestion or fullness in the stomach, or by a sensation of discomfort in the chest or mild dyspnea. The patient has a history of angina pectoris paroxysms frequently. True visceral pain is characterized by early pain that is deep, central, anterior, and occasionally posterior. It lasts anywhere from a few minutes to several hours. Most patients describe it as tightening, compressing, or squeezing, or as "a band across the chest." This type of pain is central and is often felt behind the lower sternum, on the epigastrium, or in both places less frequently. In certain patients, the pain is limited to the posterior region, while in others, it coexists with central back pain. Pain is frequently accompanied by diffuse sweating, nausea, and vomiting. This severe pain is frequently accompanied by a strong alarm response and, on occasion, a sense of impending death.

A later stage occurs when the pain becomes parietal, taking on the features of referred pain, and lasts anywhere from 10 minutes to several hours. It might be the first pain that you feel. This pain tends to radiate and is commonly described as pressing or constricting. Compared to visceral pain, the spatial localization is more accurate; sweating is frequently experienced along with it, but nausea and vomiting are less common. Usually referred below the sternum or in the precordial region, this pain can occasionally spread to the anterior chest's two sides or, in rare instances, just to the right. Radiation-induced sensations include numbness, cramping, and a squeezing sensation in the elbow or wrist. The pain usually radiates to the left arm in its entirety, to both arms or to the left hand and forearm; in a small number of cases, it only affects the right arm. Radiation to the jaw, neck, and temporomandibular joint simultaneously on both sides is another unusual occurrence. Seldom does a posterior pain that originates in the interscapulovertebral area radiate to the left arm's ulnar aspect. The duration of parietal pain in patients who are not receiving medication varies from 30 minutes to 12 hours or longer. It is always more persistent than actual visceral pain.

This pain develops first, and muscle tenderness develops after a few hours to a full day. The pectoralis major, the deep muscles of the interscapular region, the forearm muscles, and, less commonly, the trapezius and deltoid muscles are the main muscles involved.

Some patients experience localized, superficially referred pain that is restricted to the dermatomes C8–T1, or the ulnar side of the arm and forearm. Rarely is this pain the only initial sign. It is strong, stabbing, or lancinating, and it lasts anywhere from 30 minutes to 6 hours. It is common to find cutaneous hyperalgesia in the reference areas. The 122 pattern of pain does not appear to be correlated with the type of infarction (inferior, anterior, transmural, or non-transmural).

7.1.4. Pain in Angina Pectoris

The pain is usually deep, rarely superficial, and has characteristics and radiations similar to myocardial infarction, but it is less intense and lasts shorter. There is rarely nausea or vomiting associated with pain, nor is there a sense of impending death. Compared to a myocardial infarction, the alarm response and its accompanying symptoms are less severe. Deep muscle soreness in these patients is persistent and unrelated to pain episodes; it is located in the same regions as infarction. Stable angina, unstable angina, and variant angina (Prinzmetal's) are the three anginal syndromes that are distinguished in contemporary angina pectoris classifications.

- **Stable Angina:** Individuals who have stable angina typically experience angina during exertion, exercise, or other circumstances that raise the heart's oxygen demand. The nature of the feeling can occasionally be characterized as numbness or a slight pressure-like discomfort. "Equivalents" of an angel (i.e., breathlessness, dizziness, exhaustion, and belching—symptoms of myocardial ischemia other than angina—have also been documented (Gersh et al., 1997). The disappearance of pain following nitroglycerine use or amyl nitrite inhalation is a hallmark of stable angina.
- **Unstable Angina:** The term unstable angina, previously also known as preinfarction angina, acute coronary insufficiency, and intermediate coronary syndrome, indicates angina pectoris characterized by one or more of the following features:
  - Crescendo angina (more severe, prolonged or frequent) superimposed on a pre-existing pattern of relatively stable, exertion-related angina pectoris
  - Angina pectoris at rest as well as with minimal exertion
  - Angina pectoris of new onset (usually within 1 month), which is brought on by minimal exertion (Gersh et al., 1997).

The chest pain associated with unstable angina is comparable to that of chronic stable angina, but it is typically more severe, described as pain, and can sometimes wake the patient up from sleep. It can also last up to 30 minutes. It's important to suspect an infarction if it lasts longer than 30 minutes. This pain's ability to range widely in intensity from extremely mild to (usually) intermediate to occasionally reaching maximal intensity, similar to that of an infarction, is one of its distinguishing features.

The doctor should be made aware of a shifting anginal pattern by multiple indicators. These include a sudden drop in the threshold of physical activity that causes angina; an increase in the frequency, intensity, and duration of angina; radiation of the pain to a new location; the onset of new pain-related features, such as nausea; and a reduction in the amount of pain relief that nitroglycerine provides.

- **Variant Angina:** The uncommon syndrome of cardiac pain known as "variant" or "Prinzmetal's" angina is almost exclusively experienced at rest, typically not brought on by physical activity or psychological stress, and is linked to elevated S-T segments on an ECG (Prinzmetal et al., 1959). It has been conclusively shown that coronary artery spasm is the cause of this syndrome. Nonetheless, Maseri et al. (1978) found that in many patients, the coronary vasospasm that happened during an anginal attack was linked to elevation or depression of the S-T segment in arteriographic studies, making it difficult to distinguish between unstable angina and variant angina (Prinzmetal's). Variant angina is regarded by Selwyn and Braunwald (1998) as a distinct variety of unstable angina.

7.1.5. Syndrome X

Some studies have included a variety of patients with chest pain who have angiographically normal coronary arteries and a pattern of chronic stable angina under the broad definition of syndrome X (Kemp, 1973). On the other hand, some patients' symptoms might not have originated from their hearts (Maseri, 1995). While in some subjects, ischemia is undetectable by currently available techniques, in others ischemia-appearing S-T segment responses are evident with exercise tests (Maseri, 1995). It was suggested (Gersh et al., 1997) that patients with cardiac syndrome X have an amplification of the small response of the coronary arteries to vasoconstrictor stimuli.

Other causes of chest pain have come to light as a result of some syndrome X patients' lack of conclusive evidence of ischemia. E.g., when experiencing esophageal pain. Compared to patients with coronary artery obstructions, women with typical angina and normal coronary arteries showed decreased tolerance to forearm tourniquets and electrical skin stimulation, as well as an increased sensitivity to potentially painful cardiac stimuli. Additionally, there was an overlap between increased sensitivity to cardiac and esophageal pain, as reported by Maseri in 1995. Therefore, a common feature among patients with syndrome X appears to be a generalized increase in somatic and visceral pain sensitivity. It is unclear if this phenomenon is the result of aberrant processing of afferent neural impulses or aberrant activation of somatic and visceral receptors.

7.1.6. The Problem of Painless Coronary Heart Diseases

It is commonly known that in patients without a history of a clearly defined episode of chest pain, myocardial infarction has been discovered during electrocardiographic studies or postmortem examinations. The location, size, age, or patient's age of the infarction have not been linked to the incidence of painless infarctions (Rinzler, 1951; Friedberg, 1956; Teodori & Galletti, 1962; Stern, 1998). In the Framingham Study, which involved long-term follow-up, 25% of patients experienced "unrecognized" myocardial infarction, which was only discovered during a routine 2-year ECG. Of these, about 50% of the episodes were actually silent (Kannel & Abbott, 1984). According to other population studies, 20 to 60% of myocardial infarctions that do not result in death go undetected by the patient and are only identified during a routine electrocardiogram or postmortem examination (Antman & Braunwald, 1997). These variations can be partially attributed to the various approaches taken in examining and comprehending the symptoms. A brief episode of chest discomfort, sudden and unusual thoracic paresthesias (tingling, pricking, numbness) radiating to the left arm, a minor pain that the patient felt was not bothersome, or an episode of nausea and vomiting that was thought to be caused by gastric fullness or indigestion could all be discovered if, in fact, we gather an accurate history of patients in whom a diagnosis of asymptomatic previous myocardial infarction is suspected during a routine examination (Procacci et al., 1976). Since patients frequently underestimate and forget these episodes, the history needs to be extremely accurate. When these variables are taken into consideration, the incidence of asymptomatic myocardial infarction is decreased.

To encompass all types of painless myocardial ischemia, the term and concept of silent myocardial ischemia have recently been introduced. Patients with diabetes have a higher incidence of silent myocardial ischemia, most likely due to neuropathy affecting the visceral afferent fibers.

There are two recognized types of silent myocardial ischemia (Gersh et al., 1997). Patients with obstructive coronary artery disease, sometimes severe, who never experience angina or even pain during myocardial infarction, are said to have the first and less common form of the condition. Patients with the typical forms of unstable angina, variant angina, and chronic stable angina experience the second, more common form. These patients show some episodes of ischemia linked to chest discomfort and other episodes that are not when their dynamic ECG is monitored, i.e., periods of silent ischemia without symptoms.

7.1.7. Painful Complications of Myocardial Infarction

Angina could develop into a heart attack. Angina may become stable or unstable following myocardial infarction.

Pericarditis may be the cause of chronic pain following myocardial infarction, particularly transmural pain. It is crucial to accurately diagnose the chest pain associated with pericarditis, as misdiagnosing it could result in the mistreatment of anticoagulants, nitrates, β-adrenergic blocking agents, narcotics, or an incorrect diagnosis of recurrent ischemic pain and/or infarction extension. Leaning forward relieves the pain, while deep breathing exacerbates it. This characteristic pericardial pattern helps differentiate the pain from that of an extending infarction.

A few people may experience pleuropericardial chest pain and fever 1–6 weeks following myocardial infarction. Dressler's syndrome, also known as postmyocardial infarction syndrome, is believed to be brought on by pericarditis and pleuritis, potentially as a result of an autoimmune mechanism (Dressler, 1956; Lorell, 1997). Treatment for the syndrome usually involves corticosteroids or aspirin-like medications. When treating Dressler's syndrome, anticoagulants should be stopped because the effusions they cause can be hemorrhagic.

Left scapulohumeral periarthritis may 124
exacerbate certain cases of persistent angina and 5% of myocardial infarction cases. It presents as a frozen shoulder, with pain, stiffness, and a noticeable limitation of shoulder joint motion. There are instances where a progressive reflex dystrophy of the left arm starts 3–6 weeks following myocardial infarction. Shoulder–hand syndrome primarily affects the hand, wrist, and shoulder. Advanced stages of osteoporosis, muscular and cutaneous atrophy, glossy skin, hair loss, vasomotor abnormalities, and other symptoms could indicate a very serious evolution. Similar to other reflex dystrophies, stellate ganglion blocks frequently lead to improvement.

7.1.8. Functional or Psychogenic Chest Pain

It is common to observe patients with chest pain who do not exhibit instrumental signs of ischemic heart disease. Many anxious patients, often with a depressive trait, worry about a precordial pain that radiates with characteristics similar to angina. They frequently visit doctors and get checked out, and while this is normal, it doesn't give them much comfort.

Many adjectives are used to characterize pain, including stabbing, piercing, burning, dull, squeezing, irritating, slight, intense, fluctuating, and synchronous with heartbeats, among others. The doctor must first rule out other possible reasons for the patient's chest pain.

Some features set this pain apart from true angina: it lasts anywhere from a few minutes to several days; it is frequently unrelated to exertion; patients experience restlessness and anxiety, whereas during an angina attack, they are largely immobile. When asked where they feel pain, patients frequently behave differently: angina patients place their open hand on their sternum, while anxious patients touch their left submammary region or frequently areas of the precordial area with their index finger.

Despite these distinctions, considerable care should be taken when diagnosing functional or psychogenic chest pain because it can be challenging to distinguish between anxious depressive syndrome and true angina.

7.1.9. Other Causes of Heart Pain

7.1.9.1. Aortic Stenosis and Insufficiency

About two thirds of cases of symptomatic aortic stenosis have been reported to have angina pectoris. In comparison to other valvular lesions, angina pectoris is more common in patients with aortic stenosis. Usually, the pain is angina that is typical of effort. Cardiovascular symptoms usually do not appear in patients with severe chronic aortic stenosis until relatively late in the course of the condition. The average survival time after a patient develops symptoms is two to five years (Braunwald, 1997). It is obvious that following angioplasty or heart surgery, the course of this illness changes. Usually, a coronary narrowing or myocardial hypertrophy with an elevated oxygen demand is the cause of the pain. It is commonly known that aortic insufficiency has long been thought to be the cause of angina pectoris. Friedberg (1956) states that angina pectoris is rare in patients with simple aortic insufficiency, but it can happen as a result of coronary atherosclerosis or when the aortic valve becomes calcified over time, causing stenosis in the coronary arteries.

7.1.9.2. Mitral stenosis

It has been noted by Braunwald (1997) that approximately 15% of patients with mitral stenosis experience pain that resembles angina pectoris. Since the advent of cardiac surgery, it is now uncommon to observe pain in cases of mitral stenosis.

7.1.9.3. Mitral Valve Prolapse

Chest pain is occasionally reported in cases of mitral valve prolapse. A common anginal pain is present in certain cases where mitral valve prolapse is linked to coronary heart disease.

7.1.9.4. Inflammatory Disease of the Heart

All inflammatory heart diseases can cause pain, i.e., myocarditis, endocarditis, and pericarditis. However, pericarditis pain is much more common than myocarditis or endocarditis pain; for this reason, we will only discuss pericarditis pain.

Since pericarditis does not cause pain as frequently as pleurisy does, pleural involvement should be suspected when pain is present. For these reasons, compared to the pleura, the pericardium is thought to be less sensitive to pain (Teodori & Galletti, 1962).

The onset of pain in acute pericarditis frequently corresponds with fever, though it can also happen after a chill. Pain is usually continuous, lasting anywhere from a few hours to three days, and it usually affects the upper two-thirds of the sternum. It is also frequently deep and substernal. It might show up again, but only for short bursts of time. Coughing, deep inspiration, and lateral chest movements all exacerbate it. Leaning forward and sitting upright helps to relieve pain.

In roughly 50% of cases, there is also a superficially referred pain present in addition to the deep pain. The left shoulder, scapula and arm, neck, and epigastrium may all experience radiating pain. It could feel like angina when you're exerting yourself.

Although chronic pericarditis is frequently painless, the patient may report a deep, dull, mild pain or a feeling of fullness or heaviness in the chest upon careful questioning.

7.1.9.5. Cor Pulmonale

A true visceral pain with characteristics and radiation similar to myocardial infarction, including a strong alarm reaction, is seen in many cases of acute Cor pulmonale (pulmonary embolism).

Angina-like pain is very similar to the pain experienced by some patients with chronic Cor pulmonale. All conditions that cause pulmonary hypertension, such as idiopathic pulmonary hypertension, chronic Cor pulmonale, mitral stenosis, and certain congenital heart diseases, can cause pain. The location, radiation, quality, and intensity of angina pectoris and angina related pain are similar in patients with pulmonary hypertension. However, a thorough examination will reveal that while the patient in coronary angina is pale (Angor pallidus), the severity of cyanosis (Angor coeruleus) increases during spontaneous or exertional pain in pulmonary hypertension.

7.1.10. Causes of Chest Pain (From Organs Other Than the Heart)

7.1.10.1. Diseases of the Aorta

- **Aneurysms:** Thoracic aortic aneurysms are the source of chest pain, whereas abdominal aortic aneurysms are typically asymptomatic but can occasionally cause low back and abdominal pain (Isselbacher et al., 1997).

  The excitation of the aortic end organs as well as the compression and erosion of the surrounding musculoskeletal structures are likely the causes of pain in thoracic aortic aneurysms. It is typically monotonous and constant, though it occasionally pulses.

- **Aortic Dissection:** Severe pain is by far the most common presenting symptom of aortic dissection, occurring in 74–90% of cases, according to Isselbacher et al., (1997). Dissection frequently causes excruciating pain, making the patient writhe in agony or pace frantically in an effort to feel some relief. Although the pain seems similar to a myocardial infarction, there are a few characteristics that could lead one to suspect an aortic dissection. The patient's description of the pain is frequently strikingly accurate to what actually happened. It's common to use adjectives like "tearing," "ripping," and "stabbing." The propensity of the aortic dissection pain to spread from its site of origin to different locations along the dissecting haematoma's path as it passes through the aorta is another feature of the condition. While pain that is most severe in the interscapular area is much more common when a distal site is involved, pain felt maximally in the anterior thorax is more common with proximal dissection. The pain is often accompanied by nausea and vomiting, diffuse sweating, fainting, and hiccups that do not go away with medication or conventional measures.

7.1.10.2. Pleurisy

Due to the pleura's extreme sensitivity to pain, chest pain is commonly seen during pleurisy.

First, we'll talk about what kind of stimulus causes pleuritis pain. There are two components: a mechanical component that results from stretching of the parietal pleura during inspiration and friction between the two adjacent pleural surfaces (especially when they are covered in fibrinous exudate); the other component is chemical and results from the pleural liquid's high algogenic power, which is rich in substances that cause pain (Procacci, 1969).

The pain is usually specific to a particular area. It often starts suddenly rather than gradually, sometimes occurring before other symptoms like fever, shortness of breath, and cough, and typically lasts for a few days. The specific location of the pain depends on where and how much inflammation is present (Teodori & Galletti, 1962).

1. In effusive pleurisy, it is felt in a region corresponding to the site of inflammation and frequently referred to the submammary area.
2. In diaphragmatic pleurisy, pain is often felt on the trapezius ridge and on the base of the affected side of the chest.
3. In apical pleurisy, pain is in the interscapulovertebral region.

In effusive pleurisies, pain is almost always constant and made worse by coughing, deep inspiration, 126 chest movements, and lying on the side that is afflicted. Interscapulovertebral pain with apical pleurisy and shoulder pain with diaphragmatic pleurisy are less constrictive, less localized, and unaffected by movement, coughing, or deep inspiration. When effusive pleurisy occurs, particularly in the submammary region, empyema, pleurisy following a pulmonary or subdiaphragmatic abscess, or pleurisy complicating pneumonia or lung cancer, the pain is extremely severe.

7.1.10.3. Diseases of the Oesophagus

Both experimental and spontaneous esophageal pain exhibits the usual features of visceral pain, including poor localization, autonomic reflexes, emotions, and referability.

The fundamental algogenic stimuli for the esophagus are:

1. strong mechanical stimulation from esophageal stenosis and motor disorders, such as cancer, achalasia, diffuse esophageal spasm, nutcracker esophagus (symptomatic peristalsis), and aspecific motor disorders (Goyal, 1998)
2. gastro-oesophageal reflux and inflammation. In patients with gastro-oesophageal reflux, the most common symptom is heartburn. The term 'burning' rather than 'pain' is usually used, although heartburn can increase in intensity until it is perceived as pain. Pain can be longlasting or present during swallowing (odynophagia).

Esophageal discomfort can be caused during standard medical tests by infusing the esophagus with 0.1 N hydrochloric acid (Bernstein test) or by inflating a balloon.

The higher sternum refers to disorders of the proximal third of the esophagus, while the lower sternum refers to disorders of the distal third. Pain that is localized in one or more areas is a result of diseases affecting the intermediate third. There are numerous radiating zones for pain, some of which may be shared by disorders affecting the upper and lower esophagus. The neck, ear, jaw, precordium, shoulders, upper limbs, epigastrium, and interscapular and central dorsal areas at the level of the sixth and seventh thoracic vertebrae are the most commonly observed (Teodori & Galletti, 1962).

Pain in the esophagus can imitate the pain of a heart attack. Relief is often achieved with nitroglycerin or calcium antagonists, and unlike angina, can also be alleviated by consuming milk or antacids. Certain acute abdominal conditions like peptic ulcers, acute cholecystitis, and pancreatitis can mimic heart pain, just as heart pain can mimic the symptoms of these diseases. Sometimes, a combination of factors may contribute to the pain experienced.

7.1.11. Complex Problems

Angina from other structures often coexists with heart pain (angors coronariens intriqués) (Froment & Gonin, 1956). For example, cervicothoracic osteoarthritis (vertebrocoronary syndrome), chest fibromyalgias, or numerous gastrointestinal tract disorders, including esophageal diseases, hiatus hernia, gastroduodenitis, peptic ulcers, and calculous and non-calculous cholecystitis (cholecystocoronary syndrome), may coexist with myocardial ischemia. It is challenging to determine whether these complex conditions result from somatovisceral and viscerosomatic reflexes that may create a traditional "vicious circle" between various structures, or from the simple addition of impulses from various sources within the central nervous system (Procacci et al., 1986). Pain can range from standard angina pectoris to irregularly patterning chest pain.

7.1.12. Mechanisms of Cardiac Pain

Heart pain mechanisms appear to share some similarities with visceral pain and some similarities with skeletal muscle pain. For example, a cat's left ventricular wall injected with a 5% solution of NaCl, a well-known algogenic stimulus for the skeletal muscles, causes a strong release of A-δ afferent fibers from the heart (Brown, 1967). There is much discussion surrounding the issue of coronary spasm during excruciating attacks. In both stable and unstable angina, the coronary artery spasm is a characteristic feature of variant angina. Some cases of syndrome X are thought to be caused by constriction of a small coronary vessel (Maseri, 1995).

According to Aviado and Schmidt (1955), the necessary stimuli in the heart for the onset of pain and of reflex phenomena were the following:

1. reduced coronary arterial pressure distal to an occlusion, acting on coronary arterial pressoreceptors
2. ischemia, stimulating the myocardial pressoreceptors and chemoreceptors
3. release of pain-producing substances formed by tissue breakdown or platelet disintegration.

There is ongoing discussion regarding the existence of genuine cardiac nociceptors (Cervero, 1994, 1995). Malliani and his group (Malliani & Lombardi, 1982; Malliani, 1995) saw that animals would discharge more cardiac afferent C-fibers in response to strong stimuli, like intracoronary bradykinin injections. However, they never saw that the administration of bradykinin or coronary occlusion would cause a recruitment of silent afferents. According to Malliani (1995), the most plausible explanation for the characteristics of the neural substrate supporting cardiac nociception is the "intensity mechanism."

The biochemical aspect of cardiac pain in ischemic heart disease is significant in addition to mechanical factors. This component is multifactorial; it is necessary to take into account the rise in lactic acid, the release of potassium ions, the synthesis of kinins, and the production of other substances that cause pain. Adenosine has drawn attention recently as a possible biochemical mediator of anginal pain (Cannon, 1995). Adenosine has the ability to increase the excitation caused by myocardial ischemia on the impulse activity of the ventricular afferent fibers, according to research done by Malliani (1995). It's likely that several drugs that cause pain work together.

We think that the development of an ischemic neuropathy of the heart's nerves is another significant mechanism. According to Lewis (1942), the pain in this type of neuropathy is similar to that of effort angina (claudicatio cordis) and is associated with atherosclerotic artery disease of the legs presenting with intermittent claudication (claudicatio intermittens). Different cardiac pain mechanisms coexist, with one or more of them being more common in certain patient populations and conditions (Procacci et al., 1986; Maseri, 1995). We can agree with Malliani (1986) and Cervero (1994) that there is neither a clear nor strong correlation between myocardial ischemia and cardiac pain because both conditions can occur in the absence of ischemia and, on the other hand, myocardial ischemia episodes can occur without pain.

7.1.13. Mnemonic Traces

The central nervous system has the capacity to store and recall learned experiences at every level. Research has shown that the mnemonic process is enhanced when an experience is repeated repeatedly or when it is accompanied by either positive or negative emotions. Pain is, at least partially, a learned experience, just like other sensory modalities (Melzack, 1973). Melzack (1973) referred to the processes of painful memories as memory-like processes. Nathan (1962) noted that various stimuli could evoke memories of past pain experiences in certain subjects.

Patients who had previously experienced a myocardial infarction but had normal sensibility as determined by a precise examination participated in our experiments. Using the method from our school, two pneumatic cuffs were used to induce ischemia in the upper limbs (Procacci et al., 1986). The majority of patients experienced pain from ischemia that was akin to the pain experienced during the infarction episode. Common symptoms including sweating, nausea, tachycardia, and tachypnea were experienced by a few patients along with an alarm reaction. There were no changes to the ECG. As soon as these symptoms appeared, the test was promptly stopped. Patients who had previously experienced a painless myocardial infarction were also evaluated. While some patients' histories were entirely silent, others remembered an episode that was variously described as nausea, indigestion, or stomach fullness. The majority of patients experienced diffuse unpleasant common sensations, frequently accompanied by autonomic and emotional reactions, as a result of upper limb ischemia (Procacci et al., 1976).

Patients with angina pectoris were also subjected to ischemia of the upper limbs. The majority of patients whose left arm was affected by anginal pain reported pain in the same limb as their spontaneous pain, and with the same radiation. When anginal pain was limited to the chest or extended to both upper limbs, the majority of patients complained of pain in both limbs (Procacci et al., 1986). These findings imply that ischemic pain generated in the extremities may trigger memory traces associated with myocardial pain.

7.1.14. Therapy

Certain medications that are ineffective for treating other types of pain are used to treat angina pectoris pain. Amyl nitrite (Brunton, 1867) and nitroglycerine (a few years later) were the first medications used. When using nitrates, pain is frequently dramatically reduced. To stop ischemic attacks, other medications are used, such as calcium antagonists, long-lasting organic nitrates, and β-blocking agents. The way these medications work is just as debatable as how pain is caused.

It is also important to note the beneficial correlation between aspirin and antianginal medications, which may directly affect cardiac pain and aid in the removal of the algogenic summation from myalgic spots, which are frequently seen in angina patients. This latent afferent input might play a significant part in reflexes that help angina attacks occur. Aspirin's ability to inhibit platelet aggregation confers an antithrombotic effect. Patients with unstable angina have had their myocardial ischemia controlled with intravenous heparin (Neri

Serneri et al., 1995). Morphine is the preferred medication for myocardial infarction because it typically results in good sedation and pain relief. In myocardial infarction, morphine not only reduces pain but also centrally blocks reflexes that could exacerbate the condition of the heart or cause potentially fatal arrhythmias.

Intracoronary thrombolysis using urokinase, streptokinase, and other medications is helpful in the initial hours following the onset of symptoms in myocardial infarction. Intravenous thrombolysis is used when intracoronary thrombolysis is not possible.

Back in 1955, White and Sweet provided a thorough explanation of how to inject procaine and alcohol into each of the four upper thoracic sympathetic ganglia to relieve chronic pain in angina pectoris. Patients with acute myocardial infarction or severe unstable angina have demonstrated to benefit greatly from epidural blockade of the upper thoracic sympathetic segments in terms of pain relief (Blomberg et al., 1990; Kirnö et al., 1994; Olausson et al., 1997). Given that both sympathetic and visceral afferent fibers are blocked, the mode of action of the therapy is undoubtedly complex.

It is common knowledge in cardiac surgery that following coronary angioplasty or aortocoronary bypass, the majority of angina patients experience significant pain relief. A decrease in coronary flow is typically linked to the absence of pain. Nonetheless, it should be remembered that certain cardiac afferent fibers that supply sympathetic nerves are severed during coronary bypass surgery. The alleviation of heart pain might be related to this denervation (Rosenwasser, 1996; Selwyin & Braunwald, 1998).

7.2. Vascular Pain

Vascular pain is a multifaceted field. It can be separated into three categories: venous pain, pain resulting from lesion or malfunction of the microvessels (small venules, capillaries, and arterioles), and arterial pain. It goes without saying that a variety of traumas that occur frequently in daily life can harm the vascular tree in different ways.

7.2.1. Arterial Pain

Pain in the arteries can be caused by a variety of conditions, including atherosclerosis, arterial thrombosis, arteritis, arteriolitis, and arteriole dysfunction.

7.2.1.1. Atherosclerosis and/or Thrombosis of the Arterial Bed

Atherosclerosis and/or thrombosis in the coronary vessels lead to the pain associated with angina pectoris and myocardial infarction. In diseases affecting arterial flow in the limbs, it causes intermittent claudication or rest pain. Intermittent claudication is described as pain, cramping, numbness in the muscles during activity that is alleviated by rest. Similar to angina pectoris, the onset of pain in intermittent claudication is key to understanding the severity of the condition. A stable condition is indicated by a consistent free interval before pain begins, while a decreasing interval is indicative of an unstable condition, similar to unstable angina. This observation is vital for determining appropriate medical or surgical treatment.

Ipotence, atrophy of the limbs, pallor of the skin on the feet and legs, intermittent claudication of the low back, buttocks, and thigh or calf muscles, and other characteristic clinical manifestations are the result of isolated aortoiliac occlusive arterial disease, the cause of Leriche's syndrome. Angina abdominis occurs in a small percentage of patients when abdominal vessels are affected by atherosclerotic processes. Chronic mesenteric insufficiency pain is similar to angina pectoris in that it arises when there is a greater need for splanchnic blood flow.

After eating, there is typically sporadic dull or cramping midabdominal pain. The coeliac axis, superior or inferior mesenteric arteries, or both are occluded or have high-grade stenosis, according to arteriographic studies of angina abdominis.

7.2.1.2. Arteritis or Arteriolitis

Certain illnesses are well-known, including systemic giant cell arteritis, Takayasu's syndrome, and thromboangiitis obliterans (Rosenwasser, 1996; Fauci, 1998).

Thromboangiitis obliterans, also known as Bürger's disease, is an obstructive arterial disease brought on by proliferative and segmental inflammatory lesions in the limbs' medium and small arteries and veins (Kontos, 1996). The primary cause of the symptoms is a disturbance in the arterial blood supply to the tissues, although local venous insufficiency also plays a role. Intermittent claudication, pain during rest when severe tissue ischemia has developed, pain from ulcerations and gangrene, and pain from ischemic neuropathy—which is a crucial symptom—are the symptoms. Both migratory superficial thrombophlebitis and Raynaud's phenomenon are frequent.

Aortic arc syndrome, also known as Takayasu's syndrome, is caused by arteriolitis and arteritis of the upper body's vessels, including the arterioles in the eyes. It is common in young women and adolescent girls. Approximately two-thirds of the patients experience limb-girdle stiffness, arthralgia, fever, and malaise during a prodromic phase. This prodromic phase is comparable to that of systemic lupus erythematosus, giant cell arteritis, and rheumatic diseases. Localized pain over the afflicted arteries, along with erythema nodosum and erythema induratum, frequently follow this. Angina pectoris or myocardial infarction are the disease's evolving symptoms in certain cases.

Large and medium arteries can become inflamed with giant cell arteritis, also known as temporal arteritis. The term "cranial" or "temporal" arteritis refers to the characteristic of involving one or more carotid artery branches, specifically the temporal artery. It primarily affects people over the age of 55 and is more common in women than in men. A headache is frequently so severe as to be intolerable. The temporal arteries are the arteries that are usually affected by headaches, though they can also occur in the occipital region. There is visible induration and typical tenderness along the vessels. The vascular environment is extremely sensitive to pressure. Up to two thirds of patients experience claudication in the jaw muscles during chewing.

Large cell arteritis can affect arteries in several different places and is regarded as a systemic illness (Fauci, 1998). The patient frequently reports experiencing severe malaise, a slight fever, and myalgia, with an initial illness similar to "flu syndrome." The neck, shoulder girdle, and pelvic girdle are the primary areas affected by the muscle pain, which can progress and worsen. The trunk and distal limbs are also somewhat affected; the involvement is bilateral but may not always be of equal intensity. There have been reports of myocardial infarctions, visceral organ infarctions, and intermittent claudication. This syndrome is categorized as a rheumatic disease because it is thought to be exclusively linked to polymyalgia rheumatica.

It can be difficult to distinguish between giant cell arteritis and Takayasu's syndrome. Both of them are now recognized as connective tissue disorders. Rosenwasser (1996) divides giant cell arteritides into subgroups that include Takayasu's arteritis and cranial or temporal arteritis.

7.2.1.3. Dysfunction of Arterioles

The hallmark of Raynaud's phenomenon is episodes of severe pallor in the fingers and toes (ischemic phase), which are typically followed by cyanosis and rubor. An abrupt constriction of the arteriolar lumen, followed by a paralyzed phase, is the cause of the phenomenon. During the ischemic phase, patients typically experience a sharp, burning, or throbbing pain; during the cyanotic phase, they typically experience a less severe pain along with paresthesias. This condition can be categorized as secondary to other diseases, trauma, or medications, or as primary or idiopathic Raynaud's phenomenon (Raynaud's disease). Several changes to the arterioles that are indicative of various types of arteriolitis have been reported in relation to Raynaud's disease. Raynaud's phenomenon is thought to be specifically treated with calcium antagonists, adrenergic blockers, and other sympathicolytic medications (Creager & Dzau, 1998).

The syndrome known as erythromelalgia, also known as erythermalgia, is typified by the following symptoms in the extremities: deep and superficial burning pain, frequently accompanied by tingling and prickling; red discoloration and elevated skin temperature; and in many cases, edema. The distal portion of the lower limbs and, less frequently, the upper limbs are affected by the symptoms at the same time. Erythromelalgia attacks are brought on by elevated temperatures, either locally or in the environment, and they are made worse by a dependent posture. Attacks can last anywhere from a few minutes to several hours. Primary or secondary erythromelalgia may run in families. Thrombocytosis brought on by essential thrombocythemia or other myeloproliferative disorders (see Pain in Haemopathies, below) is the most frequently identified cause of secondary erythromelalgia (Ball, 1996). Diabetes mellitus has also been linked to erythromelalgia in reports. Skin punch biopsy samples revealed thrombotic occlusions and artery inflammation. Aspirin inhibits platelet aggregation for three or four days following a single dose, during which time erythromelalgia caused by thrombocytosis goes away. It is relevant to inquire about the possibility of classifying primary erythromelalgia under reflex sympathetic dystrophies. In fact, local anesthetic blocks of the sympathetic chain were shown to produce excellent results, including the complete disappearance of symptoms (Zoppi et al., 1985).

7.2.1.4. Mechanisms of Arterial Pain

The mechanisms of pain in arterial diseases are many and often intermingle.

1. Ischemia per se. The most evident examples of diseases due to this mechanism are angina at rest, pain occurring in arterial embolism, and Raynaud's phenomenon. Ischemia can give rise to a continuous pain in the limb when:
    - the ischemia is very severe
    - myalgic spots with the characteristics of trigger points are present in the limbs (Dorigo et al., 1979)
    - a reflex sympathetic dystrophy arises, which contributes to pain and dystrophy through different mechanisms: vasomotor changes; fast and slow changes in permeability of microvessels and tissue imbibition; release of active substances; direct control of some enzymatic reactions; and direct modulation of sensory receptors (Procacci, 1969; Maresca et al., 1984; Geppetti & Holzer, 1996; Jänig, 1996).

2. Ischemia occurring during muscular exercise because of a discrepancy between the supply and demand of oxygen carried to muscles. This mechanism, according to Lewis (1942), is typical of effort angina pectoris (stable chronic angina) and intermittent claudication of the limbs. Typical myalgic spots are found in many patients with intermittent claudication and are a component of pain (Procacci, 1969; Dorigo et al., 1979; Maresca et al., 1984).
3. Ischemia plus inflammation and/or metabolic disorders, typical of thromboangiitis obliterans, inflammatory arteriolitis and diabetic arteriolitis.

Vascular thrombosis is typically thought of as a common point of arrival for various pathways. However, as is evident from clinical observations, the two mechanisms—thrombosis and inflammation—in many vascular diseases partially overlap: thromboangiitis obliterans, angina, or infarction, which can sporadically occur in thrombophlebitis, giant cell arteritis, and other conditions.

7.2.2. Pain Due to Dysfunction of Microvessels

For pathophysiological and clinical reasons, pain originating from microvessels needs to be differentiated from traditional arterial and venous pain.

First off, certain classic syndromes like Raynaud's phenomenon, pernio (chilblains), and erythromelalgia (erythermalgia) are associated with both venous and arterial vessels (Kontos, 1996; Creager & Dzau, 1998). According to Zimmermann (1979) and Jänig (1996), there is undoubtedly a change in capillary filtration in these situations as well, and the onset of pain is significantly influenced by alterations in the microenvironment. Numerous substances have the potential to cause pain. Just a few of these, including substance P, kinins, histamine, and 5-hydroxytriptamine, have been identified. It is unknown what temporal correlations are involved in the release of active ingredients in various scenarios. neural inflammation, that is the antidromic release from substance P, calcitonin gene-related peptide (CGRP), neurokin-A, and possibly other substances from afferent C-fibers (Geppetti & Holzer, 1996), likely contributes to many microvessel diseases; neurogenic phenomena are undoubtedly significant in erythromelalgia and Raynaud's phenomenon. It should be mentioned that Raynaud's phenomenon is frequently brought on by cold, but it usually affects the face rather than the hands; this suggests that there may be a problem with the hypothalamic centers of thermoregulation.

7.2.3. Venous Pain

A characteristic vein pain is seen in cases of thrombophlebitis. A red, sensitive cord may be visible as the vein in superficial thrombophlebitis. Pain is frequently felt when at rest. Approximately 50% of patients with deep vein thrombophlebitis may not exhibit any symptoms. One may notice pain during voluntary dorsiflexion of the foot and tenderness to palpation (Kontos, 1996; Creager & Dzau, 1998). Numerous elements, including mechanical and biochemical ones, particularly venous stasis, can cause pain. Venous pain is much more painful than arterial pain because it involves inflammation in the perivascular tissues, muscles, and tendons. The fact that a postphlebitis pain frequently persists in the limbs after thrombopherebitis resolves highlights the significance of these extra factors. We have noticed that, frequently, myalgic spots—which are frequently accompanied by skin hyperalgesia—as well as the vein, which continues to cause pain, are the primary sources of pain. Finally, a postphlebitic myofascial pain syndrome is noted, which can occasionally be helped by medications that resemble aspirin. Reflex sympathetic dystrophy can occur in all vascular diseases and in myocardial infarction. In this instance, the limbs exhibit obvious vasomotor and sudomotor phenomena, muscle atrophy, osteoporosis, and skin dystrophy (glossy skin). It may be appropriate to use sympathetic blocks in conjunction with the traditional treatment of reflex sympathetic dystrophies (Procacci & Maresca, 1987b, Bonica, 1990).

7.2.4. Pain Management in Patients with Vascular Disease

The term "vascular disease" refers to a broad category of complex medical conditions, such as aneurysms, venous diseases (such as varicose veins and thromboembolic disease), lymphatic diseases, Buerger's disease, Raynaud's phenomenon, and peripheral arterial disease (PAD). Pain is taken into consideration for the purposes of this review in the context of patients with vascular disease treated for non-cardiac vascular problems, even though cardiac disease is a major contributor to morbidity and mortality.

Table 7.1. Main Risk Factors for CVD Diagnosis and Prediction

Method	Dataset	Best Rated Features	Feature Description
Diagnosis	Cleveland	cp	Chest Pain Type
		thalach	Maximum heart rate
		ca	Number of vessels colored by fluoroscopy
		oldpeak	Exercise-induced ST-segment depression
	Faisalabad	Serum creatinine	Level of creatinine in the blood
		Ejection fraction	Percentage of blood leaving the heart at each heart beat
		Age	Patient age
		Platelets	Platelets in the blood
Prediction	Framingham	sysBP	Systolic blood pressure
		BMI	Body Mass Index
		Age	Age at exam time
		totChol	Total Cholesterol
	South African Hearth	Tobacco	Cumulative tobacco
		Age	Age at onset
		Ldl	Low-density lipoprotein cholesterol
		Adiposity	Adiposity

Source: Guarneros-Nolasco LR, Cruz-Ramos NA, Alor-Hernández G, Rodríguez-Mazahua L, Sánchez-Cervantes JL. Identifying the Main Risk Factors for Cardiovascular Diseases Prediction Using Machine Learning Algorithms. *Mathematics*. 2021; 9(20):2537. https://doi.org/10.3390/math9202537.

Vascular disease is characterized by pain, which has a significant influence on function and quality of life. Pain management in this patient group is frequently complicated by pre-existing chronic pain and a number of related co-morbidities, including impaired renal function, obesity, diabetes mellitus, cognitive impairment, and ischemic heart disease. Numerous patients with vascular disease have undergone numerous surgeries as well as repeated hospital stays. Acute or chronic pain that is not under control will lead to pathophysiological alterations, such as an heightened stress response and autonomic system activation. These changes may be especially harmful to individuals suffering from vascular disease.

Patients with vascular disease experience a variety of complex and poorly understood pain mechanisms. Understanding these mechanisms is crucial for directing focused, efficient pain management, which includes a multimodal strategy for analgesia. We give an overview of the key pain mechanisms associated with vascular disease and then go over how pain is managed in different vascular disease scenarios.

7.2.5. Pain Mechanisms Relevant to Vascular Disease

Patients with vascular disease experience pain due to a variety of intricate mechanisms. There may be neuropathic, inflammatory, and nociceptive mechanisms. Successful pain management in patients with vascular disease requires identification of the predominant pathophysiological process causing their pain, as different mechanisms require different approaches to analgesic selection.

7.2.5.1. Nociceptive Pain

After thermal, chemical, or mechanical stimulation of peripheral nociceptors on small, myelinated Aδ fibers or unmyelinated C fibers, nociceptive pain is felt. It represents the typical adaptive functioning of the somatosensory nervous system and is a physiological reaction to actual or potential non-neuronal tissue damage. When the insult is removed, the pain usually goes away and is reversible. One important factor in intermittent claudication (pain and cramping after repeated muscle action or exercise) in vascular patients is nociceptive pain. Nociceptive pain is produced by a variety of peripheral receptors, including G-protein-coupled receptors and ion channels, which are located on Aά and C fibers. These comprise the transient receptor potential (TRP) channel family, responsive to calcium, and acid-sensing ion channels. The development of analgesic drugs may target the acid-sensing ion channels because they are crucial for both the initial pain response and the transition to chronic pain states.

7.2.5.2. Inflammatory Pain

This kind of pain is the somatosensory nervous system's reaction to inflammation and tissue damage. Peripheral sensitization is the process by which local nociceptors become more sensitive to elevated inflammatory mediators, such as chemokines and cytokines, thereby reducing their threshold for responsiveness. This heightened reactivity can lead to exaggerated reactions to unpleasant stimuli and the possible activation of pain pathways in response to benign input.

The activation of several receptors and ion channels, interactions between peripheral immune cells, modifications to local blood flow, and adjustments to the chemical and electrical activity of peripheral afferent neurones are all involved in the modulation of pain by the inflammatory response.

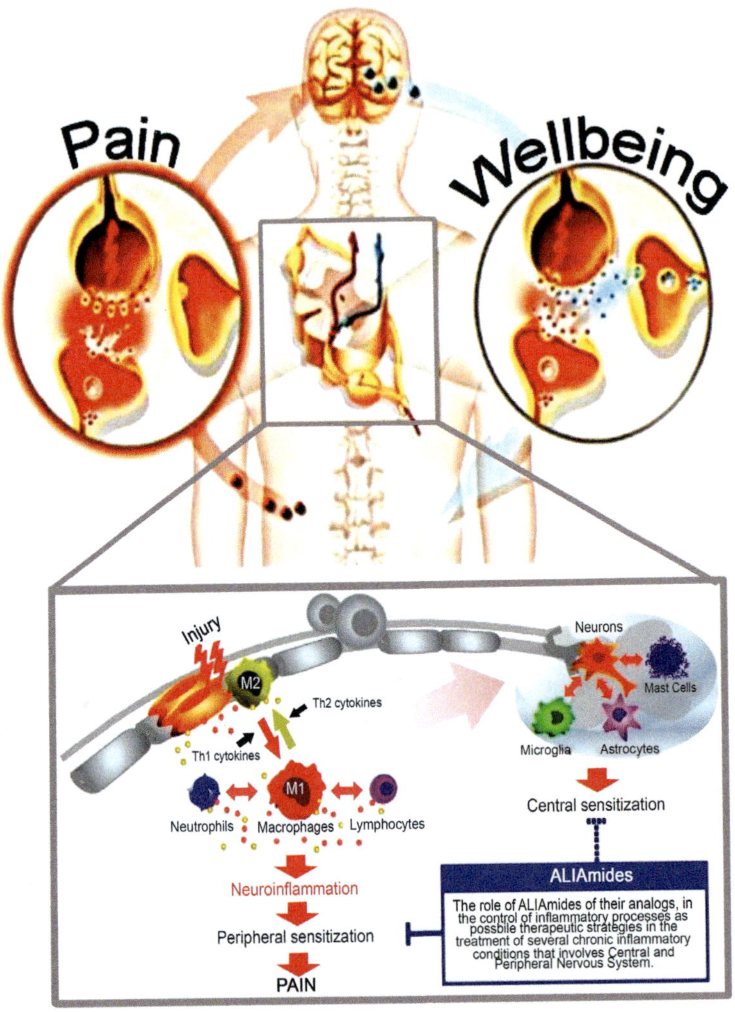

Figure 7.1. Mediators of inflammatory pain.

Source. D'Amico R, Impellizzeri D, Cuzzocrea S, Di Paola R. ALIAmides Update: Palmitoylethanolamide and its formulations on management of peripheral neuropathic pain. *International Journal of Molecular Sciences*. 2020; 21(15):5330. https://doi.org/10.3390/ijms21155330.

Note: Local inflammatory cells and infiltrating cells release mediators including pro-inflammatory cytokines [tumor necrosis factor (TNF; formerly known as TNFα), bradykinin, prostaglandins, interleukin-1β (IL-1β), and interleukin-6 (IL-6)], H^+, ATP, nerve growth factors (NGFs), and pro-inflammatory chemokines [CC-chemokine ligand 2 (CCL2), CXC-chemokine ligand 1 (CXCL1) and), CXC-chemokine ligand 5 (CXCL5)]. Receptors for these inflammatory mediators, including G-protein-coupled receptors (GPCRs), ionotropic receptors, and tyrosine kinase receptors, are expressed on nociceptive neurones. Stimulation causes generation of second messengers, such as cyclic AMP and Ca^{2+}, and downstream activation of kinases [protein kinase A (PKA), protein kinase C (PKC), extracellular signal-regulated kinase (ERK), phosphoinositide 3-kinase (PI3K), calcium/calmodulin-dependent protein kinase (CaMK), and the mitogen-activated protein kinases (MAPKs), p38 MAPK, and JUN N-terminal kinase (JNK)]. Activation of these kinases causes peripheral sensitization by modulating transduction molecules (e.g., transient receptor potential cation channel subfamily A member 1 (TRPA1) and TRPV1) and conduction (voltage-gated sodium channels Nav1.7–1.9). Activated nociceptors release substance P and calcitonin gene-related peptide (CGRP), involved in the generation of neurogenic inflammation and (CGRP) regulation of lymphadenopathy. Bacterial infection with Staphylococcus aureus induces neuronal hyperexcitability by releasing bacterial N-formylated peptides (FPs) and the formation of the pore-forming toxin α-hemolysin (α-HL). The bacteria can also directly activate nociceptors.

Underlying these changes is a rapid (minutes) plasticity that is nearly always the result of tissue trauma and surgery. This increased nociception should typically subside as the wound heals. Maladaptive reactions, such as insufficient resolution of these alterations following inflammation, are probably crucial in the transition from acute to chronic pain conditions.

7.2.5.3. Neuropathic Pain

Neuropathic pain is the term used to describe pain resulting from a somatosensory nervous system lesion or disease. The lesion may affect the structure and function of the somatosensory nervous system and manifest at the molecular, cellular, or tissue level. Increased sensitivity to both harmful and benign stimuli and sensory loss are the outcomes. Common clinical features of neuropathic pain include positive phenomena like hyperalgesia (heightened pain after painful stimuli), hyperpathia (an eruptive pain that extends beyond the duration of a stimulus), and allodynia (pain after non-painful stimuli). Neuropathic mechanisms may account for a large portion of the chronicity in pain presentations in vascular patients. Neuropathic pain in particular plays a significant role in critical limb ischemia, the associated ischemic pain, and the chronic pain that may persist following surgery. Neuropathic pain is characterized by modifications in G-protein-coupled receptors, ion channels, neurotransmitters, and central activation.

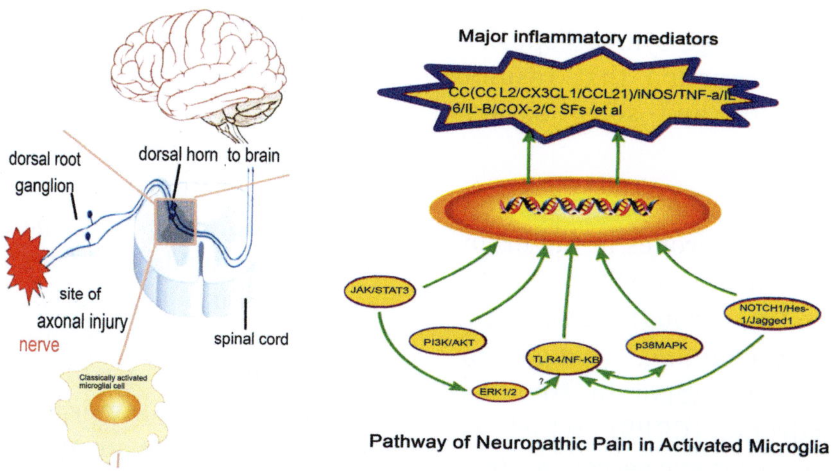

Figure 7.2. *Europathic pain and microglia signal transduction pathway.*

Source. Ji A, Xu J. Neuropathic Pain: Biomolecular intervention and imaging via targeting microglia activation. *Biomolecules.* 2021; 11(9):1343. https://doi.org/10.3390/biom11091343.

Note: DRG: dorsal root ganglia; CC: chemokines; IL: interleukin; CSFs: colony stimulating factors; TNF: tumor necrosis factor; iNOS: inducible nitric oxide synthase; COX-2: cyclooxygenase 2; p38MAPK: p38 mitogen-activated protein kinase; ERK: extracellular signal-regulated kinase; TLR4: toll-like receptor 4; NF-κB: nuclear factor-kappa B; PI3K: phosphatidylinositide 3-kinase; AKT: proteinkinaseB; JAK: c-Jun N-terminal kinase; STAT3: Signal Transducer In addition, Activator Of Transcription 3; NICD: notch intracellular domain); RBP-Jκ: recombination signal binding protein-Jκ; TACE: tumor necrosis factor-α converting enzyme.

7.2.5.4. Involvement of the Autonomic Nervous System in Neuropathic Pain

Primary sensory neurones and the sympathetic nervous system do not communicate with one another under normal circumstances. The two systems may link during conversion to chronic pain through a mechanism called sympathetic–afferent coupling. The expression of adrenergic receptors on afferent nociceptive neurones, the sprouting of sympathetic axons into dorsal root ganglia, and elevated local inflammatory mediators (e.g., sympathetically induced local vasoconstriction that results in nociceptor activation and sensitization maintains interleukin-8.

Central sensitization, or the enhanced reactivity of nociceptive neurones in the brain and spinal cord to normal or subthreshold afferent input, can be brought about by sympathetic–afferent coupling. Changes in vascular reactivity are evident in complex regional pain syndrome (CRPS), which is primarily caused by sympathetic nervous system alterations. PLP, orphan limb pain, may also be impacted by these changes (Rosenwasser, 1996; Selwyin & Braunwald, 1998).

7.2.6. Pain in the Acute Vascular (Surgical) Setting

Procedures performed in vascular surgery range widely, from simple varicose vein surgery to intricate open abdominal aortic aneurysm (AAA) repair. For elective infrarenal AAA repair, the associated morbidity is negligible to 2%, and for emergency ruptured AAA surgery, it is approximately 50%. The usage of anticoagulant medication may restrict the options for managing pain following certain surgeries. Here, we address areas where pain management may be difficult to manage and provide evidence-based treatment options for important vascular procedures.

7.2.6.1. Aortic Aneurysm Repair

Aortic aneurysm repair can be open or endovascular (EVAR), involve the thoracic or abdominal cavity, or both, and be elective or emergency. Acute aortic syndromes are more common in the past 10 years and typically manifest as pain. Strong research has been done on mortality and long-term survival rates when comparing open repair to EVAR. Pain was not a target outcome in any of these sizable, carefully planned trials.

During the same time period, three smaller studies examined physical pain in relation to quality-of-life evaluations following aortic aneurysm repair. These studies revealed that EVAR had no longer-term pain advantage over open repair, aside from a quicker return to baseline quality-of-life scores following surgery. A more recent study examining the long-term quality of life in 171 postoperative patients with ruptured AAA (26 emergency rupture repair, 98 elective open repair, and 47 EVAR) revealed that patients experienced significant pain in the long run, even though their overall quality of life was better than that of a general population with similar characteristics.

Table 7.2. Current Pharmacotherapies Used in Neuropathic Pain Treatment

Class of Drug	Nature of Action	Undesired Effects	Contraindication
Tricyclic antidepressants (Nortriptyline, Desipramine)	Inhibition of serotonin as well as norepinephrine reuptake, sodium channel blockade, anticholinergic	Sleeplessness, anticholinergic effects (e.g., xerostomia or ischuria, obesity)	Cardiovascular disease, epilepsy, glaucoma
Serotonin–norepinephrine reuptake inhibitors (Duloxetine, Venlafaxine)	Inhibition of both serotonin and norepinephrine reuptake	Nausea	Hepatic malfunction, impaired renal function, alcohol use disorder
Calcium channel α2-δ ligands (Gabapentin, Pregabalin)	Diminishes the release of glutamate, norepinephrine as well as substance P, with α2-δ subunit ligands of voltage-gated calcium channel	Somnolence, lightheadedness, peripheral edema	Impaired renal function
Opioid agonist (Morphine)	Agonist action on μ-receptor	Nausea, emesis, improper bowel movement, vertigo	History of substance abuse increased suicidal risk

Source: Shinu P, Morsy MA, Nair AB, Mouslem AKA, Venugopala KN, Goyal M, Bansal M, Jacob S, Deb PK. Novel therapies for the treatment of neuropathic pain: Potential and pitfalls. *Journal of Clinical Medicine*. 2022; 11(11):3002. https://doi.org/10.3390/jcm11113002.

Only one retrospective study comparing a locoregional technique with general anesthesia (GA) in elective EVAR and case reports regarding paravertebral blocks in thoracic or thoraco-abdominal aortic aneurysm repairs provide specific investigations of anesthetic or analgesic choice for aortic aneurysm repair. Asakura and colleagues' retrospective observational work examining the locoregional technique in EVAR does not include pain as an outcome measure. It is still unknown how locoregional use in EVAR affects pain scores or short- or long-term analgesic requirements in comparison to GA. Published case reports on the repair of thoracic aortic aneurysms indicate that paravertebral block or paravertebral catheter insertion, along with postoperative local anesthetic (LA) infusion, are useful for mitigating pain during the surgical and postoperative phases. These publications do not report outcomes related to long-term pain. A well-conducted study examining the effects of epidural anesthesia on morbidity and mortality outcomes in high-risk patients undergoing major surgery provides the only conclusive evidence regarding anesthetic and analgesic techniques for aortic aneurysm repair. 142 of the 915 patients in this cohort underwent aortic aneurysm repair; they were randomly assigned to receive either GA with opioid analgesia or GA with an epidural. Throughout the entire cohort, pain scores three days following surgery were substantially lower in the epidural group. All other outcomes were comparable between the groups, except respiratory failure, which was also significantly lower in the epidural group.

In conclusion, the best pain management strategies for aortic aneurysm repair are currently not well supported by the available data. More investigation is required into the established significance of pain results for patients following aortic aneurysm repair, as well as the known risks of transitioning to chronic pain states following complex surgery.

7.2.6.2. Carotid Endarterectomy

Under either general or regional anesthesia, a carotid endarterectomy (CEA) can be carried out. Cervical plexus blocks can be used for regional anesthesia, though some argue that the superficial kind is safer and offers superior analgesia. The GALA trial, which compared general anesthesia to local anesthesia for carotid surgery, did not show a significant advantage of RA over GA in terms of cost-effectiveness, myocardial infarction, stroke, or mortality. Pain was only taken into account in this trial when determining why a patient would convert from RA to GA during surgery. There was no assessment of chronic pain performed. Subgroup analysis that looked at early postoperative cognitive outcomes did not specifically measure postoperative pain, but it did support the use of RA over GA in terms of cognitive function. According to a survey, 89% of anesthetists primarily located in the USA still use GA for CEA procedures.

A recent Cochrane review aimed to evaluate pain indirectly as part of reported patient satisfaction outcomes by comparing stroke outcomes after GA or RA in CEA. Four of the 14 included studies (a total of 4596 patients) evaluated patient satisfaction; none of them revealed that patients had a preference for one approach over another. That review did not contain any studies that measured pain directly.

Just two studies directly examined the analgesic effects following CEA. A more recent study compared GA plus surgical wound infiltration with ropivacaine 0 point 75%, 20 ml, with GA plus surgical saline infiltration. The first study, published prior to the GALA trial, examined GA with superficial plexus block or placebo. Both demonstrated reduced opioid use in the recovery area, and the groups receiving LA had lower pain scores.

All things considered, there is a slim chance that extra LA infiltration—by surgeons or through a superficial plexus block—will enhance analgesia during the first few hours following CEA. Regarding the long-term effects of pain following CEA, there is no data.

7.2.6.3. Revascularization Procedures

When revascularization techniques prove ineffective or unsuitable, limb amputation is carried out for peripheral artery disease (PAD) in the context of vascular surgery. There isn't much information on how to manage pain during revascularization procedures. This is demonstrated by the lack of information discovered in a recent Cochrane review on neuraxial block for revascularization procedures concerning postoperative pain or patient satisfaction in this group of patients. Pain is a major characteristic of PAD both before and after surgery, which could be one of the confounding factors contributing to this. Unplanned hospital readmission following revascularization surgery is in fact caused in part by pain at rest, though it's unclear if this is due to postoperative or illness-related pain. The trial by Rigg and colleagues, which was previously discussed, provides some limited support for the use of epidurals in revascularization procedures. Aorto-femoral bypass graft surgery was performed on 3% of this cohort, which helped the trial's overall outcomes, which showed lower pain scores three days after surgery. Otherwise, there is no precise data available regarding the best analgesic method for this procedure.

7.2.6.4. Limb Amputation

There are several studies evaluating analgesic approaches for amputation surgery, in contrast to the paucity of studies on pain management for revascularization procedures. This could be connected to the difficulties in managing pain for this particular patient population, who is recognized to be highly susceptible to chronic postoperative pain (stump and phantom pain). Studies evaluating intra- and postoperative analgesic regimens and investigations into preemptive analgesia, which can be initiated up to two days before surgery, comprise the majority of the evidence regarding analgesic management for limb amputation.

Evaluation of preventive pain management strategies is connected to established pain pathways that produce pain following amputation. Preoperative epidurals that were continued after surgery were found to lower the risk of developing post-operative pain syndrome (PLP) in original research on preemptive analgesia. That study, however, had a number of methodological problems. Despite showing good postoperative pain control, subsequent randomized controlled trials did not find a decrease in PLP from epidural analgesia (either preemptive or administered right before surgery). In the review by Ypsilantis and Tang, the evidence supporting preemptive analgesia for persistent post-amputation pain is summarized. The authors conclude that while preemptive analgesia is useful in the short postoperative period, there is no proof that pain following amputation will lessen over the long run. This is in contrast to a more recent single-center study that found amputees receiving pre-emptive fentanyl patient-controlled analgesia or epidural analgesia had less pain than those receiving routine non-pre-emptive preoperative analgesia before, after, and at six months. The study's findings must be validated in a larger patient population.

Research on the implantation of intraoperative perineural catheters and postoperative local anesthetic infiltration protocols indicates a reduction in pain during the first postoperative phase. However, long-term data on the results of pain are lacking. The retrospective design of these studies, as well as the absence of blinding and control groups, pose limitations.

Because PAD amputees have a high mortality rate, evaluating long-term analgesic outcomes presents significant challenges. As a result, research on this topic is still underpowered due to issues with patient dropout or recruitment. Short- and long-term pain reduction may be achieved with analgesia initiated ~2 days before amputation. There is, however, a lack of conclusive evidence to support the claim that any particular intra- or postoperative analgesic method affects long-term results.

7.2.7. Conversion of Pain from Acute to Chronic in Vascular Patients

Maladaptive inflammatory and neuropathic pain syndromes are among the mechanisms that cause acute pain in vascular patients to become chronic. Analgesic decisions made during the perioperative period and possibly even earlier, when the patient first presents with pain related to blood vessels, may have an impact on these processes. The effectiveness of regional anesthesia in preventing chronic postoperative pain was evaluated in a recent meta-analysis. The four amputation studies that were found did not allow for statistical data pooling due to methodological heterogeneity. There was insufficient data to conclusively support the use of epidural and paravertebral analgesia in the non-vascular surgeries covered by the meta-analysis to prevent chronic pain following surgery. The risk factors that lead to the development of chronic pain are thoroughly explained. High levels of acute, baseline, or preoperative pain, psychosocial factors like catastrophizing, female sex, and vague genetic susceptibility are a few of them. A significant contributing factor to the conversion rate to chronic pain states in vascular patients is the high level of baseline pain.

When considered collectively, the data point to the potential benefits of minimizing the conversion to chronic pain states in subgroups of vascular patients, such as PAD patients, by using preemptive analgesic strategies.

7.2.8. Chronic Pain in Vascular Patients

Many anesthetists treat vascular disease patients who need surgery because they already have chronic pain. The following describes the prevalence, etiology (where known), and available treatments for common chronic pain conditions in patients with vascular disease.

7.2.8.1. Phantom Limb Pain and Stump Pain

Out of all amputees, 50–80% experience phantom limb pain. The mechanisms underlying the development of PLP can be classified into two categories: peripheral mechanisms that influence afferent transmission, and central mechanisms that affect efferent signaling. Regenerative axon sprouting occurs peripherally as a result of nerve transection during amputation. These increase the risk of developing neuromas and having maladaptive reactions to chemical and mechanical stimuli. The typical symptoms of neuropathic pain are caused by the ectopic nerve impulses that ensue. Furthermore, there is a chance of sympathetic afferent coupling, which results in sympathetically maintained pain. After limb loss, dorsal horn neurons and somatosensory cortices reorganize centrally, resulting in modifications that modify efferent signaling and preserve PLP. Cortical remapping has been shown by neuroimaging research to be a crucial part of PLP maintenance. Recent research indicates that one of the primary components of the fundamental changes maintaining PLP is pain catastrophizing, which is distinct from anxiety and depression.

The intricate mechanisms underlying PLP necessitate multimodal management, which is reflected in the treatment options available. Topical therapies such as lidocaine or capsaicin patches, injections of botulin toxin at neuroma sites, and transcutaneous electrical nerve stimulation of the stump can target peripheral mechanisms, though the evidence for these treatments is not very strong. To target central changes, a wide range of agents have been employed, with evidence of varying quality. In the early acute phase of PLP presentation, these include gabapentinoids, ketamine, opioids, topiramate (a new-generation antiepileptic), and memantine.

PLP has been used as a context for studying various psychological therapies, such as biofeedback, mirror therapy, mental imagery, hypnosis, and meditation. These therapies may be applied as part of the multimodal approach to PLP management, along with pharmaceutical interventions. We refer readers to two recent reviews for additional reading on PLP management options.

7.2.8.2. Complex Regional Pain Syndrome

About 20 out of every 100,000 patients experience the crippling pain syndrome known as complex regional pain syndrome. With a mean age of occurrence between 37 and 52 years old and a higher female-to-male distribution ratio, the incidence is very low in childhood. Types I and II of complex regional pain syndrome are distinguished by clinical and scientific consensus, not by pathophysiological mechanisms. Patients who meet the "Budapest" criteria and undergo a physical examination are the basis for the diagnosis of CRPS.

Vascular reactivity changes significantly as a result of autonomic dysfunction, one of the complex pathophysiological mechanisms underlying CRPS. Treatments that work focus on established pathophysiological pathways. The use of bisphosphonates or immunoglobulins in CRPS patients has drawn attention recently. Even though CRPS is obviously neuropathic, there isn't enough evidence to support the use of the three analgesics that are commonly used to treat neuropathic pain: gabapentinoids, antidepressants, and opioids. Repetitive transcranial magnetic stimulation appears to help treat CRPS, according to some research. The National Institute for Health and Care Excellence (NICE), UK, has recommended the use of spinal cord stimulation for both intractable CRPS and ischemic pain (PAD). This recommendation is supported by available evidence. Changes in endothelial nitric oxide concentrations and modified spinal processing are just two of the intricate mechanisms underlying the analgesic effects of spinal cord stimulation. The best available data support the use of physical therapies in the treatment of CRPS. Graded motor imagery, a physical therapy that employs mirror therapy and imagined movement, also has some evidence supporting it within this category (Rosenwasser, 1996; Selwyin & Braunwald, 1998).

7.2.8.3. Ischemic Pain in Peripheral Arterial Disease

In the general adult population, the prevalence of PAD is approximately 12%. A disease can be asymptomatic, and approximately 17.8% of people who are at low risk of cardiovascular disease are believed to have asymptomatic PAD. One of the main indicators of PAD is pain, and increasing pain is linked to the disease's advancement. While the onset of critical limb ischemia is preceded by pain at rest, intermittent claudication manifests as pain during exercise that is relieved by rest.

These alterations are related to atherosclerotic blood flow obstruction pathophysiological mechanisms. Due to insufficient oxygen delivery to peripheral tissue, this causes muscle ischemia, a rise in inflammatory mediators, and the eventual degeneration and remodeling of nearby nerve endings. Sensitization to inflammatory pain cascades leads to peripheral and ultimately central sensitization.

Exercise is advised in the management of intermittent claudication for PAD in its earlier stages, though it's not clear how best to administer exercise therapy. Though the prevalence of critical limb ischemia and advanced PAD is rising, little is known about the best ways to manage these conditions. Recent reviews of spinal cord stimulation in ischemic pain are encouraging, indicating that patients with Parkinson's disease (PAD) who are not responding to traditional analgesic regimens may find success with this treatment option. Patients with severe ischemic pain, in particular, appear to benefit greatly from spinal cord stimulator implantation. But if revascularization treatments and analgesics don't work, amputation is still the only option. As was previously mentioned, there is a significant risk of PLP with amputation.

7.2.8.4. Thoracic Outlet Syndrome

Because major veins and arteries are involved, thoracic outlet syndrome (TOS) is a complex chronic pain syndrome associated with vascular disease. Three related syndromes are referred to as thoracic outlet syndrome: vascular TOS (compression of the major blood vessels in the upper chest), neurogenic TOS (compression of the brachial plexus), and painful non-specific or disputed TOS. There is insufficient data on incidence and prevalence, and the diagnostic criteria for TOS are not standardized. Severe pain is linked to thoracic outlet syndrome and can be attributed to both neuropathic and ischemic mechanisms. First rib resection is the only treatment option that has been shown to be clearly associated with improved pain. Despite having a mixed evidence base in TOS, other treatments (such as standard neuropathic pain treatments, exercise and physiotherapy, and local anesthetic scalene muscle injections) are still used either in addition to or instead of surgical intervention.

7.3. Pain in Hemopathies

Pain can be seen in many hemopathies for various reasons. Four hemophilic disorders, sickle cell disease, essential thrombocythemia, which frequently exhibits an erythromelalgia syndrome, hemophilic disorders, and multiple myeloma, which frequently exhibits bone pain, all have pain as a primary symptom. We will go into great detail about these four syndromes.

7.3.1. Pain in Sickle Cell Disease

Sickle cell disease is a genetic illness that is more common in some African populations and is inherited in an autosomal recessive pattern. The sickle cell gene provides a selective advantage to these individuals. e. resistance to malarial infection. In America and other places where the presence of African groups is significant, the disease affects black populations with African ancestry.

Hemolytic anemia and various complications arising from rheologic abnormalities, such as haematuria due to renal papillary necrosis, stroke due to cerebral infarction, and painful crises due to infarctions of different organs, are the primary clinical manifestations of sickle cell disease (Ballas, 1998). Acute pain is the most common complication following the newborn period and is frequently the initial indicator of a disease. According to Embury (1996), the frequency of pain peaks in the third and fourth decades, and after the second decade, frequent pain is linked to higher mortality rates. Precipitating factors that include cold, infection, fever, dehydration, menstruation, alcohol consumption, and exposure to low oxygen tension can cause painful crises. The majority of painful episodes, however, lack a distinct cause. Aside from these variables, each patient experiences painful crises at a significantly different rate.

Different body parts may experience localized pain (Ballas, 1998). Embury (1996) describes an acute chest syndrome that manifests as dyspnea, fever, chest pain, leucocytosis, and pulmonary infiltrates on radiography. The syndrome is typically brought on by infection and Vaso-occlusion. During painful episodes, the abdomen, back, and limbs are frequently affected as well. It is challenging to differentiate between painful episodes of sickle cell disease and other acute processes like appendicitis, biliary colic, and perforated viscus because pain during abdominal crises mimics intra-abdominal disorders. Increased red cell sickling on peripheral blood smears and signs of hemolysis provide a clue to the differential diagnosis.

After a few hours to weeks, the episodes end and the baseline is restored. Resolution and onset can occur suddenly or gradually. Certain patients might be in constant, chronic pain. Bone infarctions are associated with severe skeletal pain. Arthritic pain, swelling, and effusion can all be brought on by periarticular infarctions. Regular pain can lead to psychosocial issues like poor family relationships and social isolation as well as feelings of hopelessness, depression, and apathy. According to Shapiro et al. (1995), children and adolescents with sickle cell disease may find it difficult to attend school due to the negative effects of pain on psychosocial functioning.

Steroid and non-steroidal anti-inflammatory medicine (NSAIDs) is the mainstay of treatment for painful episodes of sickle cell disease; in more severe cases, mild or strong opioids are added. Infection-related conditions such as acute chest syndrome also require antibiotic treatment. The incidence of painful episodes may be reduced by hydroxycarbamide (hydroxyurea) therapy, which also improves other clinical manifestations of sickle cell disease. Antidepressant medication and psychosocial support are two components of a comprehensive strategy for addressing pain in sickle cell disease patients (Ballas, 1998).

7.3.2. Pain in Essential Thrombocythemia

Thrombocytosis is the main disease manifestation in essential thrombocythemia; this condition is also seen in other acute or chronic myeloproliferative disorders, including polycythemia vera and granulocytic leukemia (Tefferi & Silverstein, 1996). Erythromelalgia is by far the most common painful condition, though myocardial infarction, headache, and angina are also possible. Acute pain attacks in the lower limbs without any cutaneous manifestation were observed in some of the cases we observed, while others exhibited a true case of erythromelalgia. When aspirin was given, the symptoms vanished in every instance.

7.3.3. Pain in Hemophilic Disorders

A class of blood coagulation disorders is known as hemophilia. Deficits in factor VIII and IX, respectively, cause Christmas disease (hemophilia B) and classic hemophilia (hemophilia A). Both hemophilia A and hemophilia B are linked to traumatic and recurrent hemarthroses.

Pain may complicate hemophiliac arthropathy in different ways:

1. Hemarthroses are characterized by load pain and joint swelling: the most involved joints are the 132 knees, ankles, elbows, and shoulders.
2. Septic arthritis: this complication is not rare and is accompanied by fever and allodynia in the affected joints (Rasner & Bhogal, 1991; Gilliland, 1998).
3. Subacute or chronic arthritis with intraarticular effusion and synovitis whose typical symptom is morning stiffness and pain on awakening in the morning, lasting up to 2–3 h.
4. End-stage hemophiliac arthritis: pain, in this case, is continuous and exacerbated by little movements of the joints; the joint appears enlarged and 'knobby' owing to osteophytic bony overgrowth. Pain is due to severe restriction of motion, fibrous ankylosis, subluxation, joint laxity, and malalignment. The joint changes stimulated by repeated intraarticular bleeding resemble those of rheumatoid arthritis (Gilliland, 1998).
5. Muscle and soft tissue hemorrhage: bleeding into muscles and soft tissues is common and provokes spontaneous pain, which worsens on moving the affected muscle. The most frequently

involved muscles are the iliopsoas and the volar forearm muscles: if the pressure remains elevated for several hours cramp-like pain worsens and the normal function of muscles and nerves is compromised, and over time, muscle infarction and nerve injury lead to Volkman's ischemic contracture accompanied by a continuous very intense pain on the volar surface of the hand which interferes with sleep (Heck, 1997).

The best therapy is an infusion of recombinant factor VIII to stop bleeding. Non-steroidal anti-inflammatory drugs are contraindicated as they may worsen bleeding (York, 1998).

7.3.4. Pain in Multiple Myeloma

A single clone can produce multiple myeloma, which is a cancerous proliferation of plasma cells. Numerous organ dysfunctions and symptoms are caused by the tumor, its byproducts, and the host's reaction to them. About 70% of patients experience bone pain, which is the most common symptom resulting from bone destruction. In contrast to the pain of metastatic carcinoma, which is frequently worse at night, myeloma pain is typically in the back and ribs and is triggered by movement. When a myeloma patient experiences persistent localized pain, it typically indicates a pathologic fracture (Longo, 1998). Loss of bladder and bowel control, radicular pain, and cord compression can result from bone damage and collapse. Sensorimotor mono- and polyneuropathies, including carpal tunnel syndrome, may be brought on by amyloid infiltration of peripheral nerves.

A Closer Look

Algogenic Process

An algogenic process refers to any biological mechanism or pathway that leads to the generation or modulation of pain signals within the body. These processes can involve various physiological and biochemical changes in tissues, nerves, and the central nervous system, ultimately resulting in the perception of pain. Understanding algogenic processes is crucial for elucidating the mechanisms underlying pain conditions and developing effective treatments.

One common algogenic process involves tissue injury or inflammation. When tissues are damaged or inflamed due to trauma, infection, or disease, a cascade of events is triggered, including the release of inflammatory mediators such as prostaglandins, cytokines, and histamine. These substances sensitize nerve endings, particularly nociceptors, specialized sensory neurons that detect potentially harmful stimuli, leading to heightened pain sensitivity and the generation of pain signals.

Another important algogenic process involves the activation of peripheral and central nervous system pathways. Nociceptors transmit pain signals from the site of injury or inflammation to the spinal cord and brain, where they are processed and perceived as pain. Peripheral sensitization occurs when nociceptors become more responsive to stimuli, lowering the threshold for pain perception. Central sensitization, on the other hand, involves changes in the spinal cord and brain that amplify pain signals and prolong pain perception, even after the initial stimulus is removed.

Neuropathic pain, which arises from dysfunction or damage to the nervous system itself, involves distinct algogenic processes. Nerve injury or compression can lead to aberrant signaling patterns, such as spontaneous firing or increased excitability of neurons, resulting in chronic pain conditions like neuropathic pain.

Psychological factors, including stress, anxiety, and depression, can also modulate pain perception through complex interactions with the nervous system. These factors can influence neurotransmitter levels, pain processing pathways, and pain modulation systems, contributing to the development or exacerbation of pain conditions.

Treatment of pain often involves targeting specific algogenic processes to alleviate symptoms and improve quality of life. This may include pharmacological interventions such as analgesic medications, anti-inflammatory drugs, or neuromodulators, as well as non-pharmacological approaches like physical therapy, cognitive-behavioral therapy, and interventional procedures. By addressing the underlying algogenic processes involved in pain generation and modulation, healthcare providers can tailor treatments to the individual needs of patients and enhance pain management outcomes.

Summary

- Heart, vascular, and hemopathic pain collectively refer to a spectrum of pain syndromes originating from the cardiovascular system and blood-related disorders.
- Chest wall pain may also accompany or follow herpes zoster, chest injury, or Tietze's syndrome (i.e., discomfort localized in swelling of the costochondral and costosternal joints, which are painful to palpation).
- The pain is generally deep, more rarely superficial, with the same qualities and radiations as those described in myocardial infarction, but the intensity and duration are less.
- Angina may evolve into myocardial infarction. After myocardial infarction, stable or unstable angina may develop.
- A precordial pain, often radiating with characteristics that resemble those of angina, worries many anxious patients, often with a depressive trait.
- Vascular pain is a complex area. It may be divided into three sections: arterial pain; pain due to lesion or dysfunction of the microvessels (arterioles, capillaries, small venules); and venous pain.
- Pain originating from microvessels must be distinguished from classic arterial and venous pain for pathophysiological and clinical reasons.
- A typical venous pain is observed in thrombophlebitis. In superficial thrombophlebitis the vein may be apparent as a red, tender cord.
- In four hemopathies, pain is a fundamental symptom: sickle cell disease, in which strong pain crises in trunks and limbs are frequent; essential thrombocythemia, in which an erythromelalgic syndrome is frequently observed; hemophilic disorders; and multiple myeloma, in which bone pain can be observed.
- Haemophilia is a group of disorders of blood coagulation. Classic hemophilia (hemophilia A) and Christmas disease (hemophilia B) are deficiencies of factor VIII and IX, respectively.

References

1. Antman, E. M., & Braunwald, E. (1997). Acute myocardial infarction. In E. Braunwald (Ed.), *Heart Disease* (5th ed., pp. 1184–1288). Saunders, Philadelphia.
2. Aviado, D. M., & Schmidt, C. F. (1955). Reflexes from stretch receptors in blood vessels, heart and lungs. *Physiological Reviews, 35*, 247–300.
3. Ball, E. V. (1996). Erythromelalgia. In J. C. Bennett & F. Plum (Eds.), *Cecil Textbook of Medicine* (20th ed., p. 1528). Saunders, Philadelphia.
4. Ballas, S. K. (1998). *Sickle Cell Pain*. IASP Press, Seattle.
5. Blomberg, S., Emanuelsson, H., Kvist, H., et al. (1990). Effects of thoracic epidural anesthesia on coronary arteries and arterioles in patients with coronary artery disease. *Anesthesiology, 75*, 840–847.
6. Bonica, J. J. (1990). Causalgia and other reflex sympathetic dystrophies. In J. J. Bonica (Ed.), *The Management of Pain* (2nd ed., pp. 220–243). Lea & Febiger, Philadelphia.
7. Braunwald, E. (1997). Valvular heart disease. In E. Braunwald (Ed.), *Heart Disease* (5th ed., pp. 1007–1076). Saunders, Philadelphia.

8. Brown, A. M. (1967). Excitation of afferent cardiac sympathetic nerve fibers during myocardial ischaemia. *Journal of Physiology, 190*, 35–53.

9. Brunton, T. L. (1867). On the use of nitrite of amyl in angina pectoris. *Lancet, 2*, 97.

10. Cannon, R. O. (1995). Cardiac pain. In G. F. Gebhart (Ed.), *Visceral pain* (pp. 373–389). IASP Press, Seattle.

11. Cervero, F. (1994). Sensory innervation of the viscera: Peripheral basis of visceral pain. *Physiological Reviews, 74*, 95–137.

12. Cervero, F. (1995). Mechanisms of visceral pain: Past and present. In G. F. Gebhart (Ed.), *Visceral Pain* (pp. 25–40). IASP Press, Seattle.

13. Creager, M. A., & Dzau, V. J. (1998). Vascular diseases of the extremities. In A. S. Fauci, E. Braunwald, K. J. Isselbacher, et al. (Eds.), *Harrison's Principles of Internal Medicine* (14th ed., pp. 1398–1406). McGraw-Hill, New York.

14. Dorigo, B., Bartoli, V., Grisillo, D., & Beconi, D. (1979). Fibrositis myofascial pain in intermittent claudication. Effect of anesthetic block of trigger points on exercise tolerance. *Pain, 6*, 183–190.

15. Dressler, W. (1956). Post-myocardial infarction syndrome; preliminary report of a complication resembling idiopathic, recurrent, benign pericarditis. *Journal of the American Medical Association, 160*, 1379–1383.

16. Embury, S. H. (1996). Sickle cell anemia and associated hemoglobinopathies. In J. C. Bennett & F. Plum (Eds.), *Cecil Textbook of Medicine* (20th ed., pp. 882–893). Saunders, Philadelphia.

17. Fauci, A. S. (1998). The vasculitis syndromes. In A. S. Fauci, E. Braunwald, K. J. Isselbacher, et al. (Eds.), *Harrison's Principles of Internal Medicine*. McGraw-Hill, New York, pp. 1910–1922.

18. Friedberg, C. K. (1956). *Disease of the Heart* (2nd ed.). Saunders, Philadelphia.

19. Froment, R., & Gonin, A. (1956). *Les angors coronariens intriqués*. Expansion Scientifique Française, Paris.

20. Geppetti, P., & Holzer, P. (Eds.). (1996). *Neurogenic Inflammation*. CRC Press, Boca Raton.

21. Gersh, B. J., & Braunwald, E. (1997). Chronic coronary artery disease. In E. Braunwald (Ed.), *Heart Disease* (5th ed., pp. 1289–1365). Saunders, Philadelphia.

22. Gilliland, B. C. (1998). Relapsing polychondritis and other arthritides. In A. S. Fauci, E. Braunwald, K. J. Isselbacher, et al. (Eds.), *Harrison's Principles of Internal Medicine* (14th ed., pp. 1951–1963). McGraw-Hill, New York.

23. Goyal, R. K. (1998). Diseases of the esophagus. In A. S. Fauci, E. Braunwald, K. J. Isselbacher, et al. (Eds.), *Harrison's Principles of Internal Medicine* (14th ed., pp. 1588–1596). McGraw-Hill, New York.

24. Heck, L. V., Jr. (1997). Arthritis associated with hematologic disorders, storage diseases, disorders of lipid metabolism and dysproteinemias. In W. J. Koopman (Ed.), *Arthritis and Allied Conditions* (13th ed., pp. 1697–1717). Williams & Wilkins, Baltimore.

25. Isselbacher, E. M., Eagle, K. A., & Desanctis, R. W. (1997). Diseases of the aorta. In E. Braunwald (Ed.), *Heart Disease* (5th ed., pp. 1546–1581). Saunders, Philadelphia.

26. Jänig, W. (1996). The puzzle of 'reflex sympathetic dystrophy': Mechanisms, hypotheses, open questions. In W. Jänig & M. Stanton-Hicks (Eds.), *Reflex Sympathetic Dystrophy: A Reappraisal* (pp. 1–24). IASP Press, Seattle.

27. Kannel, W. B., & Abbott, R. D. (1984). Incidence and prognosis of unrecognized myocardial infarction. *New England Journal of Medicine, 311*, 1144–1147.

28. Kemp, H. G. (1973). Left ventricular function in patients with the anginal syndrome and normal coronary arteriograms. *American Journal of Cardiology, 32*, 375–376.

29. Kirnö, K., Friberg, P., Grzegorczyk, A., et al. (1994). Thoracic epidural anesthesia during coronary artery bypass surgery: Effects on cardiac sympathetic activity, myocardial blood flow and metabolism, and central hemodynamics. *Anesthesia and Analgesia, 79*, 1075–1081.

30. Kontos, H. A. (1996). Vascular diseases of the limbs. In J. C. Bennett & F. Plum (Eds.), *Cecil Textbook of Medicine* (20th ed., pp. 346–357). Saunders, Philadelphia.

31. Lewis, T. (1942). *Pain*. Macmillan, New York.

32. Longo, D. L. (1998). Plasma cell disorders. In A. S. Fauci, E. Braunwald, K. J. Isselbacher, et al. (Eds.), *Harrison's Principles of Internal Medicine* (14th ed., pp. 712–718). McGraw-Hill, New York.

33. Lorell, B. H. (1997). Pericardial diseases. In E. Braunwald (Ed.), *Heart Disease* (5th ed., pp. 1478–1534). Saunders, Philadelphia.

34. Malliani, A. (1986). The elusive link between transient myocardial ischaemia and pain. *Circulation, 73*, 201–204.

35. Malliani, A. (1995). The conceptualization of cardiac pain as a nonspecific and unreliable alarm system. In G. F. Gebhart (Ed.), *Visceral Pain* (pp. 63–74). IASP Press, Seattle.

36. Malliani, A., & Lombardi, F. (1982). Considerations of fundamental mechanisms eliciting cardiac pain. *American Heart Journal, 103*, 575–578.

37. Maresca, M., Nuzzaci, G., & Zoppi, M. (1984). Muscular pain in chronic occlusive arterial diseases of the limbs. In C. Benedetti, C. R. Chapman, & G. Moricca (Eds.), *Recent Advances in the Management of Pain* (pp. 521–527). Raven Press, New York.

38. Maseri, A. (1995). *Ischemic Heart Disease*. Churchill Livingstone, New York.

39. Maseri, A., Severi, S., Nes, M. D., et al. (1978). 'Variant' angina: One aspect of a continuous spectrum of vasospastic myocardial ischemia. Pathogenetic mechanisms, estimated incidence and clinical and arteriographic findings in 138 patients. *American Journal of Cardiology, 42*, 1019–1035.

40. Melzack, R. (1973). *The Puzzle of Pain*. Penguin, Harmondsworth.

41. Nathan, P. W. (1962). Pain traces left in the central nervous system. In C. A. Keele & R. Smith (Eds.), *The Assessment of Pain in Man and Animals* (pp. 129–134). Livingstone, Edinburgh.

42. Neri Serneri, G. G., Modesti, P. A., Gensini, G. F., et al. (1995). Randomized comparison of subcutaneous heparin, intravenous heparin, and aspirin in unstable angina. *Lancet, 345*, 1201–1204.

43. Olausson, K., Magnusdottir, H., Lurje, L., et al. (1997). Anti-ischemic and anti-anginal effects of thoracic epidural anesthesia versus those of conventional medical therapy in the treatment of severe refractory unstable angina pectoris. *Circulation, 96*, 2178–2182.

44. Prinzmetal, M., Kennamer, R., Merliss, R., et al. (1959). A variant form of angina pectoris. *American Journal of Medicine, 27*, 375–388.

45. Procacci, P. (1969). A survey of modern concepts of pain. In P. J. Vinken & G. W. Bruyn (Eds.), *Handbook of Clinical Neurology* (Vol. 1, pp. 114–146). North-Holland, Amsterdam.

46. Procacci, P., & Maresca, M. (1987a). Clinical aspects of heart pain. In M. Tiengo, J. Eccles, A. C. Cuello, & D. Ottoson (Eds.), *Advances in Pain Research and Therapy* (Vol. 10: Pain and mobility, pp. 127–133). Raven Press, New York.

47. Procacci, P., & Maresca, M. (1987b). Reflex sympathetic dystrophies and algo dystrophies: Historical and pathogenic considerations. *Pain, 31*, 137–146.

48. Procacci, P., Zoppi, M., & Maresca, M. (1986). Clinical approach to visceral sensation. In F. Cervero & J. F. B. Morrison (Eds.), *Visceral Sensation* (pp. 21–28). Elsevier, Amsterdam.

49. Procacci, P., Zoppi, M., Padeletti, L., & Maresca, M. (1976). Myocardial infarction without pain. A study of the sensory function of the upper limbs. *Pain, 2*, 309–313.

50. Rasner, S. M., & Bhogal, R. S. (1991). Infectious arthritis in a hemophiliac. *Journal of Rheumatology, 8*, 519–523.

51. Rinzler, S. H. (1951). *Cardiac Pain*. Thomas, Springfield, IL.

52. Rogers, W. J. (1996). Angina pectoris. In J. C. Bennett & F. Plum (Eds.), *Cecil Textbook of Medicine* (20th ed., pp. 296–301). Saunders, Philadelphia.

53. Rosenwasser, L. J. (1996). The vasculitic syndromes. In J. C. Bennett & F. Plum (Eds.), *Cecil Textbook of Medicine* (20th ed., pp. 1490–1495). Saunders, Philadelphia.

54. Selwyin, A. P., & Braunwald, E. (1998). Ischemic heart disease. In A. S. Fauci, E. Braunwald, K. J. Isselbacher, et al. (Eds.), *Harrison's Principles of Internal Medicine* (14th ed., pp. 1365–1375). McGraw-Hill, New York.

55. Shapiro, B. S., Dinges, D. F., Orne, E. C., et al. (1995). Home management of sickle cell-related pain in children and adolescents: Natural history and impact on school attendance. *Pain, 61*, 139–144.

56. Stern, S. (1998). *Silent Myocardial Ischemia*. Martin Dunitz, London.

57. Tefferi, A., & Silverstein, M. N. (1996). Chronic myeloproliferative diseases. In J. C. Bennett & F. Plum (Eds.), *Cecil Textbook of Medicine* (20th ed., pp. 922–925). Saunders, Philadelphia.

58. Teodori, U., & Galletti, R. (1962). *II Dolore Nelle Affezioni Degli Organi Interni Del Torace*. Pozzi, Roma.

59. White, J. C., & Sweet, W. H. (1955). *Pain. Its Mechanisms and Neurosurgical Control*. Thomas, Springfield, IL.

60. York, J. R. (1998). Endocrine and hemoglobin-related arthropathies and storage diseases. In J. H. Klippel & P. A. Dieppe (Eds.), *Rheumatology* (2nd ed., pp. 8–24). Mosby, London.

61. Zimmermann, M. (1979). Peripheral and central nervous mechanisms of nociception, pain and pain therapy: Facts and hypotheses. In J. J. Bonica, J. C. Liebeskind, & D. Albe-Fessard (Eds.), *Proceedings of the Second World Congress on Pain* (pp. 3–32). Raven Press, New York.

62. Zoppi, M., Zamponi, A., Pagni, E., & Buoncristiano, U. (1985). A way to understand erythromelalgia. *Journal of the Autonomic Nervous System, 13*, 85–89.

Chapter

8

GENITOURINARY PAIN

Contents

Introduction

Genitourinary pain refers to a wide variety of pain syndromes that impact the kidneys, bladder, ureters, urethra, prostate, and reproductive organs, among other organs and structures within the genitourinary system. These illnesses, which can affect people of all ages and genders, can significantly reduce quality of life and cause significant discomfort. It is crucial to comprehend the underlying causes, mechanisms, and management techniques of genitourinary pain in order to effectively care for patients with urologic and reproductive health concerns.

Genitourinary pain refers to any discomfort that affects the kidneys, bladder, ureters, urethra, and genital organs as well as the urinary and reproductive systems. It is caused by a range of illnesses, including inflammation, infections, structural irregularities, and functional issues. Urinary tract infections (UTIs), kidney stones, prostatitis, pelvic floor dysfunction, endometriosis, interstitial cystitis/bladder pain syndrome (IC/BPS), and prostatitis are among the common causes.

Urinary urgency, frequency, lower abdominal or pelvic pain, pain during urination, and sexual dysfunction are all possible signs of genitourinary pain. A complete medical history, a physical examination, and frequently diagnostic tests like imaging studies, urine analyzes, and specialized procedures are all part of the diagnosis process. The goals of management techniques are to treat the underlying cause, reduce symptoms, and enhance general reproductive and urologic health. Medication, dietary adjustments, pelvic floor therapy, lifestyle modifications, and occasionally surgical procedures may be necessary for this. Effective management and enhanced quality of life for patients with genitourinary pain necessitate collaborative care among urologists, gynecologists, nephrologists, pain specialists, and other medical specialists.

Orientation and Directional Terms

Genitourinary pain	Genitourinary pain syndromes present at the confluence of pain, infection, and urinary symp- toms.	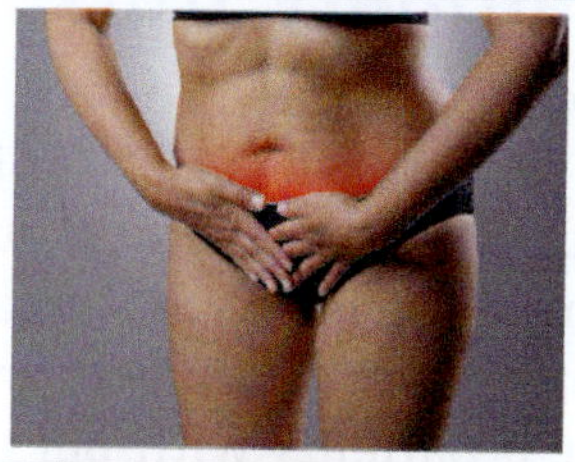
Urinary tract infections	Urinary tract infections are more common in women. They usually occur in the bladder or urethra, but more serious infections involve the kidney.	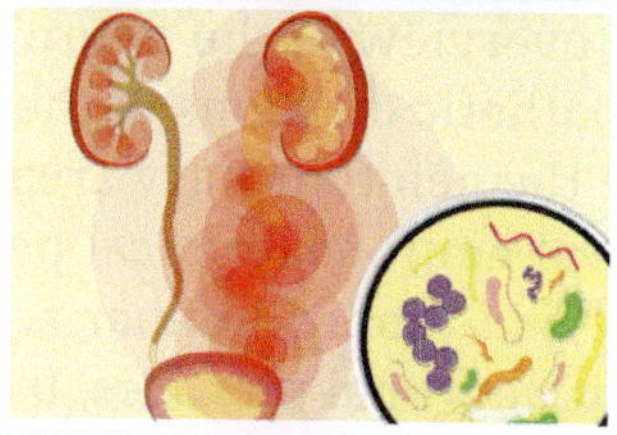
Sexual dysfunction	Sexual dysfunction is a problem that prevents a person or couple from enjoying or having sex, and it can affect any stage of sexual activity.	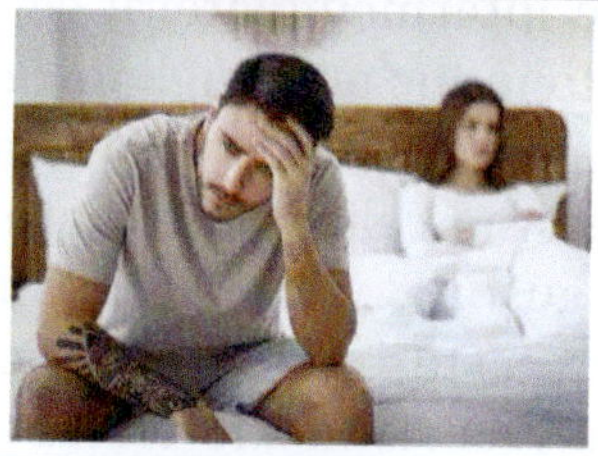
Micturition	Micturition (urination) is the process of urine excretion from the urinary bladder.	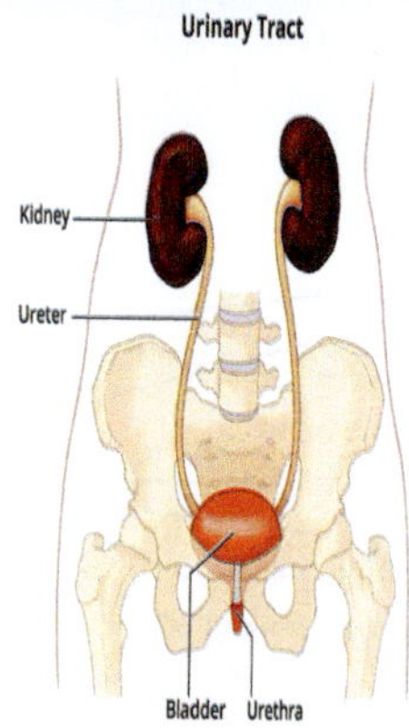
Hypogastric plexus	The hypogastric plexus is the target of sympathetic neurolysis for painful lesions involving the pelvic viscera.	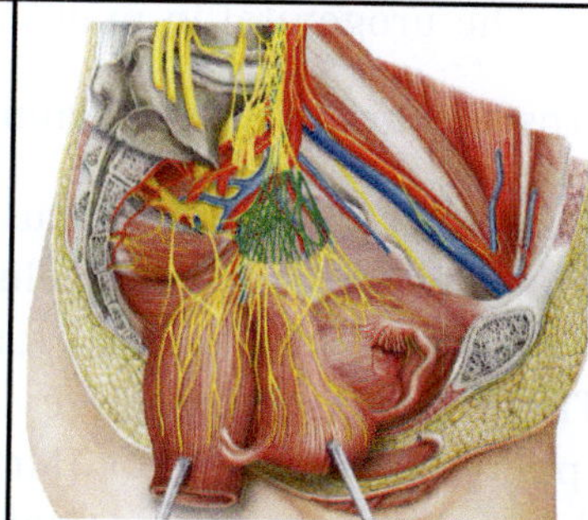

8.1. Neurobiology of the Genitourinary Tract

The genitourinary tract and the pelvic region together constitute the highly specialized area of the body that performs a variety of fundamental biological functions, such as copulation, reproduction, and micturition. Precise nervous system control, in conjunction with endocrine and other local control mechanisms, is necessary for the display of these various functions. A brief review of genitourinary neurobiology is provided in this paragraph, aimed at medical professionals who assess and manage patients with persistent urogenital pain. Burnett and Wesselmann (1999) provide a thorough overview of the neurobiology of the pelvis and genitourinary tract. The sympathetic and parasympathetic divisions of the autonomic nervous system, as well as the somatic nervous system, innervate the genitourinary area (Morrison, 1987; de Groat et al., 1993, de Groat, 1994). According to a general neuroanatomical perspective, this innervation is carried out by dual projections from the sacral and thoracolumbar segments of the spinal cord. These projections mostly converge into peripheral neuronal plexuses, from which nerve fibers ramify throughout the pelvic floor. At sacral levels, the intermediolateral cell column—also known as the sacral parasympathetic nucleus—is where autonomic preganglionic efferents primarily originate, while the cell bodies of corresponding afferents are located within dorsal root ganglia. Preganglionic projections to the superior hypogastric plexus and the celiac plexus are part of the sympathetic thoracolumbar outflow to the urogenital tract (Ferguson & Bell, 1993; Lincoln & Burnstock, 1993). The ureter, kidney, adrenal gland, renal pelvis, and testes receive most of their autonomic innervation from the celiac plexus. The internal spermatic vessels in the testes also receive some sympathetic input.

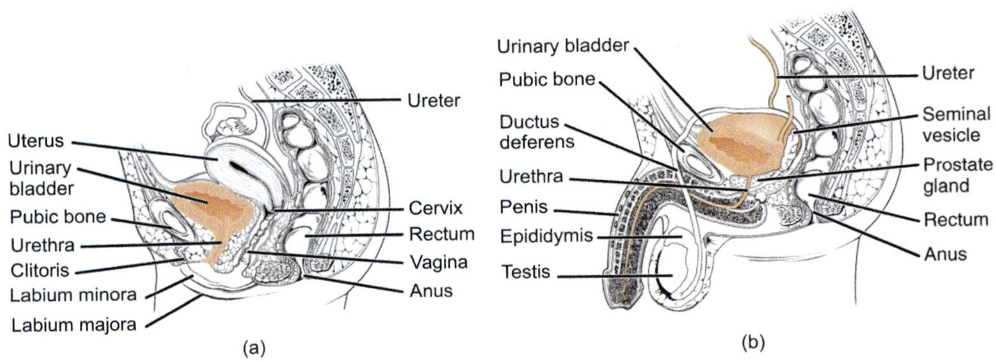

Figure 8.1. The urogenital in males and females.

Source: https://courses.lumenlearning.com/suny-ap2/chapter/gross-anatomy-of-urine-transport/.

The superior hypogastric plexus receives most of the sympathetic input to the genital tract and pelvic urinary organs. Thoracolumbar preganglionic nerves not only supply pelvic structures through this route, but they also form synapses on postganglionic nerves in sympathetic chain ganglia. These synapses converge with autonomic sacral nerve projections and with somatic neuronal pathways in the pelvis (McKenna & Nadelhaft, 1986). Preganglionic nerves, also known as the pelvic splanchnic nerves, make up the parasympathetic sacral outflow (S2-S4). The pelvic splanchnic nerve and the S2–S4 dorsal root ganglia are home to parasympathetic afferent cell bodies. According to Lincoln and Burnstock (1993), the primary neuronal coordinating center supplying the pelvic floor and visceral structures of the pelvis is the inferior hypogastric plexus. The inferior hypogastric plexus receives input from the parasympathetic nervous system (pelvic splanchnic nerve) and the sympathetic nervous system (superior hypogastric plexus and its caudal extension, the hypogastric plexus, the sympathetic chain ganglia) (de Groat, 1994). These sympathetic and parasympathetic projections carry both efferent and afferent fibers (Jänig & Koltzenburg, 1993).

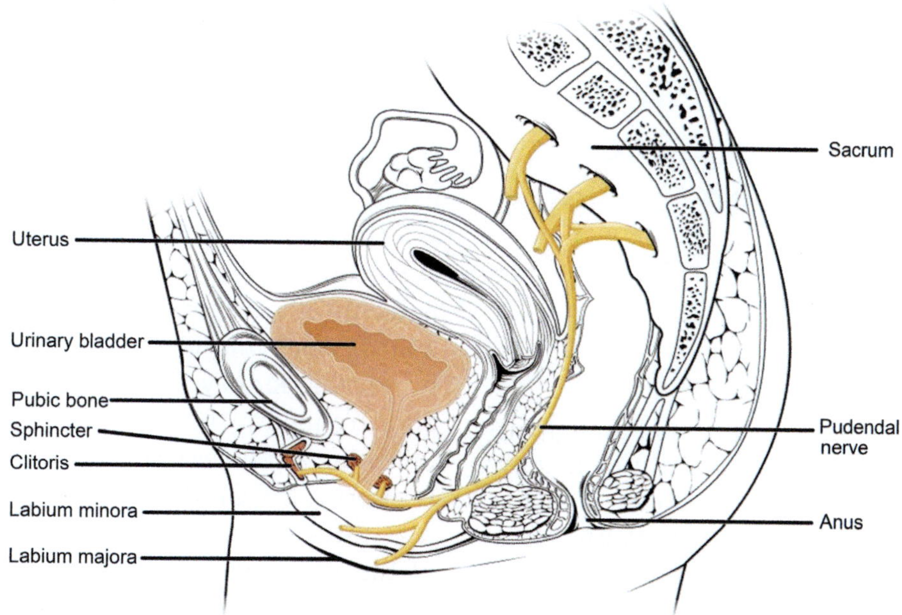

Figure 8.2. The innervation of the urogenital and rectal area in females.

Source: https://courses.lumenlearning.com/suny-ap2/chapter/gross-anatomy-of-urine-transport/.

Sacral spinal cord levels (S2–S4) are the source of somatic efferent and afferent innervation to the pelvic floor. At these levels, somatic efferents originate in the ventral horn's Onuf nucleus, while afferents' cell bodies are found in the dorsal root ganglia (Lincoln & Burnstock, 1993). The coordination of visceral and somatic motor activity has been proposed to be explained by the overlap of somatic afferents with pelvic splanchnic nerve afferents at the spinal cord level (McKenna & Nadelhaft, 1986). The sacral plexus is made up of sacral nerve roots. The pelvic viscera and the pelvic floor muscles are the two main efferent and afferent somatic distributions that branch off of the pudendal nerve, which originates from the sacral plexus (Elbadawi, 1996). Terminations of postganglionic axons from the caudal sympathetic chain ganglia are also received by the pudendal nerve (de Groat, 1994). The posterior perineal muscles are supplied by nerve branches primarily originating from sacral level S4, while the anterior perineal musculature is primarily supplied by branches originating from sacral level S3. The coccygeal plexus, which supplies the perineal, perianal, and scrotal/labial skin, is formed by branches of the S4–S5 nerve roots.

The sacral afferent parasympathetic system primarily transmits pelvic floor sensations, with a much smaller afferent supply from afferents traveling with the thoracolumbar sympathetics (Jänig & Koltzenburg, 1993). Nonetheless, thoracolumbar afferents may be primarily involved in testicular and epididymal sensations (Jänig & Koltzenburg, 1993). According to Vodusek and Light (1983), cholinergic nerve release most likely controls the somatic mechanisms of the perineal musculature. Perineal sensations seem to be explained by neuropeptide release (Jänig & Koltzenburg, 1993).

8.2. Chronic Pain Syndromes of the Genitourinary Tract: Clinical Presentation, Etiology, Differential Diagnosis, and Treatment Strategies

8.2.1. Kidney and Ureter Pain

Few upper urinary tract chronic non-malignant pain syndromes exist. The majority of kidney and ureter pain syndromes are acute, colicky, and brought on by acute distension from an infection or obstructing lesion. Cases of idiopathic nephralgia, which were commonly diagnosed earlier this century (Harris & Harris, 1930), have become extremely rare due to improved diagnostic techniques. Patients with diseases of the kidney and/or ureter present with true visceral pain and visceral pain referred to somatic structures, just like in other visceral diseases. Usually, the referred pain radiates laterally from the costovertebral angle, into the lower quadrant, and into the labia or testicles.

Patients who experience recurrent episodes of either unilateral or bilateral loin pain combined with microscopic or macroscopic hematuria for which there is no known cause are diagnosed with loin pain/hematuria syndrome (Little et al., 1967; Editorial, 1992). Women experience the syndrome at a higher rate than men do (Little et al., 1967; Bultitude et al., 1998). Renal specimens have not shown any consistent histological changes (Editorial, 1992; Weisberg et al., 1993). Since there is currently no aetiological treatment available, the diagnosis is made by exclusion, and pain relief is achieved through symptomatic treatment. Occasionally, the syndrome resolves on its own. For pain relief, the majority of patients need high dosages of analgesics, typically opioids (Bultitude, 1995). Some women have found relief from birth control pill side effects when using transcutaneous electrical nerve stimulation (TENS), and several patients have found relief from bleeding disorders when using anticoagulation (Burden et al., 1975; Aber & Higgins, 1982). Renal denervation and even nephrectomy or autotransplantation have been used as surgical techniques (with the aim of achieving complete denervation while preserving kidney function). Nevertheless, the pain frequently returns on the opposite side following a nephrectomy or autotransplantation (Editorial, 1992). Bultitude et al. (1998) found that after several months of local irrigation of the renal pelvis and ureter with capsaicin solution, symptomatic pain relief was observed in 65% of patients with loin pain/hematuria syndrome. Degeneration of the ureter's afferent fibers and the renal pelvis is the result of this treatment (Allan et al., 1997).

8.2.2. Interstitial Cystitis

The etiology and pathophysiology of interstitial cystitis (IC), a chronic, painful, and frequently incapacitating disease, are mainly unknown (for review see Hanno et al., 2001). It is characterized by pain in the pelvis and suprapubic area, symptoms related to the urination process, such as urgency and frequency, and in females, dyspareunia that can be alleviated by voiding. Based on cystoscopic findings of either Hunner's ulcer or glomerulations without ulcer on the bladder wall, IC is classified as either ulcerative or non-ulcerative (Johansson & Fall, 1994; Elbadawi, 1997; Messing et al., 1997; Nigro et al., 1997). The number of Americans with IC or conditions similar to it has been estimated to be between 450 000 (Slade et al., 1997) and 1 million (Jones & Nyberg, 1997), although prevalence estimates vary greatly. The Nurses' Health Study (NSH) I and II cohort was utilized as the study population in the most recent study on the epidemiology of IC, which found that the prevalence of IC was 52/100 000 in NSH I and 67/100 000 in NSH II (Curhan et al., 1999). One characteristic that sets IC apart is the enormous burden that women report experiencing. According to estimates of population prevalence, there are nine women for every one male (Jones & Nyberg, 1997).

The following aetiologies have been considered: infection (Ratliff et al., 1994; Warren, 1994; Duncan & Schaeffer, 1997), lymphatic or vascular obstruction (Ratliff et al., 1994), immunological deficiencies (Ratliff et al., 1994), deficiency of the glycosaminoglycan layer (Ratliff et al., 1994; Mobley & Baum, 1996; Parsons, 1997), alterations in bladder epithelial regeneration (Keay et al., 2001), presence of toxic urogenous substance (Ratliff et al., 1994), neural factors, and primary mast cell disorders (Elbadawi, 1997; Theoharides et al., 2001; Wesselmann, 2001). Additionally, it has been suggested that the underlying factor that caused IC has disappeared, leaving a persistent visceral pain syndrome in its wake (Wesselmann, 2001). This is in line with the findings of Baskin and Tanagho's (1992) report, which showed that in multiple instances, bladder removal in individuals with IC did not result in pain relief. There have been isolated reports of vulvodynia and IC coexisting, and it has been suggested that these syndromes are caused by a generalized disorder of the epithelium derived from the urogenital sinus (Fitzpatrick et al., 1993). There may be a connection between IC or a related illness in 60% of men who have prostate pain but do not have bacteriuria (Miller et al., 1995; Berger et al., 1998). A variety of treatment options have been suggested for the management of IC, including oral, intravesical, surgical, local, and behaviorally based treatments. Surgical interventions may involve bladder removal or modification. Local treatments such as laser therapy, hydrodistension, and urethral dilatation have also been proposed. Additionally, infusions of substances like DMSO, silver nitrate, heparin, chlorpactin, and hyaluronic acid into the bladder have been considered. Oral medications, ranging from amitriptyline to calcium channel blockers, have been used to manage IC. Other medications targeting possible allergic mechanisms, such as hydroxyzine and antihistamines, have also been recommended. Pentosan polysulfate sodium, an anticoagulant with glycosaminoglycan properties, has been utilized based on the theory that a defect in the glycosaminoglycan layer contributes to IC pathogenesis. Non-medical treatments like TENS, acupuncture, and behavioral interventions such as voiding diaries and pelvic floor muscle training have been suggested. However, there is a lack of consensus on what defines an IC case and limited valid outcome data. The National Institutes of Health in the USA have undertaken significant research initiatives on IC. Several ongoing multicenter controlled trials are comparing different treatment strategies for IC management, with the hope of establishing more logical and systematic approaches to treatment in the future.

8.2.3. Urethral Syndrome

Many women have painful micturition but no sign of an organic disease when they visit their family doctor, gynecologist, or urologist, and standard procedures yield a negative urine culture. Gallagher et al. (1965) coined the term "urethral syndrome" to characterize this issue. According to his report, 41% of women who presented with symptoms of a urinary tract infection in general practice actually had sterile urine. In the absence of objective urological findings, the urethral syndrome is defined as a condition characterized by urinary urgency, frequency, dysuria, and occasionally suprapubic and back pain as well as urinary hesitancy. According to Peters-Gee (1998), the urethral syndrome is thought to be the cause of up to 5 million office visits annually in the US.

The urethral syndrome usually affects women who are fertile, although it has also been documented in men and children (Barbalias, 1990; Kaplan et al., 1980).

It's unclear what causes the urethral syndrome. Nonetheless, a number of theories have been put forth with scant proof. According to a widely held belief, urethral obstruction is the cause of the symptoms and can be treated surgically (Davis, 1955; Bergman et al., 1989; Sand et al., 1989). While excellent outcomes are claimed for surgical procedures intended to relieve urethral obstructions, it should be noted that diagnostic criteria were sadly not well documented (Splatt & Weedon, 1981). Above all, an anatomically obstructive etiology is rarely supported by evidence (Mabry et al., 1981). These treatments have an unknown and typically transient efficacy, along with a small risk of incontinence (Mabry et al., 1981; Schmidt & Tanagho, 1981). Numerous research have examined the part infection plays in the urethral syndrome; however, the idea that the urethral syndrome has an inflammatory or infectious etiology is not well supported by the available data (reviewed in Messinger, 1992). Patients with urethral syndrome frequently report urinary hesitancy, which may be caused by external urethral sphincter spasms. In patients with urethral syndrome, uroflowmetry revealed a staccato or prolonged flow phase, and urethral pressure profilometry revealed an increase in external sphincter tone (Raz & Smith, 1976; Kaplan et al., 1980; Schmidt & Tanagho, 1981). Because these urodynamic results can also be produced voluntarily in a neurologically intact individual, it is challenging to interpret them in favor of a neurogenic etiology of the urethral syndrome (Messinger, 1992). Compared to other non-malignant genitourinary pain syndromes, this patient population has extremely high rates of spontaneous remission (85% in Carson et al., 1980; 100% in Zufall, 1978).

An extensive diagnostic assessment is essential. The urethral syndrome is an exclusion diagnosis, meaning that other conditions need to be ruled out in order to distinguish the symptoms from those of urinary infections, tumors, stones, interstitial cystitis, and many other conditions. Urine analysis, culture, and cytology are all part of a comprehensive urological examination that serves as the initial diagnostic step. More radiographic, urodynamic, and cystoscopy investigations are required in a subset of patients (Messinger, 1992). It is necessary to rule out a gynecological issue in females. The signs and symptoms of systemic diseases that impact the innervation of the urogenital area, such as diabetes mellitus, multiple sclerosis, and collagen diseases, can overlap with those of the urethral syndrome. The multidisciplinary evaluation should include a psychological assessment to rule out a psychogenic etiology and screen for depression symptoms linked to chronic pain syndrome.

Patients with the urethral syndrome have been offered a range of invasive and non-invasive treatment options (reviewed in Messinger, 1992). There have been reports of endoscopic and open surgical procedures performed to remove a suspected urethral stenosis. It has been suggested that cystoscopically visible urethritis can be completely eradicated by fulguration, scarification, resection, or cryosurgery. Several anti-inflammatory or cauterizing agents have been used for bladder instillations, and anticholinergics, α-adrenergic blockers, and muscle relaxants have been used for systemic therapy. It has been suggested that biofeedback and electrical stimulation can address neurogenic causes. Skeletal muscle relaxants or electrostimulation in conjunction with biofeedback techniques have been shown to have high success rates (Kaplan et al., 1980; Schmidt & Tanagho, 1981). A conservative approach is advised when it comes to invasive and irreversible therapeutic procedures, as they are typically less risky, less expensive, and just as effective as surgery.

8.2.4. Vulvodynia (Vulvar Dysesthesia)

Remarkably, nineteenth-century American (Thomas, 1880) and European (Pozzi, 1897) gynecological textbooks gave a thorough description of hyperesthesia of the vulva. Surprisingly, until the early 1980s, there was minimal attention paid to chronic vulvar pain, despite early thorough reports. A task force was established in 1982 by the International Society for the Study of Vulvar Disease (ISSVD) to investigate vulvar pain syndromes. The term vulvodynia was first used by this task force in 1984 to describe chronic vulvar discomfort, which is characterized by burning (and occasionally stinging, irritation, or rawness) in the vulvar area as reported by the patient. The term "vulvodynia" encompassed a number of conditions, including vulvar dermatosis, vulvar vestibulitis, vulvar papillomatosis, cyclic vulvovaginitis, and dysesthetic vulvodynia (McKay, 1988, 1989). All of these conditions cause persistent vulvar pain. A new classification scheme for vulvar dysesthesia was proposed at the 1999 World Congress of the ISSVD. It divided the condition into two main categories: (1) generalized vulvar dysesthesia and (2) localized vulvar dysesthesia, which includes vestibulodynia, clitorodynia, and other conditions. However, the majority of vulvar pain studies to date have used the term vulvodynia, and this new classification system has not been fully published in the peer-reviewed literature. Therefore, from now on in this chapter, we will refer to it as vulvodynia. Definitions, however, will likely change as our understanding of the etiology and management of vulvar dysesthesia advances and takes into account new insights into the underlying pathophysiological mechanisms. Appropriate evaluation and treatment of vulvodynia depend on the identification of several factors in its etiology.

Although the incidence and prevalence of vulvodynia are unknown, Thomas (1880) has already noted that this pain syndrome is likely more common than is generally believed. According to data analyzed from the National Health and Social Life Survey, a study on sexual dysfunction in the USA found that 16% of women in American households between the ages of 18 and 59 report experiencing pain during sex (Laumann et al., 1999). This study did not analyze the location or cause of pain. 18% of 303 women between the ages of 20 and 59 in a small sample reported having experienced lower genital tract discomfort in the past; the cause of the pain was not disclosed, though (Harlow et al., 2001). Vulvodynia affects people primarily in their twenties through their late sixties (Lynch, 1986; Paavonen, 1995a, b).

Uncertainty surrounds the vulvodynia's genesis. Although numerous etiological theories have been put forth, the majority of these explanations are based on clinical case reports, which limits our current understanding of vulvodynia. The possibility of a genetic predisposition is raised by the fact that 25–33% of women with vulvodynia are aware of a female relative who has dyspareunia or tampon intolerance (Goetsch, 1991; Bergeron et al., 1997). It has been reported that vulvodynia and interstitial cystitis coexist, and it has been suggested that these syndromes are indicative of a generalized disorder of the epithelium derived from the urogenital sinus (Fitzpatrick et al., 1993). Although vulvodynia frequently has an abrupt onset, patients occasionally cannot recall any related events. The onset is frequently associated with vaginal infection episodes, local treatments (such as the application of steroid or antimicrobial cream, cryotherapy, or laser surgery), or alterations in the sexual activity pattern. To determine whether a history of vaginal infection, irritation, or trauma is associated with the development of chronic vulvar discomfort, controlled prospective studies are required because many of these parameters are already quite common in women. One theory is that some women's vaginal tissue is more sensitive to these events than others.

Punch biopsies of the vulvar vestibule in patients with vestibulitis were subjected to histopathological analyzes in relation to control cases. These studies revealed that patients with vulvar vestibulitis had abnormalities related to a chronic inflammatory reaction of the vestibule mucosa, the cause of which was still unknown. Studies employing molecular techniques were unable to corroborate early reports that the human papilloma virus (HPV) is a major factor in the pathophysiology of vulvar vestibulitis (De Deus et al., 1995). Women with vulvar vestibulitis have a distinct distribution of interleukin 1 receptor antagonist alleles, which implies that a polymorphism in this gene may influence a person's susceptibility to this pain syndrome (Jeremias et al., 2000). Anatomical research shows that women with vulvar vestibulitis have different vestibule innervation than controls, and patients with vulvar dysaesthesia have vestibular neural hyperplasia (BohmStarke et al., 1998; Weststrom & Willen, 1998).

Patients with vulvodynia typically appear normal during physical examinations. A straightforward "Swabtest" (Goetsch, 1991; Paavonen, 1995a, b) can easily cause or worsen pain in patients with vulvar vestibulitis: touching the vulvar vestibule with a cotton swab causes sharp, burning pain. Psychophysical evaluations have quantified the allodynia and hyperalgesia reported by women with vulvodynia, supporting the theory of nocicepetor sensitization (Sonni et al., 1995; Bohm-Starke et al., 2001). Before a diagnosis of vulvodynia is considered, chronic infections of the vulvar area should be treated. Furthermore, when assessing a patient with vulvodynia, iatrogenic causes need to be ruled out. When local agents are applied to the vulvar region, they may cause irritant reactions. These reactions go away when the irritant agent is stopped. Vulvodynia is therefore an exclusionary diagnosis.

Finding and removing potential allergens and local irritants is the first step in treating vulvodynia. Oral treatments for neuropathic pain management, such as antidepressants, anticonvulsants, membrane-stabilizing agents, and opioids, are beneficial for a large number of patients. Topical treatment regimens such as aspirin, steroids, estrogen, or creams containing local anesthetics may help patients with vulvar vestibulitis, a condition where pain is localized. Glazer et al. (1995) found that electromyo168 graphic biofeedback of the pelvic floor muscles relieved pain in more than 80% of vulvar vestibulitis patients. In patients with vulvar vestibulitis, surgical procedures to remove the hyperalgesic skin area have been recommended (for a review, see Wesselmann et al., 1997; Bergeron et al., 2001). The most often performed operation is perineoplasty. Goetsch (1996) has recommended a less invasive surgical revision in place of this more involved surgical intervention, in which the painful area is removed under local anesthesia.

8.2.5. Clitoral Pain

Few reports exist regarding clitoral pain, in contrast to the growing body of research regarding chronic pain syndromes of the vulva/vagina. In clinical practice, clitoral pain is occasionally observed as a component of the vulvodynia pain syndrome complex. Touch aggravates the patients' burning, stinging sensation, according to Wesselmann's unpublished data. Female circumcision, which involves the excision of the clitoris and labia minora, is still performed on young girls in many parts of the world where it is preferred as a means of controlling female sexuality and upholding cultural pride. Chronic pain has been identified as one of the complications of this procedure (Dirie & Lindmark, 1992; Hanly & Ojeda, 1995; Briggs, 1998). A growing number of these women have relocated to western nations. An estimated 2,000 young women in the UK are thought to participate in this ritual annually (Hanly & Ojeda, 1995). The prevalence of pain among these women is unknown, though, as few of them seek medical care.

8.2.6. Testicular Pain

For men and their treating physician, orchialgia, or chronic testicular pain, can be one of the most frustrating pain conditions. Similar to women who experience vulvodynia, men with testicular pain are typically embarrassed to discuss it because genital pain syndromes are frequently viewed as taboo in our society. It is unknown what the incidence and prevalence are. Chronic testicular pain has been reported in patients ranging in age from adolescence to old age (Zvieli et al., 1989; Davis et al., 1990; Costabile et al., 1991); most of these patients are in their mid- to late-thirties. Many patients report having no memory of the trigger that caused their chronic pain syndrome to start (Costabile et al., 1991; Wesselmann & Burnett, 1996). Persistent testicular pain can be either bilateral or unilateral, localized to the contents of the scrotum, or radiating to the back, legs, groin, penis, and perineum. Some patients experience pain all the time, while others only experience it occasionally. In some cases, the pain is caused by pressure or specific movements applied to the testis. Chronic orchialgia is typically not accompanied by sexual dysfunction (Davis et al., 1990; U. Wesselmann and AL. Burnett, unpublished observation).

Upon conducting a thorough history, physical examination, urological evaluation, and specific imaging studies, the majority of secondary causes of persistent testicular pain can be identified. Understanding the nerve supply of the testis is crucial for the doctor assessing a patient with persistent testicular pain because it allows the functional neuroanatomy, which includes the referred pain pattern, to guide the diagnostic evaluation. Nonetheless, the scrotum, testis, epididymis, and spermatic cord all appear perfectly normal upon physical examination in a large number of these patients. Despite a very thorough diagnostic work-up, the cause of the pain is still unknown (Davis et al., 1990). Infection, tumor, testicular torsion, varicocele, hydrocele, spermatocele, trauma (like a bicycle accident), and prior surgical procedures are among the secondary causes of chronic orchialgia (Davis et al., 1990; Costabile et al., 1991). Testicular pain may indicate entrapment neuropathies of the ilioinguinal or genitofemoral nerves (Yeates, 1985; Bennini, 1992) or referred pain from the hip or ureter (Goldberg & Witchell, 1988; Holland et al., 1994). There are case reports (Ali, 1983; McGee, 1993) of referred testicular pain resulting from pressure on the genitofemoral nerve caused by aneurysms of the common iliac artery or aorta; however, typically this pain is acute rather than chronic.

Intervertebral disc protrusion may be the cause of testicular pain (White & Leslie, 1986). Men with diabetic neuropathy have been reported to experience neuropathic testicular pain (Hagen, 1993). Vasectomy is probably far more common than is recognized and can cause chronic orchialgia (Selikowitz & Schned, 1985; McCormack, 1988; McMahon et al., 1992; Hayden, 1993). Although some have questioned this theory (Silber, 1981; McCormack, 1988), it has been proposed that sperm granuloma impairment of the genital branch of the genitofemoral nerve is the cause of this postvasectomy pain syndrome (Yeates, 1985). One sign of retroperitoneal fibrosis is chronic testicular pain, which is typically accompanied by low back and abdominal pain (Mitchinson, 1972; Baker et al., 1987). Two case reports that describe episodic testicular pain as an epileptic symptom can be found in the neurological literature (York et al., 1979; Bhaskar, 1987). Schneiderman and Voytovich (1988) described a patient who repeatedly felt his testis because he was too worried about getting testicular cancer; this led to "self-palpation orchitis.."

A comprehensive urological evaluation should be part of the diagnostic work-up. Additional gastroenterological evaluations may be required to rule out referred pain from the lower pelvic organs and to assess for hernias if the urological evaluation yields no information. Herniography is recommended by Ekberg et al. (1988) for patients who present with testicular pain in order to check for an occult hernia. A neurological examination targets the genitofemoral, pelvic, pudendal, ilioinguinal, and lumbosacral roots. Differentiating which nerves are mediating the chronic pain issue may be made easier with placebo-controlled nerve blocks mixed with local anesthetic. To determine whether a protruding disc is the source of the pain, a discogram may be useful. To screen for depression or other psychological problems, a multidisciplinary comprehensive work-up should include a psychological evaluation. It's crucial to understand that, in approximately 25% of cases, an etiology for the pain cannot be determined despite extensive evaluations (Davis et al., 1990). If there is an underlying etiology, it is the focus of treatment for persistent testicular pain. We concur that hydrocele, varicocele, or spermatocele are typically not the cause of chronic testicular pain; rather, they are a coincidental finding, as noted by Holland et al. (1994). We have seen numerous patients with chronic testicular pain who had undergone unsuccessful testicular surgery in the past for similar conditions (U. Wesselmann and AL. Burnett, unpublished observation). It is crucial that the doctor is not pressured to perform more invasive procedures in an attempt to diagnose a pathological condition that does not exist due to a lack of results (Costabile et al., 1991). For the treatment of chronic orchialgia, drastic surgical procedures such as epididymectomy (Davis et al., 1990; Chen & Ball, 1991) and orchiectomy (Davis et al., 1990) have been recommended. In lieu of an orchiectomy for persistent testicular pain, a number of studies have recently proposed microsurgical denervation of the spermatic cord (Choa & Swami, 1992; Levine et al., 1996). However, medical pain management should be tried before considering any invasive or irreversible measures for pain relief. In the past, urologists would only recommend an antibiotic and nonsteroidal anti-inflammatory drug trial to men who complained of persistent testicular pain in an attempt to treat an underlying inflammatory process that may be present (Davis et al., 1990). Clinical reports show that patients with chronic testicular pain frequently experience excellent pain relief from medications used for other chronic pain syndromes (Galer, 1995), such as low-dose antidepressants, anticonvulsants, membrane-stabilizing agents, and opiates (Costabile et al., 1991; Hagen, 1993; Hayden, 1993; Wesselmann et al., 1996). It could be beneficial to use TENS (Hayden, 1993; Holland et al., 1994). A subgroup of men with chronic testicular pain has experienced significant pain relief from sympatholytic procedures, such as lumbar sympathetic block with local anesthetic or phentolamine infusions (Wesselmann et al.,

1995; Wesselmann & Burnett, 1996). The testes have a rich sympathetic innervation.

8.2.7. Prostatodynia (Chronic Prostatitis/Chronic Pelvic Pain Syndrome)

According to Drach et al. (1978), prostodynia is the term for persistent complaints of dysuria, poor urine flow, urgency, and discomfort in the perineal area without any sign of bacteria or purulence in the prostatic fluid. Patients report pain during ejaculation as well as in the groin, suprapubic area, lower back, and perineum. Typically, they are between the ages of 20 and 60 (Moul, 1993). Frequently, any unexplained symptom or illness that may potentially have its origins in the prostate gland is referred to as "prostatitis" (Nickel, 1998). Prostatitis is diagnosed in about 25% of male patients' office visits in the USA for genitourinary tract issues (Lipsky, 1989; Meares, 1992). Four categories of prostatitis were defined by the National Institutes of Health (Nickel et al., 1999), along with research guidelines for chronic prostatitis.

1. acute bacterial prostatitis
2. chronic bacterial prostatitis
3. chronic prostatitis/chronic pelvic pain syndrome
    - inflammatory
    - non-inflammatory
4. asymptomatic inflammatory prostatitis.

The category chronic prostatitis/chronic pelvic pain syndrome has taken the place of the previous term "prostatodynia" (Drach et al., 1978) in these updated definitions. About 30% of patients who present with prostatitis have prostodynia (Brunner et al., 1983).

Physical examinations usually reveal a normal prostate with no palpable signs of tenderness (Orland et al., 1985). Urinalysis, urine culture, urine cytology, and urethral cultures should all be part of a comprehensive urological evaluation (de la Rosette et al., 1992). Urodynamic evaluation should be carried out in selected patients, as multiple studies 170 have shown that patients with prostatodynia have abnormalities in urethral closing pressure, urethral narrowing, and detrusor striated sphincter dyssynergy (Segura et al., 1979; Barbalias et al., 1983; Barbalias, 1990). When no identifiable inflammatory prostatic process can be found, prostatodynia is a diagnosis of exclusion, meaning that it is presumed that the chronic pain syndrome is related to the prostate. Other illnesses that can resemble prostatodynia should be taken into account when making a differential diagnosis. In the event that referred pain from the colon or rectum is suspected, a gastroenterological examination is recommended. The focus of the neurological examination is the prostate's nerve supply. Prostatodynia can be confused with osteoitis pubis, a well-known condition that affects people who engage in intense sports and exercise regularly. Osteitis pubis is confirmed by a bone scan and pelvic X-ray (Buck et al., 1982). Prostatodynia is one of the presenting symptoms of interstitial cystitis in certain patients.

For those with prostatodynia, a number of invasive and medical treatment options have been proposed; however, the majority of these are anecdotal reports. Antibiotics are the most commonly recommended treatment for prostatodynia patients, even though no infection can be demonstrated in them (Brunner et al., 1983). This is likely due to the possibility that an infection is present but has not been diagnosed. De la Rosette et al. (1992) examined the diagnostic and treatment outcomes of 409 patients who had been diagnosed with prostate pain. Treatment with antibiotics led to the resolution of complaints in 36% of the patients and a cure in 24% of the patients. Interestingly, though, comparable outcomes were observed even in the absence of antibiotic administration: 32% of patients reported relief and 30% reported cure. Since certain patients with prostatodynia exhibit urodynamic abnormalities that point to increased sympathetic activity (Barbalias et al., 1983), treating the abnormalities in voiding and pain with oral α-adrenergic blockers has been suggested. The most commonly used medications are doxazosin, terazosin, and prazosin (Orland et al., 1985; Moul, 1993; Barbalias et al., 1998). However, side effects, most commonly hypotension, frequently prevent these medications from being used.

Retrograde transurethral balloon dilatation of the prostate has been proposed when urodynamic testing demonstrates a functional obstruction of the urinary outlet. The voiding symptomatology significantly improved as a result, but no information was provided about how it affected the pain scores (Lopatin et al., 1990). For non-bacterial prostatitis and prostatodynia, transurethral microwave hyperthermia has been proposed (Montorsi et al., 1993; Nickel & Sorenson, 1994). Pelvic floor relaxation techniques (Segura et al., 1979) and muscle-relaxing drugs (Moul, 1993) have been shown to reduce pain.

8.2.8. Penile Pain

Chronic penile pain appears to be extremely rare, in contrast to other chronic pain syndromes of the genitourinary tract. Treatment for the underlying condition (herpes genitalis, priapism, paraphimosis, Peyronie's disease) is typically effective in managing a patient's persistent penile pain (see Gee et al., 1990). The intracavernous injection of medication for the treatment of erectile dysfunction is one of the most commonly reported acute penile pain events (Godschalk et al., 1996). Penile prosthesis and acute penile pain have been studied (Althof et al., 1987; Pedersen et al., 1988; Tiefer et al., 1988). According to patients having surgery for penile prostheses, one of the worst side effects of the procedure is postoperative pain (Tiefer et al., 1988). There are no reports, nevertheless, suggesting that these acute noxious events lead to the development of a chronic pain syndrome. Furthermore, there does not appear to be a persistent penile pain syndrome following surgical trauma to the penis, such as that sustained during a routine circumcision. A man with recurrent penile pain attacks was the subject of a case report published in British literature (Corder, 1989). An inguinal hernia was discovered during a physical examination and surgically repaired. Since there was no sign of a recurrence of his episodic episodes of penile pain, the ilioinguinal nerve, which supplies the ventral base of the penis, was thought to be irritated in this instance. Men who suffer from pudendal nerve injuries experience sensory loss over the shaft and bulb of the penis as well as difficulties achieving an erection; however, no reports of chronic pain linked to the nerve injury have been made (Goodson, 1981; Hofmann et al., 1982).

8.2.9. Perineal Pain

The perineal region may experience pain that radiates to other parts of the body. Some of the more specific genitourinary pain syndromes that are covered here include interstitial cystitis, urethral syndrome, clitoral pain, vulvodynia, testicular pain, and prostatodynia. Chronic perineal pain, however, is frequently a distinct entity despite being ill-defined. Excluding gastroenterological, proctological, urological, gynecological, and neurological pathology is necessary in the broad differential diagnosis of chronic perineal pain. Perineal pain can be a symptom of systemic diseases like diabetes mellitus or AIDS that are linked to painful peripheral neuropathies. Up to 91% of patients with perineal pain who are referred to a pain clinic have pudendal nerve entrapment, according to French studies (Bensignor et al., 1996). 67% of the patients experienced pain relief following surgical neurolysis-transposition (Robert et al., 1993). Patients with an early diagnosis of pudendal nerve entrapment showed the best outcomes. To confirm the diagnosis, local anesthetic blocks of the pudendal nerve, electromyography, and studies of the pelvic floor's nerve conduction may be useful (Beck et al., 1994). When perineal pain is suspected to be caused by meningeal cysts (Van De Kleft & Van Vyve, 1993) or meningiomas (Pagni & Canavero, 1993), imaging studies of the thoracolumbosacral spine may be warranted. In 10 out of 12 patients with perineal pain, surgical resection of sacral meningeal cysts has been reported to result in complete resolution of symptoms (Van de Kleft & Van Vyve, 1993). There have been a few documented instances of plexiform neurofibromas affecting the perineum's nerves causing perineal pain (Batta et al., 1989). Perineal pain was identified by Ford et al. (1994, 1996) as a sign of movement disorders.

8.2.10. Psychological Aspects of Chronic Genitourinary Pain

Numerous theories regarding the psychogenic origin of chronic non-malignant genitourinary pain have been entertained, similar to other chronic pain syndromes in the absence of obvious organic pathology (review available; Wesselmann et al., 1997). An important predictor of pain assessments, affective responses, and pain complaint disclosure could be the location of the pain. This is probably going to be a big deal when it comes to genitourinary pain syndromes, which are taboo. It is not surprising that when asked to imagine experiencing pain in their genitalia, participants said they would be more anxious, depressed, and ashamed of such pain than they would be in any other area. They would also be less likely to disclose such pain. Compared to when asked to imagine the pain in the head, stomach, chest, or mouth, they evaluated themselves as being more ill (Klonoff et al., 1993). The majority of genitourinary pain syndromes have been the subject of preliminary psychological research; however, most of these studies have been limited by small sample sizes, significant self-selection factors, retrospective designs, inadequate control groups, and a lack of standardized measures. The fact that the majority of studies have not evaluated whether the psychological findings in genitourinary pain patients were likely to be reactive or pre-existing is a serious cause for concern (review Wesselmann et al., 1997). While the traditional psychosocial view of sexual pain disorders has concentrated on marital and sexual issues, conflicts, and experiences and has attempted to distinguish between psychological and physiological factors as the etiology, recent psychological literature has proposed a pain-centered approach that focuses on the primary symptom of these issues, pain (Binik et al., 1999).

Moreover, a history of physical and/or sexual abuse has been linked to several different pain syndromes (Kinzl et al., 1995), with a particularly strong correlation seen with chronic gynecological pain (Walker & Stenchever, 1993). These studies, however, might erroneously infer a cause-and-effect relationship between a history of abuse and the onset of chronic pain. Sexual and physical abuse are frequently signs of multiproblem families, which are marked by disorder, drug and alcohol misuse, and general neglect, leaving children without enough protection. The link between childhood victimization and pain symptoms in adulthood is more complicated than previously thought, according to a recent prospective study that sought to determine whether childhood victimization increases the risk for adult pain complaints. According to Raphael et al. (2001), there was no significant correlation found between the likelihood of reporting unexplained pain symptoms and childhood victimization. However, there was a significant correlation with retrospective self-reports of all specific types of childhood victimization.

8.3. Retroperitoneal Causes of Genitourinary Pain Syndromes

In clinical practice, female patients frequently describe their perceived pelvic pain as coming from their "ovaries," "vagina," "uterus," or "bladder." These reports frequently result in a differential diagnosis that is commonly linked to visceral genitourinary pain syndromes, however, the symptoms could also be brought on by pelvic and abdominal musculoskeletal disorders. For diagnosis and treatment, it is prudent to comprehend the musculoskeletal and neuroanatomical aspects that may contribute to genitourinary pain.

The pelvic myofascial support, or pelvic diaphragm, as well as the lower anterior abdominal nerves, sacral nerve plexus, and pelvic nerves, are the main structures covered in this review.

The posterior cervical region, the uterine fundus, the uterine body, and the anterior dome of the bladder are all covered by the pelvic peritoneum and its ligamentous attachments. The uterosacral ligaments, the lateral inferior hypogastric nerve plexus, and the pelvic nerve traveling along the lateral pelvic side wall are all covered by the peritoneal covering, which then reflects posteriorly to cover the upper half of the rectum and extends laterally to form the lateral pelvic peritoneum. The retroperitoneal structures, which are located behind that single layer of mesothelial cells, are capable of producing pain signals that reach the spinal cord and brain cortex's sensory centers via somatic and visceral afferent neurons.

Clinicians should be aware of the pathophysiology of pain and central nervous system sensitization in cases of chronic pain, as these conditions can exacerbate treatment complications. Inadequate physical examinations and incomplete history taking by the physician can result in incorrect diagnoses and unsuccessful treatments. A clinical case of a patient receiving care at a women's health clinic is presented now as an example. This complicated case shows how the patient's symptoms were multifactorial and needed a multidisciplinary approach for prompt and effective treatment. The patient presented with symptoms of vulvar burning, dysuria, frequency of urination, and nocturia. This case emphasizes how crucial it is to conduct a thorough history and physical examination, as well as to possess a clinical understanding of common genitourinary pain syndromes and pelvic neuroanatomy. The most common neuropathic and musculoskeletal causes of both acute and persistent pelvic pain are then discussed, along with complex, multimodal treatment options.

A 65-year-old menopausal woman sought medical attention after experiencing a worsening vulvar burning sensation for three months, which was accompanied by frequent, burning, burning nocturia. Sitting for longer than an hour and at night made the pain worse. She confirmed that she had low back pain that shot down her anterior thighs like needles and pins. She was evaluated for vaginal yeast infection and possible urinary tract infection. She received partial relief from vaginal estrogen treatment, leading to a working diagnosis of urogenital syndrome of menopause.

The patient was referred to a gynecologist because the relief was insufficient. The results of the external vulvar examination were normal upon a thorough pelvic examination. The Q-tip test caused a burning sensation in the labia minora on the medial and lateral aspects of the left and right, as well as in the labia majora. A pelvic floor examination revealed bilateral ischial spine tenderness and left-sided pelvic floor tenderness, along with a positive Tinel sign suggestive of pudendal neuralgia. Overlying the left lower extremity at the L3 and L4 distribution at the medial thigh, paresthesia was also observed. After undergoing a bilateral pudendal block via the vaginal approach, the patient's vulvar pain completely disappeared for a full day. In light of this finding, a request for lumbar and pelvic magnetic resonance imaging was made to rule out a pathologic process that could lead to peripheral neuropathy and nerve entrapment.

Table 8.1. Definition, Classification, Histology, Diagnosis, and Treatment Show Differences Between Interstitial Cystitis/Bladder Pain Syndrome (IC/BPS): Hunner (Ulcerative) Type IC/BPS (HIC/BPS) or Non-Hunner (Nonulcerative) Type IC/BPS (NHIC/BPS)

Item		HIC/BPS	NHIC/BPS
Definition		IC/BPS with Hunner lesions	IC/BPS without Hunner lesions
Classification		Hunner-type (Ulcerative) type	Non-Hunner-type (Unulcerative) type
Histopathology	Subepithelial chronic inflammation	Present	Absent or minimal
	Types of infiltrating inflammatory cells	Lymphocytes and plasma cells are dominant.	Plasma cells are few.
	Lymphoid follicles	Often present	Extremely rare
	Urothelium	Frequently denuded	Full layer is preserved
	Mast cell	Often present	Extremely rare
Diagnosis	Cystoscopy	Hunner lesions: presence	Hunner lesions: absence
	Bladder capacity	Low	Low
	Bladder biopsy	Dense inflammatory infiltration and epithelial denudation	Slight inflammation
Treatment	Fulguration/Distension	Fulguration/Distension	Distension
	Intravesical instillation	HA, chondroitin sulfate, Botulinum toxin, steroid	HA, chondroitin sulfate, Botulinum toxin, steroid
	Medicine	Necessary	Necessary

Source: Lin H-Y, Lu J-H, Chuang S-M, Chueh K-S, Juan T-J, Liu Y-C, Juan Y-S. Urinary biomarkers in interstitial cystitis/bladder pain syndrome and its impact on therapeutic outcome. *Diagnostics*. 2022; 12(1):75. https://doi.org/10.3390/diagnostics12010075.

Table 8.2. Clinical Symptom, Histopathology, Biomarkers, Diagnosis, and Treatment Exhibit Differences Between IC/PBS and OAB

Item	IC/PBS	OAB
Clinical symptom	Bladder pain (suprapubic pain), urinary frequency, nocturia, and urgency	Daytime frequency of micturition ≥8 times, nocturia ≥1 times, urgency ≥1 time, or urgency incontinence ≥1 time.
Histopathology	Mast cell infiltration	
Urothelial defects	Present in Hunner-type IC/PBS	Absent or minimal
Biomarkers	The levels of NGF in urine and bladder tissue, serum cytokines, and serum CRP were elevated.	
Diagnosis	Cystoscopy, bladder capacity, 3-day urinary diary	Uroflowmetry, bladder capacity, 3-day urinary diary,
Symptom score	O'Leary–Sant Problem Index (ICSI and ICPI), VAS	OABSS, ICIQ-SF, UDI-6, and IIQ-7
Medical therapy	BoNT-A intravesical injection, LiESWT, PRP	ß3 agonist, BoNT-A intravesical injection, LiESWT

Note: BoNT-A, Onabotulinumtoxin A (botulinum toxin A); CRP, C-reactive protein; IC/BPS, interstitial cystitis/bladder pain syndrome; ICSI, Interstitial Cystitis Symptom Index; ICPI, Interstitial Cystitis Problem Index; ICIQ-SF, International Consultation on Incontinence Questionnaire-Short Form; IIQ-7, Incontinence Impact Questionnaire-7 score LiESWT, Low-intensity extracorporeal shock wave therapy; NGF, nerve growth factor; OAB, overactive bladder; OABSS, Overactive Bladder Symptom Scores; PRP, platelet-rich plasma; UDI-6, Urogenital Distress Inventory-Short Form; VAS, visual analog scale.

Source: Lin H-Y, Lu J-H, Chuang S-M, Chueh K-S, Juan T-J, Liu Y-C, Juan Y-S. Urinary biomarkers in interstitial cystitis/bladder pain syndrome and its impact on therapeutic outcome. Diagnostics. 2022; 12(1):75. https://doi.org/10.3390/diagnostics12010075.

A 3.3 × 4.4 cm left ovarian mass and uterine fibroids were found on imaging, which may help to explain the L2-L5 radiculopathy. A cystic mass in the right midabdomen was discovered by lumbar magnetic resonance imaging, prompting the recommendation for additional testing using computed tomography (CT).

Concerns about retroperitoneal sarcoma led to the patient's referral for gynecologic oncology and surgery assessments. The tumor marker values for epithelial ovarian cancer were normal. Except an inexplicable rise in dopamine levels, catecholamine research yielded no meaningful results. The patient had bilateral salpingo-oophorectomy, retroperitoneal tumor excision, and exploratory surgery. A retroperitoneal Schwannoma with cystic degeneration and a left ovarian fibromatosis were identified by pathologic analysis. Her vulvar burning and urine symptoms completely resolved, and her postoperative course was uneventful and asymptomatic. She experienced a recurrence of vulvar burning symptoms six months following her surgery; there were no problems with her back, thighs, or urine. At that point, vaginal estrogen therapy had been discontinued.

The patient was directed to the physical medicine and rehabilitation department after receiving counseling regarding pudendal neuralgia. Her pain was temporarily relieved after undergoing bilateral pudendal nerve blocks using triamcinolone and bupivacaine under ultrasound guidance. Pregabalin was given to the patient, who experienced some relief. Reevaluation results suggested hormone-mediated vestibulitis, and topical estrogen and testosterone cream for the vulvar was recommended. She claimed that her symptoms had significantly improved. However, six months later, the patient complained of vulvar discomfort that was relieved by lying down and that was triggered by sitting or standing. A reassessment revealed widespread varicosities in the lower extremities. For the purpose of ruling out a retroperitoneal tumor recurrence, her primary care physician ordered a follow-up CT scan. According to her symptoms, a CT scan revealed a distended left ovarian vein and a confluence of vascular congestion in the vulva, suggesting the presence of pelvic congestion syndrome. The patient was referred to the department of interventional radiology for coiling and sclerotherapy management.

8.3.1. Pelvic Pathologic Processes That Alter Neural Function or Integrity

Neuropathic pain is thought to affect 8% of people at some point, and it can be brought on by acute nerve damage, diseases, or degenerative conditions. Chronic pain is characterized by different mechanisms than acute pain, such as pathologic activation of microglia, impaired inhibitory modulation, or peripheral and central sensitization, in which abnormal ectopic activity in nociceptive nerves triggers pain signals instead of the noxious stimulus. Common terms used to characterize pain include allodynia, pain triggered by a normally non-painful stimulus (e.g., skin-to-clothing contact), and hyperalgesia, an exaggerated reaction to pain that would otherwise be felt.

Pain can be radicular or peripheral, depending on where the injury to the nerve is anatomically located. The pain will travel down the nerve dermatome and radiate from the back if the irritation of the nerve is at the level of the spinal nerve roots, or radius. Extrinsic causes frequently include neoplastic growths (e.g., schwannomas, as seen in our case study) or degenerative disease of the intervertebral disc.

Schwannomas, which account for 6% of retroperitoneal tumors, are derived from Schwann cells found in the nerve sheath. They are common in the head, neck, or thoracic region and grow slowly. Schwaannomas only rarely originate in the pelvis and typically manifest later in life and in larger sizes. Although they are rarely malignant, they could resemble malignant neoplasms radiologically.

Different symptoms of pain can arise depending on the specific peripheral nerve involved. For example, in a documented case of a schwannoma developing in the right parametrium, the patient experienced a combination of increasing abdominal distension and persistent pain in the lower right abdominal quadrant. The patient also reported suffering from symptoms including vomiting, nausea, increased urinary frequency, and incontinence.

Positive staining for the proteins S100 and SOX10, which are specific to tumors derived from the neural crest, confirms the pathological diagnosis of schwannomas. These tumors are uncommon, and regardless of the imaging modality used, preoperative diagnosis can be challenging.

Other iatrogenic causes of extrinsic neuropathic pain include suture entrapment and surgical scarring. Operations utilizing an incision in the lower transverse abdomen (e.g., Pfannenstiel, inguinal herniorrhaphy, or appendectomy) and abdominoplasty may be linked to genitofemoral or ilioinguinal nerve damage (5% incidence rate), which can lead to chronic pelvic and lower abdominal pain syndromes, as iscovered later. surgical procedures for sacrospinal fixation with mesh in pelvic prolapse repair (e.g.due to their anatomical proximity, sacrocollipomexy, rectopexy, and others) may also raise the risk of pudendal nerve damage. While damage to the left S2 nerve root is more frequently sustained following vaginal uterosacral ligament suspension (McCall procedure), damage to the right S2 nerve root is most frequently sustained during laparoscopic sacral colpopexy and rectopexy. A low threshold for evaluating iatrogenic pelvic neuropathy in the differential diagnosis should be applied by clinicians treating patients with pelvic pain and a history of comparable surgical procedures.

Deep infiltrating endometriosis (DIE) is becoming more widely acknowledged in the literature as a contributing factor to the pathophysiology of both cyclic and acyclic pelvic pain. The traditional theories of the pathophysiology of pain associated with endometriosis have focused only on inflammatory and visceral infiltrative factors. Additional ways that endometriosis causes pain are associated with its restrictive or infiltrative effects on nerve integrity.

Because endometriosis excision procedures often require surgical dissection of the pelvic side wall or parametria, there is a higher risk of harm to the somatic pelvic nerves during these procedures. If the inferior hypogastric plexus is harmed, hysterectomy and laparoscopic uterosacral nerve ablations may also result in visceral pelvic pain. Ironically, presacral neurolysis—which is done to treat persistent pelvic pain—may cause harm to the superior hypogastric plexus and induce new pelvic pain.

Changes in pelvic vein circulation may also be facilitated by pelvic vascular interventions and thrombosis, which could ultimately lead to the development of pelvic varicose veins. Such varicosities can induce pelvic congestion syndrome, which can lead to sacral compartment syndrome or vascular entrapment. In addition to childbirth-related trauma, other potential risk factors for pelvic pain include muscle or ligamentous entrapment or irritation, such as in sacrospinous ligament entrapment or pelvic floor muscle spasms. In less frequent instances, intrinsic neurotropic factors (e.g., either infiltrative (invasive neoplasia) or multiple sclerosis.

Damage to or irritation of the pelvic visceral afferent nerve fibers, also known as the pelvic splanchnic nerves, can also cause pelvic pain. These nerves, along with their somatic counterparts, transmit signals to the spinal cord through the dorsal root ganglia. Referred pain patterns arise from such damage, which the patient primarily attributes to the bladder, deep vagina, uterus, or ovaries. The clinical picture and management approach are complicated by the overlap between somatic pain distribution and visceral referred pain patterns (Burnett & Wesselmann, 1999).

8.3.2. Typical Presentation of the Most Common Pelvic Neuropathic Pain Syndromes

8.3.2.1. Vulvodynia, Coccygodynia, and Pudendal Neuralgia Pain Syndromes

Because symptoms of diseases affecting the sacral nerve roots can overlap with those of common genitourinary visceral disorders, diagnosing these conditions can be difficult. The posterior aspect of the thigh is affected by sciatica-like symptoms that are caused by lesions affecting the sacral nerve roots L5, S1, and S2. Sacral schwannomas frequently cause irritation to sacral nerve roots L5, S1, and S2 collectively. This contributes to the explanation of the clinical presentation of sciatica, vulvodynia, coccygodynia, and pudendal nerve pain.

Where symptoms start on the growth curve of a tumor depends on where it is along the nerve; smaller and earlier tumors can cause significant pudendal neuropathy (e.g., should the tumor be located in the Alcock canal. At that level, nerve involvement may first manifest as pain referred to the rectum and vaginal region, then progress to include the gluteal region and medial thigh. The dorsal nerve of the clitoris may be affected by irritation of the nerve prior to its entry into the canal, which can result in clitorodynia in addition to the usual vulvodynia symptoms.

Table 8.3. Gynecological Causes of Acute Pelvic Pain

Not Pregnant Women	Pregnant Woman
Ovarian torsion	Ectopic pregnancy
Ovarian follicle rupture/ hemorrhage	Uterine rupture
Pelvic inflammatory disease (PID)	Uterine torsion
Uterine myomas degeneration/ torsion	Placental disorders
Endometriosis	Spontaneous abortion
Endometriosis cyst rupture	
Ovarian hyperstimulation syndrome	
Gynecological cancers	
Ovarian vein thrombosis	

Source: *Franco PN, García-Baizán A, Aymerich M, Maino C, Frade-Santos S, Ippolito D, Otero-García M. Gynaecological causes of acute pelvic pain: Common and not-so-common imaging findings. Life. 2023; 13(10):2025. https://doi.org/10.3390/life13102025.*

A unilateral or bilateral burning sensation in the vulvar, perineal, or rectal areas can be a symptom of pudendal neuralgia pain. Pudendal neuralgia may manifest as progressive, refractory perineal pain that worsens with sitting. This pain may last the entire day. Pain is reduced when pressure is applied to the ischial tuberosities instead of the pelvic floor muscles, as when using a toilet seat. Pudendal nerve injury may cause the bladder's C-fiber pathway to become more active, which may result in urgency and frequency of urination similar to symptoms of genitourinary syndrome of menopause or bladder pain syndrome. In addition to the typical pudendal nerve symptoms caused by irritation of the pelvic splanchnic nerve in a referred pain pattern, some patients may also experience pain outside the pudendal dermatome. Patients frequently describe feeling pressured, as well as sitting on a tiny ball or having a foreign body in their vagina. The pudendal and pelvic visceral nerve afferent fibers transmit the sensation of a "hot poker" in the vagina or rectum, which can also be described. Genitopelvic dysesthesia, which has significant psychosocial ramifications, or symptoms of persistent genital arousal may be present in some patients with pelvic nerve injury or irritation.

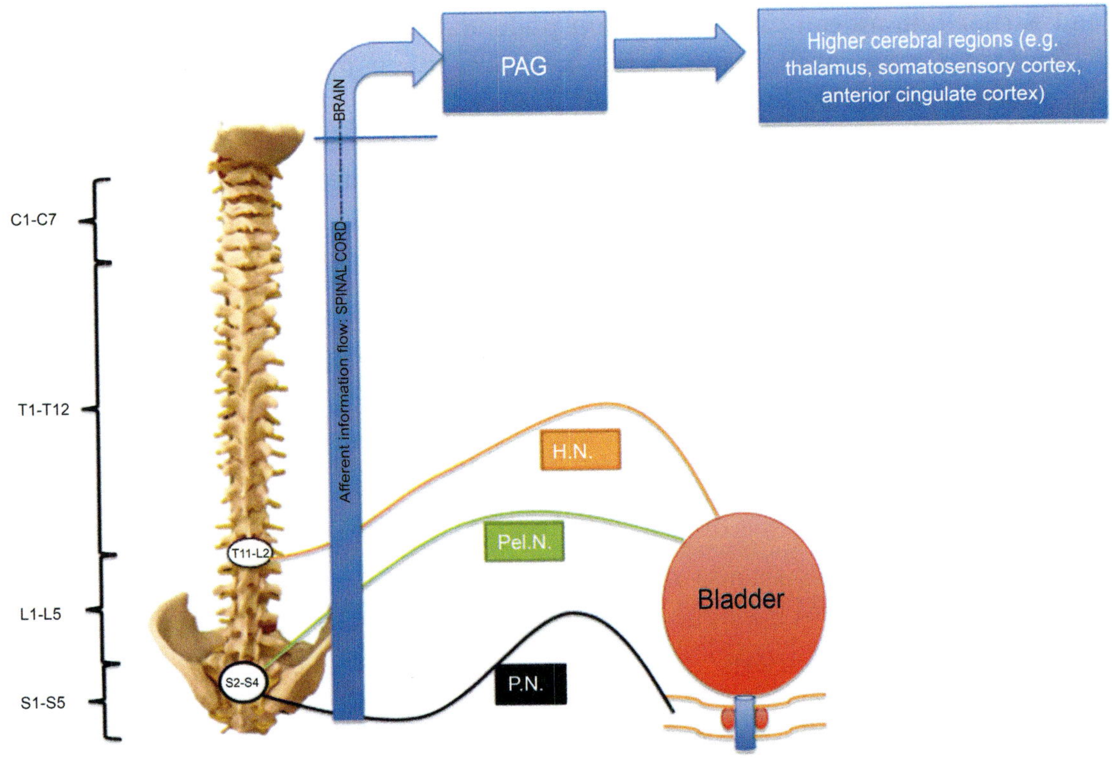

Figure 8.3. *Bladder innervation.*

Source. Roy H, Offiah I, Dua A. Neuromodulation for pelvic and urogenital pain. *Brain Sciences.* 2018; 8(10):180. https://doi.org/10.3390/brainsci8100180.

8.3.2.2. Ilioinguinal and Genitofemoral Nerve Entrapment Syndromes

When tissue planes cross and abruptly change direction at specific anatomical landmarks, peripheral nerves are susceptible to mechanical irritation; this is frequently the case for nerves supplying the anterior abdominal wall. Acute pain syndromes resulting in perineal, one-sided lower quadrant abdominal pain, and suprapubic pain can be caused by entrapment of the genitofemoral or ilioinguinal nerve. It may be chronic or acute. Because hormones can cause fluid retention or redistribution in the abdominal wall, pregnancy and the use of oral contraceptives may increase the risk of nerve entrapment at the locations of prior abdominal surgeries.

Due to the mechanical irritation of the abdominal wall muscles, young and active adults are most vulnerable. Because the symptoms resemble other acute gynecologic emergencies, these individuals frequently worry about their kidneys or ovaries. Therefore, cautious assessment is required to prevent needless diagnostic procedures and costly testing.

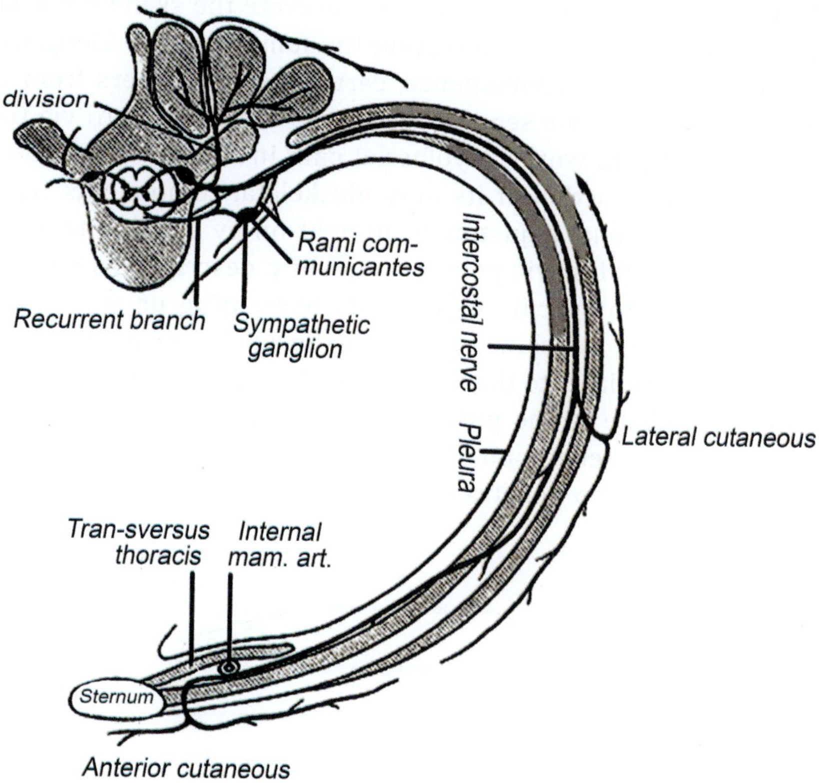

Figure 8.4. *Intercostal nerve fibers.*

Source: By Henry Vandyke Carter – Henry Gray (1918) Anatomy of the Human Body (See "Book" section below) Bartleby.com: Gray's Anatomy, Plate 819, Public Domain, https://commons.wikimedia.org/w/index.php?curid=541675.

The referred pain pathway, which is mediated by the visceral afferent fibers of the bladder, may be linked to bladder irritative symptoms that are brought on by irritation of these nerves. The thoracolumbar region (T12-L2), where these fibers project, is in charge of the spinal reflex that causes the bladder to fill. Therefore, in addition to keeping in mind anterior abdominal wall nerve entrapment syndromes, which are frequently overlooked, it is crucial to take into account retroperitoneal conditions that may irritate the pelvic nerves when pelvic pain is linked to sensory dysfunction of the bladder.

8.3.2.3. Musculoskeletal Syndromes That Present with Pelvic Pain

Over time, there has likely been a rise in the awareness and identification of musculoskeletal syndromes that manifest as pelvic pain. Myofascial pain syndromes are typically more common in adults 30 to 60 years of age, and more common in adults 65 and older, at 85%. Patients with myofascial pain frequently have trigger points, which are tender foci that are present in particular muscle groups and are brought on by either acute or repeated microtrauma to the muscle. Furthermore, referred pain—a distant site of pain that is felt but is not unique to the trigger point origin itself—may manifest as a result of these trigger points.

The spinal cord sends out motor fibers that innervate the skeletal muscles of the pelvic floor, pelvic walls, and perineum, thereby innervating the female pelvis. Along with afferents from the pelvic organs via viscerosomatic convergence, certain sensory fibers from these musculoskeletal organs and the parietal peritoneum send sensations to the spinal cord via the sacral nerve plexus. This clarifies how visceral pain works. Myofascial pain in the pelvis may be caused by overuse or trauma-related primary dysfunction of its musculoskeletal components (e.g., tendons, or nerves) or could result from a functional adjustment brought on by conditions of the hips or spine (e.g., misalignment). Muscle-skeletal pelvic pain is frequently described as vague and poorly localized, and it is frequently linked to specific movements like sitting or standing. One may experience unilateral pain that manifests as aching, throbbing, heaviness, or pelvic pressure. They frequently exhibit low back pain that radiates to the sacrum, the location of the levator ani muscle attachment. Additionally, pain may radiate to the posterior thigh and hip, which is indicative of a piriformis muscle spasm or neuropathy. Pelvic pain may be caused by hypertonicity of the pelvic floor muscles, which can also account for deep penetration sexual pain symptoms.

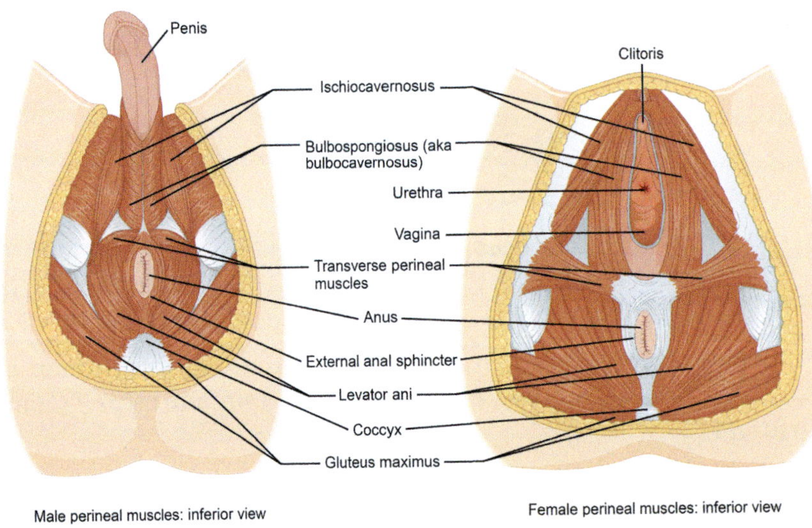

Figure 8.5. Pelvic floor muscles.

Source: By OpenStax – https://cnx.org/contents/FPtK1zmh@8.25:fEI3C8Ot@10/Preface, CC BY 4.0, https://commons.wikimedia.org/w/index.php?curid=30131691 (Burnett & Wesselmann, 1999).

8.4. Diagnostic Approach to Evaluation of Pelvic Pain

It is crucial to rule out surgical emergencies when treating pelvic pain syndromes because they are difficult and complex. In order to prevent needless treatment delays, pointless diagnostic procedures, or surgery that yields insignificant results, a methodical approach to evaluation and management should be followed.

It is crucial to listen to patients with chronic pelvic pain with empathy, to recognize that bias is ingrained in human nature, and to avoid the trap of satisfying one's own curiosity. A comprehensive review of the medical history should always be a part of the evaluation process to determine the source of pain. It is important to acknowledge the pathologic mechanisms affecting the spinal cord, cervical spine, and central nervous system. When taking a history, it's important to evaluate the location, duration, intensity, characteristic quality, and factors that aggravate or relieve the pain.

Furthermore, it's critical to find out how the medication is functioning in relation to daily activities, mood, and sleep; responses to previous treatment attempts and medication usage—whether beneficial or not—should also be carefully recorded. The presence of coexisting or past alcohol or drug use disorders should be noted due to potential treatment consequences and dependence risk. Details regarding previous pelvic trauma (e.g., falls, birth instruments, car crashes, sports injuries), medical procedures, or diagnoses that came on before the pain (e.g., endometriosis, herniorrhaphy, and Pfannenstiel incision) are also significant. Finally, because physical or psychological abuse has been linked to chronic pelvic floor pain, it is imperative to find out if there has been any history of this type of abuse.

8.4.1. Quality of Pain

Neuropathic pain patients typically describe their pain as electrical shock-like, burning (hot), tingling, prickling, or shooting. Visceral pelvic pain, which is felt through the pelvic splanchnic nerve afferents, is more ill-defined; it is dull, poorly localized, and may even be more of a general malaise than actual pain. Additionally, it frequently radiates along the midline to the lower back. Somatic pelvic pain, on the other hand, is best defined as localized pain that can be either chronic or intermittent. It frequently has distal radiation in the corresponding dermatomes. This pain is felt via the pelvic somatic nerve afferents. There is typically a trigger point at the irritability level for somatic pain. Increased sensitivity, throbbing, cramping, gnawing, stabbing, aching, or pinching are possible symptoms, as well as changes in the perception of temperature.

8.4.2. Location of Pain

Deep vaginal pain can be attributed to irritation of the pelvic nerves that transmit their signals through the afferent nerve fibers, or to irritation of the inferior hypogastric plexus (a portion of the pelvic splanchnic nerve plexus), which results in visceral, poorly localized pain with vegetative symptoms like nausea and vomiting. The presence of groin pain along with anterior vulvar pain, whether or not it radiates to the thigh, suggests genitofemoral nerve (or lumbar plexus) pathology. Symptoms of irritation of the pudendal nerve include perianal, vulvar, and perineal pain.

8.4.3. Associated Symptoms

Pudendal pain associated with leg pain (sciatica), low back pain, or gluteal pain indicates a sacral plexus pathology, while pain radiating to the anterior thigh indicates a spinal-vertebral disorder. Visceral pain frequently coexists with diaphoresis, pallor, tachycardia, nausea, and vomiting. In addition to bowel-related symptoms like constipation/dyschezia or decreased awareness of defecating, other symptoms like urinary hesitancy, frequency, or urgency may be related to pelvic nerve afferents or ilioinguinal nerve irritation. Pelvic pain syndromes are frequently linked to sexual dysfunction, including loss of libido. Loss of movement in the hip, knee, and foot flexion is a characteristic of large lesions of the sacral nerve roots, or plexopathy. Bladder irritative symptoms can occur in any sacral nerve root irritation or damage due to the parasympathetic supply (pelvic splanchnic nerves) to the bladder in sacral nerve roots S3–S5. Loss of sensitivity or even numbness in the corresponding dermatomes is observed in cases of axonal nerve damage. When the sacral nerve is involved, urodynamic testing can confirm bladder hyposensitivity and increased bladder capacity, as well as detrusor hypotonia or atonia.

8.4.4. Exacerbating Factors

Musculoskeletal dysfunction is characterized by pain that gets worse with prolonged sitting or standing, physical activity, bowel movements, sexual activity, or anxiety, especially if the pain gets worse throughout the day. Levator ani syndrome is a possibility. Some exacerbating factors, like a sedentary lifestyle, poor ergonomics, wearing high heels frequently, or long driving hours with inadequate back support, may be related to the patient's work or way of life. Pudendal neuralgia patients find that sitting makes their pain worse and that standing, lying down, or sitting on a toilet seat makes their pain go away. Pelvic nerve entrapment caused by endometriosis causes pain that worsens during menstruation and may go down in response to gonadotropin-releasing hormone analogs. Increases in pelvic venous pressure (from standing or sitting for extended periods of time, or straining to pass gas) can irritate the pelvic nerves due to vascular entrapment or compression (sacral compartment syndrome), which in turn triggers a pain response. Furthermore, there are circumstances in which a strong pulsation of the pelvic veins can cause pain, such as tricuspid insufficiency or a close anatomical relationship between the nerve and the arterial vasculature.

8.4.5. Careful and Focused Physical Examination

Observing the patient's gait or sitting posture, which may point to bad sitting habits, is the first step in the examination process. To prevent pressure on one side of the pelvis, which could exacerbate their pain, patients may choose to sit in a specific way. A thorough physical examination starts with a head and neck examination to rule out adenopathy. Then, the heart and lungs are examined to rule out any abnormal heart murmurs that could indicate valvular heart disease. Along with evaluating the curvature, asymmetry, and hypertrophy of the muscles or changes in range of motion, evaluation of the lumbar spine and pelvic joints is also crucial. Along with the anterior superior iliac joints for asymmetry, which would indicate pelvic misalignment, and lower extremity range of motion, the pubic symphysis and sacroiliac joints are evaluated for palpable tenderness. Hernias, trigger points, and scars from prior surgeries should all be evaluated on the abdomen. Pain believed to have ovarian or visceral origins could be replicated with careful evaluation along the course of the ilioinguinal and genitofemoral nerve, superior and medial to the anterior superior iliac spine. It is essential to assess the inferior rib cage margin, particularly the point where the rectus abdominis joins the costal margin. Patients experiencing pelvic or lower abdominal pain may benefit from an unexpected diagnosis provided by thoracic nerves 11 and 12, which supply the dermatomes of the lower abdomen. A comprehensive neurological assessment ought to encompass skin visualization, muscle strength, sensation, and reflex testing.

It is possible to evaluate sensory abnormalities using affordable and easily accessible methods. A soft brush, a piece of cotton, or light finger pressure can be used to evaluate beta touch fibers; a sharp object, like a pin, can be used to evaluate A delta (fast) pain fibers; and a warm object is the best tool for evaluating C (slow) pain fibers.

Patients experiencing pelvic or lower abdominal pain should have a proper pelvic examination, which should include the Q-tip test (pelvic floor reflex testing) for anal winking. The medial thigh and the mons pubis should be included in the sensory function assessment.

Pelvic prolapse has been linked to persistent pelvic pain, so it's important to properly evaluate the condition with a Sims speculum exam to check for pelvic floor organ bulging. If clinically indicated, additional testing should involve examining all genital organs, getting a vaginal culture, a urine sample, a vaginal pH test, a Papanicolaou test, and a biopsy of any abnormal vulvar areas.

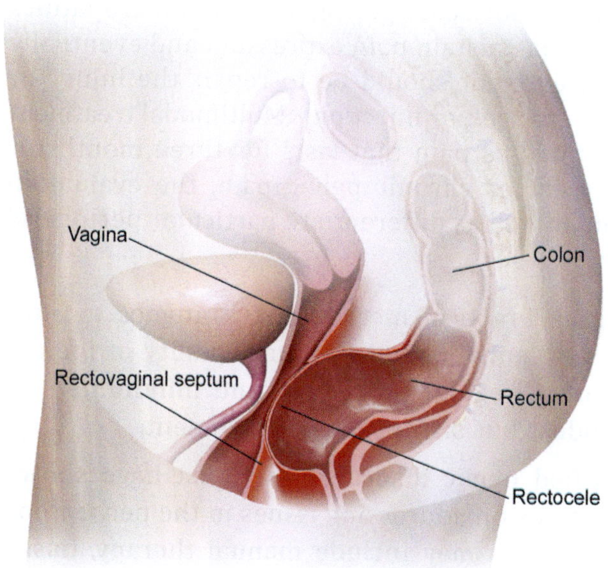

Figure 8.6. A rectocele is a bulge, or herniation, of the front wall of the rectum into the back of the vagina.

Source. By BruceBlaus - Own work, CC BY-SA 4.0, https://commons.wikimedia.org/w/index.php?curid=61278372.

Assessing the internal pelvic musculature is crucial next. Examiners should pay close attention to the patient's pain perception for signs of increased muscle tone, introital tenderness, spasm, or an inability of the muscles to relax. It is important to evaluate the quality and coordination of pelvic floor contraction and relaxation. The parametria, rectovaginal space, pudendal nerves, and low sacral nerve roots are all evaluated by rectal palpation. Patients with pudendal neuralgia may exhibit tenderness in the genitoanal area upon transrectal/vaginal palpation of the pudendal nerve at the sacrospinous ligament, along with a positive Tinel sign. The low sacral nerve roots are reachable a few centimeters to the left and right of the midline sacral bone. Individuals who meet the criteria for central nervous system pathology should be referred to a neurologist for a thorough evaluation of their neurologic and neuropsychiatric conditions.

8.4.6. Imaging

In some cases, it may be advised to make prudent use of imaging to support treatment planning or to confirm retroperitoneal pathologic processes. Vaginal ultrasonography is taken into account when evaluating the structures and organs found in the female pelvis. Moreover, pelvic varicosities—defined as >7-mm dilated vessels with reflux—and bladder wall thickness can be assessed with ultrasonography in addition to postvoid residual urine volume. For women with pelvic endometriosis, kidney ultrasonography may be advised as a screening for ureteral obstructive uropathy, which can be asymptomatic.

To rule out soft-tissue neoplasms suspected of exacerbating pelvic pain symptoms, such as in patients with suspected lumbosacral radicular symptoms or DIE affecting the sacral plexus or parametria, magnetic resonance imaging is frequently required. In cases of suspected DIE, pudendal nerve entrapment syndromes, or Tarlov cysts, special protocols are typically requested.

In order to determine whether a patient is a candidate for coil embolization or sclerotherapy, vascular evaluation for patients suspected of having pelvic congestion syndrome and vulvar varices typically uses duplex studies of the lower extremities to rule out venous insufficiency or

CT venography to rule out communication of the deep and superficial veins. Pudendal nerve blocks may be used as a therapeutic or diagnostic tool. They can be performed vaginally or through a transgluteal approach with ultrasound guidance. If the pain completely goes away after receiving a local anesthetic injection, the diagnosis of entrapment neuropathy is verified.

8.5. Nonsurgical Treatment of Neuropathic Pelvic Pain

Treating the presumed cause of neuropathic pelvic pain should be the primary treatment strategy. With a few notable exceptions, peripheral mononeuropathies such as genitofemoral neuralgia, pudendal neuralgia, ilioinguinal, iliohypogastric, and abdominal cutaneous nerve entrapment can be treated similarly to other mononeuropathies. Treatment for acute peripheral mononeuropathies generally aims to stop the formation of cortical changes that sustain pain expression and eventually lead to chronic pain. The goal of the first course of treatment should be to repair the injury or adequately manage the pain with medication, behavioral changes, or injections. Multimodal treatment works best for chronic neuropathic pain, which is defined as pain that lasts for three months or longer. In order to better customize the treatment plan for chronic pelvic pain, the evaluation process aims to determine treatable causes of the pain as well as differentiate particular peripheral causes from overlapping centralized pain syndromes.

Nonsurgical methods have demonstrated potential. Practical methods or strategies to alter physical activity, lessen anxiety and catastrophizing, and enhance function and quality of life are all part of cognitive behavior therapy. Encouragement of regular movement and mindfulness to prevent patient fixation on the site may lead to a modest but significant improvement.

Patients receiving physical therapy from a certified pelvic disorders therapist have shown improvement in their outcomes. The therapy sessions focus on addressing issues in the pelvic floor, hip, back, and abdominal wall muscles. Treatment methods may include manual therapy, tissue mobilization, biofeedback, acupressure, and ultrasound treatments. Therapists also incorporate pain education and cognitive-behavioral techniques like mindfulness strategies. In a study of 60 patients with chronic pelvic pain, those who received conventional therapy along with yoga experienced a greater reduction in pain intensity and improved quality of life after 8 weeks compared to those who only received therapy.

NSAIDs, tricyclic antidepressants (TCAs), gabapentinoids, selective serotonin reuptake inhibitors, serotonin-norepinephrine reuptake inhibitors, muscle relaxants, and topical analgesics are among the medications used in pharmacologic treatment. Compared to swallowed drugs, topical creams or suppositories are typically more well tolerated and have a more focused effect with fewer systemic side effects.

Nerve blocks, radiofrequency ablation, and neuromodulation procedures can be beneficial when addressing a particular pathology and after more conventional treatment options have been used up. For some pathologic processes, additional targeted treatments may be used, as explained in the paragraphs that follow.

Table 8.3. Best Evidence for Lifestyle Interventions for Women with Pelvic Girdle Pain According to Systematic Reviews Following PRISMA

Lifestyle Factor	First Author Year Published Type of Data Synthesis	Included Population PGP/LPP/LBP	Pregnancy/Postpartum Number of SR/RCT Number of Participants	Detail of Lifestyle Factor/Intervention Assessed	Quality of Studies (Tool and Results)	Main Results on Interventions	Summary of Evidence
Physical activity and/or Exercise	Weis et al., 2020 [55] SR and meta-analysis	PGP/LPP LBP	Pregnancy Six SRs based on nine RCTs **PGP**: Four SRs based on three RCTs **LPP**: Nine SRs based on four RCTs **LBP**: Five SRs based on seven RCTs	land or water-based exercise in group or individual	Modified version of Scottish Intercollegiate Guideline Network **PGP**: high-quality, low risk of bias (1 SR) acceptable-quality, moderate risk of bias (1 SR) low-quality, high risk of bias (2 SR) **LPP**: high-quality, low risk of bias (1 SR) acceptable-quality, moderate risk of bias (7 SR) low-quality, high risk of bias (1 SR) **LBP**: high-quality, low risk of bias (1 SR) acceptable-quality, moderate risk of bias (3 SR) low-quality, high risk of bias (1 SR)	**PGP**: decreased pain intensity and disability **LPP**: improved function and reduced prevalence from most SRs **LBP**: 4/5 SRs reduced pain intensity and disability	**PGP**: inconclusive, evidence with favorable outcomes **LPP**: moderate strength evidence with unclear outcomes **LBP**: inconclusive, strength with favorable outcomes

Physical activity and/or Exercise	Weis et al., 2020 **[42]** SR and meta-analysis	PGP/LPP	Postpartum Two SRs based on six RCTs **PGP**: Two SRs based on four RCTs **LPP**: Two SRs based on two RCTs **LBP**: 0 SR	exercise in group or individual	Modified version of Scottish Intercollegiate Guideline Network **PGP**: Acceptable-quality, moderate risk of bias **LPP**: Acceptable-quality, moderate risk of bias	**PGP**: One of three SRs stated additional effect of exercises at reducing pain and disability. **LPP**: no firm conclusions could be drawn	**PGP**: moderate strength of evidence with unclear outcomes. **LPP**: inconclusive strength of evidence and unclear outcomes
Physical activity and/or Exercise	Davenport et al., 2019 **[56]** SR and meta-analysis	PGP/LPP LBP	Pregnancy and postpartum 3 studies (n = 52297) out of 23 RCTs (13 exercise only and 10 exercise +co-interventions) **pregnancy** -pooled estimates prevalence 12 RCTs (n = 1987) -pooled estimates severity 10 RCTs (n = 784). **postpartum** -pooled estimates prevalence 3 RCTs (n = 491) -severity 1 RCTs (n = 257)	result presented from 'exercise only' or 'exercise with co-intervention' (yoga, aerobic exercise, general muscle strengthening or muscle strengthening specific to one body region and combination of aerobic and resistance training)	GRADE criteria **pregnancy** Prevalence: very low-quality Serious risk of bias, serious directness of the interventions and serious imprecision. Severity: very low-quality Serious risk of bias, serious inconsistency, and serious indirectness of the interventions. **postpartum**: Prevalence: low-quality Serious indirectness of the interventions and serious imprecision. Severity: low quality Serious risk of bias and serious inconsistency.	**pregnancy** PGP/LPP/LBP: no reduced odds (OR 0.78, 95% CI 0.60, 1.02) lower pain severity (standardized mean difference −1.03, 95% CI −1.58, −0.48) **postpartum** PGP/LPP/LBP: no reduced odds (OR 0.89, 95% CI 0.51, 1.56) decreased severity of LBP (p = 0.034) (only 1 RCT)	**pregnancy** PGP/LPP/ LBP: very low to moderate quality evidence **postpartum** PGP/LPP/ LBP: low quality to moderate evidence low quality evidence

Physical activity and/or Exercise	Almousa et al., 2018 **[57]** SR	PGP	Pregnancy and postpartum Five RCTs + 1 follow up (n between 44 and 330) **pregnancy** Two RCTs (n = 426) **postpartum** Two RCTs (n = 125) +1 follow up (n = 65) pregnancy and postpartum One RCT (n = 103)	stabilizing exercises	Pedro scale Scores range 5–8, i.e., 5 studies good-quality and 1 study fair-quality	**pregnancy** decrease pain (2 RCTs) and improved quality of life (1 RCT) **postpartum** contradictory results	insufficient evidence
Physical activity and/or Exercise	Shiri et al., 2018 **[58]** SR and meta-analysis	PGP LBP	Pregnancy pooled 11 RCTs (n = 2347) **PGP**: Four RCTs (n = 565) **LPP**: Eight RCTs (n = 1737); out of only three RCTs (n = 1168) evaluating sick leave) **LBP**: Seven RCTs (n = 1175) out of only two RCTs (n = 349) evaluating sick leave	exercise of different type and in different combinations	Cochrane Collaboration's tool. Low heterogeneity in meta-analyzes * Low publication bias *	**PGP**: no protective effect (RR 0.99, 95% CI 0.81–1.21 **LPP**: no protective effect (RR 0.96, 95% CI 0.90–1.02) but prevented new episodes of sick leave (RR 0.79, 95% CI 0.64–0.99) **LBP**: reduced risk 9% (pooled RR) 0.91, 95% CI 0.83–0.99) prevented new episodes of sick leave (RR 0.67, 95% CI 0.40–1.12)	Exercise appears to reduce risk of LBP and sick leave due to LPP but no clear evidence on PGP

Physical activity and/or Exercise	Liddle and Pennick 2015 [**4**] SR and meta-analysis	PGP/LPP LBP	pregnancy Thirty-four RCTs (*n* = 5121) **PGP**: Six RCTs (*n* = 889) pooled two RCTs (*n* = 374) **LPP**: Thirteen RCTs (*n* = 2385) pooled four RCTs (*n* = 1176) **LBP**: Fifteen RCTs (*n* = 1847) pooled seven RCTs (*n* = 645)	exercises on land/in water	Cochrane Collaboration's tool GRADE criteria Clinical heterogeneity precluded pooling results in many cases. Statistical heterogeneity was substantial in all but three meta-analyzes, not improving following sensitivity analyzes. Publication bias and selective reporting cannot be ruled out.	**PGP**: no effect on prevalence of PGP **LPP**: reduced prevalence and pain (RR 0.66; 95% CI 0.45 to 0.97) reduced sick leave (RR 0.76; 95% CI 0.62 to 0.94.) **LBP**: no effect on prevalence (RR 0.97; 95% CI 0.80 to 1.17) reduced pain (SMD −0.64; 95% CI −1.03 to −0.25) and reduced functional disability (SMD −0.56; 95% CI −0.89 to −0.23)	**PGP**: Low quality evidence **LPP**: Moderate-quality evidence Low-quality evidence **LBP**: Low-quality evidence

Physical activity and/or Exercise	Tseng et al., 2015 **[59]** SR	LPP	postpartum Four RCTs n = 251	exercise programs to strengthen deep local muscles and global muscles in the lumbopelvic regions	Cochrane Collaboration's tool Pedro scale Scores range 4–8, i.e., three studies good-quality and one study fair quality. All studies except one were at low risk of bias on key domains such as sequence generation, allocation concealment, blinding of participants and personnel, completeness of outcome data for each main outcome, and selective reporting.	inconclusive on pain intensity and disability	no evidence

PGP: pelvic girdle pain; LPP: lumbopelvic pain; LBP: low back pain; RR: risk ratio; SMD: standardized mean difference; CI: 95% confidence interval; SR: systematic reviews; RCT: randomized controlled trials; * for details on risk of bias, refer to original study.

Source: Gutke A, Sundfeldt K, De Baets L. Lifestyle and Chronic Pain in the Pelvis: State of the Art and Future Directions. *Journal of Clinical Medicine*. 2021; 10(22):5397. https://doi.org/10.3390/jcm10225397.

8.5.1. Pudendal Neuralgia

Early on in the treatment plan, it is important to incorporate behavioral modifications specific to pudendal neuralgia, such as using an offloading cushion, avoiding cycling, and avoiding prolonged sitting. Pudendal neuralgia frequently causes excessive pelvic floor muscle spasm, so techniques to ease tension, like physical therapy, are beneficial. Physical therapy can help release the tension or compression on the irritated nerve and help train the overactive pelvic muscles.

NSAIDs, TCAs, anticonvulsants, and topical or oral muscle relaxants are examples of pharmacologic treatments. According to a retrospective study, pudendal nerve blocks were successful in 31% of patients, sitting pads and conservative treatment led to slight to moderate improvements, and surgical decompression worked for 60% of patients. 29 A different study demonstrated the efficacy of hyaluronidase or botulinum toxin. 20 out of the 27 patients who received spinal cord stimulation of the conus medullaris experienced long-term relief. However, because of anatomical structures and conus movement, treatment failures involving lead placement at the conus medullaris have been documented. It has also been demonstrated that other methods, such as radiofrequency ablation of the pudendal nerve, peripheral nerve stimulation, and sacral nerve stimulation, reduce pain.

8.5.2. Ilioinguinal, Iliohypogastric, and Genitofemoral Neuralgia and Anterior Cutaneous Nerve Entrapment

Wearing less-restrictive clothing and staying away from exercises that put undue strain on the area of the nerve entrapment are behavioral management strategies for ilioinguinal, genitofemoral, and abdominal cutaneous nerve entrapment. NSAIDs, TCAs, anticonvulsants, and topical or oral local analgesics are examples of pharmacologic treatments.

Both anterior neuronectomy techniques and trigger point injections produced noticeably better results in a 2016 systematic review of 7 studies that specifically addressed abdominal cutaneous nerve entrapment. If all other conservative options have been exhausted and nerve blocks are unable to produce long-lasting relief, then pulsed radiofrequency ablation may be a possibility. In a recent randomized controlled trial, patients with anterior cutaneous nerve entrapment syndrome who received a neurectomy (17 of 28 patients) or pulsed radiofrequency (12 of 32 patients) experienced pain reductions of more than 50%. In a retrospective study, the average length of time patients experienced relief from chronic inguinal neuralgia following pulsed radiofrequency treatment was 12.5 months, as opposed to 11.6 months for conventional nerve block using anesthetic and corticosteroid. Patients with genitofemoral neuralgia experienced a 70% reduction in pain upon peripheral nerve stimulation.

8.5.3. Pelvic Floor Dysfunction

Given that active trigger points can arise from localized trauma, psychological stressors, and viscerosomatic reflexes (such as in endometriosis and interstitial cystitis), pelvic floor dysfunction should be evaluated and treated if it is present. Injections of botulinum toxin, trigger point injections, physical therapy, cognitive behavior therapy, and muscle relaxants are among the available treatment options.

Diazepam and Baclofen are frequently used vaginal muscle relaxants that improve the ability of γ-aminobutyric acid to relieve skeletal muscle spasms. Comparable serum levels can be obtained with topical vaginal diazepam and oral administration. Because baclofen can still intensify opioid-related central nervous system depression, which raises the risk of overdose, it is only advised as a diazepam substitute for patients who are already taking opioids.

Abdominal wall or pelvic musculature trigger points linked to pelvic pain can result in motor, sensory, and autonomic dysfunction. Anesthetic-only trigger point injections appear to be just as effective as those that also include corticosteroid. Additionally, smaller focal areas of pain appear to respond better to trigger point injections than widespread pain that can be palpated.

Apart from trigger point injections, mechanically modifying the muscle dynamics can be achieved through dry-needling and injection of botulinum toxin. Inhibiting the target tissue's cholinergic innervation, botulinum toxin blocks nociceptive transmission not only at the neuromuscular junction but also in the parasympathetic or sympathetic neural synopsis. 44 Vaginal manometry measures lower resting pressures and maximum contraction pressures, demonstrating that botulinum toxin reduces both muscle hyperactivity and tenderness to palpation. Before proceeding, it is advisable to have a discussion with the patient regarding the possible side effects of botulinum toxin injections in the pelvic region. These effects may include urinary retention, incontinence, constipation, vulvar irritation, urinary tract infection, and flulike symptoms. Therefore, it would be best to consider botulinum toxin after a patient has not responded to trigger point injections, medications, or physical therapy.

Routine follow-up is crucial for patients with neuropathic pain in order to rule out or treat other underlying medical conditions, in addition to pursuing and achieving symptom control. In order to help patients understand what to expect from their treatments, treating physicians should talk to them about the limitations of the current treatments as well as the natural history of the neuropathic condition. Because some patients will respond well to less invasive, safer, and more affordable treatment options, a stepwise approach to treatment is advised. Early detection and evaluation of co-occurring mental health and drug use disorders may facilitate prompt referral to other specialists within the multidisciplinary treatment team (Aber & Higgins, 1982; Beck, Fowler, & Mathias, 1994).

A Closer Look

Hypogastric Plexus

The hypogastric plexus is a complex network of nerves located in the pelvic region, specifically in the lower abdomen near the sacral vertebrae. It plays a crucial role in the autonomic nervous system (ANS) and serves as a major center for the regulation of various visceral functions, including those of the reproductive and urinary systems. Composed of sympathetic and parasympathetic fibers, the hypogastric plexus integrates sensory information from pelvic organs and modulates their activity to maintain homeostasis.

The sympathetic fibers within the hypogastric plexus originate from the lumbar and sacral segments of the spinal cord, forming connections with preganglionic neurons in the sympathetic chain ganglia. These fibers innervate pelvic organs such as the bladder, uterus, and rectum, regulating functions such as smooth muscle contraction, blood flow, and glandular secretion. Sympathetic activation of the hypogastric plexus can lead to responses such as bladder relaxation and inhibition of peristalsis, whereas sympathetic inhibition can induce bladder contraction and enhance peristalsis.

Parasympathetic fibers also contribute to the hypogastric plexus, originating from the sacral segments of the spinal cord and forming connections with ganglia located within or near the plexus. Parasympathetic innervation plays a key role in promoting activities such as bladder emptying, sexual arousal, and bowel movements. Stimulation of parasympathetic pathways within the hypogastric plexus leads to increased bladder contraction and relaxation of the internal urethral sphincter, facilitating urine expulsion.

The hypogastric plexus is involved in the transmission and modulation of pain signals arising from pelvic organs, a process known as visceral nociception. Sensory neurons within the plexus relay pain signals to the central nervous system, where they are integrated with other sensory inputs and contribute to the perception of visceral pain. Dysregulation of the hypogastric plexus can lead to various pelvic pain syndromes, including conditions such as interstitial cystitis, endometriosis, and chronic pelvic pain.

The hypogastric plexus plays a critical role in regulating visceral functions within the pelvis through its intricate network of sympathetic and parasympathetic fibers. Understanding the anatomy and function of the hypogastric plexus is essential for elucidating the pathophysiology of pelvic disorders and developing targeted interventions for their management.

Summary

- Genitourinary pain encompasses a diverse range of pain syndromes affecting the organs and structures of the genitourinary system, including the kidneys, bladder, ureters, urethra, prostate, and reproductive organs.
- The pelvic region including the genitourinary tract is a highly specialized area of the body, responsible for carrying out a host of basic biological functions including micturition, copulation, and reproduction.
- Somatic efferents originate within Onuf's nucleus in the ventral horn and afferents have their cell bodies located within dorsal root ganglia at these levels.
- Interstitial cystitis (IC) is a chronic, painful, and often debilitating disease, whose etiology and pathophysiology are largely unknown.
- Chronic testicular pain (orchialgia) can be one of the most vexing pain problems for men and their treating physicians.
- Prostatodynia is defined as persistent complaints of urinary urgency, dysuria, poor urinary flow, and perineal discomfort, without evidence of bacteria or purulence in the prostatic fluid.
- Perineal pain can be part of one of the more specific genitourinary pain syndromes discussed here, such as interstitial cystitis, urethral syndrome, clitoral pain, vulvodynia, testicular pain, or prostatodynia, all of which might present with pain radiating into the perineal region.
- Endometriosis excision procedures commonly performed for DIE cases pose an increased risk of damage to the somatic pelvic nerves because of the necessary surgical dissection of the pelvic side wall or parametria.
- Patients with neuropathic pain usually describe their pain as burning (hot), pins and needles, tingling, prickling, or shooting (electrical shock-like).

References

1. Aber, G. M., & Higgins, P. M. (1982). The natural history and management of the loin pain/haematuria syndrome. *British Journal of Urology, 54*, 613–615.
2. Ali, M. S. (1983). Testicular pain in a patient with aneurysm of the common iliac artery. *British Journal of Urology, 55*, 447–448.
3. Allan, J. D. D., Bultitude, M. I., Bultitude, M. F., Wall, P. D., & McMahon, S. B. (1997). The effect of capsaicin on renal pain signaling systems in humans and Wistar rats. *Journal of Physiology, 505*, 39P.
4. Althof, S. E., Turner, L. A., Levine, S. B., et al. (1987). Intracavernosal injection in the treatment of impotence: A prospective study of sexual, psychological, and marital functioning. *Journal of Sex and Marital Therapy, 13*, 155–167.
5. Baker, L. R., Mallinson, W. J., Gregory, M. C., et al. (1987). Idiopathic retroperitoneal fibrosis. A retrospective analysis of 60 cases. *British Journal of Urology, 60*, 497–503.
6. Barbalias, G. A. (1990). Proctodynia or painful male urethral syndrome? *Urology, 36*, 146–153.

7. Barbalias, G. A., Meares, E. M. Jr., & Sant, G. R. (1983). Proctodynia: Clinical and urodynamic characteristics. *Journal of Urology, 130*, 514–517.

8. Barbalias, G. A., Nikiforidis, G., & Liatsikos, E. N. (1998). Alpha-blockers for the treatment of chronic prostatitis in combination with antibiotics. *Journal of Urology, 159*, 883–887.

9. Barker, S. B., Matthews, P. N., Philip, P. F., & Williams, G. (1987). Prospective study of intravesical dimethyl sulphoxide in the treatment of chronic inflammatory bladder disease. *British Journal of Urology, 59*, 142–144.

10. Baskin, L. S., & Tanagho, E. A. (1992). Pain without pelvic organs. *Journal of Urology, 147*, 683–686.

11. Batta, A. G., Gundian, J. C., & Myers, R. P. (1989). Neurofibromatosis presenting as perineal pain and urethral burning. *Urology, 33*, 138–140.

12. Beck, R., Fowler, C. J., & Mathias, C. J. (1994). Genitourinary dysfunction in disorders of the autonomic nervous system. In D. N. Rushton (Ed.), *Handbook of Neuro-Urology* (pp. 281–301). Marcel Dekker, New York.

13. Bennini, A. (1992). Die Ilioinguinalis- und Genitofemoralisneuralgie. *Schweizerische Rundschau der Medizin, 81*, 1114–1120.

14. Bensignor, M. F., Labat, J. J., Robert, R., & Ducrot, P. (1996). Diagnostic and therapeutic pudendal nerve blocks for patients with perineal non-malignant pain. *Abstract, 8th World Congress on Pain*, p 56.

15. Berger, R. E., Miller, J. E., Rothman, I., Krieger, J. N., & Muller, C. H. (1998). Bladder petechiae after cystoscopy and hydrodistension in men diagnosed with prostate pain. *Journal of Urology, 159*, 83–85.

16. Bergeron, S., Binik, Y. M., Khalife, S., Pagidas, K., Glazer, H. I., Meana, M., & Amsel, R. (2001). A randomized comparison of group-cognitive behavioral therapy, surface electromyographic biofeedback, and vestibulectomy in the treatment of dyspareunia resulting from vulvar vestibulitis. *Pain, 91*, 297–306.

17. Bergeron, S., Bouchard, C., Fortier, M., & Binik, Y. M., Khalife, S. (1997). The surgical treatment of vulvar vestibulitis syndrome: A follow-up study. *Journal of Sex and Marital Therapy, 23*, 317–325.

18. Bergman, A., Karram, M., & Bhatia, N. N. (1989). Urethral syndrome: A comparison of different treatment modalities. *Journal of Reproductive Medicine, 34*, 157–160.

19. Bhaskar, P. A. (1987). Scrotal pain with testicular jerking: An unusual manifestation of epilepsy. *Journal of Neurology, Neurosurgery and Psychiatry, 50*, 1233–1234.

20. Binik, Y. M., Meana, M., Berkley, K., & Khalife, S. (1999). The sexual pain disorders: Is the pain sexual or is the sex painful. *Annual Reviews of Sex Research, 10*, 210–235.

21. Bohm-Starke, N., Hilliges, M., Brodda-Jansen, G., Rylander, E., & Torebjörk, E. (2001). Psychophysical evidence of nociceptor sensitization in vulvar vestibulitis syndrome. *Pain, 94*, 177–183.

22. Bohm-Starke, N., Hilliges, M., Falconer, C., & Rylander, E. (1998). Increased intraepithelial innervation in women with vulvar vestibulitis syndrome. *Gynecologic and Obstetric Investigation, 46*, 256–260.

23. Briggs, L. A. (1998). Female circumcision in Nigeria—Is it not time for government intervention. *Health Care Analysis, 6*, 14–23.

24. Brunner, H., Weidner, W., & Schiefer, H. C. (1983). Studies on the role of Ureaplasma urealyticum and Mycoplasma hominis in prostatitis. *Journal of Infectious Diseases, 126*, 807–813.

25. Buck, A. C., Crean, M., & Jenkins, I. L. (1982). Osteitis pubis as a mimic of prostatic pain. *British Journal of Urology, 54*, 741–744.

26. Bultitude, M. I. (1995). Capsaicin in treatment of loin pain/hematuria syndrome. *Lancet, 345*, 921–922.

27. Bultitude, M., Young, J., Bultitude, M., & Allan, J. (1998). Loin pain hematuria syndrome: Distress resolved by pain relief. *Pain, 76*, 209–213.

28. Burden, R. P., Booth, L. J., Ockenden, B. G., Boyd, W. N., Higgins, P. McR., & Aber, G. M. (1975). Intrarenal vascular changes in adult patients with recurrent hematuria and loin pain: A clinical, histological and angiographic study. *Quarterly Journal of Medicine, 175*, 433–447.

29. Burnett, A. L., & Wesselmann, U. (1999). Neurobiology of the pelvis and perineum: Principles for a practical approach. *Journal of Pelvic Surgery, 5*, 224–232.

30. Carson, C. C., Segura, J. W., & Osborne, D. M. (1980). Evaluation and treatment of the female urethral syndrome. *Journal of Urology, 124*, 609–610.

31. Cervero, F. (1994). Sensory innervation of the viscera: Peripheral basis of visceral pain. *Physiological Reviews, 74*, 95–138.

32. Chaiken, D. C., Blaivas, J. G., & Blaivas, S. T. (1993). Behavioral therapy for the treatment of refractory interstitial cystitis. *Journal of Urology, 149*, 1445–1448.

33. Chen, T. F., & Ball, R. Y. (1991). Epididymectomy for post-vasectomy pain: Histological review. *British Journal of Urology, 68*, 407–413.

34. Childs, S. J. (1994). Dimethyl sulfone in the treatment of interstitial cystitis. *Urologic Clinics of North America, 21*, 85–88.

35. Choa, R. G., & Swami, K. S. (1992). Testicular denervation: A new surgical procedure for intractable testicular pain. *British Journal of Urology, 70*, 417–419.

36. Corder, A. P. (1989). Penile pain and direct inguinal hernia. *British Journal of Hospital Medicine, 42*, 238.

37. Costabile, R. A., Hahn, M., & McLeod, D. G. (1991). Chronic orchialgia in the pain prone patient: The clinical perspective. *Journal of Urology, 146*, 1571–1574.

38. Curhan, G. C., Speizer, F. E., Hunter, D. J., Curhan, S. G., & Stampfer, M. J. (1999). Epidemiology of interstitial cystitis: A population-based study. *Journal of Urology, 161*, 549–552.

39. Davis, B. E., Noble, M. J., Weigel, J. W., Foret, J., & Mebust, W. K. (1990). Analysis and management of chronic testicular pain. *Journal of Urology, 143*, 936–939.

40. Davis, D. M. (1955). Vesicle orifice obstruction in women and its treatment by transurethral resection. *Journal of Urology, 73*, 112–117.

41. De Deus, J. M., Focchi, J., Stavale, J. N., & De Lima, G. R. (1995). Histologic and biomolecular aspects of papillomatosis of the vulvar vestibule in relation to human papillomavirus. *Obstetrics and Gynecology, 86*, 758–763.

42. De Groat, W. C. (1994). Neurophysiology of the pelvic organs. In D. N. Rushton (Ed.), *Handbook of Neuro-Urology* (pp. 55–93). Marcel Dekker, New York.

43. De Groat, W. C., Booth, A. M., & Yoshimura, N. (1993). Neurophysiology of micturition and its modification in animal models of human disease. In C. A. Maggi (Ed.), *Nervous Control of The Urogenital System* (pp. 227–290). Harwood Academic, Chur, Switzerland.

44. De la Rosette, J. J. M. C. H., Hubregtse, M. R., Karhaus, H. F. M., & Debruyne, F. M. J. (1992). Results of a questionnaire among Dutch urologists and general practitioners concerning diagnostics and treatment of patients with prostatitis syndrome. *European Journal of Urology, 22*, 14–19.

45. Dirie, M. A., & Lindmark, G. (1992). The risk of medical complications after female circumcision. *East African Medical Journal, 69*, 479–482.

46. Drach, G. W., Fair, W. R., Meares, E. M., & Stamey, T. A. (1978). Classification of benign diseases associated with prostatic pain: Prostatitis or proctodynia? *Journal of Urology, 120*, 266.

47. Editorial. (1992). Loin pain/hematuria syndrome. *Lancet, 340*, 701–702.

48. Ekberg, O., Abrahamsson, P.-A., & Kesek, P. (1988). Inguinal hernia in urological patients: The value of herniorrhaphy. *Journal of Urology, 139*, 1253–1255.

49. Elbadawi, A. (1996). Functional anatomy of the organs of micturition. *Urologic Clinics of North America, 23*, 177–210.

50. Elbadawi, A. (1997). Interstitial cystitis: A critique of current concepts with a new proposal for pathologic diagnosis and pathogenesis. *Urology, 49*, 14–40.

51. Fall, M., & Lindstrom, S. (1994). Transcutaneous electrical nerve stimulation in classic and nonulcer interstitial cystitis. *Urologic Clinics of North America, 21*, 131–139.

52. Ferguson, M., & Bell, C. (1993). Autonomic innervation of the kidney and ureter. In C. A. Maggi (Ed.), *Nervous Control of The Urogenital System* (pp. 1–31). Harwood Academic, Chur, Switzerland.

53. Fitzpatrick, C. C., Delancey, J. O. L., Elkins, T. E., & McGuire, E. J. (1993). Vulvar vestibulitis and interstitial cystitis: A disorder of urogenital sinus-derived epithelium? *Obstetrics and Gynaecology, 81*, 860–862.

54. Fleischmann, J. (1994). Calcium channel antagonists in the treatment of interstitial cystitis. *Urologic Clinics of North America, 21*, 107–112.

55. Ford, B., Greene, P., & Fahn, S. (1994). Oral and genital tardive pain syndromes. *Neurology, 44*, 2115–2119.

56. Ford, B., Louis, E. D., Greene, P., & Fahn, S. (1996). Oral and genital pain syndromes in Parkinson's disease. *Movement Disorders, 11*, 421–426.

57. Fowler, J. E. (1981). Prospective study of intravesical dimethyl sulphoxide in treatment of suspected early interstitial cystitis. *Urology, 18*, 21–26.

58. Fritjofsson, A., Fall, M., Juhlin, R., Persson, E., & Ruutu, M. (1987). Treatment of ulcer and nonulcer interstitial cystitis with sodium pentosanpolyphosphate: A multicenter trial. *Journal of Urology, 138*, 508–512.

59. Galer, B. S. (1995). Neuropathic pain of peripheral origin: Advances in pharmacologic treatment. *Neurology, 45*, S17–S25.

60. Gallagher, D. J. A., Montgomerie, J. Z., & North, J. D. K. (1965). Acute infections of the urinary tract and the urethral syndrome in general practice. *British Medical Journal, 1*, 622–626.

61. Gee, W. F., Ansell, J. S., & Bonica, J. J. (1990). Pelvic and perineal pain of urologic origin. In J. J. Bonica (Ed.), *The Management of Pain, vol 2* (pp. 1368–1394). Lea & Febiger, Philadelphia.

62. Geirsson, G., Wang, Y. G., Lindstrom, S., & Fall, M. (1993). Traditional acupuncture and electrical stimulation of the posterior tibial nerve. A trial in chronic interstitial cystitis. *Scandinavian Journal of Urology and Nephrology, 27*, 67–70.

63. Glazer, H. I., Rodke, G., Swencionis, C., Hertz, R., & Young, A. W. (1995). Treatment of vulvar vestibulitis syndrome with electromyographic biofeedback of pelvic floor musculature. *Journal of Reproductive Medicine, 40*, 283–290.

64. Godschalk, M., Gheorghiu, D., Katz, P. G., & Mulligan, T. (1996). Alkalization does not alleviate penile pain induced by intracavernous injection of prostaglandin E1. *Journal of Urology, 156*, 999–1000.

65. Goetsch, M. F. (1991). Vulvar vestibulitis: Prevalence and historic features in a general gynecologic practice population. *American Journal of Obstetrics and Gynecology, 164*, 1609–1616.

66. Goetsch, M. F. (1996). Simplified surgical revision of the vulvar vestibule for vulvar vestibulitis. *American Journal of Obstetrics and Gynecology, 174*, 1701–1707.

67. Goldberg, S. D., & Witchell, S. J. (1988). Right testicular pain: Unusual presentation of obstruction of the ureteropelvic junction. *Canadian Journal of Surgery, 31*, 246–247.

68. Goodson, J. D. (1981). Pudendal neuritis from biking. *New England Journal of Medicine, 304*, 365.

69. Hagen, N. A. (1993). Sharp, shooting neuropathic pain in the rectum or genitals: Pudendal neuralgia. *Journal of Pain and Symptom Management, 8*, 496–501.

70. Hanly, M. G., & Ojeda, V. J. (1995). Epidermic inclusion cysts of the clitoris as a complication of female circumcision and pharaonic infibulation. *Central African Journal of Medicine, 41*, 22–24.

71. Hanno, P. M. (1994). Diagnosis of interstitial cystitis. *Urologic Clinics of North America, 21*, 63–66.

72. Hanno, P. M. (1997). Analysis of long-term elmiron therapy for interstitial cystitis. *Urology, 49*, 93–99.

73. Hanno, P. M., Ratner, V., Sant, G., & Wein, A. J. (Eds.). (2001). *Interstitial Cystitis 2001: An evolving clinical syndrome.* Urology, 57 (suppl 6a).

74. Harlow, B. L., Wise, L. A., & Stewart, E. G. (2001). Prevalence and predictors of lower genital tract discomfort. *American Journal of Obstetrics and Gynecology, 185*, 545–550.

75. Harris, S. H., & Harris, R. G. S. (1930). Sympathicotonus, renal pain and renal sympathectomy. *British Journal of Urology, 2*, 367–374.

76. Hayden, L. J. (1993). Chronic testicular pain. *Australian Family Physician, 22*, 1357–1365.

77. Hofmann, A., Jones, R. E., & Schoenvogel, R. (1982). Pudendal nerve neurapraxia as a result of traction on the fracture table. *Journal of Bone and Joint Surgery, 64*, 136–138.

78. Holland, J. M., Feldman, J. L., & Gilbert, H. C. (1994). Phantom orchalgia. *Journal of Urology, 152*, 2291–2293.

79. Irwin, P. P., & Galloway, N. T. M. (1994). Surgical management of interstitial cystitis. *Urologic Clinics of North America, 21*, 145–152.

80. Jänig, W., & Koltzenburg, M. (1993). Pain arising from the urogenital tract. In C. A. Maggi (Ed.), *Nervous Control of the Urogenital System* (pp. 525–578). Harwood Academic, Chur, Switzerland.

81. Jänig, W., Schmidt, M., Schnitzler, A., & Wesselmann, U. (1991). Differentiation of sympathetic neurons projecting in the hypogastric nerve in terms of their discharge patterns in cats. *Journal of Physiology (London), 437*, 157–179.

82. Jepsen, J. V., Sall, M., Rhodes, P. R., Schmid, D., Messing, E., & Bruskewitz, R. C. (1998). Long-term experience with pentosanpolysulfate in interstitial cystitis. *Urology, 51*, 381–387.

83. Jeremias, J., Ledger, W. J., & Witkin, S. S. (2000). Interleukin 1 receptor antagonist gene polymorphism in women with vulvar vestibulitis. *American Journal of Obstetrics and Gynecology, 182*, 283–285.

84. Johansson, S. L., & Fall, M. (1994). Pathology of interstitial cystitis. *Urologic Clinics of North America, 21*, 55–62.

85. Jones, C. A., & Nyberg, L. M. (1997). Epidemiology of interstitial cystitis. *Urology, 49*, 2–9.

86. Kaplan, W. E., Firlit, C. F., & Schoenberg, H. W. (1980). The female urethral syndrome: External sphincter spasm as etiology. *Journal of Urology, 124*, 48–49.

87. Keay, S. K., Zhang, C.-O., Shoenfelt, J., Erickson, D. R., Whitmore, K., Warren, J. W., Marvel, R., & Chai, T. (2001). Sensitivity and specificity of antiproliferative factor, heparin-binding epidermal growth factor-like growth factor, and epidermal growth factor as urine markers for interstitial cystitis. *Urology, 57* (Suppl 6A), 9–14.

88. Kinzl, J. F., Traweger, C., & Biebl, W. (1995). Family background and sexual abuse associated with somatization. *Psychotherapy and Psychosomatics, 64*, 82–87.

89. Klonoff, E. A., Landrine, H., & Brown, M. (1993). Appraisal and response to pain may be a function of its bodily location. *Journal of Psychosomatic Research, 37*, 661–670.

90. Laumann, E. O., Paik, A., & Rosen, R. C. (1999). Sexual dysfunction in the United States. Prevalence and Predictors. *Journal of American Medical Association, 281*, 537–544.

91. Levine, L. A., Matkov, T. G., & Lubenow, T. R. (1996). Microsurgical denervation of the spermatic cord: A surgical alternative in the treatment of chronic orchialgia. *Journal of Urology, 155*, 1005–1007.

92. Lincoln, J., & Burnstock, G. (1993). Autonomic innervation of the urinary bladder and urethra. In C. A. Maggi (Ed.), *Nervous Control of The Urogenital System* (pp. 33–68). Harwood Academic, Chur, Switzerland.

93. Lipsky, B. A. (1989). Urinary tract infections in men. *Annals of Internal Medicine, 110*, 138.

94. Little, P. J., Sloper, J. S., & de Wardener, H. E. (1967). A syndrome of loin pain and haematuria associated with disease of peripheral renal arteries. *Quarterly Journal of Medicine, 36*, 253–259.

95. Lopatin, W. B., Martynik, M., Hickey, D. P., Vivas, C., & Hakala, T. R. (1990). Retrograde transurethral balloon dilation of prostate: Innovative management of abacterial chronic prostatitis and proctodynia. *Urology, 36*, 508–510.

96. Lynch, P. J. (1986). Vulvodynia: A syndrome of unexplained vulvar pain, psychologic disability and sexual dysfunction. *Journal of Reproductive Medicine, 31*, 773–780.

97. Mabry, E. W., Carson, C. C., & Older, R. A. (1981). Evaluation of women with chronic voiding discomfort. *Urology, 18*, 244–246.

98. Malloy, T. R., & Shanberg, A. M. (1994). Laser therapy for interstitial cystitis. *Urologic Clinics of North America, 21*, 141–144.

99. McCormack, M. (1988). Physiologic consequences and complications of vasectomy. *Canadian Medical Association Journal, 138*, 223–225.

100. McGee, S. R. (1993). Referred scrotal pain: Case reports and review. *Journal of General Internal Medicine, 8*, 694–701.

101. McKay, M. (1984). Burning vulva syndrome. *Journal of Reproductive Medicine, 29*, 457.

102. McKay, M. (1988). Subsets of vulvodynia. *Journal of Reproductive Medicine, 33*, 695–698.

103. McKay, M. (1989). Vulvodynia. A multifactorial problem. *Archives of Dermatology, 125*, 256–262.

104. McKenna, K. D., & Nadelhaft, I. (1986). The organization of the pudendal nerve in the male and female cat. *Journal of Comparative Neurology, 248*, 532–549.

105. McMahon, A. J., Buckley, J., Taylor, A., LLoyd, S. N., Deane, R. F., & Kirk, D. (1992). Chronic testicular pain following vasectomy. *British Journal of Urology, 69*, 188–191.

106. Meares, E. M. J. (1992). Prostatitis and related disorders. In P. C. Walsh, A. B. Retik, T. A. Stanley, & E. D. J. Vaughan (Eds.), *Campbell's urology, 6th edn.* (pp. 807–822). Saunders, Philadelphia.

107. Messing, E., Pauk, D., Schaeffer, A., et al. (1997). Associations among cystoscopy findings and symptoms and physical examination findings in women enrolled in the interstitial cystitis data base study. *Urology, 49*, 81–85.

108. Messinger, E. M. (1992). Urethral syndrome. In P. C. Walsh, A. B. Retik, T. A. Stanley, & E. D. J. Vaughan (Eds.), *Campbell's Urology, 6th edn.* (pp. 997–1005). Saunders, Philadelphia.

109. Miller, J. L., Rothman, I., Bavendam, T. G., & Berger, R. E. (1995). Proctodynia and interstitial cystitis: One and the same? *Urology, 45*, 587–589.

110. Mitchinson, M. J. (1972). Some clinical aspects of idiopathic retroperitoneal fibrosis. *British Journal of Surgery, 59*, 58–60.

111. Mobley, D. F., & Baum, N. (1996). Interstitial cystitis: When urgency and frequency mean more than routine inflammation. *Postgraduate Medicine, 99*, 201–208.

112. Montorsi, F., Guazzoni, G., Bergamaschi, F., et al. (1993). Is there a role for transrectal microwave hyperthermia of the prostate in the treatment of abacterial prostatitis and prostatodynia. *Prostate, 22*, 139–146.

113. Morales, A., Emerson, L., & Nickel, J. C. (1997). Intravesical hyaluronic acid in the treatment of refractory interstitial cystitis. *Urology, 49*, 111–113.

114. Morrison, J. F. B. (1987). Role of higher levels of the central nervous system. In M. Torrens & J. F. B. Morrison (Eds.), *The Physiology of The Lower Urinary Tract* (pp. 237–274). Springer-Verlag, London.

115. Moul, J. W. (1993). Prostatitis: Sorting out the different causes. *Postgraduate Medicine, 94*, 191–194.

116. Nickel, J. C. (1998). Prostatitis—Myths and realities. *Urology, 51*, 363–366.

117. Nickel, J. C., & Sorenson, R. (1994). Transurethral microwave thermotherapy of nonbacterial prostatitis and prostatodynia: Initial experience. *Urology, 44*, 458–460.

118. Nickel, J. C., Nyberg, L. M., & Hennenfent, M. (1999). Research guidelines for chronic prostatitis: Consensus report from the first National Institutes of Health International Prostatitis Collaborative Network. *Urology, 54*, 229–233.

119. Nigro, D. A., Wein, A. J., Foy, M., et al. (1997). Associations among cystoscopy and urodynamic findings for women enrolled in the interstitial cystitis data base study. *Urology, 49*, 86–92.

120. Orland, S. M., Hanno, P. M., & Wein, A. J. (1985). Prostatitis, prostatitis, and prostatodynia. *Urology, 25*, 439–459.

121. Paavonen, J. (1995a). Diagnosis and treatment of vulvodynia. *Annals of Medicine, 27*, 175–181.

122. Paavonen, J. (1995b). Vulvodynia—A complex syndrome of vulvar pain. *Acta Obstetricia et Gynecologica Scandinavica, 74*, 243–247.

123. Pagni, C. A., & Canavero, S. (1993). Paroxysmal perineal pain resembling tic douloureux, only symptom of a dorsal meningioma. *Italian Journal of Neurological Sciences, 14*, 323–324.

124. Parkin, J., Shea, C., & Sant, G. R. (1997). Intravesical dimethyl sulfoxide for interstitial cystitis—A practical approach. *Urology, 49*, 105–107.

125. Parsons, C. L. (1997). Epithelial coating techniques in the treatment of interstitial cystitis. *Urology, 49*, 100–104.

126. Pedersen, B., Tiefer, L., Ruiz, M., & Melman, A. (1988). Evaluation of patients and partners 1 to 4 years after penile prosthesis surgery. *Journal of Urology, 139*, 956–958.

127. Peeker, R., Aldenborg, F., & Fall, M. (1998). The treatment of interstitial cystitis with supratrigonal cystectomy and ileocystoplasty—Difference in outcome between classic and nonulcer disease. *Journal of Urology, 159*, 1479–1482.

128. Peters-Gee, J. M. (1998). Bladder and urethral syndromes. In J. F. Steege, D. A. Metzger, & B. S. Levy (Eds.), *Chronic Pelvic Pain* (pp. 197–204). Saunders, Philadelphia.

129. Pontari, M. A., Hanno, P. M., & Wein, A. J. (1997). Logical and systematic approach to the evaluation and management of patients suspected of having interstitial cystitis. *Urology, 49*, 114.

130. Pranikoff, K., & Constantino, G. (1998). The use of amitriptyline in patients with urinary frequency and pain. *Urology, 51* (suppl 5A), 179–181.

131. Raphael, K. G., Spatz Widom, C., & Lange, G. (2001). Childhood victimization and pain in adulthood: A prospective investigation. *Pain, 92*, 283–293.

132. Ratliff, T. L., Klutke, C. G., & McDougall, E. M. (1994). The etiology of interstitial cystitis. *Urologic Clinics of North America, 21*, 21–30.

133. Raz, S., & Smith, R. B. (1976). External sphincter spasticity syndrome in female patients. *Journal of Urology, 115*, 443–446.

134. Robert, R., Brunet, C., Faure, A., et al. (1993). La chirurgie du nerf pudental lors de certaines algies perineales: Evolution et resultats. *Chirurgie, 119*, 535–539.

135. Sand, P. K., Bowen, L. W., Ostergard, D. R., Bent, A., & Panganibaum, R. (1989). Cryosurgery

versus dilation and massage for treatment of recurrent urethral syndrome. *Journal of Reproductive Medicine, 34*, 499–504.

136. Sant, G. R., & LaRock, D. R. (1994). Standard intravesical therapies for interstitial cystitis. *Urologic Clinics of North America, 21*, 73–84.
137. Schmidt, R. A., & Tanagho, E. A. (1981). Urethral syndrome or urinary tract infection? *Urology, 18*, 424–427.
138. Schneiderman, H., & Voytovich, A. (1988). Self-palpation orchitis. *Journal of General Internal Medicine, 3*, 97.
139. Segura, J. W., Opitz, J. L., & Greene, L. F. (1979). Prostatitis, prostatitis or pelvic floor tension myalgia? *Journal of Urology, 122*, 168–169.
140. Selikowitz, S. M., & Schned, A. R. (1985). A late post-vasectomy syndrome. *Journal of Urology, 134*, 494–497.
141. Silber, S. J. (1981). Reversal of vasectomy and the treatment of male infertility: Role of microsurgery, vasoepididymostomy, and pressure-induced changes of vasectomy. *Urologic Clinics of North America, 8*, 53–62.
142. Simmons, J. L., & Bunce, P. L. (1958). On the use of antihistamine in the treatment of interstitial cystitis. *American Journal of Surgery, 24*, 664–667.
143. Slade, D., Ratner, V., & Chalker, R. (1997). A collaborative approach to managing interstitial cystitis. *Urology, 49*, 10–13.
144. Sonni, L., Cattaneo, A., De Marco, A., De Magnis, C., Carli, P., & Marabini, S. (1995). Idiopathic vulvodynia clinical evaluation of the pain threshold with acetic acid solutions. *Journal of Reproductive Medicine, 40*, 337–341.
145. Splatt, A. J., & Weedon, D. (1981). The urethral syndrome: Morphological studies. *British Journal of Urology, 53*, 263–265.
146. Theoharides, T. C., & Sant, G. R. (1997). Hydroxyzine therapy for interstitial cystitis. *Urology, 49*, 108–110.
147. Theoharides, T. C., Kempuraj, D., & Sant, G. R. (2001). Mast cell involvement in interstitial cystitis: A review of human and experimental evidence. *Urology, 57* (Suppl 6A), 47–55.
148. Thomas, T. G. (Ed.). (1880). *Practical Treatise on the Diseases of Woman*. Henry C. Lea's Son, Philadelphia, pp. 145–147.
149. Tiefer, L., Pederson, B., & Melman, A. (1988). Psychosocial follow-up of penile prosthesis implant patients and partners. *Journal of Sex and Marital Therapy, 14*, 184–201.
150. Van de Kleft, E., & Van Vyve, M. (1993). Sacral meningeal cysts and perineal pain. *Lancet, 341*, 500–501.
151. Vodusek, D. B., & Light, J. K. (1983). The motor nerve supply of the external sphincter muscles: An electrophysiological study. *Neurourology and Urodynamics, 293*, 193–200.
152. Walker, E. A., & Stenchever, M. A. (1993). Sexual victimization and chronic pelvic pain. *Obstetrics and Gynecology Clinics of North America, 20*, 795–807.
153. Warren, J. W. (1994). Interstitial cystitis as an infectious disease. *Urologic Clinics of North America, 21*, 31–40.

154. Weisberg, L. S., Bloom, P. B., Simmons, R. L., & Viner, E. D. (1993). Loin pain haematuria syndrome. *American Journal of Nephrology, 13*, 229–237.

155. Wesselmann, U. (1987). Untersuchungen der Impulsübertragung im Ganglion Mesentericum Inferius. Dissertation, Medizinische Fakultät der Christian-Albrechts-Universität zu Kiel, Germany, pp. 1–244.

156. Wesselmann, U. (2001). Interstitial cystitis: A chronic visceral pain syndrome. *Urology, 57* (Suppl 6A), 32–39.

157. Wesselmann, U., & Burnett, A. L. (1996). Treatment of neuropathic testicular pain. *Neurology, 46* (Suppl), 206.

158. Wesselmann, U., & Lai, J. (1997). Mechanisms of referred visceral pain: Uterine inflammation in the adult virgin rat results in neurogenic plasma extravasation in the skin. *Pain, 73*, 309–317.

159. Wesselmann, U., Burnett, A. L., & Campbell, J. N. (1995). The role of the sympathetic nervous system in chronic visceral pain. *Society for Neuroscience (Abstracts), 21*, 1157.

160. Wesselmann, U., Burnett, A. L., & Heinberg, L. J. (1996). Chronic testicular pain—A neuropathic pain syndrome: Diagnosis and treatment. Abstract, *8th World Congress on Pain*, p. 256.

161. Wesselmann, U., Burnett, A. L., & Heinberg, L. J. (1997). The urogenital and rectal pain syndromes. *Pain, 73*, 269–294.

162. Westrom, L. V., & Willen, R. (1998). Vestibular nerve fiber proliferation in vulvar vestibulitis syndrome. *Obstetrics and Gynecology, 91*, 572–576.

163. White, S. H., & Leslie, I. J. (1986). Pain in scrotum due to intervertebral disc protrusion. *Lancet, 1*, 504.

164. Whitmore, K. E. (1994). Self-care regimens for patients with interstitial cystitis. *Urologic Clinics of North America, 21*, 121–130.

165. Yeates, W. K. (1985). Pain in the scrotum. *British Journal of Hospital Medicine, 33*, 101–104.

166. York, G. K., Gabor, A. J., & Dreyfus, P. M. (1979). Paroxysmal genital pain: An unusual manifestation of epilepsy. *Neurology, 29*, 516–519.

167. Zimmern, P. E. (1995). Hydrodistension in suspected interstitial cystitis patients: Diagnosis and therapeutic benefits. *Urology, 153*, 290A.

168. Zufall, R. (1978). Ineffectiveness of treatment of urethral syndrome in women. *Urology, 12*, 337–339.

169. Zvieli, S., Vinter, L., & Herman, J. (1989). Nonacute scrotal pain in adolescents. *Journal of Family Practice, 28*, 226–228.

Chapter

9

THE MANAGEMENT OF CANCER PAIN

Contents

Introduction

A vital component of all-encompassing cancer care is the management of cancer pain, which attempts to lessen suffering and improve the quality of life for cancer patients. Pain associated with cancer is a broad category that can result from the illness itself, various forms of treatment, or coexisting conditions. This presents a variety of difficulties for medical professionals. An estimated large percentage of cancer patients experience pain at some point during their illness; the intensity of the pain varies, and it can have an impact on a patient's social, emotional, and physical well-being.

A customized, multidisciplinary strategy is used to manage cancer pain, taking into account both the psychosocial and underlying pathophysiology of pain. This usually involves adjuvant drugs, opioids, nonsteroidal anti-inflammatory drugs (NSAIDs), and neurolytic techniques, as well as pharmacological interventions like nerve blocks. Acupuncture, physical therapy, radiation therapy, and psychological support are examples of non-pharmacological modalities that are essential to pain management.

Close coordination between oncologists, pain specialists, nurses, palliative care teams, and other medical professionals is necessary for effective cancer pain management. Patients and their caregivers must also actively participate in the decision-making process regarding their course of treatment. The management of cancer pain not only increases comfort but also supports overall treatment outcomes and improves the quality of life for those facing cancer by offering comprehensive pain relief and attending to patients' holistic needs.

Understanding a variety of therapeutic options, such as antineoplastic therapies, analgesic pharmacotherapy, and anesthetic, neurosurgical, psychological, and rehabilitation techniques, is essential for the best management of cancer pain. Implementing the techniques that have the most favorable therapeutic index for the current situation and allowing for recurrent evaluations to maintain a favorable balance between pain relief and side effects are hallmarks of successful pain management. For most patients, the existing methods that employ particular analgesic strategies can offer sufficient relief. If a patient's pain relief is insufficient, they should consider neurosurgical and anesthetic methods. These therapies must always be expertly combined with the management of other symptoms.

Orientation and Directional Terms

Term	Definition	Illustration
Cancer pain	Cancer pain can be a common symptom of cancer, and can be caused by the cancer itself, cancer treatments, or a combination of factors.	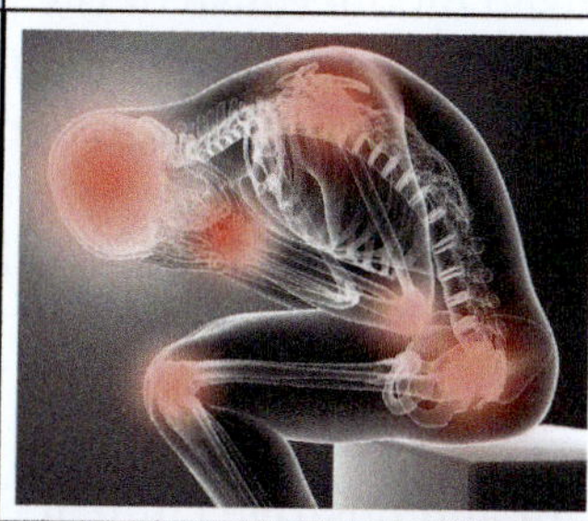
Chemotherapy	Chemotherapy is the type of cancer treatment that uses one or more anti-cancer drugs in a standard regimen.	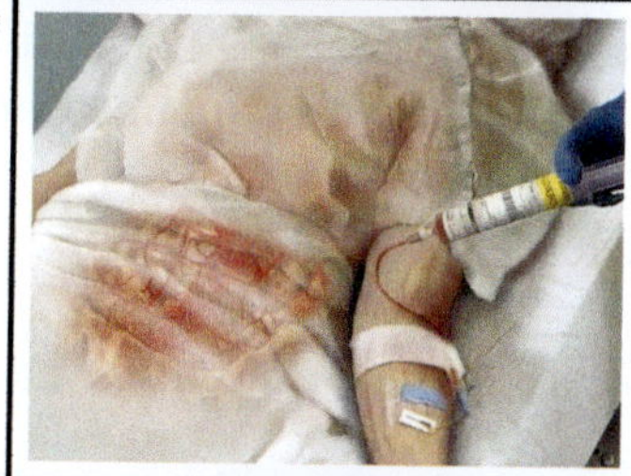
Radiotherapy	Radiotherapy, also known as radiation therapy, is a cancer treatment that uses high doses of radiation to kill or slow the growth of cancer cells.	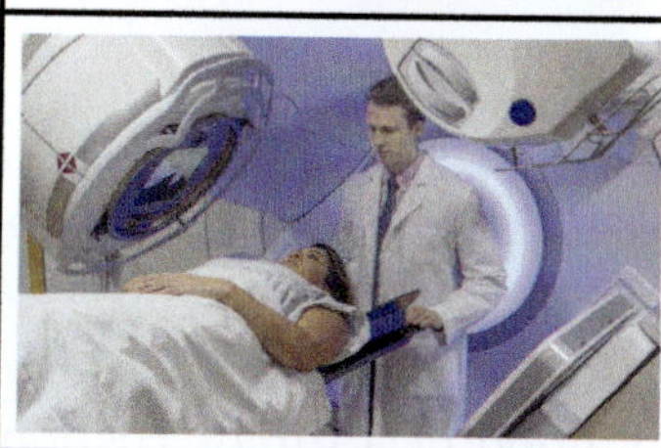
Cerebral metastases	Cerebral metastases, also known as brain metastases or metastatic brain cancer, are tumors that form when cancer cells spread from another part of the body to the brain.	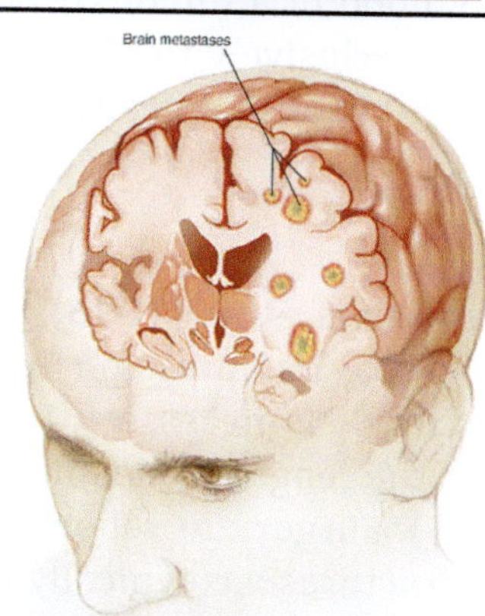
Gastroduodenal morbidity	Gastroduodenal morbidity may refer to the effects of gastroduodenal disorders on morbidity and mortality.	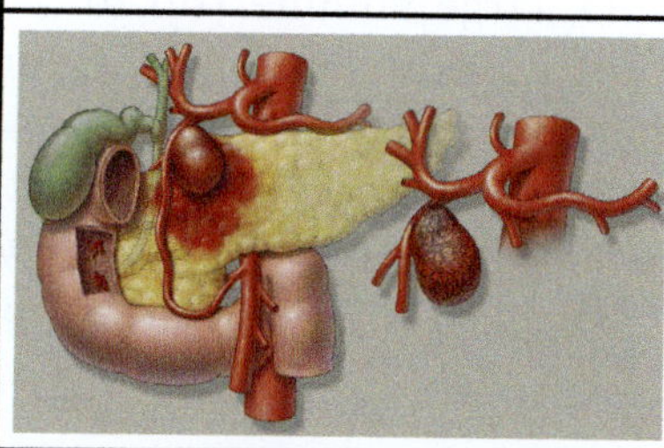

9.1. Primary Therapy

The evaluation procedure might identify a pain source that responds well to initial therapy (i.e., treatment focused on the cause of the pain). This treatment might increase survival time, comfort, or functionality. For instance, antineoplastic treatments such as surgery, radiotherapy, or chemotherapy may be used to treat pain brought on by tumor infiltration, while antibiotic therapy or drainage techniques may be used to treat pain brought on by infections. In most cases, specialized analgesic therapies are needed in addition to the main therapy.

9.1.1. Radiotherapy

A wealth of data and positive clinical experience in treating painful bone metastases (Janjan, 1997), epidural neoplasms (Bates, 1992), and headaches caused by cerebral metastases (Vermeulen, 1998) attest to the analgesic effectiveness of radiation therapy. On the other hand, little information is available and most reports of radiotherapy use are anecdotal in other contexts. For instance, the prognosis for low sacral plexopathy-related perineal pain appears promising (Dobrowsky & Schmid, 1985), and hepatic radiotherapy (e.g., 2000–3000 cGy) can be well tolerated and useful in 50–90% of patients for the relief of hepatic capsular distension pain (Leibel et al., 1987).

9.1.2. Chemotherapy

Although there is a lack of information regarding the precise analgesic effects of chemotherapy, there is a strong clinical impression that pain relief is typically linked to tumor shrinkage. While some reports (Thatcher et al., 1995; Rothenberg, 1996) indicate analgesic value even in the absence of significant tumor shrinkage, the likelihood of a positive effect on pain is typically correlated with the likelihood of a tumor response. Under no circumstances should the choice to administer chemotherapy exclusively to treat symptoms be made without first giving careful thought, unless the patient exhibits a manifestly favorable balance between benefit and side effects.

9.1.3. Surgery

According to Harris et al. (1996), surgery may be necessary to relieve symptoms brought on by certain issues like compression of neural tissues, unstable bone structures, and obstruction of a hollow viscus. It is necessary to balance the possible advantages against the risks associated with surgery, the length of hospital stay and recovery period, and the expected length of benefit (Boraas, 1985). Surgery to relieve intestinal obstructions, drain symptomatic ascites, or stabilize pathological fractures has typically resulted in the best clinical outcomes (Algan & Horowitz, 1996). For example, large volume (up to 5–10 L) paracentesis may relieve the pain and discomfort of tense ascites quickly and for an extended period of time (Ross et al., 1989). However, there is a slight risk of hypotension (Cruikshank & Buchsbaum, 1973; Ross et al., 1989) or hypoproteinemia (Lifshitz & Buchsbaum, 1976). In patients without signs of metastatic spread, radical surgery to remove locally advanced disease may be palliative and even improve some patients' chances of survival (Estes et al., 1993; Avradopoulos et al., 1996).

9.1.4. Antibiotic Therapy

Infections can cause pain, in which case antibiotics can also act as an analgesic. Examples that serve as illustrations include pyonephrosis, cellulitis, pelvic abscesses, chronic sinus infections, and osteitis pubis. Sometimes the only way to determine whether an infection is present is to treat it empirically with these medications to alleviate symptoms (Coyle & Portenoy, 1991).

9.2. Analgesic Drug Therapy

There is universal agreement that analgesic pharmacotherapy remains the mainstay of cancer pain management.

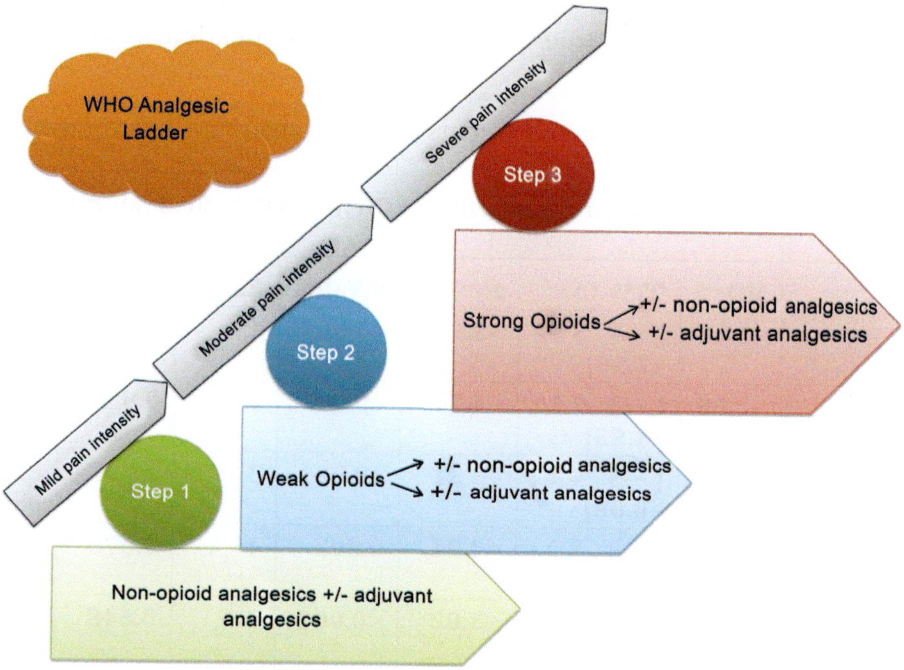

Figure 9.1. WHO analgesic ladder.

Source: V. Subramaniam A, Salem Yehya AH, Oon CE. Molecular basis of cancer pain management: an updated review. *Medicina*. 2019; 55(9):584. https://doi.org/10.3390/medicina55090584.

The World Health Organization's "three-step analgesic ladder," which recommended three basic stages of therapy based on the severity of the presenting pain problem, has, however, generated controversy regarding its applicability and validity (World Health Organization, 1986). A review of these studies found no evidence for the long-term efficacy of this approach (Jadad & Browman, 1995), despite data from a series of validation studies showing that this approach, in conjunction with appropriate dosing guidelines, provides adequate relief to 70–90% of patients. These studies included Takeda 1985; Ventafridda et al., 1987; Walker et al., 1988; Goisis et al., 1989; Schug et al., 1990; and Grond et al., 1991. Furthermore, it is now difficult to distinguish between Steps 2 and 3 due to the development of low-dose versions of pure opioid agonists that were previously only used for extremely severe pain and the introduction of other medications like tramadol.

9.2.1. Systemic Analgesic Pharmacotherapy

9.2.1.1. Non-opioid Analgesics

According to Eisenberg et al. (1994), non-opioid analgesics such as aspirin, acetaminophen, and non-steroidal anti-inflammatory drugs (NSAIDs) are effective when taken alone for mild to moderate pain (Step 1 of the analgesic ladder) and when combined with opioid medications for more severe pain, they provide additive analgesia. They are helpful in a wide variety of pain syndromes with various mechanisms, but other than inflammation, there is no evidence to support their therapeutic superiority over other options (Eisenberg et al., 1994). The non-opioid analgesics have a "ceiling" effect on analgesia and do not cause tolerance or physical dependence, in contrast to opioid analgesics.

Table 9.1. Effects of Intravenous Non-opioid Agents and Adjuvants on Postoperative Pain

VAS at the End of Surgery	**$\tau^2 = 0.4460$; $\tau = 0.6678$; $I^2 = 76\%$ [58.0%; 86.3%]; $p < 0.001$ at Q Test**						
Drug	**MD**	**95% CI**	**z**	***p* Value**	**Rank**	**P Score**	**QoE**
Ibuprofen	**-3.27**	**[-4.39; -2.16]**	**-5.79**	**<0.001**	**1**	**0.954**	⊕⊕⊕⊖ Moderate §
Gabapentin	**-2.65**	**[-3.75; -1.55]**	**-4.74**	**<0.001**	**2**	**0.838**	⊕⊕⊕⊖ Moderate §
Lidocaine	**-2.16**	**[-3.44; -0.88]**	**-3.31**	**<0.001**	**3**	**0.727**	⊕⊕⊕⊖ Moderate §
Ketamine + clonidine	**-2.00**	**[-3.33; -0.66]**	**-2.94**	**0.003**	**4**	**0.679**	⊕⊕⊕⊖ Moderate §
Acetminophen	**-1.88**	**[-2.84; -0.91]**	**-3.82**	**<0.001**	**5**	**0.648**	⊕⊕⊕⊖ Moderate §
Clonidine	-1.51	[-3.37; 0.34]	-1.60	0.109	6	0.554	⊕⊕⊖⊖ Low §#
Ketamine	-0.68	[-1.50; 0.13]	-1.63	0.103	7	0.334	⊕⊕⊖⊖ Low §#
Dexmedetomidine	-0.53	[-1.32; 0.24]	-1.35	0.178	8	0.278	⊕⊕⊖⊖ Low §#
Pregabalin	-0.20	[-1.77; 1.37]	-0.25	0.803	9	0.202	⊕⊕⊖⊖ Low §#
Ketamine + magnesium	-0.17	[-1.54; 1.18]	-0.25	0.799	10	0.182	⊕⊕⊖⊖ Low §#
Placebo	-	-	-	-	11	0.099	
VAS 30 min	**$\tau^2 = 1.65$; $\tau = 1.28$; $I^2 = 88.5\%$ [77.6%; 94.1%]; $p < 0.001$ at Q test**						
Drug	**MD**	**95% CI**	**z**	***p* value**	**Rank**	**P score**	**QoE**
Ketamine + clonidine	-2.00	[-4.54; 0.54]	-1.54	0.123	1	0.765	⊕⊕⊖⊖ Low §#
Dexmedetomidine	**-1.36**	**[-2.59; -0.12]**	**-2.15**	**0.031**	**2**	**0.639**	⊕⊕⊕⊖ Moderate §

Magnesium	−1.00	[−3.63; 1.63]	−0.74	0.457	3	0.498	⊕⊕⊖⊖ Low §
Ketamine	−0.89	[−2.90; 1.10]	−0.88	0.380	4	0.472	⊕⊕⊖⊖ Low §#
Placebo	-	-	-	-	5	0.124	
VAS 60 min	**τ^2 = 1.3943; τ = 1.18; I^2 = 88.7% [82.7%; 92.6%]; *p* < 0.001 at Q test**						
Drug	**MD**	**95% CI**	**z**	***p* value**	**Rank**	**P score**	QoE
Lidocaine	**−2.23**	**[−3.61; −0.85]**	**−3.17**	**0.001**	**1**	**0.836**	⊕⊕⊕⊖ Moderate §
Gabapentin	−2.20	[−4.59; 0.19]	−1.80	0.072	2	0.764	⊕⊕⊖⊖ Low §#
Ketamine	**−1.31**	**[−2.33; −0.29]**	**−2.53**	**0.011**	**3**	**0.546**	⊕⊕⊕⊖ Moderate §
Dexmedetomidine	**−1.24**	**[−2.16; −0.33]**	**−2.67**	**0.007**	**4**	**0.519**	⊕⊕⊕⊖ Moderate §
Ketamine + clonidine	−1.00	[−3.34; 1.34]	−0.83	0.403	5	0.453	⊕⊕⊖⊖ Low §#
Pregabalin	−0.20	[−2.93; 2.53]	−0.14	0.885	6	0.264	⊕⊕⊖⊖ Low §#
Placebo	-	-	-	-	7	0.115	
VAS 2 h	**τ^2 = 0.1162; τ = 0.3408; I^2 = 50.5% [0.0%; 76.0%]; *p* < 0.001 at Q test**						
Drug	**MD**	**95% CI**	**z**	***p* value**	**Rank**	**P score**	**QoE**
Ibuprofen	**−2.37**	**[−3.32; −1.41]**	**−4.85**	**<0.001**	**1**	**0.988**	⊕⊕⊕⊖ Moderate §
Acetaminophen	**−1.53**	**[−2.48; −0.57]**	**−3.16**	**0.001**	**2**	**0.785**	⊕⊕⊕⊖ Moderate §
Ketamine	**−1.03**	**[−1.65; −0.40]**	**−3.23**	**0.001**	**3**	**0.624**	⊕⊕⊕⊖ Moderate §
Dexmedetomidine	**−0.87**	**[−1.69; −0.05]**	**−2.10**	**0.035**	**4**	**0.545**	⊕⊕⊕⊖ Moderate §
Gabapentin	−0.60	[−1.80; 0.60]	−0.98	0.328	5	0.418	⊕⊕⊖⊖ Low §#
Lidocaine	−0.28	[−1.25; 0.67]	−0.59	0.557	6	0.278	⊕⊕⊖⊖ Low §#
Magnesium	−0.17	[−1.32; 0.98]	−0.29	0.773	7	0.237	⊕⊕⊖⊖ Low §#
Placebo	-	-	-	-	8	0.121	
VAS 4 h	**τ^2 = 0.2421; τ = 0.4921; I^2 = 59% [10.4%; 81.2%]; *p* < 0.001 at Q test**						
Drug	**MD**	**95% CI**	**z**	***p* value**	**Rank**	**P score**	**QoE**
Dexmedetomidine	**−3.10**	**[−5.35; −0.84]**	**−2.70**	**0.006**	**1**	**0.925**	⊕⊕⊕⊖ Moderate §
Magnesium	**−2.06**	**[−3.58; −0.53]**	**−2.65**	**0.008**	**2**	**0.783**	⊕⊕⊕⊖ Moderate §

Ibuprofen	**−1.63**	**[−2.88; −0.37]**	**−2.54**	**0.011**	**3**	**0.688**	⊕⊕⊕⊖ Moderate §
Gabapentin	**−1.19**	**[−2.09; −0.29]**	**−2.59**	**0.009**	**4**	**0.540**	⊕⊕⊕⊖ Moderate §
Ketamine	−1.17	[−2.57; 0.23]	−1.63	0.103	5	0.537	⊕⊕⊖⊖ Low §#
Acetaminophen	−1.10	[−2.34; 0.14]	−1.73	0.083	6	0.496	⊕⊕⊖⊖ Low §#
Ketamine + magnesium	−0.34	[−1.75; 1.07]	−0.47	0.637	7	0.248	⊕⊕⊖⊖ Low §#
Lidocaine	0.04	[−1.53; 1.61]	0.05	0.960	8	0.161	⊕⊕⊖⊖ Low §#
Placebo	-	-	-	-	9	0.118	
VAS 6 h	**$\tau^2 = 0$; $\tau = 0$; $I^2 = 0\%$ [0.0%; 74.6%]; $p = 0.568$ at Q test**						
Drug	**MD**	**95% CI**	**z**	***p* value**	**Rank**	**P score**	**QoE ‡**
Lidocaine	**−2.27**	**[−2.92; −1.63]**	**−6.93**	**<0.001**	**1**	**0.944**	⊕⊕⊕⊖ Moderate §
Clonidine	**−1.73**	**[−2.98; −0.48]**	**−2.71**	**0.006**	**2**	**0.814**	⊕⊕⊕⊖ Moderate §
Ketamine + clonidine	−1.00	[−3.04; 1.04]	−0.96	0.338	3	0.571	⊕⊕⊖⊖ Low §#
Dexmedetomidine	**−0.44**	**[−0.75; −0.12]**	**−2.74**	**0.006**	**4**	**0.474**	⊕⊕⊕⊖ Moderate §
Ketamine	−0.36	[−0.77; 0.04]	−1.75	0.080	5	0.395	⊕⊕⊖⊖ Low §#
Gabapentin	−0.20	[−0.40; 0.01]	−1.88	0.060	6	0.258	⊕⊕⊖⊖ Low §#
Placebo	-	-	-	-	7	0.041	
VAS 8 h	**$\tau^2 = 0$; $\tau = 0$; $I^2 = 0\%$ [10.4%; 89.6%]; $p = 1.000$ at Q test**						
Drug	**MD**	**95% CI**	**z**	***p* value**	**Rank**	**P score**	**QoE ‡**
Ibuprofen	**−2.50**	**[−2.87; −2.12]**	**−13.16**	**<0.001**	**1**	**0.926**	⊕⊕⊕⊖ Moderate §
Gabapentin	**−2.44**	**[−3.17; −1.70]**	**−6.50**	**<0.001**	**2**	**0.896**	⊕⊕⊕⊖ Moderate §
Acetaminophen	**−1.80**	**[−2.19; −1.40]**	**−8.96**	**<0.001**	**3**	**0.677**	⊕⊕⊕⊖ Moderate §
Ketamine	−0.34	[−1.17; 0.49]	−0.80	0.423	4	0.426	⊕⊕⊖⊖ Low §#
Placebo	-	-	-	-	5	0.284	
Ketamine + magnesium	−0.00	[−0.84; 0.84]	−0.00	1.000	6	0.274	⊕⊕⊖⊖ Low §#
Magnesium	0.77	[0.23; 1.30]	2.81	0.005	7	0.013	⊕⊕⊖⊖ Low §#
VAS 12 h	**$\tau^2 = 0.1162$; $\tau = 0.3408$; $I^2 = 50.5\%$ [0.0%; 76.0%]; $p = 0.033$ at Q test**						

Drug	MD	95% CI	z	*p* value	Rank	P score	QoE
Ibuprofen	**-2.23**	**[-2.87; -1.58]**	**-6.79**	**<0.001**	**1**	**0.964**	⊕⊕⊕⊖ Moderate §
Lidocaine	**-1.90**	**[-2.72; -1.08]**	**-4.55**	**<0.001**	**2**	**0.878**	⊕⊕⊕⊖ Moderate §
Acetaminophen	**-1.63**	**[-2.27; -0.98]**	**-4.93**	**<0.001**	**3**	**0.801**	⊕⊕⊕⊖ Moderate §
Clonidine	-0.77	[-2.00; 0.44]	-1.25	0.212	4	0.580	⊕⊕⊖⊖ Low §#
Ketamine	**-0.43**	**[-0.85; -0.00]**	**-1.97**	**0.048**	**5**	**0.502**	⊕⊕⊕⊖ Moderate §
Gabapentin	-0.30	[-1.11; 0.51]	-0.72	0.468	6	0.411	⊕⊕⊖⊖ Low §#
Dexmedetomidine	-0.19	[-0.71; 0.31]	-0.76	0.450	7	0.354	⊕⊕⊖⊖ Low §#
Ketamine + clonidine	0.00	[-0.76; 0.76]	0.00	1.000	8	0.268	⊕⊕⊖⊖ Low §#
Placebo	-	-	-	-	9	0.231	
Ketamine + magnesium	1.06	[0.20; 1.92]	2.43	0.015	10	0.007	⊕⊕⊖⊖ Low §#
VAS 24 h	**τ^2 = 0.1535; τ = 0.3918; I^2 = 61.8% [35.4%; 77.4%]; p < 0.001 at Q test**						
Drug	**MD**	**95% CI**	**z**	***p* value**	**Rank**	**P score**	**QoE**
Ibuprofen	**-1.00**	**[-1.57; -0.43]**	**-3.45**	**<0.001**	**1**	**0.919**	⊕⊕⊕⊖ Moderate §
Pregabalin	-0.80	[-1.94; 0.34]	-1.37	0.171	2	0.771	⊕⊕⊖⊖ Low §#
Acetaminophen	-0.45	[-0.91; 0.03]	-1.95	0.051	3	0.649	⊕⊕⊖⊖ Low §#
Clonidine	-0.39	[-1.73; 0.94]	-0.57	0.566	4	0.564	⊕⊕⊖⊖ Low §#
Ketamine	-0.28	[-0.70; 0.12]	-1.36	0.173	5	0.543	⊕⊕⊖⊖ Low §#
Gabapentin	-0.12	[-1.01; 0.77]	-0.26	0.792	6	0.409	⊕⊕⊖⊖ Low §#
Dexmedetomidine	-0.12	[-0.64; 0.39]	-0.46	0.646	7	0.393	⊕⊕⊖⊖ Low §#
Lidocaine	0.10	[-0.93; 1.13]	0.19	0.849	8	0.291	⊕⊕⊖⊖ Low §#
Placebo	-	-	-	-	9	0.278	
Ketamine + magnesium	0.28	[-0.62; 1.19]	0.62	0.536	10	0.179	⊕⊕⊖⊖ Low §#
VAS 48 h	**τ^2 = 0.2421; τ = 0.4921; I^2 = 59% [10.4%; 81.2%]; p = 0.017 at Q test**						
Drug	**MD**	**95% CI**	**z**	***p* value**	**Rank**	**P score**	**QoE**

Dexmedetomidine	**−0.80**	**[− 1 . 5 8 ; −0.02]**	**−2.03**	**0.042**	**1**	**0.771**	⊕ ⊕ ⊕ ⊖ Moderate §
Lidocaine	−0.65	[− 1 . 4 0 ; 0.10]	−1.69	0.090	2	0.650	⊕⊕⊖⊖ Low §#
Acetaminophen	−0.60	[− 1 . 9 0 ; 0.70]	−0.90	0.366	3	0.575	⊕⊕⊖⊖ Low §#
Ketamine	−0.38	[− 0 . 9 9 ; 0.23]	−1.21	0.224	4	0.411	⊕⊕⊖⊖ Low §#
Placebo	-	-	-	-	5	0.090	
VAS POD7	**τ^2 = 0.6176; τ = 0.7859; I^2 = 67.6% [0.0%; 90.6%]; p = 0.045 at Q test**						
Drug	**MD**	**95% CI**	**z**	***p* value**	**Rank**	**P score**	**QoE**
Dexmedetomidine	−1.05	[− 2 . 1 3 ; 0.02]	−1.91	0.056	1	0.915	⊕⊕⊖⊖ Low §#
Ketamine	0.00	[− 1 . 5 7 ; 1.57]	0.00	1.000	2	0.320	⊕⊕⊖⊖ Low §#
Placebo	-	-	-	-	3	0.264	

Source. Carron M, Tamburini E, Linassi F, Pettenuzzo T, Boscolo A, Navalesi P. Non-Opioid Analgesics and Adjuvants after Surgery in Adults with Obesity: Systematic Review with Network Meta-Analysis of Randomized Controlled Trials. *Journal of Clinical Medicine*. 2024; 13(7):2100. https://doi.org/10.3390/jcm13072100.

VAS: visual analog scale (range from 0 ["no pain"] to 10 ["worst pain possible"]), assessed at various time points; POD7: seventh postoperative day; MD: mean difference; 95% CI: 95% confidence interval; I2 measures percentage variation across studies due to heterogeneity; $\tau 2$: the between-study variance in the random-effects meta-analysis; τ: the standard deviation estimate of effect sizes in the random-effects meta-analysis; Q test: Cochran's Q test assesses heterogeneity among the study results; z: the Z-score measures how many standard deviations a data point is from the mean; rank: the effectiveness-based order of treatments; QoE: quality of evidence; §: downgraded one level for inconsistency (such as heterogeneity of estimates of effects across trials) [11]. #: downgraded one level for imprecision (e.g., 95% confidence intervals are wide and include or are close to null effect) [11]. Moderate QoE: the authors are moderately confident in the effect estimate. The true effect is likely to be close to the estimate of the effect, but there is a possibility that it is substantially different. Low QoE: the authors' confidence in the effect estimate is limited. The true effect may be substantially different from the estimate of the effect [11]. ‡: the heterogeneity was considered uncertain. This uncertainty arises from a broad confidence interval for I2, suggesting the possibility of undetected heterogeneity. This concern remains despite the reported absence of between-study variance ($\tau 2$ = 0), no variation in effect estimates (τ = 0), and a reported I2 value of 0%.

The non-opioid analgesics are a diverse class of drugs with varying molecular structures but similar pharmacological effects. Cyclooxygenase is competitively blocked by NSAID medications. Recent research has revealed that cyclooxygenase has at least two isoforms, each of which plays a different role in toxicity and analgesia (Vane et al., 1998). While cyclooxygenase-2 is an induced enzyme involved in inflammation, pain, and fever, cyclooxygenase-1 is in charge of synthesizing the protective prostaglandins that maintain normal renal function not just in a compromised but in a healthy kidney also, but their physiological role in maintaining renal blood flow and GFR is not dominate. (Weir M.R., Froch L. Weighing the renal effects of NSAIDs and COX-2 inhibitors. Clin. Dilemmas. 2000, 1:3–12.) and preserve the integrity of the stomach lining. A variety of comparatively selective cyclooxygenase-2 inhibitors, such as celecoxib, meloxicam, nimesulide, and rofecoxib, have recently been approved for use as analgesics. According to preliminary findings, these medications have less gastroduodenal morbidity and are equianalgesic when compared to non-selective inhibitors (Brooks & Day, 2000; Watson et al., 2000). Other side effects resemble those of non-selective NSAIDs, including the potential to cause renal dysfunction in patients with impaired renal function and interference with antihypertensive medications (Brooks & Day, 2000; Perazella & Eras, 2000; Eras & Perazella, 2001).

Understanding the possible side effects of non-opioid analgesics is necessary for safely administering them (Brooks & Day, 1991; Bennett et al., 1996; Laine, 1996; Lehmann et al., 1997). While there is a wide range of possible side effects from aspirin and other NSAIDs, the most frequent ones are renal impairment, gastroduodenopathy (including peptic ulcer disease), and bleeding diathesis brought on by inhibition of platelet aggregation (Lehmann et al., 1997). Some less frequent side effects include worsening hypertension, confusion, and the beginning of heart failure. Although hepatic toxicity is possible and patients with chronic alcoholism and liver disease can develop severe hepatotoxicity at the usual therapeutic doses, acetaminophen rarely causes gastrointestinal toxicity and has no negative effects on platelet function (Makin & Williams, 1997). Patients who are more susceptible to negative outcomes, such as the elderly, people with blood clotting disorders, people who are more likely to develop peptic ulcers, people with impaired renal function, and people receiving concurrent corticosteroid therapy, should be administered these agents with extra caution. The choice of medication and the application of peptic cytoprotective agents can affect the risk of gastrointestinal bleeding (Lanas & Hirschowitz, 1999; Wolfe et al., 1999). The nonacetylated salicylates (choline magnesium trisalicylate and salsalate) (Johnson & Miller, 1994) or the relatively selective cyclooxygenase-2 inhibitors (nabumetone, nimesulide, and meloxicam) (Lancaster, 1995; Masferrer et al., 1996) are preferred among NSAIDs in patients who tend to bleeding or peptic ulceration; at the recommended clinical doses, these medications have little effect on platelet aggregation and have no effect on bleeding time. The recommended treatment for preventing NSAID-related peptic ulceration is either omeprazole (Hawkey, 1998), pantoprazole, misoprostol (Valentini et al., 1995), or high-dose famotidine (80 mg/day) (Taha et al., 1996). These recommendations are based on data from randomized trials. A convenient and affordable option, a combination formulation of diclofenac and misoprostol is available in certain countries (McKenna, 1998; Plosker & Lamb, 1999).

Understanding the clinical pharmacology of non-opioid analgesics is necessary for their optimal administration. For each patient with cancer-related pain, there is no known minimum effective analgesic dose, ceiling dose, or toxic dose. These dosages might be greater or less than the typical ranges advised for the medication in question. The majority of the time, recommended doses are based on research done on relatively healthy patients with inflammatory diseases—a population that is very different from that of cancer patients, who frequently have coexisting organ failure and may be on multiple medications. The lowest effective analgesic dose in the cancer population is unknown because the effects of these medications are (at least in part) dose-dependent. These findings back up a method of administering NSAIDs that combines dose titration with low starting doses. The risk of significant toxicity may be decreased and the ceiling dose may be determined by a process of gradual dose escalation.

An upper limit for dose titration is typically set at 1.5–2 times the standard recommended dose of the drug in question, based on clinical experience. Sequential trials of multiple NSAIDs may be helpful to find a medication with a favorable balance between analgesia and side effects because failure with one NSAID can be followed by success with another.

9.2.1.2. Opioid Analgesics—Basic Pharmacology

All cancer patients, regardless of the mechanism causing their pain, should receive a trial of systemic opioid therapy if their pain is moderate or more severe. Even though neuropathic pain does not seem to be as responsive to opioid analgesics as somatic and visceral pain, a neuropathic mechanism does not confer "opioid resistance," and many neuropathic pain patients can find adequate relief with appropriate dose escalation (Portenoy et al., 1990; Hanks & Forbes, 1997).

The best way to use opioid analgesics is to have a solid understanding of the general principles of opioid pharmacology, the pharmacological properties of each commonly used medication, and the principles of administration, which include choosing the right medication, administering it via the right route, titrating the dosage and drug selection, and preventing and managing side effects.

9.2.1.3. Important Principles in Opioid Drug Therapy

- **Classification:** The way that opioid compounds interact with different receptor subtypes allows them to be classified into three classes: agonist, agonist–antagonist, and antagonist. When it comes to treating cancer pain, pure agonists are most frequently utilized. Because of the existence of a ceiling effect for analgesia, the possibility of precipitating withdrawal in patients physically dependent on opioid agonists, and—in the case of mixed agonist–antagonists—the issue of dose-dependent psychotomimetic side effects that surpass those of pure agonist drugs, these opioids—both partial agonist and mixed agonist—play a minor role in the management of cancer pain (Hanks, 1987).
- **Dose–Response Relationship:** There is no maximum dosage for pure agonist medications; instead, as the dose is increased, the patient experiences an increase in analgesic effects in a semi-logarithmic manner until either analgesia is reached or dose-limiting side effects like nausea, vomiting, dizziness, sedation, myoclonus, or respiratory depression occur.

Table 9.2. Major Types of Opioid Receptors

Receptor Nomenclature [1]	Gene	Most Common Location in the CNS [2]	Most Common Roles and Functions	Selective Agonist [3]	Selective Antagonist [4]
μ, mu, MOP	OPRM1	Thalamus, amygdala, dorsal horn, cerebral cortex, striatum, hippocampus, locus coeruleus	Analgesia, intestinal transit, feeding, mood, hormone secretion, thermoregulation, cardiovascular function	DAMGO, sufentanil, PL017	CTAP, CTOP, β-FNA
δ, delta, DOP	OPRD1	Olfactory bulb, thalamus, cortex, caudate putamen, nucleus accumbens (NAc), amygdala, dorsal horn	Analgesia, mood, gastrointestinal motility, behavior, cardiovascular regulation	DPDPE, [D-Ala^2] deltorphin I, [D-Ala^2] deltorphin II SNC80	Naltrindole, TIPP, Naltriben
κ, kappa, KOP	OPRK1	Olfactory bulb, NAc, cerebral cortex, claustrum, amygdala, caudate nucleus, hypothalamus, subthalamic nucleus, thalamus, corpus callosum.	Analgesia in inflammation, diuresis, feeding, neuroprotection, neuroendocrine functions	Enadoline, U50488, U69593, salvinorin A	norBNI, GNTI
N/OFQ, NOP	OPRL1	Hippocampus, hypothalamus, amygdala, substantia nigra, dorsal horn, lateral septum	Spinal analgesia, anxiety, mood, memory, feeding, locomotor activity	UFP-102, Ro64–6198, N/OFQ-(1–13)-NH_2, UFP-112	UFP-101, SB 612111, J-113397, JTC-801

Source. Paul AK, Smith CM, Rahmatullah M, Nissapatorn V, Wilairatana P, Spetea M, Gueven N, Dietis N. Opioid analgesia and opioid-induced adverse effects: A review. *Pharmaceuticals*. 2021; 14(11):1091. https://doi.org/10.3390/ph14111091.

[1,2,3,4] Further detailed information can be obtained from IUPHAR/BPS guide to pharmacology (http://www.guidetopharmacology.org; accessed on: 26 October 2021) and Alexander and colleagues [14]. Abbreviations: β-funaltrexamine (β-FNA), [D-Ala2, N-MePhe4, Gly-ol]-enkephalin (DAMGO), norbinaltorphimine (norBNI), [D-Pen2, D-Pen5] enkephalin (DPDPE), nociceptin/orphanin-FQ (N/OFQ), H-Tyr–Tic–Phe–Phe-OH (TIPP).

- **The Equianalgesic Dose Ratio:** The equianalgesic dose ratio is a commonly used measure of the relative analgesic potency of opioids. This represents the proportion of two analgesic doses needed to have the same analgesic effect. Conventionally, a comparison to 10 mg of parenteral morphine is used to determine the relative potency of each opioid that is frequently used (Houde et al., 1966). Guidelines for choosing a dose when the medication or administration method is altered are provided by equianalgesic dose information.

When interpreting the information shown in equianalgesic dose tables, a few key concepts are important to remember. The widely reported values are not indicative of the significant variability that has been noted in cross-over studies involving both single and multiple doses.

Table 9.3. Genetic Variants Analyzed on the Effectiveness and Safety of the Administered Treatment

Analgesics	Study Type	Genetic Variants	Side Effect	References
Morphine	Non-randomized clinical trial	Multidrug resistance-1 gene (MDR-1)	Moderate or severe drowsiness and confusion or hallucinations.	[Ross, J.R.;et. al. 2008]
		Catechol-O-methyltransferase (COMT) enzyme		
		Single nucleotide polymorphisms (SNPs) in intron 1		
	In vitro study-breast cancer cell lines	NET1 gene expression (mediating the direct effect of morphine on breast cancer cell migration)		[Ecimovic, P.; et al. 2011]
Codeine	Non-randomized clinical trial	CYP2D6 gene	Sedation, addiction, dizziness and constipation	[Kirchheiner, J.; et al. 2007]
Hydrocodone	Observational study	CYP2D6 gene	Dizziness and constipation	[Agarwal, D.; et al. 2017, Raji, M.A.; et al. 2018]
Hydromorphone	Non-randomized clinical trial	CYP2D6 gene	Dizziness and constipation	[Agarwal, D.; et al. 2017, Oldenmenger, W.H.; et al. 2012]
Fentanyl	Non-randomized clinical trial	CYP3A5 and ABCB1 gene polymorphisms	Dry mouth, wheal and flare	[Takashina, Y.; et al. 2012]
	Observational study	Genetic variants rs12948783 (RHBDF2) and rs7016778 (OPRK1)		[Oosten, A.W.; et al. 2016]
Methadone	Randomized double-blind study	ABCB1, OPRM1 gene polymorphisms	Constipation, nausea, dizziness and delirium	[Bruera, E.;et al. 2004, Li, Y.; et al. 2008]

Levorphanol	Non-randomized clinical trial	-	Nausea and vomiting	[Portenoy, R.K.; et al. 1986]
Buprenorphine	Non-randomized clinical trial	Polymorphisms in OPRD1	Dizziness, dry mouth, thirst and nausea	[Clarke, T.-K.; et al. 2014, Sittl, R. 2006]
Oxycodone	Non-randomized clinical trial	CYP3A5	Nausea, vomiting, constipation, lightheadedness, dizziness or drowsiness	[Naito, T.; et al. 2011]
Tramadol	Randomized double-blind placebo controlled cross over study	CYP2D6	Dizziness, headache, drowsiness, nausea, vomiting, constipation, lack of energy, sweating and dry mouth	[Arbaiza, D.; et al. 2019]
Tapentadol	Non-randomized clinical trial	No genetic variation	Nausea, vomiting, constipation, fatigue, dizziness, sleepiness, drowsiness and dry mouth	[Galiè, E.; et al. 2017]
Paracetamol (Acetaminophen)	Randomized double-blind placebo controlled parallel group study	COX-3	Low fever with nausea, stomach pain and loss of appetite	[Wiffen, P.J.; et al. 2017]
Non-steroidal Anti-Inflammatory Drugs (NSAID)	Randomized, double-blind, placebo-controlled	COX-1/COX-2	Stomach pain, heartburn, stomach ulcers, a tendency to bleed, headaches, dizziness and ringing in the ears	[Portenoy, R.K.; et al. 2019, Eisenberg, E.; et al. 1994]

Source: V. Subramaniam A, Salem Yehya AH, Oon CE. Molecular Basis of Cancer Pain Management: An Updated Review. *Medicina*. 2019; 55(9):584. https://doi.org/10.3390/medicina55090584.

A multitude of factors can impact the suitable dosage for a given patient, such as the intensity of pain, age, the route of administration, the degree of cross tolerance acquired from previous opioid exposure, the degree of consciousness, and genetic heterogeneity in metabolism or receptors. The equianalgesic dose relationship to morphine for the majority of agents is linear; however, for methadone, the relationship appears to be curvilinear, with the equianalgesic dose ratio decreasing as the dose of previous morphine increases: at low doses of morphine (30–300 mg oral morphine), the equianalgesic ratio for oral methadone to oral morphine is 1:10–1:12, and at high doses (> 300 mg oral morphine) 1:10–1:12 (Ripamonti et al., 1998).

9.2.1.4. Selecting an Appropriate Opioid

Several factors play a role in determining which opioid is selected for chronic pain management, including the level of pain, pharmacokinetics, formulation, past adverse reactions, and any other underlying medical conditions.

A combination product comprising acetaminophen or aspirin plus codeine, dihydrocodeine, hydrocodone, oxycodone, and propoxyphene has historically been used to treat patients with moderate pain. The non-opioid co-analgesic's maximum dose can be reached by increasing the doses of these combination products (e.g., acetaminophen (4,000 mg). New opioid formulations have proliferated in recent years, potentially making medication administration more convenient for patients experiencing mild to moderate pain. Codeine, dihydrocodeine, oxycodone, morphine, and tramadol in controlled release formulations at dosages suitable for mild to moderate pain are among them.

Patients who arrive in severe pain are typically treated with methadone, oxycodone, hydromorphone, morphine, or fentanyl. Among these, the opioid agonists with short half-lives (morphine, hydromorphone, fentanyl, oxycodone, or oxymorphone) are typically preferred due to their ease of titration in comparison to those with long half-lives, which take longer to reach steadystate plasma concentrations. Since it can be easily titrated in its immediate release form and has a short half-life, morphine is typically recommended. It is also available in a controlled release preparation that permits an 8–12 hour dosing interval.

Unless there are issues with dose titration or the necessary dose cannot be conveniently administered, the patient's well-tolerated opioid prescription is usually continued. If the patient experiences dose-limiting toxicity that prevents them from receiving enough pain relief without experiencing too many side effects, or if a particular formulation that isn't available with the current medication is either required or could significantly increase the convenience of administering opioids, switching to an alternative opioid is taken into consideration.

Before a medication that is both efficient and well-tolerated is found, some patients may need to undergo successive trials of multiple opioids (Cherny et al., 1995; de Stoutz et al., 1995). This tactic has been referred to as opioid-switching or opioid-rotation in different contexts. These consecutive trials may be useful because people are not fully cross-tolerated to all opioid effects, including side effects and analgesia. When switching between opioid medications, it is highly advised that clinicians understand at least three of the medications and be able to compute the proper starting doses using equianalgesic dosing data.

9.2.1.5. Selecting the Appropriate Route of Systemic Opioid Administration

9.2.1.5.1. Non-Invasive Routes

The least invasive and safest method for administering opioids that can still produce sufficient analgesia should be used. Oral administration is typically recommended. Patients who require an extremely quick onset of analgesia, have impaired swallowing or gastrointestinal dysfunction, or are unable to handle the logistics or side effects of the oral route must use alternative routes. The invention of transdermal fentanyl has made oral administration of the drug more convenient and non-invasive. There are transdermal patches that can deliver 25, 50, 75, and 100 µg/h. Each patch should be taken every 72 hours (Varvel et al., 1989), however some patients need to be taken every 48 hours (Jeal and Benfield, 1997). According to recent data from controlled trials, transdermal fentanyl administration is frequently preferred over oral morphine because it is linked to a lower incidence of constipation (Donner et al., 1996; Ahmedzai & Brooks, 1997; Payne et al., 1998).

Other non-invasive methods are not as frequently employed. Controlled-release morphine tablets can also be given intrarectally, as can reconstituted rectal suppositories containing oxycodone, hydromorphone, oxymorphone, and morphine (Maloney et al., 1989; Kaiko et al., 1992). When given rectally, the potency of opioids is roughly equal to what is obtained orally (European Association for Palliative Care, 1996).

Because there are few formulations available, most drugs absorb poorly under the tongue, and the sublingual route cannot deliver large doses or stop the patient from swallowing their medication, its usefulness is limited. Fentanyl has recently received approval for use in the treatment of breakthrough pain in an oral transmucosal formulation that dissolves the medication into a candy base (Simmonds, 1997).

9.2.1.5.2. Invasive Routes

When the oral route is not an option, when analgesia must start quickly, or when a more convenient regimen is required, a parenteral route may be taken into consideration. Parenteral bolus injections are given repeatedly; these can be given intravenously (IV. V. intermuscular (I. M.) or sublingual (S. C. routes, offer the quickest start and lengthiest duration of action. Parenteral boluses are most frequently used to treat extremely severe pain. In this situation, doses can be repeated as often as necessary, as long as the time-to-peak effect dictates, until the patient experiences sufficient relief (Hagen et al., 1997). With an indwelling I, repeated bolus doses can be administered without the need for frequent skin punctures. V. or SdotC. a 25–27-gauge infusion device, also known as a "butterfly," that can be inserted beneath the skin and left there for up to seven days (Coyle et al., 1994).

For many patients who cannot be kept on oral opioids, continuous parenteral infusions are helpful. One may give long-term infusions I. V. or S.C. In actuality, patients who are unable to swallow or absorb opioids are the main candidates for continuous infusion. Some patients whose high opioid requirement makes oral treatment unfeasible also use continuous infusion. Continuous S.C is easily utilizable by ambulatory patients. blending. As an addition to a continuous basal infusion, a variety of pumps are available, differing in complexity, price, and capacity to deliver patient-controlled "rescue doses" (Coyle et al., 1994). Opioids appropriate for ongoing S.C. The infusion needs to be easily absorbed, soluble, and non-irritating. There have been numerous reports of extensive experience with heroin, fentanyl, hydromorphone, oxymorphone, and morphine. It is not advised to use methadone because it seems to be somewhat irritating. The S.C aims to preserve an infusion site's comfort. No more than 3–5 cc/h should be infused at a time. Concentrated solutions may be beneficial for patients who need high doses. Commercially available is a high-concentration hydromorphone (10 mg/cc), and in certain nations, morphine tartrate—the organic salt of morphine—is available as an 80 mg/cc solution.

9.2.1.5.3. *Changing Routes of Administration*

To prevent overdosing or underdosing later on, the transition between the oral and parenteral routes should be guided by an understanding of relative potency. The potencies of the I. in equianalgesic dosage calculation. V. SdotC., as well as me. M. routes are regarded as being comparable. Given the uncertainty surrounding the recommended equianalgesic dosages and the potential for overdose toxicity, it is prudent to reduce the dose of the analgesic by a modest amount.

9.2.1.6. Scheduling of Opioid Administration

To achieve the best possible balance between patient comfort and convenience, the opioid administration schedule should be customized for each patient. Both "as needed" and "around the clock" dosing have a role in clinical practice.

9.2.1.6.1. *'Around the Clock' Dosing with 'Rescue Doses'*

"Around the clock" dosing keeps the patient's pain from coming back, giving them constant relief. Opioid controlled release formulations can reduce the inconvenience of using "around-the-clock" drug administration for short-acting medications. In addition, patients ought to receive a "rescue dose," which is an additional dosage given "as needed" to address pain that interferes with the prescribed course of care (Cleary, 1997).

The route of administration and the drug's time-to-peak effect determine how frequently the rescue dose can be administered. Parenteral doses can be administered as frequently as every 15–30 minutes, while oral rescue doses are typically administered up to every 1–2 hours. Based on clinical experience, the initial size of the rescue dose should be roughly 50–100% of the dose given every 4 hours for parenteral or oral bolus drugs, or 50–100% of the hourly infusion rate for patients on continuous infusions. An alternative calculation method would be to use 5–15% of the 24-hour baseline dose. It is important to determine the exact amount of rescue medication for each patient, as some may need much higher doses in cases of severe exacerbations despite having low baseline pain (Lyss, 1997). The medication used for the rescue dosage is typically the same as what is taken on a regular basis.

This strategy offers a stepwise dose escalation method that is safe and sensible and can be used with any opioid administration route. Patients who need more than four to six rescue doses in a day should usually have their baseline dose increased. The dose increase can be guided by the amount of the rescue medication consumed. As an alternative, you can set each dose increment between 33 and 50% of the previous dose. To ensure that the size of the supplemental dose stays a constant percentage of the fixed dose, increasing the baseline dose should always be accompanied by an equal increase in the rescue dose.

9.2.1.6.2. *'As-needed' (PRN) Dosing*

When starting opioid therapy, administering opioids "as needed" rather than following a "around the clock" dosing schedule may increase safety. This is especially true when starting therapy with a long-half-life opioid like methadone or levorphanol or when rapid dose escalation is required. Patients with rapidly decreasing analgesic requirements or those with intermittent pain interspersed with pain-free intervals may also benefit from "as needed" dosing.

9.2.1.6.3. *Patient-Controlled Analgesia (PCA)*

Patient-controlled analgesia (PCA) is a method of administering pain medication where the patient controls the delivery of the drug through an infusion device. Typically used in cancer patients on a long-term basis, PCA is often administered subcutaneously using a portable infusion device. It is usually used in conjunction with a continuous baseline infusion and serves as an additional dose for breakthrough pain. In some cases, PCA may be used as the sole method of managing sudden, intense pain that cannot be managed effectively with oral medication.

9.2.1.7. Dose Selection and Titration

9.2.1.7.1. *Selecting a Starting Dose*

An opioid usually used for severe pain should usually be started at a dose equivalent to 5–10 mg of morphine in a patient who is relatively non-tolerant and has only had limited exposure to an opioid typically used on the second rung of the "analgesic ladder" for moderate pain. M. As per the European Association for Palliative Care (1996), every 4 hours. When using morphine, a P. O. I. M. The standard ratio for relative potency is 2:1–3:1. (European Association for Palliative Care, 1996).

9.2.1.7.2. *Dose Adjustment*

When there is insufficient relief, the dosage should be gradually increased until either sufficient analgesia is reported or severe side effects occur. Less than a 30–50% dose increment is unlikely to significantly improve analgesia because the opioid response grows linearly with the log of the dose. As long as administration is not jeopardized by severe side effects, inconvenience, discomfort, or expense, the exact dosage is irrelevant.

9.2.1.7.3. *Rate of Dose Titration*

The degree of pain, the patient's health, and the treatment objectives all influence how quickly a dose should be titrated. Sometimes the best course of action for patients who present with extremely severe pain is to administer a dose parenterally repeatedly every 15 to 30 minutes until the patient's pain is partially relieved. Instead of starting with a loading dose of the opioid, patients with moderate pain may benefit from a regular dose that is gradually increased with rescue doses. In this case, dose increases of 30–50% can be given at intervals longer than what is needed to achieve steady state after each modification. Every 24 to 48 hours, the dose of transdermal fentanyl or controlled release oral morphine can be increased. The doses of morphine (tablets or elixir), hydromorphone, and oxycodone can be increased twice daily.

9.2.1.7.4. *The Problem of Tolerance*

True analgesic tolerance is far less common when the need for dose escalation arises than disease progression (Paice, 1988; Schug et al., 1992), rising psychological distress, or changes in the pharmacokinetics of an analgesic drug. The presence of increasing opioid doses in the absence of other factors (e.g., patient compliance) is a sign of true analgesic tolerance, which may jeopardize the effectiveness of treatment e. g., progressive illness, which could account for the rise in pain.

9.2.2. Management of Opioid Adverse Effects

For opioid therapy to be effective, analgesia's advantages must manifestly surpass the side effects of the treatment. This suggests that everyone involved in cancer pain management needs to have a thorough awareness of the negative effects of opioids and the techniques used to prevent and manage them. Table 9.4 provides an overview of the side effects that are commonly seen in patients receiving oral morphine and other opioids. There is a lot of variation in the dose-response relationship among side effects. When it comes to the negative effects of sedation on the central nervous system, such as respiratory depression, myoclonus, hallucinations, and cognitive impairment, a dose-response relationship is most frequently apparent. However, many of these effects have very significant interindividual variability even among them. Furthermore, the range of negative effects changes with continued use as tolerance to some effects grows. Patients with extended exposure to opioids typically experience less sedation or respiratory depression, with delirium and myoclonus being the most common neuroexcitatory effects on the central nervous system. The dose-response relationship for adverse effects related to the digestive system is typically weaker. Certain side effects, such as nausea and vomiting, are typical when therapy first starts, but they can then vary widely among patients, sometimes going away and sometimes persisting. Constipation is almost a universal condition with a very poor dose response.

9.2.2.1. Factors Predictive of Opioid Adverse Effects

9.2.2.1.1. Drug Side Effects

All things considered, there is hardly any consistent data indicating that a particular pure opioid agonist has a significantly better adverse effect profile than any other. Meperidine's side effect profile raises concerns, so it is not advised for the treatment of chronic cancer pain. According to recent data from controlled studies, fentanyl administered transdermally is linked to a lower incidence of constipation than morphine taken orally (Donner et al., 1996; Ahmedzai & Brooks, 1997; Payne et al., 1998).

Table 9.4. Common Opioid-Induced Adverse Effects

Oral Opioid					Placebo			
	Number of patients		**Event rate (%)**		**Number of Patients**		**Event Rate (%)**	
Adverse Event	**With AE**	**Total**	**Average**	**95% CI**	**With AE**	**Total**	**Average**	**95% CI**
Patients experiencing any adverse event	1387	2743	51	49–53	122	404	30	26–34
Withdrawals								
Adverse event withdrawal	933	4221	22	21–23	51	721	7.1	5 . 2 – 8.9
Lack of efficacy withdrawal	177	2719	6.5	5 . 6 – 7.4	135	679	20	17–23
Specific adverse events								
Dry mouth	100	399	25	21–29	3	94	3.2	0–6.7

Nausea	902	4314	21	20–22	40	718	5.6	3.9–7.2
Constipation	606	4043	15	14–16	32	643	5.0	3.3–6.7
Dizziness	530	3899	14	13–15	28	623	4.5	2.9–6.1
Drowsiness or somnolence	425	3078	14	13–15	21	531	4.0	2.3–5.6
Pruritus	106	794	13	11–16	7	336	2.1	0.6–3.6
Vomiting	345	3330	10	9.3–11	12	497	2.4	1.1–3.8

1. AE, adverse event; CI, 95% confidence interval.

Source. Moore, R.A., McQuay, H.J. Prevalence of opioid adverse events in chronic non-malignant pain: systematic review of randomized trials of oral opioids. Arthritis Res Ther., 7, R1046 (2005). https://doi.org/10.1186/ar1782.

9.2.2.1.3. Route Related

There is not much data to support the idea that different systemic administration routes have different side effects. Small studies have shown reduced nausea and vomiting with rectal (Babul et al., 1998) and subcutaneous (McDonald et al., 1991) morphine administration compared to oral morphine administration. In three trials, patients who received transdermal fentanyl experienced less constipation than those who received oral morphine. The effect's relationship to the drug or the route is unclear (Donner et al., 1996; Ahmedzai & Brooks, 1997; Payne et al., 1998).

9.2.2.1.4. Patient Related

There is a remarkable interindividual variability in the sensitivity to side effects from morphine and other opioid drugs, for reasons that remain poorly understood. Preclinical research has demonstrated that genetic variability influences opioid sensitivity, and it is logical to believe that genetic background has a similar significant effect in clinical settings.

Comorbidity has a role in some of this variability. Pharmacokinetics are known to be altered with age, with decreased clearance and volume of distribution being two prominent characteristics. For morphine (Baillie et al., 1989) and fentanyl (Bentley et al., 1982; Holdsworth et al., 1994), this has been thoroughly examined.

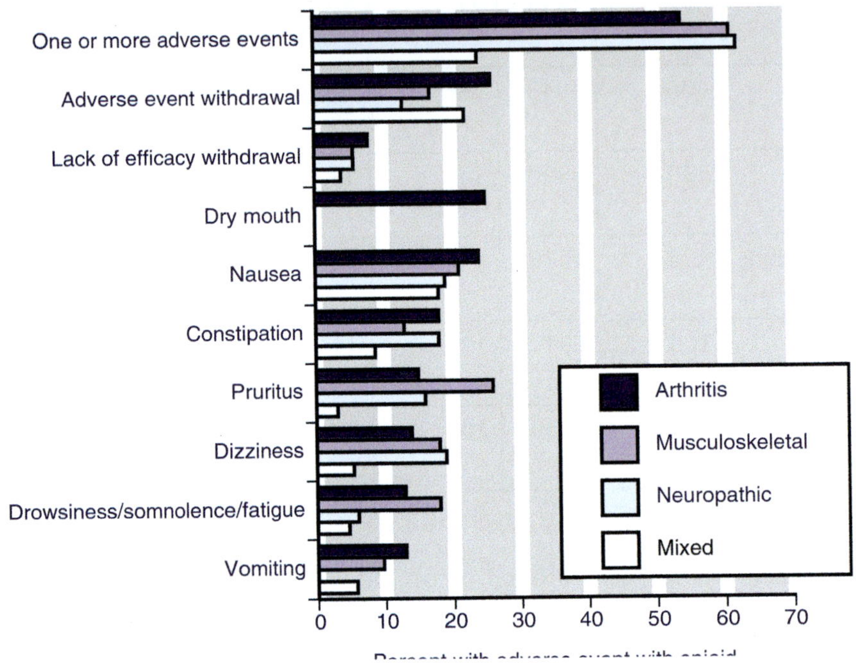

Figure 9.2. Adverse event rates in patients with different etiology of chronic non-malignant pain treated with opioids.

Source. Moore, R.A., McQuay, H.J. Prevalence of opioid adverse events in chronic non-malignant pain: systematic review of randomized trials of oral opioids. Arthritis Res Ther 7, R1046 (2005). https://doi.org/10.1186/ar1782.

In general, older patients needed lower doses of morphine than younger patients in a study on the treatment of chronic cancer pain in the elderly, and they did so without showing an increased risk of opioid-induced side effects (Rapin, 1989). Morphine-6-glucuronide, an active metabolite of morphine, is cleared more slowly in patients with reduced renal function (Osborne et al., 1993). High M6G concentrations have been anecdotally linked to toxicity (Osborne et al., 1986; Hagen et al., 1991; Sjogren et al., 1993); however, no correlation with renal function was noted in a prospective study of patients with opioid-induced delirium or myoclonus (Tiseo et al., 1995).

The coadministration of medications that may have cumulative toxicity or other concurrent comorbidity are additional patient-related factors that may increase the risk of adverse effects.

9.2.2.1.5. Opioid Initiation and Dose Escalation

Some side effects occur momentarily and then go away on their own when an opioid is started or when the dosage is increased. A prospective study on the impact of increasing the dosage of morphine on cognitive function provides a clear demonstration of this phenomenon (Bruera et al., 1989). This study showed that after seven days, cognitive impairment typically improved. Despite being frequently reported, this phenomenon has not been thoroughly investigated in relation to other negative effects.

9.2.2.2. Differential Diagnosis

Not all adverse changes in a patient's well-being among opioid users can be attributed to the drug itself. It's important to distinguish adverse effects from medication interactions and other potential causes of comorbidity in the patient receiving treatment.

In fact, the opioid is rarely the cause of a new, detrimental change in a patient's well-being that appears in the context of stable opioid dosing; instead, a different explanation needs to be actively pursued. Given that patients with advanced cancer frequently take multiple medications, it is critical to carefully review medication records and patient reports to look for potential drug interactions or other drug-related explanations for the symptoms that have been reported.

9.2.2.3. Overview of the Alternative Approaches to Treating Opioid Adverse Effects

In general, four different approaches to the management of opioid adverse effects have been described:

1. Dose reduction of systemic opioid
2. Specific therapy to reduce the adverse effect
3. Opioid rotation
4. Change the route of administration

9.2.2.3.1. Dose Reduction of Systemic Opioid

The majority of the time, dosage-related side effects disappear when administered opioid dosages are decreased. Gradually reducing the opioid dose in patients with well-controlled pain frequently resolves dose-related adverse effects while maintaining sufficient pain relief (Fallon and O'Neill, 1998).

When opioid doses cannot be reduced without the loss of pain control, dose reduction must be accompanied by the addition of an accompanying synergist approach. Extensive experience has been reported with four accompanying approaches:

1. The addition of a non-opioid coanalgesic. The analgesia achieved from non-opioid coanalgesics from the non-steroidal anti-inflammatory class of agents is additive and often synergistic with that achieved by opioids. This is supported from a number of prospective studies (Sevarino et al., 1992; Bjorkman et al., 1993; Joishy & Walsh, 1998; Minotti et al., 1998) and from one retrospective drug utilization survey (Zech et al., 1995).
2. The addition of an adjuvant analgesic that is appropriate to the pain syndrome and mechanism. Adjuvant analgesics (see below) may be combined with primary analgesics to improve the outcome for patients who cannot otherwise attain an acceptable balance between relief and side effects (Portenoy, 1996). There is great interindividual variability in the response to all adjuvant analgesics and, for most, the likelihood of benefit is limited. Furthermore, many of the adjuvant analgesics have the potential to cause side effects that may be additive to the opioid-induced adverse effects already problematic. In evaluating the utility of an adjuvant agent in a particular patient setting, one must consider the likelihood of benefit, the risk of adverse effects, the ease of administration, and patient convenience.
3. The application of a therapy targeting the cause of the pain. Specific antitumor therapies, such

as radiotherapy, chemotherapy, or surgery targeting the cause of cancer-related pain can provide substantial relief and thus lower the need for opioid analgesia. Radiotherapy is of established benefit in the treatment of painful bone metastases (Bates, 1992; Hoskin, 1995; Janjan, 1997), epidural neoplasm (Bates, 1992), and headache due to cerebral metastases (Coia, 1992; Sneed et al., 1996; Vermeulen, 1998). In other settings there is a lack of well-established supportive data, and the use of radiotherapy is largely anecdotal. Despite a paucity of evidence concerning the specific analgesic benefits of chemotherapy (Queisser, 1984; Rubens et al., 1992), there is a strong clinical impression that tumor shrinkage is generally associated with relief of pain. Although there are some reports of analgesic value even in the absence of significant tumor shrinkage (Patt et al., 1985; Thatcher et al., 1995; Rothenberg, 1996), the likelihood of a favorable effect on pain is generally related to the likelihood of tumor response. Surgery may have a role in the relief of symptoms caused by specific problems, such as obstruction of a hollow viscus (Jong et al., 1995; Mainar et al., 1996; Parker & Baines, 1996; Barbalias et al., 1997), unstable bony structures (Braun & Rohe, 1984; Tarn & Lee, 1994; Algan & Horowitz, 1996), and compression of neural tissues (Sucher et al., 1994; Gokaslan, 1996; Harris et al., 1996).

4. The application of a regional anesthetic or neuroablative intervention (see below). The results of the WHO 'analgesic ladder' validation studies suggest that 10–30% of patients with cancer pain do not achieve a satisfactory balance between relief and side effects using systemic pharmacotherapy alone without unacceptable drug toxicity (Takeda, 1985; Ventafridda et al., 1987; Walker et al., 1988; Goisis et al., 1989; Schug et al., 1990; Grond et al., 1991). Anesthetic and neurosurgical techniques may reduce or eliminate the requirement for systemically administered opioids to achieve adequate analgesia. In general, regional analgesic techniques such as intraspinal opioid and local anesthetic administration or intrapleural local anesthetic administration are usually considered first because they can achieve this end without compromising neurological integrity. Neurodestructive procedures, however, are valuable in a small subset of patients, and some of these procedures, such as celiac plexus blockade in patients with pancreatic cancer, may have a favorable enough risk: benefit ratio that early treatment is warranted.

9.2.2.3.2. Symptomatic Management of the Adverse Effect

Symptomatic medications are frequently used to stop or manage the negative effects of opioids. The majority of these methods rely on a collection of anecdotal evidence. The literature outlining these methods is primarily anecdotal or "expert opinion," with very few exceptions. There are very few studies that have assessed efficacy prospectively, and none that have assessed the long-term toxicity of these methods. This method typically entails adding a new medication, which increases the burden of medications and the risks of side effects or drug interactions.

9.2.2.3.3. *Opioid Rotation*

Changes to alternative opioids have successfully reduced the side effects of opioids, according to multiple clinicians and cancer pain services over the past 10 years (Galer et al., 1992; Bruera et al., 1995, 1996; Cherny et al., 1995; de Stoutz et al., 1995; Paix et al., 1995; Thomas & Bruera, 1995; Maddocks et al., 1996; Vigano et al., 1996; Fitzgibbon & Ready, 1997; Hagen & Swanson, 1997; Lawlor et al., 1997; Makin & Ellershaw, 1998; Ripamonti et al., 1998; Ashby et al., 1999). There have been numerous reports of improvements in myoclonus, sedation, hallucinations, nausea, and vomiting in addition to cognitive impairment. To use this method, one must be conversant with a variety of opioid agonists and understand how to convert doses when switching between opioids using equianalgesic tables. Although reducing polypharmacy is a practical benefit of this strategy, results are unpredictable and fluctuating. Because each patient is different, even with careful application of equianalgesic tables, patients may under- or overdose when alternating between opioids.

The intraindividual variability in sensitivity to opioid analgesia and adverse effects is attributed to a complex biological basis. According to preclinical research (de Stoutz et al., 1995; Pasternak and Standifer, 1995; Zadina et al., 1995; Rossi et al., 1997), opioids can act on a variety of receptors or subtypes of receptors, and the analgesic effects and side effects may vary depending on the specific receptor profile. According to several studies (Brosen et al., 1993; Sindrup et al., 1993; Fromm et al., 1995; Sindrup & Brosen, 1995; Poulsen et al., 1996; Kirkwood et al., 1997; Heiskanen et al., 1998), analgesia for some opioids is significantly influenced by an individual's genetic composition. Similar phenomena may also contribute to variation in adverse effect sensitivity.

9.2.2.3.4. *Switching Route of Systemic Administration*

There is insufficient evidence to suggest that changing the admission route to subcutaneous morphine can alleviate some of the negative side effects experienced by patients on oral morphine. This phenomenon was linked to nausea and vomiting in one small study (McDonald et al., 1991); in another, constipation, drowsiness, and nausea were less common (Drexel et al., 1989).

9.2.2.4. Initial Management of the Patient Receiving Opioids Who Presents with Adverse Effects

In the early management of adverse effects in patients receiving opioid analgesic therapy, there are two important steps. First and foremost, the clinician needs to differentiate between side effects of morphine and comorbidity or drug interactions. If other conditions exist, they ought to be addressed. Treatment for metabolic problems, dehydration, or sepsis is necessary; non-essential medications that might be causing an adverse interaction should be stopped. It can be necessary to take symptomatic measures up until an effect is seen.

Second, lowering the dosage of an opioid should be taken into consideration if it appears that there is a genuine negative effect. If the patient is managing their pain well, cut back on the morphine dosage by 25%.

9.2.2.4.1. *Adverse Drug Interactions*

Drug combinations frequently cause side effects in patients with advanced cancer. It is important to be aware of the possibility of severe toxicity and additive side effects from drug combinations. An opioid's sedative effect may compound the effects of many other centrally acting medications, including antidepressants, anxiolytics, and neuroleptics (Pies, 1996). Similarly, anticholinergic medications likely exacerbate the constipating effects of opioids. As previously mentioned, meperidine treatment for patients receiving monoamine oxidase inhibitors has been associated with a serious adverse reaction that can include excitation, hyperpyrexia, convulsions, and even death (Browne & Linter, 1987).

9.2.2.4.2. Gastrointestinal Side Effects

Opioids frequently cause adverse effects in the gastrointestinal tract. They are typically distinguished by a poor dose-response relationship. According to Fallon and O'Neill (1997), the most frequent side effect of long-term opioid therapy is constipation. Most patients should be prescribed laxative medications as a preventive measure because of the high likelihood of opioid-induced constipation. Opioids can cause vomiting and nausea via peripheral as well as central mechanisms. These medications have effects on the gastrointestinal tract, such as increased gastric antral tone, decreased motility, and delayed gastric emptying. They also increase vestibular sensitivity and stimulate the medullary chemoreceptor trigger zone. When starting opioid therapy, patients should be made aware that nausea is common, usually fleeting, and under control. Patients should have access to an antiemetic at the beginning of therapy if necessary, but routine prophylactic administration of one is not required, with the exception of those who have a history of severe opioid-induced nausea and vomiting. According to anecdotal evidence, prochlorperazine and metoclopromide have typically been adequate.

9.2.2.4.3. Central Nervous System Side Effects

The side effects on the CNS are typically dose-related. The duration of opioid exposure, dosage, and individual patient factors all affect the specific pattern of CNS adverse effects.

9.2.2.4.4. Sedation

When opioid therapy is started or a large dose is increased, sedation is often the first side effect and lasts for days or weeks until tolerance to the effect sets in. Patients should be made aware of this possibility in order to lower their anxiety and encourage them to refrain from potentially hazardous activities like driving (Vainio et al., 1995). Some patients, especially those with additional complicating factors, struggle with sedation for an extended period of time. These include coexisting conditions like dementia, metabolic encephalopathy, or brain metastases, as well as the use of additional sedatives. Methylphenidate and dextroamphetamine have both been extensively used to treat opioid-induced sedation (Portenoy, 1994). Methylphenidate or dextroamphetamine treatment is usually started with 2.5 to 5 mg in the morning and continued at midday if needed to keep the effects going into the evening. If necessary, doses are then gradually increased. Few patients need more than 40 mg in divided doses per day. Patients with paranoid personality, agitated delirium, cardiac arrhythmias, or history of amphetamine abuse should generally avoid this treatment.

9.2.2.4.5. Confusion and Delirium

When opioid treatment or dosages are started, mild cognitive impairment is frequently experienced. Pure opioid-induced encephalopathy, on the other hand, seems to be temporary in most patients, lasting anywhere from a few days to a few weeks, much like sedation. The etiology of persistent delirium is typically related to the combined effect of the opioid and other contributing factors, such as electrolyte disorders, neoplastic involvement of the central nervous system, sepsis, vital organ failure, and hypoxemia, even though persistent confusion attributable to opioids alone occurs (Portenoy, 1994). A neuroleptic medication trial is frequently the last step in a step-by-step management strategy. Low dosages of haloperidol (0–5–1–0 mg P. O. or 0.25–0.05 milligram I. V. or myself. M. is most frequently advised due to its effectiveness and low risk of anticholinergic and cardiovascular side effects.

9.2.2.4.6. Respiratory Depression

Respiratory depression is rare when sedation is used as a clinical indicator of CNS toxicity and appropriate measures are implemented. When it does, however, always comes with other symptoms of depression of the central nervous system, such as drowsiness and confusion. Tachypnea and anxiety coupled with respiratory compromise is never a primary opioid event.

Table 9.5. Non-Pharmacological Interventions for Delirium Management

Minimize the use of immobilizing catheters, intravenous lines, and physical restraints
Avoid immobility, early mobilization
Monitor nutrition
Provide visual and hearing aids
Monitor closely for dehydration
Control pain
Monitor fluid-electrolyte balance
Monitor bowel and bladder functioning
Review medications
Reorient communications with the patient
Place orientation board, clock, or familiar objects (family photos, etc) in the room
Encourage cognitively stimulating activities such as word puzzles
Facilitate sleep hygiene, including relaxation music at bedtime, warm drinks, and gentle massage
Minimize noise and interventions at bedtime (reschedule medications, do not interrupt sleep for checking temperature, etc.)

Source: Bramati P, Bruera E. Delirium in Palliative Care. *Cancers.* 2021; 13(23):5893. https://doi.org/10.3390/cancers13235893.

Clinically significant respiratory depression is an extremely uncommon occurrence in cancer patients whose opioid dosage has been adjusted to manage pain because tolerance to the respiratory depressant effects of opioids appears to develop quickly with repeated administration.

The stimulus-related impact of pain on breathing is also correlated with the capacity to withstand high opioid doses, but this relationship is counterbalanced by the depressant effects of opioids. However, if the pain is abruptly removed (as may happen after neurolytic procedures) and the opioid dosage is not decreased, opioid-induced respiratory depression may occur (Wells et al., 1984).

When naloxone, a particular opioid antagonist, is administered to patients receiving chronic opioid therapy, respiratory depression usually improves. This holds true even in cases where a concomitant cardiac or pulmonary process rather than the opioid itself was the main cause of the respiratory event. Therefore, a naloxone response shouldn't be interpreted as evidence that the event was caused solely by the opioid; instead, these other processes should be evaluated.

Naloxone should only be used when clearly necessary because it can cause a severe abstinence syndrome. The opioid should be stopped and the patient closely watched until they improve if they are bradypneic but easily aroused and the last opioid dose's peak plasma level has already been reached. Naloxone should be given if the patient experiences severe hypoventilation (regardless of any concomitant conditions that may be causing respiratory compromise) or if they are unconscious and bradypneic. When administering opioids, diluted naloxone (1:10) should be used at doses adjusted to the patient's respiratory rate and consciousness level to lessen the chance of severe withdrawal. After administering naloxone to a comatose patient, it might be wise to insert an endotracheal tube to prevent aspiration.

9.2.2.4.7. Multifocal Myoclonus

Myoclonus can be caused by any opioid analgesic. Myoclonus which is mild and sporadic is frequent. However, myoclonus can occasionally be upsetting or exacerbate breakthrough pain that comes with uncontrollable movement. Consideration should be given to either switching to an alternative opioid (Cherny et al., 1995) or symptomatic treatment with a benzodiazepine (especially clonazepam or midazolam), dantrolene, or an anticonvulsant if the dose cannot be reduced due to persistent pain (Portenoy, 1994).

9.2.2.4.8. Other Effects

- Urinary Retention: Opioid analgesics cause an increase in smooth muscle tone, which can sometimes increase sphincter tone and bladder spasms. This is an uncommon issue that is typically seen in older male patients. Although tolerance can grow quickly, catheterization might be required to treat temporary issues.

9.2.3. Adjuvant Analgesics

A medication that is analgesic in certain circumstances but has a primary indication other than pain is referred to as an adjuvant analgesic. These medications can be used in any of the three steps of the "analgesic ladder" in conjunction with primary analgesics in the cancer population to help patients who would not otherwise be able to achieve an acceptable balance between side effects and relief. When a drug has a non-analgesic effect, it may still be useful as an adjuvant analgesic, as indicated by the nature of the pain or the presence of another symptom.

Every adjuvant analgesic has a wide range of effects on different individuals. While certain patient characteristics, like advanced age or coexisting major organ failure, may raise the chance of certain responses, most of which are adverse, it is impossible to predict with any degree of accuracy which benefits or side effects a particular patient may experience. Additionally, there exists notable interindividual variation in the way that the body reacts to various medications, even those that belong to the same class. These findings point to the possible benefit of testing adjuvant analgesics one after the other in succession. To improve compliance and lessen the potential for distress in the event that treatments are unsuccessful, patients should be informed about the sequential drug trial process, including dose titration and the use of low starting doses, at the beginning of therapy.

In the management of cancer pain, adjuvant analgesics can be broadly classified based on conventional use. Four groups are distinguished:

1. Multipurpose adjuvant analgesics.
2. Adjuvant analgesics used for neuropathic pain.
3. Adjuvant analgesics used for bone pain.
4. Adjuvant analgesics used for visceral pain.

9.2.3.1. Multipurpose Adjuvant Medications

9.2.3.1.1. Corticosteroids

Among the most popular adjuvant analgesics are corticosteroids (Watanabe & Bruera, 1994). Research has shown that they can provide analgesic effects, greatly enhance quality of life, and positively impact appetite, nausea, mood, and malaise in cancer patients. Raised intracranial pressure headaches, acute spinal cord compression, superior vena cava syndrome, metastatic bone pain, neuropathic pain from tumor infiltration or compression, symptomatic lymphedema, and hepatic capsular distension are among the painful conditions that frequently improve with corticosteroids (Watanabe & Bruera, 1994). According to Devor et al. (1985), these mechanisms of analgesia may include anti-inflammatory, anti-edema, and direct effects on the electrical activity of injured nerves. Dextamethasone is the most widely used medication; this choice is theoretically supported by the agent's comparatively low mineralocorticoid effect. Conventionally, dexamethasone has also been used to treat spinal cord compression and increased intracranial pressure.

When pain and other symptoms are present in advanced cancer patients, a comparatively small dose of corticosteroid (e.g., 1–2 mg of dexamethasone twice a day). However, a high-dose regimen might be suitable in some circumstances. For instance, a brief course of relatively high doses may have a dramatic effect on patients with spinal cord compression, an acute episode of extremely severe bone pain, or neuropathic pain that cannot be promptly reduced with opioids. e.g., dexamethasone 100 mg, first administered as divided doses of 96 mg per day (Sorensen et al., 1994). This dosage can be gradually reduced over a few weeks while other analgesic methods, like radiation therapy, are started.

While corticosteroids can have very satisfying effects on patients with advanced cancer, there is a risk of serious side effects that worsen with continued use (Twycross, 1994). Oropharyngeal candidiasis, edema, or cushingoid habitus, dyspepsia, weight gain, neuropsychological abnormalities and ecchymoses, hyperglycemia, and myopathy are among the most frequent side effects. Patients receiving chronic corticosteroid treatment have a roughly doubled risk of developing peptic ulcers; additionally, it is not advised to co-administer corticosteroids with aspirin or an NSAID due to the increased risk of gastroduodenopathy (Ellershaw & Kelly, 1994). Corticosteroids should not be used as adjuvant analgesics in patients with unstable diabetes, systemic infection, or active peptic ulcer disease.

9.2.3.1.2. Topical local Anesthetics

Topical local anesthetics can be used as a premedication before skin puncture and to treat painful cutaneous and mucosal lesions. A eutectic mixture consisting of 2.5% lignocaine (lidocaine) and 2.5% prilocaine (EMLA) works well to lessen pain after lumbar punctures, arterial punctures, and venipunctures. It has also been applied to skin lesions that cause excruciating ulcers. The treatment of oropharyngeal ulcerations often involves the use of viscous lidocaine, also known as lignocaine. Eating after oropharyngeal anesthesia requires caution, despite the seemingly low risk of aspiration.

9.2.3.2. Adjuvants Used for Neuropathic Pain

Compared to nociceptive pain, neuropathic pain is typically less responsive to opioid therapy. In many cases, adding an adjuvant analgesic to pharmacotherapy can improve its results.

9.2.3.2.1. Antidepressant Drugs

Antidepressant medications are frequently used to treat ongoing neuropathic pain, and tertiary amine tricyclic medications, such as imipramine, doxepin, and amitriptyline, have the strongest evidence for analgesic efficacy (McQuay et al., 1996). When sedation, anticholinergic effects, or cardiovascular toxicity are major concerns, secondary amine tricyclic antidepressants (like desipramine, clomipramine, and nortryptyline) are recommended because they have fewer side effects (McQuay et al., 1996). Antidepressants that block selective serotonin uptake are generally not advised for the treatment of neuropathic pain because of their significantly lower efficacy in this area.

A tricyclic antidepressant should be started at a low dose, e.g., amitriptyline 10 mg for senior citizens and 25 mg for younger individuals. Doses can be raised every few days, with the first dosage increment typically equal to the initial dose. Once dosages are within the customary range of effectiveness (e.g., amitriptyline 75–150 mg), it is wise to wait a week to see how the medication is working before titrating the dosage higher. In patients who do not show improvement and who do not experience any limiting side effects, it is reasonable to continue upward dose titration beyond the customary analgesic doses. If available, plasma drug concentration should be monitored throughout the course of treatment as it may offer helpful information.

9.2.3.2.2. Anticonvulsant Drugs

According to McCraw et al. (1995), certain anticonvulsant medications seem to have analgesic properties for the lancinating dysesthesias that are present in various forms of neuropathic pain. Due to the excellent response rate in trigeminal neuralgia (McQuay et al., 1995), most practitioners prefer to start with carbamazepine; however, this medication needs to be used carefully in cancer patients who have thrombocytopenia, those who are at risk for 654 marrow failure (e.g., after chemotherapy), and those whose blood counts need to be checked frequently to assess the progress of their condition. When using carbamazepine, a complete blood count should be taken before therapy begins, two and four weeks later, and then every three to four months after that. Treatment should be stopped if the leukocyte count falls below 4,000, which is generally regarded as contraindication to leukocyte counts below 3,000, or if the absolute neutrophil count falls below 1,500 while on therapy. Trials using gabapentin, phenytoin, clonazepam, and valproate are supported by published reports and clinical experience, and other anticonvulsant medications may also be helpful (McQuay et al., 1995). It is advised that dosage recommendations for anticonvulsant medications that are used as adjuvant analgesics adhere to the usual guidelines used when treating seizures.

9.2.3.2.3. Oral Local Anesthetic Drugs

Sometimes neuropathic pain with lancinating or continuous dysesthesias can be effectively managed with systemically administered local anesthetics. In patients with persistent dysesthesias who do not respond well to tricyclic antidepressants or who are intolerable to them, as well as in patients with excruciating pains that do not improve after trying baclofen and anticonvulsant medications, it makes sense to conduct a trial using an oral local anesthetic. Mexiletine is the preferred oral local anesthetic because it is the safest (CAST Investigators, 1989; Ruskin, 1989). The likelihood of a response to oral mexiletine may be predicted by the analgesic response to an intravenous lidocaine (lignocaine; 5 mg/kg, over 45 min) trial (Galer et al., 1996). The recommended starting dose for mexiletine is typically 100–150 mg daily. The dosage can be raised by a comparable amount every few days if intolerable side effects do not manifest, up to the standard maximum dose of 300 mg three times a day.

The use of calcitonin, baclofen, clonidine, and subcutaneous ketamine administration is supported by less convincing evidence (Lipman, 1996).

9.2.3.3. Adjuvant Analgesics Used for Bone Pain

The effective management of bone pain often necessitates the combination of opioid therapy with a variety of auxiliary strategies. Some patients seem to benefit greatly from the addition of such a drug, although a meta-analysis of NSAID therapy in cancer pain (Eisenberg et al., 1994) that examined data from 1,615 patients in 21 trials found no specific efficacy in bone pain and analgesic effects equivalent only to "weak" opioids. In challenging situations, corticosteroids are frequently recommended (Watanabe & Bruera, 1994).

- **Bisphosphonates:** Analogs of inorganic pyrophosphate, known as bisphosphonates, lower bone resorption in a range of diseases by blocking osteoclast activity. Intravenous pamidronate has been shown to significantly reduce bone pain in patients with advanced cancer in both controlled and uncontrolled trials (Strang, 1996). Pamidronate's analgesic effect appears to be schedule- and dose-dependent; at doses between 15 and 30 mg/week, a dose-response is visible, and 30 mg every two weeks is reported to be less effective than 60 mg every four weeks (Strang, 1996). When clodronate is taken orally, comparable results have been reported (Ernst et al., 1997).
- **Radiopharmaceuticals:** Potential treatments for metastatic bone disease have included the absorption of radiolabeled agents into regions with high bone turnover. Its benefits include comparatively selective absorption and coverage of all sites of involvement, thereby reducing the amount of radiation that is exposed to normal tissues. Radiopharmaceuticals have demonstrated a range of excellent clinical responses with acceptable hematological toxicity. Strontium-89 is the most extensively researched and frequently used radionuclide. Its effectiveness as a first-line therapy (Robinson et al., 1995) or as an adjuvant to external-beam radiation therapy (Porter et al., 1993) has been shown in large, prospectively randomized clinical trials. Patients with a WCC < 2.4 or a platelet count < 60 000 should not use this approach, and patients with a very poor performance status should not use it either (Schmeler & Bastin, 1996). Bone seeking radiopharmaceuticals, which combine a radioisotope and a bisphosphonate compound, have been created through an alternative method. Positive experiences with rhenium-186-hydroxyethylidene diphosphonate and samarium-153-ethylenediamine tetramethylene phosphonic acid have been documented.

9.2.3.4. Adjuvant Analgesics for Visceral Pain

The potential effectiveness of several adjuvant medications for the treatment of colicky intestinal pain, tenesmoid pain, and bladder spasms is supported by a paucity of data. Both flavoxate and oxybutynin chloride, are tertiary amines with direct muscular antispasmodic effects that are papaverine-like and anticholinergic (Paulson, 1978; Baert, 1974). For patients experiencing painful bladder spasms, an NSAID trial may be warranted based on limited clinical experience and in vitro evidence that prostaglandins contribute to bladder smooth-muscle contraction (Abrams & Fenely, 1976). A trial using intravesical capsaicin is supported by a limited amount of data (Barbanti et al., 1993; Lazzeri et al., 1996). For excruciating rectal spasms, there is currently no proven medication treatment. Nebulized salbutamol can lessen the length and intensity of attacks, according to a recent double-blind study (Eckardt et al., 1996). Trials with clonidine (Swain, 1987), diltiazem (Boquet et al., 1986; Castell, 1985), chlorpromazine (Patt et al., 1994), and benzodiazepines (Hanks, 1984) have anecdotal evidence supporting them.

Intravenous scopolamine (hyoscine) butylbromide (Baines, 1997; De Conno et al., 1991; Ventafridda et al., 1990) and sublingual scopolamine (hyoscine) hydrobromide (Baines, 1994) have been used as empirical treatments for colicky pain caused by irreversible bowel obstruction. The use of octreotide for this indication is supported by limited data (Mercadante, 1994b).

9.3. Other Non-Invasive Analgesic Techniques

9.3.1. Psychological Therapies in Cancer Pain

A key component of the care given to cancer patients who are in pain is psychological counseling. Psychological evaluation and support are beneficial for all patients, and certain patients may benefit from particular psychological interventions, such as those that are frequently used to treat pain. Through the development of new coping mechanisms and the modification of thoughts, feelings, and behaviors, cognitive-behavioral interventions can assist some patients in reducing the perception of distress caused by the pain (Spiegel & Moore, 1997). According to Arathuzik (1994), relaxation techniques may be able to improve pain tolerance, and lessen emotional arousal and muscle tension. Alternative methods lessen the distress brought on by the pain or lessen the anticipatory anxiety that could result in avoidant behaviors (Turk & Feldman, 1992). A patient who is cognitively intact and a committed, skilled physician are necessary for the successful application of these techniques in the cancer population (Fishman, 1992).

9.3.2. Physiatric Techniques

By applying modalities like electrical stimulation, heat, or cryotherapy, physiatric techniques can improve analgesia or maximize the function of the patient with chronic cancer. Pneumatic pump devices, pressure stockings, and wraps can all be used to treat lymphedema and relieve pain and fatigue while also improving function (Brennan et al., 1996; Marcks, 1997).

For patients experiencing pain brought on by weight bearing or walking, assistive devices can be extremely helpful. Orthotic devices can be used to immobilize and support painful or weak structures.

9.3.3. Transcutaneous Electrical Nerve Stimulation

There have been theories regarding the mechanisms underlying transcutaneous electrical stimulation's pain-reduction effects, including activation of the central inhibitory system and local neural blockade. Based on clinical experience, this modality may be a helpful addition to treatment for mild to moderate neuropathic or musculoskeletal pain (Sykes et al., 1997).

9.4. Invasive Analgesic Techniques

9.4.1. Anesthetic and Neurosurgical Techniques

According to the WHO's "analgesic ladder" validation studies, 10–30% of cancer patients with pain do not find that systemic pharmacotherapy alone provides a good enough balance between side effects and relief without causing unacceptable drug toxicity (World Health Organization, 1996). It may be possible to achieve adequate analgesia without systemically administered opioids by using anesthetic and neurosurgical techniques.

When thinking about invasive approaches, exercise caution. Care must be taken when interpreting data about the use of alternative analgesic methods and extrapolating to the clinical issue that is currently present. The literature is typified by irregularities in outcome evaluation, inconsistent reporting of prior analgesic therapies, inconsistent patient selection, and a dearth of long-term follow-up. Moreover, the results of a procedure carried out on a patient who is medically ill by a doctor who has less experience with the techniques involved may differ from those reported in the literature.

When necessary, the likelihood and duration of analgesic benefit, the short- and long-term risks, the expected survival time, the accessibility of local expertise, and the expected length of hospital stay should all be taken into consideration before invasive and neurodestructive procedures are used. There are a variety of theoretically applicable techniques for the majority of pain syndromes.

Table 9.6. Available Therapies for Cancer Pain Management

Treatment Options		
Analgesics		
Nonopioid	Paracetamol, NSAIDs	Every patient if indicated
Weak opioids	Codeine, hydrocodone, tramadol	Mild-to-moderate pain in association with nonopioid Tramadol: second line for neuropathic pain
Strong opioids	• First line: Morphine, oxycodone, hydromorphone • Second line: methadone, buprenorphine, tapentadol	Moderate to severe pain
Adjuvants		
Ketamine		Refractory chronic pain
Magnesium		Hypomagnesemia, refractory cancer pain
Tricyclic antidepressants (TCA)	Amitriptyline, nortriptyline	Neuropathic pain
Serotonin and norepinephrine reuptake inhibitors (SNRI)	Duloxetine, venlafaxine	Neuropathic pain
Anticonvulsant	Gabapentin, pregabalin	Neuropathic pain
Cannabis-related medicines		Chronic pain

Lidocaine infusion		Refractory neuropathic painRefractory visceral pain
Topical treatment	Lidocaine capsaicin	Localized neuropathic pain
Interventional treatments		
Photobiomodulation		Localized neuropathic pain
Neuromodulation	Deep brain stimulation, transcranial magnetic stimulation, transcranial direct current stimulation	Under research
	Spinal cord stimulation, dorsal root ganglion stimulation	Neuropathic pain
	Neuraxial drug delivery (morphine, ziconotide, local anesthetic, baclofen, clonidine, ketamine)	Refractory pain, opioids intolerance, widespread bone metastases, specific location (i.e., pancreatic cancer)
	Percutaneous neurolysis (cryoanalgesia, thermal neurotomy, pulsed radiofrequency) • Stellate ganglia • Coeliac or splanchnic plexus • Hypogastric plexus • Ganglion impar	Neuropathic refractory pain • Breast, upper limb, or posterior cervical spine cancer pain • Abdominal and epigastric cancer pain • Pelvic cancer pain • Lower rectal and perianal burns
Cordotomy		Severe nociceptive or neuropathic pain in short term survival patients
Percutaneous ablation of metastasis	Radiofrequency, cryotherapy	Metastatic bone lesions
Vertebroplasty and kyphoplasty		Vertebral instability and spinal cord compression consecutive to fracture
Botulinum toxin		Neuropathic pain
Integrative medicine		
Hypnosis		Chronic pain
Yoga **Tai Chi and Qi Gong**		Aromatase inhibitor-related joint pain Chronic pain

Mindfulness and meditation	Cancer-related symptoms
Cognitive behavioral strategies	Chronic pain
Music therapy	Chronic pain
Acupuncture	Chronic pain
Massage therapy	Chronic pain
Spiritual and religious interventions	Chronic pain
Future therapeutic approach	
Virtual reality	Under research

Source: Mestdagh F, Steyaert A, Lavand'homme P. Cancer pain management: a narrative review of current concepts, strategies, and techniques. *Current Oncology*. 2023; 30(7):6838–6858. https://doi.org/10.3390/curroncol30070500.

In choosing between a range of procedures the following principles are salient:

1. Ablative procedures are deferred as long as pain relief is obtainable by non-ablative modalities.
2. The procedure most likely to be effective should be selected. If there is a choice, however, the one with the fewest and least serious adverse effects is preferred.
3. In progressive stages of cancer, pain is likely to be multifocal, and a procedure aimed at a single locus of pain, even if completed flawlessly, is unlikely to yield complete relief of pain until death. A realistic and sound goal is a lasting decrease in pain to a level manageable by pharmacotherapy with minimal side effects.
4. Whenever possible, neurolysis should be preceded by the demonstration of effective analgesia with a local anesthetic prognostic block.
5. Since there is a learning curve with all of the procedures, performance by a physician experienced in the specific intervention may improve the likelihood of a successful outcome.

Since they can accomplish this goal without compromising neurological integrity, regional analgesic techniques like intraspinal opioids and local anesthetic administration or intrapleural local anesthetic administration are typically considered first. However, only a small percentage of patients benefit from neurodestructive procedures. Some of these procedures, like coeliac plexus blockade in pancreatic cancer patients, may have a risk: benefit ratio that is favorable enough to justify early treatment.

9.4.2. Regional Analgesia

9.4.2.1. Epidural and Intrathecal Opioids

Low opioid doses administered close to the spinal cord's sites of action may lessen side effects that are supraspinally mediated. The indications for the spinal route remain empirical and are based on the relative therapeutic index in the lack of randomized trials comparing the various intraspinal techniques with other analgesic approaches. According to a survey, only 16 out of 1,205 cancer patients who experienced pain needed intraspinal treatment (Hogan et al., 1991). Spinal opioids have the benefit of maintaining sympathetic function, strength, and sensation in contrast to neuroablative therapies. Sepsis, severe leukopenia, and bleeding diathesis are among the contraindications. Before the permanent catheter implantation, a short-term trial of spinal opioid therapy should be conducted to evaluate the possible advantages of this strategy.

Numerous factors influence the choice of opioids for intraspinal delivery. According to Brose et al. (1991), hydrophilic medications, like morphine and hydromorphone, have a considerable rostral redistribution and a prolonged half-life in cerebrospinal fluid. Since lipophilic opioids, like fentanyl and sufentanil, have less rostral redistribution, they might be a better option for spinal infusion-level segmental analgesia. It has been shown that a low concentration of a local anesthetic, such as 0% bupivacaine (0.125–0.25%), added to an intrathecal opioid (Mercadante, 1994a; Sjoberg et al., 1994; Nitescu et al., 1995) or epidural (Du Pen & Williams, 1992) can enhance the analgesic effect without increasing toxicity. Additional research is necessary to evaluate the potential utility of other agents that have been coadministered with intraspinal opioids, such as clonidine (Eisenach et al., 1995), octreotide (Penn et al., 1992), ketamine (Yaksh, 1996; Yang et al., 1996), and calcitonin (Blanchard et al., 1990).

Extensive experience has been reported with both intrathecal and epidural routes for cancer pain; however, trials comparing them have not been conducted. According to longitudinal studies (Hassenbusch et al., 1995; Gestin et al., 1997), there may be comparable risks involved with intrathecal or epidural opioid infusions for the treatment of cancer pain. The possibility of morbidity from these procedures suggests that long-term monitoring and a skilled clinician are required.

9.4.2.2. Intraventricular Opioids

An increasing body of research from around the world indicates that in certain patients, long-term analgesia may be achieved by injecting small amounts of an opioid, especially morphine, into the cerebral ventricles (Cramond & Stuart, 1993; Karavelis et al., 1996). Patients with severe diffuse pain, head pain, or upper body pain have been treated with this technique, which has generally been well tolerated. There have been two types of schedules: continuous infusion with an implanted pump (Dennis & DeWitty, 1990) and intermittent injection using an Ommaya reservoir (Cramond & Stuart, 1993; Karavelis et al., 1996).

9.4.2.3. Regional Local Anesthetic

To manage chronic post-thoracotomy pain (Symreng et al., 1989) and pain related to cancer that affects the head, neck, chest, arms, and upper abdominal viscera (Dionne, 1992; Lema et al., 1992), many authors have documented the use of intrapleural local anesthetics. Patients with chronic pain from advanced cancer have been advised to receive continuous infusions of local anesthetic, even though a single bolus may offer a prolonged analgesic (Myers et al., 1993). An interscalene brachial plexus catheter used for intermittent bupivicaine infusion may be helpful for patients with localized upper limb pain (Cooper et al., 1994).

9.4.3. Anesthetic Techniques for Sympathetically Maintained Pain and Visceral Pain

9.4.3.1. Celiac Plexus Block

When treating pain brought on by neoplastic infiltration of the upper abdominal viscera, such as the pancreas, upper retroperitoneum, liver, gall bladder, and proximal small bowel, neurolytic celiac plexus blockade may be taken into consideration (Eisenberg et al., 1995; Caraceni & Portenoy, 1996). This technique is supported not only by a wealth of anecdotal evidence but also by two controlled studies

(Mercadante, 1993; Kawamata et al., 1996) regarding the percutaneous approach and a controlled trial (Lillemoe et al., 1993) regarding intraoperative neurolysis. Patients with pancreatic cancer have reported analgesic response rates of 50–90%, with effects lasting typically 1 to 12 months (Eisenberg et al., 1995; Caraceni & Portenoy, 1996). Certain clinicians advocate for this intervention at an early stage due to the generally positive response to this approach and the supportive data from two small studies (Mercadante, 1993; Kawamata et al., 1996). However, other experts disagree, recommending celiac plexus block only for patients who do not maintain an adequate balance between analgesia and side effects from an oral opioid (Caraceni & Portenoy, 1996). Two common short-term side effects are diarrhea and postural hypotension. In rare cases, the surgery may result in paraplegia from an acute ischemic myelopathy (likely brought on by Adamkievicz's artery involvement) (Wong & Brown, 1995; Hayakawa et al., 1997). Neuropathic pain syndrome may arise from the involvement of the lower thoracic and lumbar somatic nerves caused by the posterior spread of neurolytic solution. Retroperitoneal hemorrhage and pneumothorax are two other rare complications.

9.4.3.2. Sympathetic Blocks for Pelvic Visceral Pain

There are only a few anecdotal reports of experience with these two techniques. According to reports, 40–80% of patients experience relief from chronic cancer pain originating from the descending colon and rectum as well as the lower genitourinary structures after phenol ablation of the superior hypogastric nerve plexus, which is located anterior to the sacral promontory (Plancarte et al., 1990, 1997). Nebab & Florence, 1997; Wemm & Saberski, 1995; Plancarte et al., 1993, and others have reported that neurolysis of the ganglion impar (ganglion of Walther), a solitary retroperitoneal structure at the sacrococcygeal junction that marks the termination of the paired paravertebral sympathetic chains, can alleviate visceral sensations referred to the vagina, rectum, or perineum due to locally advanced cancers of the pelvic visceral structures.

9.4.3.3. Sympathetic Blockade of Somatic Structures

Interrupting the sympathetic outflow to the afflicted area of the body can alleviate pain syndromes that are maintained by the sympathetic nervous system. Stellate ganglion blockade may be helpful for sympathetically maintained pain involving the face or arms, and lumbar sympathetic blockade should be taken into consideration for sympathetically maintained pain involving the legs (Lamacraft & Cousins, 1997).

9.4.4. Neuroablative Techniques for Somatic and Neuropathic Pain

9.4.4.1. Rhizotomy

For patients with otherwise refractory localized pain syndromes, surgical section, chemical neurolysis, or radiofrequency lesion can be used to destroy the dorsal sensory roots in one or more segments (rhizotomy). According to Patt and Reddy (1994), these methods are most frequently employed in the treatment of pain in the chest wall caused by tumor invasion of the somatic and neural structures. Refractory pain in the upper, lower, pelvic, or perineal limbs are additional indications (Saris et al., 1986). A neurolytic solution can be injected into the intrathecal or epidural space to cause chemical rhizotomy (Patt & Reddy, 1994). Chemical rhizotomies can be carried out at any level up to the mid-cervical region, after which there is an intolerable risk of cardiorespiratory collapse due to the neurolytic agent spreading to the medullary centers. Catheter tip position should be confirmed radiographically, and small volumes of phenol (1–2 ml) should be injected to reduce the risk of excessive spread and lysis beyond the target segments (Salmon et al., 1992).

About 50% of patients experience satisfactory analgesia (Patt and Reddy, 1994), and the average length of relief is 2–4 months, though there is a wide distribution in this time frame. The injection technique may have an impact on adverse effects (e.g.arachnoiditis, spinal headaches, infections, and degeneration of non-nociceptive nerve fibers. The location of neurolysis determines which complications are specific to the process. For instance, paresis (5 to 20%), sphincter dysfunction (5 to 60%), impaired touch and proprioception, and dysaesthesias are among the side effects of lumbosacral neurolysis. While neurological deficits are typically temporary, patients with limited function and pre-existing urinary diversion should be spared these techniques due to the increased risk of disability from weakness, sphincter incompetence, and loss of positional sense. It is crucial to provide patients with risk assessment counseling.

9.4.5. Neurolysis of Primary Afferent Nerves or Their Ganglia

For some patients with localized pain, neurolysis of the primary afferent nerves may also result in a significant improvement in pain relief. The possibility of concurrent motor or sphincteric dysfunction limits the usefulness of these methods. Trigeminal neurolysis (also known as gangliolysis) or glossopharyngeal neurolysis may be effective treatments for refractory unilateral facial or pharyngeal pain (Rizzi et al., 1985; Ischia et al., 1990). Blockade of the sphenopalatine ganglion may be helpful for unilateral pain involving the tongue or floor of the mouth (Prasanna & Murthy, 1993). For patients experiencing pain in their chest wall, intercostal or paravertebral neurolysis may be a better option than rhizotomy. Suprascapular neurolysis may be effective for treating unilateral shoulder pain (Meyer-Witting & Foster, 1992). Brachial plexus neurolysis can be an effective treatment for more severe arm pain, but it will cause weakness (Neill, 1979). Anecdotally, injecting 10 ml of 10% phenol into the psoas muscle sheath has been shown to relieve refractory leg pain without impairing motor function (Calava et al., 1996). Neurolysis of the S4 nerve root through the ipsilateral posterior sacral foramen is one method for treating severe somatic pain that is localized to the perineum. This procedure has a low risk of sphincter or motor dysfunction (Robertson, 1983).

Neuropathic pain can occasionally accompany the regeneration of peripheral nerves; however, the risk of postablative dysesthesia is minimal in situations where life expectancy is extremely low or intractable pain already surpasses tolerance.

9.4.5.1. Cordotomy

The anterolateral spinothalamic tract is ablated during a cordotomy, resulting in a contralateral loss of temperature sensitivity and pain perception (Stuart & Cramond, 1993; Sanders & Zuurmond, 1995). The patient most likely to benefit from this procedure is the one who has severe unilateral pain originating in the lower extremities or torso (Stuart & Cramond, 1993; Sanders & Zuurmond, 1995). Patients with pain in the chest wall have also shown impressive outcomes (Sanders & Zuurmond, 1995). According to Stuart and Cramond (1993) and Sanders and Zuurmond (1995), the percutaneous approach is typically chosen; open cordotomy is typically saved for patients who are unable to lie supine or who are not cooperative enough to undergo a percutaneous procedure.

In the immediate post-cordotomy period, over 90% of patients experience significant pain relief (Stuart & Cramond, 1993; Sanders & Zuurmond, 1995). After a year, half of the patients who make it survive experience pain again (Cowie & Hitchcock, 1982). Sometimes repeat cordotomy is beneficial. Paresis, ataxia, bladder, and "mirror-image" pain are among the neurological side effects of cordotomy (Sanders & Zuurmond, 1995). Although the problems are usually temporary, about 5% of the time they become chronic and incapacitating (Sanders & Zuurmond, 1995). Rarely, patients who survive for longer than 12 months experience dysesthetic pain with a delayed onset (Cowie & Hitchcock, 1982). The most dangerous possible side effect is respiratory dysfunction, which can be brought on by sleep or manifest as paralysis of the phrenic nerve (Chevrolet et al., 1983; Polatty & Cooper, 1986). Bilateral high cervical cordotomies or a unilateral cervical cordotomy ipsilateral to the location of the only lung that functions are not advised due to the latter worry.

9.4.5.2. Pituitary Ablation

It has been reported that diffuse and multifocal pain syndromes that have not responded to opioid therapy and are not a good candidate for any regional neuroablative procedure can be relieved by pituitary ablation by chemical or surgical hypophysectomy (Gonski & Sackelariou, 1984; Levin & Ramirez, 1984). It has been documented that tumors that are hormone-dependent or hormone-independent can both cause pain relief (Gonski & Sackelariou, 1984; Levin & Ramirez, 1984).

9.4.5.3. Cingulotomy

The effectiveness of MRI-guided stereotactic cingulotomy in treating diffuse pain syndromes that have not responded to opioid therapy is further supported by anecdotal reports (Hassenbusch et al., 1990; Wong et al., 1997). The duration of analgesia is often limited, although this procedure seems safe and has minimal neurological or psychological morbidity (Hassenbusch et al., 1990; Wong et al., 1997). The process is rarely taken into consideration, and the mode of action is unknown.

9.5. Sedation as Pain Therapy

When analgesics are used carefully, pain can often be sufficiently relieved without impairing the patient's ability to communicate or function in ways that go beyond what is necessary to treat the underlying illness. Sometimes, though, this isn't possible, and people believe that pain is "refractory" (Cherny & Portenoy, 1994). When determining whether a pain is refractory, a clinician must believe that: (1) more standard interventions won't relieve the problem adequately; (2) more standard interventions will result in unacceptable acute or chronic morbidity; or (3) more standard interventions are unlikely to relieve the pain in a reasonable amount of time. Sedation might be the only therapeutic approach that can offer sufficient relief in this case. "Sedation in the management of refractory symptoms at the end of life" is how Cherny and Portenoy (1994) define this strategy.

Sedation is justified in this situation because it is appropriate and proportionate. Even in the case of a limited therapeutic index for the required palliative treatments, adequate symptom relief must be sought toward the end of life when the primary objective of care is preserving the patient's comfort (President's Commission for the Study of Ethical Problems in Medical and Biomedical and Behavioral Research, 1983; American Medical Association, 1996; Burt, 1997). In this situation, sedation is a proportionate and medically necessary therapeutic response to refractory symptoms that cannot be relieved in any other way. The moral justification of sedation in the treatment of otherwise unbearable pain at the end of life is also supported by an appeal to patients' rights.

Recently, the Supreme Court upheld the right of patients to receive palliative care in response to unbearable suffering (Burt, 1997).

It is appropriate to offer this option to the patient or their proxy once there is a consensus among clinicians that the pain is refractory. Offering sedation to a patient who is exhibiting refractory symptoms can show that the doctor is committed to relieving their suffering. This can improve the patient-doctor relationship's trust and have an impact on how well the patient perceives their ability to cope. In fact, patients frequently refuse sedation, understanding that their pain will only be partially relieved, but feeling safe in the knowledge that they have this option available should the situation become unbearable. Some patients ask for the administration of sedation and reiterate that comfort is the most important factor.

Anecdotal reports in the published literature discuss the use of benzodiazepines, opioids, neuroleptics, propofol, and barbiturates in the treatment of refractory pain at the end of life (Cherny & Portenoy, 1994). Drug selection guidelines are empirical in the absence of relative efficacy data. Whatever the agent or agents chosen, therapy must first be administered by dose titration to provide sufficient relief, and then continuous 660 therapy must be provided to guarantee effect maintenance.

A Closer Look

Gastroduodenal Morbidity

Gastroduodenal morbidity encompasses a range of health conditions affecting the stomach (gastric) and the duodenum (the first part of the small intestine), constituting a significant burden on global public health.

Gastroduodenal morbidity encompasses various conditions, including gastritis, peptic ulcers, gastroesophageal reflux disease (GERD), and gastric cancer. These conditions collectively contribute to a substantial burden of disease worldwide, impacting individuals' quality of life and healthcare systems' resources.

Several factors contribute to the development of gastroduodenal morbidity, including infection with Helicobacter pylori bacteria, excessive alcohol consumption, smoking, non-steroidal anti-inflammatory drug (NSAID) use, stress, and dietary factors. Genetic predisposition and certain medical conditions, such as autoimmune diseases, also play a role.

Gastritis, characterized by inflammation of the stomach lining, can result from various factors, including H. pylori infection, NSAID use, alcohol consumption, or autoimmune processes. Peptic ulcers, which are open sores that develop on the lining of the stomach or duodenum, often result from H. pylori infection or NSAID use. GERD occurs when stomach acid flows back into the esophagus, leading to symptoms such as heartburn and regurgitation. Gastric cancer may develop from chronic gastritis or long-standing peptic ulcers, particularly if left untreated.

Symptoms of gastroduodenal morbidity vary depending on the specific condition but may include abdominal pain, indigestion, heartburn, nausea, vomiting, bloating, and changes in appetite or weight loss. Complications can range from mild discomfort to life-threatening conditions such as gastrointestinal bleeding, perforation of ulcers, or the development of gastric malignancies.

Management of gastroduodenal morbidity typically involves a combination of lifestyle modifications, pharmacotherapy, and, in some cases, surgical intervention. Treatment aims to alleviate symptoms, promote healing of ulcers, eradicate H. pylori infection (if present), and reduce the risk of complications. Prevention strategies include avoiding risk factors such as smoking, excessive alcohol consumption, and NSAID use, as well as practicing good dietary habits and seeking early medical intervention for symptoms.

Gastroduodenal morbidity encompasses a range of conditions affecting the stomach and duodenum, with various risk factors, pathophysiological mechanisms, symptoms, and management strategies. Effective prevention and management efforts are essential to reduce the burden of these conditions on public health.

Summary

- The management of cancer pain represents a critical aspect of comprehensive cancer care, aiming to alleviate suffering and enhance the quality of life for individuals battling cancer.
- The assessment process may reveal a cause for the pain that is amenable to primary therapy (i.e., therapy that is directed at the etiology of the pain).
- Despite a paucity of data concerning the specific analgesic benefits of chemotherapy, there is a strong clinical impression that tumor shrinkage is generally associated with the relief of pain.
- The non-opioid analgesics (aspirin, acetaminophen, and non-steroidal anti-inflammatory drugs (NSAIDs)) are useful alone for mild to moderate pain (Step 1 of the analgesic ladder) and provide additive analgesia when combined with opioid drugs in the treatment of more severe pain.
- A trial of systemic opioid therapy should be administered to all cancer patients with pain of moderate or greater severity regardless of the pain mechanism.
- Adverse changes in patient well-being among patients taking opioids are not always caused by the opioids.
- Symptomatic drugs used to prevent or control opioid adverse effects are commonly employed. Most of these approaches are based on cumulative anecdotal experience.
- Antidepressant drugs are commonly used to manage continuous neuropathic pains and the evidence for analgesic efficacy is greatest for the tertiary amine tricyclic drugs, such as amitriptyline, doxepin, and imipramine.
- Physiatric techniques can be used to optimize the function of the patient with chronic cancer or enhance analgesia through the application of modalities such as electrical stimulation, heat, or cryotherapy.

References

1. Abrams, P., Fenely, R. (1976). The action of prostaglandins on smooth muscle of the human urinary tract in vitro. British Journal of Urology, 47, 909–915.
2. Ahmedzai, S., Brooks, D. (1997). Transdermal fentanyl versus sustained-release oral morphine in cancer pain: Preference, efficacy, and quality of life. The TTS-Fentanyl Comparative Trial Group Journal of Pain and Symptom Management, 13, 254–261.
3. Algan, S. M., Horowitz, S. M. (1996). Surgical treatment of pathologic hip lesions in patients with metastatic disease. Clinical Orthopaedics, 332, 223–231.
4. American Medical Association. (1996). Good care of the dying patient. Council on Scientific Affairs, American Medical Association. Journal of the American Medical Association, 275, 474–478.
5. Arathuzik, D. (1994). Effects of cognitive-behavioral strategies on pain in cancer patients. Cancer Nursing, 17, 207–214.
6. Ashby, M. A., Martin, P., Jackson, K. A. (1999). Opioid substitution to reduce adverse effects in cancer pain management. Medical Journal of Australia, 170, 68–71.

7. Avradopoulos, K. A., Vezeridis, M. P., Wanebo, H. J. (1996). Pelvic exenteration for recurrent rectal cancer. Advances in Surgery, 29, 215–233.
8. Babul, N., Provencher, L., Laberge, F., Harsanyi, Z., Moulin, D. (1998). Comparative efficacy and safety of controlled-release morphine suppositories and tablets in cancer pain. Journal of Clinical Pharmacology, 38, 74–81.
9. Baert, L. (1974). Controlled double-blind trial of flavoxate in painful conditions of the lower urinary tract. Current Medical Research and Opinion, 2, 631–635.
10. Baillie, S. P., Bateman, D. N., Coates, P. E., Woodhouse, K. W. (1989). Age and the pharmacokinetics of morphine. Age and Ageing, 18, 258–262.
11. Baines, M. J. (1994). Management of intestinal obstruction in patients with advanced cancer. Annals, Academy of Medicine, Singapore, 23, 178–182.
12. Baines, M. J. (1997). ABC of palliative care. Nausea, vomiting, and intestinal obstruction. British Medical Journal, 315, 1148–1150.
13. Barbalias, G. A., Siablis, D., Liatsikos, E. N., Karnabatidis, D., Yarmenitis, S., Bouropoulos, K., Dimopoulos, J. (1997). Metal stents: A new treatment of malignant ureteral obstruction. Journal of Urology, 158, 54–58.
14. Barbanti, G., Maggi, C. A., Beneforti, P., Baroldi, P., Turini, D. (1993). Relief of pain following intravesical capsaicin in patients with hypersensitive disorders of the lower urinary tract. British Journal of Urology, 71, 686–691.
15. Bates, T. (1992). A review of local radiotherapy in the treatment of bone metastases and cord compression. International Journal of Radiation Oncology–Biology–Physics, 23, 217–221.
16. Bennett, W. M., Henrich, W. L., Stoff, J. S. (1996). The renal effects of nonsteroidal anti-inflammatory drugs: Summary and recommendations. American Journal of Kidney Disease, 28, S56–S62.
17. Bentley, J. B., Borel, J. D., Nenad, R. E. Jr, Gillespie, T. J. (1982). Age and fentanyl pharmacokinetics. Anesthesia and Analgesia, 61, 968–971.
18. Bjorkman, R., Ullman, A., Hedner, J. (1993). Morphine-sparing effect of diclofenac in cancer pain. European Journal of Clinical Pharmacology, 44, 1–5.
19. Blanchard, J., Menk, E., Ramamurthy, S., Hoffman, J. (1990). Subarachnoid and epidural calcitonin in patients with pain due to metastatic cancer. Journal of Pain and Symptom Management, 5, 42–45.
20. Boquet, J., Moore, N., Lhuintre, J. P., Boismare, F. (1986). Diltiazem for proctalgia fugax [letter]. Lancet, 1, 1493.
21. Boraas, M. C. (1985). Palliative surgery. Seminars in Oncology, 12, 368–374.
22. Braun, A., Rohe, K. (1984). Orthopedic surgery for management of tumor pain. Recent Results in Cancer Research, 89, 157–170.
23. Brennan, M. J., DePompolo, R. W., Garden, F. H. (1996). Focused review: Postmastectomy lymphedema. Archives of Physical Medicine and Rehabilitation, 77, S74–S80.
24. Brooks, P. M., Day, R. O. (1991). Nonsteroidal anti-inflammatory drugs—Differences and similarities. New England Journal of Medicine, 324, 1716–1725.
25. Brooks, P. M., Day, R. O. (2000). COX-2 inhibitors. Medical Journal of Australia, 173, 433–436.

26. Brose, W. G., Tanelian, D. L., Brodsky, J. B., Mark, J. B., Cousins, M. J. (1991). CSF and blood pharmacokinetics of hydromorphone and morphine following lumbar epidural administration. Pain, 45, 11–15.

27. Brosen, K., Sindrup, S. H., Skjelbo, E., Nielsen, K. K., Gram, L. F. (1993). Role of genetic polymorphism in psychopharmacology—An update. Psychopharmacology Ser, 10, 199–211.

28. Browne, B., Linter, S. (1987). Monoamine oxidase inhibitors and narcotic analgesics. A critical review of the implications for treatment. British Journal of Psychiatry, 151, 210–212.

29. Bruera, E., Franco, J. J., Maltoni, M., Watanabe, S., Suarez-Almazor, M. (1995). Changing pattern of agitated impaired mental status in patients with advanced cancer: Association with cognitive monitoring, hydration, and opioid rotation. Journal of Pain and Symptom Management, 10, 287–291.

30. Bruera, E., Macmillan, K., Hanson, J., MacDonald, R. N. (1989). The cognitive effects of the administration of narcotic analgesics in patients with cancer pain. Pain, 39, 13–16.

31. Bruera, E., Pereira, J., Watanabe, S., Belzile, M., Kuehn, N., Hanson, J. (1996). Opioid rotation in patients with cancer pain. A retrospective comparison of dose ratios between methadone, hydromorphone, and morphine. Cancer, 78, 852–857.

32. Burt, R. A. (1997). The Supreme Court speaks—Not assisted suicide but a constitutional right to palliative care. New England Journal of Medicine, 337, 1234–1236.

33. Calava, J. M., Patt, R. B., Reddy, S., Varma, D. G., Chiang, J. (1996). Psoas sheath chemical neurolysis for management of intractable leg pain from metastatic liposarcoma. Clinical Journal of Pain, 12, 69–75.

34. Caraceni, A., Portenoy, R. K. (1996). Pain management in patients with pancreatic carcinoma. Cancer, 78, 639–653.

35. Cardiac Arrhythmia Suppression Trial (CAST) Investigators. (1989). Preliminary report: Effect of encainide and flecainide on mortality in a randomized trial of arrhythmia suppression after myocardial infarction. New England Journal of Medicine, 321, 406–412.

36. Castell, D. O. (1985). Calcium-channel blocking agents for gastrointestinal disorders. American Journal of Cardiology, 55, 210B–213B.

37. Cherny, N. I., Portenoy, R. K. (1994). Sedation in the management of refractory symptoms: Guidelines for evaluation and treatment. Journal of Palliative Care, 10, 31–38.

38. Cherny, N. J., Chang, V., Frager, G., Ingham, J. M., Tiseo, P. J., Popp, B., Portenoy, R. K., Foley, K. M. (1995). Opioid pharmacotherapy in the management of cancer pain: A survey of strategies used by pain physicians for the selection of analgesic drugs and routes of administration. Cancer, 76, 1283–1293.

39. Chevrolet, J. C., Reverdin, A., Suter, P. M., Tschopp, J. M., Junod, A. F. (1983). Ventilatory dysfunction resulting from bilateral anterolateral high cervical cordotomy. Dual beneficial effect of aminophylline. Chest, 84, 112–115.

40. Cleary, J. F. (1997). Pharmacokinetic and pharmacodynamic issues in the treatment of breakthrough pain. Seminars in Oncology, 24 (Suppl 16), 13–19.

41. Coia, L. R. (1992). The role of radiation therapy in the treatment of brain metastases. International Journal of Radiation Oncology–Biology–Physics, 23, 229–238.

42. Cooper, M. G., Keneally, J. P., Kinchington, D. (1994). Continuous brachial plexus neural blockade in a child with intractable cancer pain. Journal of Pain and Symptom Management, 9, 277–281.

43. Cowie, R. A., Hitchcock, E. R. (1982). The late results of antero-lateral cordotomy for pain relief. Acta Neurochirurgia (Wien), 1, 39–50.

44. Coyle, N., Cherny, N. I., Portenoy, R. K. (1994). Subcutaneous opioid infusions at home. Oncology (Huntingt), 8, 21–27; discussion 31–32, 37.

45. Coyle, N., Portenoy, R. K. (1991). Infection as a cause of rapidly increasing pain in cancer patients. Journal of Pain and Symptom Management, 6, 266–269.

46. Cramond, T., Stuart, G. (1993). Intraventricular morphine for intractable pain of advanced cancer. Journal of Pain and Symptom Management, 8, 465–473.

47. Cruikshank, D. P., Buchsbaum, H. J. (1973). Effects of rapid paracentesis. Cardiovascular dynamics and body fluid composition. Journal of the American Medical Association, 225, 1361–1362.

48. De Conno, F., Caraceni, A., Zecca, E., Spoldi, E., Ventafridda, V. (1991). Continuous subcutaneous infusion of hyoscine butylbromide reduces secretions in patients with gastrointestinal obstruction. Journal of Pain and Symptom Management, 6, 484–486.

49. de Stoutz, N. D., Bruera, E., Suarez-Almazor, M. (1995). Opioid rotation for toxicity reduction in terminal cancer patients. Journal of Pain and Symptom Management, 10, 378–384.

50. Dennis, G. C., DeWitty, R. L. (1990). Long-term intraventricular infusion of morphine for intractable pain in cancer of the head and neck. Neurosurgery, 26, 404–407; discussion 407–408.

51. Devor, M., Govrin-Lippmann, R., Raber, P. (1985). Corticosteroids suppress ectopic neural discharge originating in experimental neuromas. Pain, 22, 127–137.

52. Dionne, C. (1992). Tumor invasion of the brachial plexus: Management of pain with intrapleural analgesia [letter]. Canadian Journal of Anesthesia, 39, 520–521.

53. Dobrowsky, W., Schmid, A. P. (1985). Radiotherapy of presacral recurrence following radical surgery for rectal carcinoma. Diseases of Colon and Rectum, 28, 917–919.

54. Donner, B., Zenz, M., Tryba, M., Strumpf, M. (1996). Direct conversion from oral morphine to transdermal fentanyl: A multicenter study in patients with cancer pain. Pain, 64, 527–534.

55. Drexel, H., Dzien, A., Spiegel, R. W., Lang, A. H., Breier, C., Abbrederis, K., Patsch, J. R., Braunsteiner, H. (1989). Treatment of severe cancer pain by low-dose continuous subcutaneous morphine. Pain, 36, 169–176.

56. Du Pen, S. L., Williams, A. R. (1992). Management of patients receiving combined epidural morphine and bupivacaine for the treatment of cancer pain. Journal of Pain and Symptom Management, 7, 125–127.

57. Eckardt, V. F., Dodt, O., Kanzler, G., Bernhard, G. (1996). Treatment of proctalgia fugax with salbutamol inhalation. American Journal of Gastroenterology, 91, 686–689.

58. Eisenach, J. C., Du Pen, S., Dubois, M., Miguel, R., Allin, D. (1995). Epidural clonidine analgesia for intractable cancer pain. The Epidural Clonidine Study Group. Pain, 61, 391–399.

59. Eisenberg, E., Berkey, C. S., Carr, D. B., Mosteller, F., Chalmers, T. C. (1994). Efficacy and safety of nonsteroidal anti-inflammatory drugs for cancer pain: A meta-analysis. Journal of Clinical Oncology, 12, 2756–2765.

60. Eisenberg, E., Carr, D. B., Chalmers, T. C. (1995). Neurolytic celiac plexus block for treatment of cancer pain: A meta-analysis. Anesthesia and Analgesia, 80, 290–295. [Erratum 1995 Anesthesia and Analgesia, 81: 213]

61. Ellershaw, J. E., Kelly, M. J. (1994). Corticosteroids and peptic ulceration. Palliative Medicine, 8, 313–319.

62. Eras, J., Perazella, M. A. (2001). NSAIDs and the kidney revisited: Are selective cyclooxygenase-2 inhibitors safe? American Journal of the Medical Sciences, 321, 181–190.

63. Ernst, D. S., Brasher, P., Hagen, N., Paterson, A. H., MacDonald, R. N., Bruera, E. (1997). A randomized, controlled trial of intravenous clodronate in patients with metastatic bone disease and pain. Journal of Pain and Symptom Management, 13, 319–326.

64. Estes, N. C., Thomas, J. H., Jewell, W. R., Beggs, D., Hardin, C. A. (1993). Pelvic exenteration: A treatment for failed rectal cancer surgery. American Surgery, 59, 420–422.

65. European Association for Palliative Care (1996). Morphine in cancer pain: Modes of administration. Expert working group of the European association for palliative care. British Medical Journal, 312, 823–826.

66. Fallon, M. T., O'Neill, B. (1998). Substitution of another opioid for morphine. Opioid toxicity should be managed initially by decreasing the opioid dose [letter; comment]. British Medical Journal, 317, 81.

67. Fallon, M., O'Neill, B. (1997). ABC of palliative care. Constipation and diarrhea. British Medical Journal, 315, 1293–1296.

68. Fishman, B. (1992). The cognitive behavioral perspective on pain management in terminal illness. Hospital Journal, 8, 73–88.

69. Fitzgibbon, D. R., Ready, L. B. (1997). Intravenous high-dose methadone administered by patient-controlled analgesia and continuous infusion for the treatment of cancer pain refractory to high-dose morphine. Pain, 73, 259–261.

70. Fromm, M. F., Hofmann, U., Griese, E. U., Mikus, G. (1995). Dihydrocodeine: A new opioid substrate for the polymorphic CYP2D6 in humans. Clinical Pharmacology and Therapeutics, 58, 374–382.

71. Galer, B. S., Coyle, N., Pasternak, G. W., Portenoy, R. K. (1992). Individual variability in the response to different opioids: Report of five cases. Pain, 49, 87–91.

72. Galer, B. S., Harle, J., Rowbotham, M. C. (1996). Response to intravenous lidocaine infusion predicts subsequent response to oral mexiletine: A prospective study. Journal of Pain and Symptom Management, 12, 161–167.

73. Gestin, Y., Vainio, A., Pegurier, A. M. (1997). Long-term intrathecal infusion of morphine in the home care of patients with advanced cancer. Acta Anaesthesiologica Scandinavica, 41, 12–17.

74. Goisis, A., Gorini, M., Ratti, R., Luliri, P. (1989). Application of a WHO protocol on medical therapy for oncologic pain in an internal medicine hospital. Tumori, 75, 470–472.

75. Gokaslan, Z. L. (1996). Spine surgery for cancer. Current Opinion in Oncology, 8, 178–181.

76. Gonski, A., Sackelariou, R. (1984). Cryohypophysectomy for the relief of pain in malignant disease. Medical Journal of Australia, 140, 140–142.

77. Grond, S., Zech, D., Schug, S. A., Lynch, J., Lehmann, K. A. (1991). Validation of World Health Organization guidelines for cancer pain relief during the last days and hours of life. Journal of Pain and Symptom Management, 6, 411–422.

78. Hagen, N. A., Elwood, T., Ernst, S. (1997). Cancer pain emergencies: A protocol for management. Journal of Pain and Symptom Management, 14, 45–50.

79. Hagen, N. A., Foley, K. M., Cerbone, D. J., Portenoy, R. K., Inturrisi, C. E. (1991). Chronic nausea and morphine-6-glucuronide. Journal of Pain and Symptom Management, 6, 125–128.

80. Hagen, N., Swanson, R. (1997). Strychnine-like multifocal myoclonus and seizures in extremely high-dose opioid administration: Treatment strategies [see comments]. Journal of Pain and Symptom Management, 14, 51–58.

81. Hanks, G. W. (1984). Psychotropic drugs. Postgraduate Medical Journal, 60, 881–885.

82. Hanks, G. W. (1987). The clinical usefulness of agonist–Antagonistic opioid analgesics in chronic pain. Drug and Alcohol Dependence, 20, 339–346.

83. Hanks, G. W., Forbes, K. (1997). Opioid responsiveness. Acta Anaesthesiologica Scandinavica, 41, 154–158.

84. Harris, J. K., Sutcliffe, J. C., Robinson, N. E. (1996). The role of emergency surgery in malignant spinal extradural compression: Assessment of functional outcome. British Journal of Neurosurgery, 10, 27–33.

85. Hassenbusch, S. J., Pillay, P. K., Barnett, G. H. (1990). Radiofrequency cingulotomy for intractable cancer pain using stereotaxis guided by magnetic resonance imaging. Neurosurgery, 27, 220–223.

86. Hassenbusch, S. J., Stanton-Hicks, M., Covington, E. C., Walsh, J. G., Guthrey, D. S. (1995). Long-term intraspinal infusions of opioids in the treatment of neuropathic pain. Journal of Pain and Symptom Management, 10, 527–543.

87. Hawkey, C. J. (1998). Progress in prophylaxis against nonsteroidal anti-inflammatory drug-associated ulcers and erosions. Omeprazole NSAID Steering Committee. American Journal of Medicine, 104, 67S–74S; discussion 79S–80S.

88. Hayakawa, J., Kobayashi, O., Murayama, H. (1997). Paraplegia after intraoperative celiac plexus block. Anesthesia and Analgesia, 84, 447–448.

89. Heiskanen, T., Olkkola, K. T., Kalso, E. (1998). Effects of blocking CYP2D6 on the pharmacokinetics and pharmacodynamics of oxycodone. Clinical Pharmacology and Therapeutics, 64, 603–611.

90. Hogan, Q., Haddox, J. D., Abram, S., Weissman, D., Taylor, M. L., Janjan, N. (1991). Epidural opiates and local anesthetics for the management of cancer pain. Pain, 46, 271–279.

91. Holdsworth, M. T., Forman, W. B., Killilea, T. A., Nystrom, K. M., Paul, R., Brand, S. C., Reynolds, R. (1994). Transdermal fentanyl disposition in elderly subjects. Gerontology, 40, 32–37.

92. Hoskin, P. J. (1995). Radiotherapy for bone pain. Pain, 63, 137–139.

93. Houde, R. W., Wallenstein, S. L., Beaver, W. T. (1966). Evaluation of analgesics in patients with cancer pain. In: Lasagna L (ed) International encyclopedia of pharmacology and therapeutics, vol 1. Pergamon Press, New York, pp 59–67.

94. Ischia, S., Luzzani, A., Polati, E. (1990). Retrogasserian glycerol injection: A retrospective study of 112 patients. Clinical Journal of Pain, 6, 291–296.

95. Jadad, A. R., Browman, G. P. (1995). The WHO analgesic ladder for cancer pain management. Stepping up the quality of its evaluation [see comments]. Journal of the American Medical Association, 274, 1870–1873.

96. Janjan, N. A. (1997). Radiation for bone metastases: Conventional techniques and the role of systemic radiopharmaceuticals. Cancer, 80, 1628–1645.

97. Jeal, W., Benfield, P. (1997). Transdermal fentanyl. A review of its pharmacological properties and therapeutic efficacy in pain control. Drugs, 53, 109–138.

98. Johnson, J. R., Miller, A. J. (1994). The efficacy of choline magnesium trisalicylate (CMT) in the management of metastatic bone pain: A pilot study. Palliative Medicine, 8, 129–135.

99. Joishy, S. K., Walsh, D. (1998). The opioid-sparing effects of intravenous ketorolac as an adjuvant analgesic in cancer pain: Application in bone metastases and the opioid bowel syndrome. Journal of Pain and Symptom Management, 16, 334–339.

100. Jong, P., Sturgeon, J., Jamieson, C. G. (1995). Benefit of palliative surgery for bowel obstruction in advanced ovarian cancer. Canadian Journal of Surgery, 38, 454–457.

101. Kaiko, R. F., Fitzmartin, R. D., Thomas, G. B., Goldenheim, P. D. (1992). The bioavailability of morphine in controlled-release 30-mg tablets per rectum compared with immediate-release 30-mg rectal suppositories and controlled-release 30-mg oral tablets. Pharmacotherapy, 12, 107–113.

102. Karavelis, A., Foroglou, G., Selviaridis, P., Fountzilas, G. (1996). Intraventricular administration of morphine for control of intractable cancer pain in 90 patients. Neurosurgery, 39, 57–61.

103. Kawamata, M., Ishitani, K., Ishikawa, K., Sasaki, H., Ota, K., Omote, K., Namiki, A. (1996). Comparison between celiac plexus block and morphine treatment on quality of life in patients with pancreatic cancer pain. Pain, 64, 597–602.

104. Kirkwood, L. C., Nation, R. L., Somogyi, A. A. (1997). Characterization of the human cytochrome P450 enzymes involved in the metabolism of dihydrocodeine. British Journal of Clinical Pharmacology, 44, 549–555.

105. Laine, L. (1996). Nonsteroidal anti-inflammatory drug gastropathy. Gastrointestinal and Endoscopy Clinics of North America, 6, 489–504.

106. Lamacraft, G., Cousins, M. J. (1997). Neural blockade in chronic and cancer pain. International Anesthesiology Clinics, 35, 131–153.

107. Lanas, A., Hirschowitz, B. I. (1999). Toxicity of NSAIDs in the stomach and duodenum. European Journal of Gastroenterology and Hepatology, 11, 375–381.

108. Lancaster, C. (1995). Effective nonsteroidal anti-inflammatory drugs devoid of gastrointestinal side effects: Do they really exist? Digestive Diseases, 13 (Suppl 1), 40–47.

109. Lawlor, P., Turner, K., Hanson, J., Bruera, E. (1997). Dose ratio between morphine and hydromorphone in patients with cancer pain: A retrospective study. Pain, 72, 79–85.

110. Lazzeri, M., Beneforti, P., Benaim, G., Maggi, C. A., Lecci, A., Turini, D. (1996). Intravesical capsaicin for treatment of severe bladder pain: A randomized placebo-controlled study. Journal of Urology, 156, 947–952.

111. Lehmann, T., Day, R. O., Brooks, P. M. (1997). Toxicity of antirheumatic drugs. Medical Journal of Australia, 166, 378–383.

112. Leibel, S. A., Pajak, T. F., Massullo, V., Order, S. E., Komaki, R. U., Chang, C. H., Wasserman, T. H., Phillips, T. L., Lipshutz, J., Durbin, L. M. (1987). A comparison of misonidazole sensitized radiation therapy to radiation therapy alone for the palliation of hepatic metastases: Results of a Radiation Therapy Oncology Group randomized prospective trial. International Journal of Radiation Oncology–Biology–Physics, 13, 1057–1064.

113. Lema, M. J., Myers, D. P., De Leon-Casasola, O., Penetrante, R. (1992). Pleural phenol therapy for the treatment of chronic esophageal cancer pain. Regional Anesthesia, 17, 166–170.

114. Levin, A. B., Ramirez, L. L. (1984). Treatment of cancer pain with hypophysectomy: Surgical and chemical. Advances in Pain Research and Therapy, 7, 631–645.

115. Lifshitz, S., Buchsbaum, H. J. (1976). The effect of paracentesis on serum proteins. Gynecological Oncology, 4, 347–353.

116. Lillemoe, K. D., Cameron, J. L., Kaufman, H. S., Yeo, C. J., Pitt, H. A., Sauter, P. K. (1993). Chemical splanchnicectomy in patients with unresectable pancreatic cancer. A prospective randomized trial. Annals of Surgery, 217, 447–455; discussion 456–457.

117. Lipman, A. G. (1996). Analgesic drugs for neuropathic and sympathetically maintained pain. Clinics in Geriatric Medicine, 12, 501–515.

118. Lyss AP: Long-term use of oral transmucosal fentanyl citrate (OTFC) for breakthrough pain in cancer patients (Meeting abstract). Proc Annu Meet Am Soc Clin Oncol, 1997;16:A144.

119. Maddocks, I., Somogyi, A., Abbott, F., Hayball, P., Parker, D. (1996). Attenuation of morphine-induced delirium in palliative care by substitution with infusion of oxycodone. Journal of Pain and Symptom Management, 12, 182–189.

120. Mainar, A., Tejero, E., Maynar, M., Ferral, H., Castaneda-Zuniga, W. (1996). Colorectal obstruction: Treatment with metallic stents. Radiology, 198, 761–764.

121. Makin, A. J., Williams, R. (1997). Acetaminophen-induced hepatotoxicity: Predisposing factors and treatments. Advances in Internal Medicine, 42, 453–483.

122. Makin, M. K., Ellershaw, J. E. (1998). Substitution of another opioid for morphine. Methadone can be used to manage neuropathic pain related to cancer [letter; comment]. British Medical Journal, 317, 81.

123. Maloney, C. M., Kesner, R. K., Klein, G., Bockenstette, J. (1989). The rectal administration of MS Contin: Clinical implications of use in end stage cancer. American Journal of Hospital Care, 6, 34–35.

124. Marcks, P. (1997). Lymphedema. Pathogenesis, prevention, and treatment. Cancer Practice, 5, 32–38.

125. Masferrer, J. L., Isakson, P. C., Seibert, K. (1996). Cyclooxygenase-2 inhibitors: A new class of anti-inflammatory agents that spare the gastrointestinal tract. Gastroenterology Clinics of North America, 25, 363–372.

126. McDonald, P., Graham, P., Clayton, M., Buhagiar, A., Stuart-Harris, R. (1991). Regular subcutaneous bolus morphine via an indwelling cannula for pain from advanced cancer. Palliative Medicine, 5, 323–329.

127. McKenna, F. (1998). Diclofenac/misoprostol: The European clinical experience. Journal of Rheumatology, 51 (Suppl), 21–30.

128. McQuay, H. J., Tramer, M., Nye, B. A., Carroll, D., Wiffen, P. J., Moore, R. A. (1996). A systematic review of antidepressants in neuropathic pain. Pain, 68, 217–227.

129. McQuay, H., Carroll, D., Jadad, A. R., Wiffen, P., Moore, A. (1995). Anticonvulsant drugs for management of pain: A systematic review. British Medical Journal, 311, 1047–1052.

130. Mercadante, S. (1993). Celiac plexus block versus analgesics in pancreatic cancer pain. Pain, 52, 187–192.

131. Mercadante, S. (1994a). Intrathecal morphine and bupivacaine in advanced cancer pain patients implanted at home. Journal of Pain and Symptom Management, 9, 201–207.

132. Mercadante, S. (1994b). The role of octreotide in palliative care. Journal of Pain and Symptom Management, 9, 406–411.

133. Meyer-Witting, M., Foster, J. M. (1992). Suprascapular nerve block in the management of cancer pain. Anesthesia, 47, 626.

134. Minotti, V., De Angelis, V., Righetti, E., Celani, M. G., Rossetti, R., Lupatelli, M., Tonato, M., Pisati, R., Monza, G., Fumi, G., Del Favero, A. (1998). Double-blind evaluation of short-term analgesic efficacy of orally administered diclofenac, diclofenac plus codeine, and diclofenac plus imipramine in chronic cancer pain. Pain, 74, 133–137.

135. Myers, D. P., Lema, M. J., de Leon-Casasola, O. A., Bacon, D. R. (1993). Interpleural analgesia for the treatment of severe cancer pain in terminally ill patients. Journal of Pain and Symptom Management, 8, 505–510.

136. Nebab, E. G., Florence, I. M. (1997). An alternative needle geometry for interruption of the ganglion impar [letter]. Anesthesiology, 86, 1213–1214.

137. Neill, R. S. (1979). Ablation of the brachial plexus. Control of intractable pain, due to a pathological fracture of the humerus. Anesthesia, 34, 1024–1027.

138. Nitescu, P., Appelgren, L., Linder, L. E., Sjoberg, M., Hultman, E., Curelaru, I. (1990). Epidural versus intrathecal morphine-bupivacaine: Assessment of consecutive treatments in advanced cancer pain. Journal of Pain and Symptom Management, 5, 18–26.

139. Nitescu, P., Sjoberg, M., Appelgren, L., Curelaru, I. (1995). Complications of intrathecal opioids and bupivacaine in the treatment of 'refractory' cancer pain. Clinical Journal of Pain, 11, 45–62.

140. Osborne, R. J., Joel, S. P., Slevin, M. L. (1986). Morphine intoxication in renal failure: The role of morphine-6-glucuronide. British Medical Journal (Clin Res Ed), 292, 1548–1549.

141. Osborne, R., Joel, S., Grebenik, K., Trew, D., Slevin, M. (1993). The pharmacokinetics of morphine and morphine glucuronides in kidney failure [see comments]. Clinical Pharmacology and Therapeutics, 54, 158–167.

142. Paice, J. A. (1988). The phenomenon of analgesic tolerance in cancer pain management. Oncology Nursing Forum, 15, 455–460.

143. Paix, A., Coleman, A., Lees, J., Grigson, J., Brooksbank, M., Thorne, D., Ashby, M. (1995). Subcutaneous fentanyl and sufentanil infusion substitution for morphine intolerance in cancer pain management. Pain, 63, 263–269.

144. Parker, M. C., Baines, M. J. (1996). Intestinal obstruction in patients with advanced malignant disease. British Journal of Surgery, 83, 1–2.

145. Pasternak, G. W., Standifer, K. M. (1995). Mapping of opioid receptors using antisense oligodeoxynucleotides: Correlating their molecular biology and pharmacology [see comments]. Trends in Pharmacologic Sciences, 16, 344–350.

146. Patt, R. B., Proper, G., Reddy, S. (1994). The neuroleptics as adjuvant analgesics. Journal of Pain and Symptom Management, 9, 446–453.

147. Patt, R. B., Reddy, S. (1994). Spinal neurolysis for cancer pain: Indications and recent results. Annals, Academy of Medicine, Singapore, 23, 216–220.

148. Patt, Y. Z., Peters, R. E., Chuang, V. P., Wallace, S., Claghorn, L., Mavligit, G. (1985). Palliation of pelvic recurrence of colorectal cancer with intra-arterial 5-fluorouracil and mitomycin. Cancer, 56, 2175–2180.

149. Paulson, D. F. (1978). Oxybutynin chloride in control of post transurethral vesical pain and spasm. Urology, 11, 237–238.

150. Payne, R., Mathias, S. D., Pasta, D. J., Wanke, L. A., Williams, R., Mahmoud, R. (1998). Quality of life and cancer pain: Satisfaction and side effects with transdermal fentanyl versus oral morphine. Journal of Clinical Oncology, 16, 1588–1593.

151. Penn, R. D., Paice, J. A., Kroin, J. S. (1992). Octreotide: A potent new nonopiate analgesic for intrathecal infusion [see comments]. Pain, 49, 13–19.

152. Perazella, M. A., Eras, J. (2000). Are selective COX-2 inhibitors nephrotoxic? American Journal of Kidney Disease, 35, 937–940.

153. Pies, R. (1996). Psychotropic medications and the oncology patient. Cancer Practice, 4, 164–166.

154. Plancarte, R., Amescua, C., Patt, R. B., Aldrete, J. A. (1990). Superior hypogastric plexus block for pelvic cancer pain. Anesthesiology, 73, 236–239.

155. Plancarte, R., de Leon-Casasola, O. A., El-Helaly, M., Allende, S., Lema, M. J. (1997). Neurolytic superior hypogastric plexus block for chronic pelvic pain associated with cancer. Regional Anesthesia, 22, 562–568.

156. Plancarte, R., Velazquez, R., Patt, R. B. (1993). Neurolytic block of the sympathetic axis. In: Patt RB (ed) Cancer Pain. Lippincott, Philadelphia, pp 377–425.

157. Plosker, G. L., Lamb, H. M. (1999). Diclofenac/misoprostol. Pharmacoeconomic implications of therapy. Pharmacoeconomics, 16, 85–98.

158. Polatty, R. C., Cooper, K. R. (1986). Respiratory failure after percutaneous cordotomy. Southern Medical Journal, 79, 897–899.

159. Portenoy, R. K. (1994). Management of common opioid side effects during long-term therapy of cancer pain. Annals, Academy of Medicine, Singapore, 23, 160–170.

160. Portenoy, R. K. (1996). Adjuvant analgesic agents. Hematology/Oncology Clinics of North America, 10, 103–119.

161. Portenoy, R. K., Foley, K. M., Inturrisi, C. E. (1990). The nature of opioid responsiveness and its implications for neuropathic pain: New hypotheses derived from studies of opioid infusions [see comments]. Pain, 43, 273–286.

162. Porter, A. T., McEwan, A. J., Powe, J. E., Reid, R., McGowan, D. G., Lukka, H., Sathyanarayana, J. R., Yakemchuk, V. N., Thomas, G. M., Erlich, L. E., et al. (1993). Results of a randomized phase-III trial to evaluate the efficacy of strontium-89 adjuvant to local field external beam irradiation in the management of endocrine resistant metastatic prostate cancer. International Journal of Radiation Oncology–Biology–Physics, 25, 805–813.

163. Poulsen, L., Brosen, K., Arendt-Nielsen, L., Gram, L. F., Elbaek, K., Sindrup, S. H. (1996). Codeine and morphine in extensive and poor metabolizers of sparteine: Pharmacokinetics, analgesic effect and side effects. European Journal of Clinical Pharmacology, 51, 289–295.

164. Prasanna, A., Murthy, P. S. (1993). Sphenopalatine ganglion block and pain of cancer [letter]. Journal of Pain and Symptom Management, 8, 125.

165. Queisser, W. (1984). Chemotherapy for the treatment of cancer pain. Recent Results in Cancer Research, 89, 171–177.

166. Rapin, C. H. (1989). The treatment of pain in the elderly patient. The use of oral morphine in the treatment of pain. Journal of Palliative Care, 5, 54–55.

167. Raskin, J. B. (1999). Gastrointestinal effects of nonsteroidal anti-inflammatory therapy. American Journal of Medicine, 106, 3S–12S.

168. Ripamonti, C., Bruera, E. (1997). Current status of patient-controlled analgesia in cancer patients. Oncology (Huntingt), 11, 373–380, 383–384; discussion 384–386.

169. Ripamonti, C., Groff, L., Brunelli, C., Polastri, D., Stavrakis, A., De Conno, F. (1998). Switching from morphine to oral methadone in treating cancer pain: What is the equianalgesic dose ratio? [see comments]. Journal of Clinical Oncology, 16, 3216–3221.

170. Rizzi, R., Terrevoli, A., Visentin, M. (1985). Long-term results of alcoholization and thermocoagulation of trigeminal nerve for cancer pain. The Pain Clinic I. In: Erdmann, W., Oyama, T., Pernak, M. J. (eds) Proceedings of the First International Symposium. Vnu Science Press, Utrecht, The Netherlands.

171. Robertson, D. H. (1983). Transsacral neurolytic nerve block. An alternative approach to intractable perineal pain. British Journal of Anesthesia, 55, 873–875.

172. Robinson, R. G., Preston, D. F., Schiefelbein, M., Baxter, K. G. (1995). Strontium 89 therapy for the palliation of pain due to osseous metastases. Journal of the American Medical Association, 274, 420–424.

173. Ross, G. J., Kessler, H. B., Clair, M. R., Gatenby, R. A., Hartz, W. H., Ross, L. V. (1989). Sonographically guided paracentesis for palliation of symptomatic malignant ascites. American Journal of Roentgenology, 153, 1309–1311.

174. Rossi, G. C., Leventhal, L., Pan, Y. X., Cole, J., Su, W., Bodnar, R. J., Pasternak, G. W. (1997). Antisense mapping of MOR-1 in rats: Distinguishing between morphine and morphine-6beta-glucuronide antinociception. Journal of Pharmacology and Experimental Therapeutics, 281, 109–114.

175. Rothenberg, M. L. (1996). New developments in chemotherapy for patients with advanced pancreatic cancer. Oncology (Huntingt), 10, 18–22.

176. Rubens, R. D., Towlson, K. E., Ramirez, A. J., Coltart, S., Slevin, M. L., Terrell, C., Timothy, A. R. (1992). Appropriate chemotherapy for palliating advanced cancer. British Medical Journal, 304, 35–40.

177. Ruskin, J. N. (1989). The cardiac arrhythmia suppression trial (CAST). New England Journal of Medicine, 321, 386–388.

178. Salmon, J. B., Finch, P. M., Lovegrove, F. T., Warwick, A. (1992). Mapping the spread of epidural phenol in cancer pain patients by radionuclide admixture and epidural scintigraphy. Clinical Journal of Pain, 8, 18–22.

179. Sanders, M., Zuurmond, W. (1995). Safety of unilateral and bilateral percutaneous cervical cordotomy in 80 terminally ill cancer patients. Journal of Clinical Oncology, 13, 1509–1512.

180. Saris, S. C., Silver, J. M., Vieira, J. F., Nashold, B. S. Jr. (1986). Sacrococcygeal rhizotomy for perineal pain. Neurosurgery, 19, 789–793.

181. Schmeler, K., Bastin, K. (1996). Strontium-89 for symptomatic metastatic prostate cancer to bone: Recommendations for hospice patients. Hospital Journal, 11, 1–10.

182. Schug, S. A., Zech, D., Dorr, U. (1990). Cancer pain management according to WHO analgesic guidelines. Journal of Pain and Symptom Management, 5, 27–32.

183. Schug, S. A., Zech, D., Grond, S., Jung, H., Meuser, T., Stobbe, B. (1992). A long-term survey of morphine in cancer pain patients. Journal of Pain and Symptom Management, 7, 259–266.

184. Sevarino, F. B., Sinatra, R. S., Paige, D., Ning, T., Brull, S. J., Silverman, D. G. (1992). The efficacy of intramuscular ketorolac in combination with intravenous PCA morphine for postoperative pain relief. Journal of Clinical Anesthesia, 4, 285–288.

185. Simmonds, M. A. (1997). Oral transmucosal fentanyl citrate produces pain relief faster than medication typically used for breakthrough pain in cancer patients (Meeting abstract). Proceedings, Annual Meeting of the American Society of Clinical Oncologists, 16, A180.

186. Sindrup, S. H., Brosen, K. (1995). The pharmacogenetics of codeine hypoalgesia. Pharmacogenetics, 5, 335–346.

187. Sindrup, S. H., Poulsen, L., Brosen, K., Arendt-Nielsen, L., Gram, L. F. (1993). Are poor metabolisers of sparteine/debrisoquine less pain tolerant than extensive metabolisers? Pain, 53, 335–339.

188. Sjoberg, M., Nitescu, P., Appelgren, L., Curelaru, I. (1994). Long-term intrathecal morphine and bupivacaine in patients with refractory cancer pain. Results from a morphine dose regimen of 0.5:4.75 mg/ml. Anesthesiology, 80, 284–297.

189. Sjogren, P., Dragsted, L., Christensen, C. B. (1993). Myoclonic spasms during treatment with high doses of intravenous morphine in renal failure. Acta Anesthesiologica Scandinavica, 37, 780–782.

190. Sneed, P. K., Larson, D. A., Wara, W. M. (1996). Radiotherapy for cerebral metastases. Neurosurgery Clinics of North America, 7, 505–515.

191. Sorensen, S., Helweg-Larsen, S., Mouridsen, H., Hansen, H. H. (1994). Effect of high-dose dexamethasone in carcinomatous metastatic spinal cord compression treated with radiotherapy: A randomized trial. European Journal of Cancer, 30A, 22–27.

192. Spiegel, D., Moore, R. (1997). Imagery and hypnosis in the treatment of cancer patients. Oncology (Huntingt), 11, 1179–1189; discussion 1189–1195.

193. Strang, P. (1996). Analgesic effect of bisphosphonates on bone pain in breast cancer patients: A review article. Acta Oncologica, 5, 50–54.

194. Stuart, G., Cramond, T. (1993). Role of percutaneous cervical cordotomy for pain of malignant origin. Medical Journal of Australia, 158, 667–670.

195. Sucher, E., Margulies, J. Y., Floman, Y., Robin, G. C. (1994). Prognostic factors in anterior decompression for metastatic cord compression. An analysis of results. European Spine Journal, 3, 70–75.

196. Swain, R. (1987). Oral clonidine for proctalgia fugax. Gut, 28, 1039–1040.

197. Sykes, J., Johnson, R., Hanks, G. W. (1997). ABC of palliative care. Difficult pain problems. British Medical Journal, 315, 867–869.

198. Symreng, T., Gomez, M. N., Rossi, N. (1989). Intrapleural bupivacaine v saline after thoracotomy—Effects on pain and lung function—A double-blind study [see comments]. Journal of Cardiothoracic Anesthesia, 3, 144–149.

199. Taha, A. S., Hudson, N., Hawkey, C. J., Swannell, A. J., Trye, P. N., Cottrell, J., Mann, S. G., Simon, T. J., Sturrock, R. D., Russell, R. I. (1996). Famotidine for the prevention of gastric and duodenal ulcers caused by nonsteroidal anti-inflammatory drugs [see comments]. New England Journal of Medicine, 334, 1435–1439.

200. Takeda, F. (1985). Japanese field-testing of WHO guidelines. PRN Forum, 4, 4, 5.

201. Tarn, T. S., Lee, T. S. (1994). Surgical treatment of metastatic tumors of the long bones, Chung Hua I Hsueh Tsa Chih (Taipei), 54, 170–175.

202. Thatcher, N., Anderson, H., Betticher, D. C., & Ranson, M. (1995). Symptomatic benefit from gemcitabine and other chemotherapy in advanced non-small cell lung cancer: Changes in performance status and tumor-related symptoms. Anticancer Drugs, 6(Suppl 6), 39–48.

203. Thomas, Z., & Bruera, E. (1995). Use of methadone in a highly tolerant patient receiving parenteral hydromorphone. Journal of Pain and Symptom Management, 10, 315–317.

204. Tiseo, P. J., Thaler, H. T., Lapin, J., Inturrisi, C. E., Portenoy, R. K., & Foley, K. M. (1995). Morphine-6-glucuronide concentrations and opioid related side effects: A survey in cancer patients. Pain, 61, 47–54.

205. Turk, D. C., & Feldman, C. S. (1992). Noninvasive approaches to pain control in terminal illness: The contribution of psychological variables. Hospital Journal, 8, 1–23.

206. Twycross, R. (1994). The risks and benefits of corticosteroids in advanced cancer. Drug Safety, 11, 163–178.

207. Vainio, A., Ollila, J., Matikainen, E., Rosenberg, P., & Kalso, E. (1995). Driving ability in cancer patients receiving long-term morphine analgesia. Lancet, 346, 667–670.

208. Valentini, M., Cannizzaro, R., Poletti, M., Bortolussi, R., Fracasso, A., Testa, V., & Grazioli, I. (1995). Nonsteroidal anti-inflammatory drugs for cancer pain: Comparison between misoprostol and ranitidine in prevention of upper gastrointestinal damage. Journal of Clinical Oncology, 13, 2637–2642.

209. Vane, J. R., Bakhle, Y. S., & Botting, R. M. (1998). Cyclooxygenases 1 and 2. Annual Review of Pharmacology and Toxicology, 38, 97–120.

210. Varvel, J. R., Shafer, S. L., Hwang, S. S., Coen, P. A., & Stanski, D. R. (1989). Absorption characteristics of transdermally administered fentanyl. Anesthesiology, 70, 928–934.

211. Ventafridda, V., Ripamonti, C., Caraceni, A., Spoldi, E., Messina, L., & De Conno, F. (1990). The

management of inoperable gastrointestinal obstruction in terminal cancer patients. Tumori, 76, 389–393.

212. Ventafridda, V., Tamburini, M., Caraceni, A., De Conno, F., & Naldi, F. (1987). A validation study of the WHO method for cancer pain relief. Cancer, 59, 850–856.

213. Vermeulen, S. S. (1998). Whole brain radiotherapy in the treatment of metastatic brain tumors. Seminars in Surgical Oncology, 14, 64–69.

214. Vigano, A., Fan, D., & Bruera, E. (1996). Individualized use of methadone and opioid rotation in the comprehensive management of cancer pain associated with poor prognostic indicators. Pain, 67, 115–119.

215. Walker, V. A., Hoskin, P. J., Hanks, G. W., & White, I. D. (1988). Evaluation of WHO analgesic guidelines for cancer pain in a hospital-based palliative care unit. Journal of Pain and Symptom Management, 3, 145–149.

216. Watanabe, S., & Bruera, E. (1994). Corticosteroids as adjuvant analgesics. Journal of Pain and Symptom Management, 9, 442–445.

217. Watson, D. J., Harper, S. E., Zhao, P. L., Quan, H., Bolognese, J. A., & Simon, T. J. (2000). Gastrointestinal tolerability of the selective cyclooxygenase-2 (COX-2) inhibitor rofecoxib compared with nonselective COX-1 and COX-2 inhibitors in osteoarthritis. Archives of Internal Medicine, 160, 2998–3003.

218. Wells, C. J., Lipton, S., & Lahuerta, J. (1984). Respiratory depression after percutaneous cervical anterolateral cordotomy in patients on slow-release oral morphine [Letter]. Lancet, 1, 739.

219. Wemm, K. Jr., & Saberski, L. (1995). Modified approach to block the ganglion impar (ganglion of Walther) [Letter]. Regional Anesthesia, 20, 544, 545.

220. Wolfe, M. M., Lichtenstein, D. R., & Singh, G. (1999). Gastrointestinal toxicity of nonsteroidal anti-inflammatory drugs. New England Journal of Medicine, 340, 1888–1899.

221. Wong, E. T., Gunes, S., Gaughan, E., Patt, R. B., Ginsberg, L. E., Hassenbusch, S. J., & Payne, R. (1997). Palliation of intractable cancer pain by MRI-guided cingulotomy. Clinical Journal of Pain, 13, 260–263.

222. Wong, G. Y., & Brown, D. L. (1995). Transient paraplegia following alcohol celiac plexus block. Regional Anesthesia, 20, 352–355.

223. World Health Organization. (1986). Cancer Pain Relief. World Health Organization, Geneva.

224. World Health Organization. (1996). Cancer Pain Relief (2nd ed.). World Health Organization, Geneva.

225. Yaksh, T. L. (1996). Epidural ketamine: A useful, mechanistically novel adjuvant for epidural morphine? Regional Anesthesia, 21, 508–513.

226. Yang, C. Y., Wong, C. S., Chang, J. Y., & Ho, S. T. (1996). Intrathecal ketamine reduces morphine requirements in patients with terminal cancer pain. Canadian Journal of Anesthesia, 43, 379–383.

227. Zadina, J. E., Kastin, A. J., Harrison, L. M., Ge, L. J., & Chang, S. L. (1995). Opiate receptor changes after chronic exposure to agonists and antagonists. Annals of the New York Academy of Science, 757, 353–361.

228. Zech, D. F., Grond, S., Lynch, J., Hertel, D., & Lehmann, K. A. (1995). Validation of World Health Organization Guidelines for cancer pain relief: A 10-year prospective study. Pain, 63, 65–76.

INDEX

D

E

L

M

N

O

T

U

V

Z

Printed and bound by CPI Group (UK) Ltd, Croydon, CR0 4YY
18/09/2026
14965061-0005